Advances in Neuroscience

Volume 2

Functional Neural Transplantation

ADVANCES IN NEUROSCIENCE
VOLUME 2

Functional Neural Transplantation

EDITORS

Stephen B. Dunnett, Ph.D.
University Lecturer
MRC Cambridge Centre
for Brain Repair, and
Department of Experimental Psychology
University of Cambridge
Cambridge, United Kingdom

Anders Björklund, M.D., Ph.D.
Professor
Department of Medical Cell Research
University of Lund
Lund, Sweden

RAVEN PRESS ✺ NEW YORK

Raven Press, Ltd., 1185 Avenue of the Americas, New York, New York 10036

Made in the United States of America

Library of Congress Cataloging-in-Publication Data

Functional neural transplantation / editors, Stephen B. Dunnett,
    Anders Björklund.
        p.   cm.—(Advances in neuroscience ; v. 2)
    Includes bibliographical references and index.
    ISBN 0-7817-0068-X
    1. Nerve grafting—Congresses.   2. Nervous system—Regeneration—
Congresses.   3. Mammals.   I. Dunnett, S. B. (Stephen B.)
II. Björklund, Anders, 1945–   .   III. Series.
    [DNLM: 1. Nerve Tissue—transplantation.   2. Brain Tissue
Transplantation.   3. Central Nervous System—physiology.   W1 AD684L
v.2 1994 / WL 102 F9794 1994]
    RD595.F84   1994
    617.4'80592—dc20
    DNLM/DLC   94-7297
    for Library of Congress   CIP

9 8 7 6 5 4 3 2 1

Contents

v

Contributing Authors

Albert J. Aguayo
Center for Research in Neuroscience
McGill University
Montreal General Hospital
1650 Cedar Avenue
Montreal, Quebec H3G 1A4
Canada

Lucy E. Annett
Department of Experimental Psychology
University of Cambridge
Downing Street
Cambridge CB2 3EB
United Kingdom

Harry F. Baker
Department of Psychiatry
Clinical Research Center
Watford Road
Harrow, Middlesex HA1 3UJ
United Kingdom

Johan Bengzon
Restorative Neurology Unit
Department of Neurology
Lund University Hospital
Lund S-221 85
Sweden

Anders Björklund
Department of Medical Cell Research
University of Lund
Biskopsgatan 5
Lund S-223 62
Sweden

Garth M. Bray
Center for Research in Neuroscience
McGill University
Montreal General Hospital
1650 Cedar Avenue
Montreal, Quebec H3G 1A4
Canada

Barbara S. Bregman
Department of Cell Biology
Division of Neurobiology
Georgetown University School of Medicine
3900 Reservoir Road NW
Washington, DC 20007

Mara Bresjanac
Department of Neurobiology and Anatomy
University of Rochester School of Medicine
*   and Dentistry*
Rochester, New York 14642

Patrik Brundin
Restorative Neurology Unit
Department of Neurology
Lund University Hospital
Lund S-221 85
Sweden

Kenneth Campbell
Department of Medical Cell Research
University of Lund
Biskopsgatan 5
Lund S-223 62
Sweden

Harry M. Charlton
Department of Human Anatomy
University of Oxford
South Parks Road
Oxford OX1 3QX
United Kingdom

Karen S. Chen
Department of Neuroscience Research
Genentech, Inc.
460 Point San Bruno Boulevard
South San Francisco, California 94080

Wei-Ming Duan
Restorative Neurology Unit
Department of Neurology
Lund University Hospital
Lund S-221 85
Sweden

Stephen B. Dunnett, Ph.D.
MRC Cambridge Centre for Brain Repair, and
Department of Experimental Psychology
University of Cambridge
Downing Street
Cambridge CB2 3EB
United Kingdom

Eskil Elmér
Restorative Neurology Unit
Department of Neurology
Lund University Hospital
Lund S-221 85
Sweden

Bryan D. Fantie, Ph.D.
Assistant Professor of Psychology and Director
Human Neuropsychology Laboratory
Department of Psychology
The American University
4400 Massachusetts Avenue, NW
Washington, DC 20001-8062

Rosemary A. Fricker
Department of Experimental Psychology
University of Cambridge
Downing Street
Cambridge CB2 3EB
United Kingdom

Fred H. Gage
Department of Neurosciences
University of California, San Diego
9500 Gilman Drive
La Jolla, California 92093-0627

Don M. Gash
Department of Anatomy and Neurobiology
University of Kentucky Medical Center
800 Rose Street, MN224
Lexington, Kentucky 40536-0084

Jeffrey A. Gray
Department of Psychology
Institute of Psychiatry
De Crespigny Park, Denmark Hill
London SE5 8AF
United Kingdom

Helen Hodges
Department of Psychology
Institute of Psychiatry
De Crespigny Park, Denmark Hill
London SE5 8AF
United Kingdom

Fred Junn
Department of Neurobiology and Anatomy
University of Rochester School of Medicine
and Dentistry
Rochester, New York 14642

Merab Kokaia
Restorative Neurology Unit
Department of Neurology
Lund University Hospital
Lund S-221 85
Sweden

Zaal Kokaia
Restorative Neurology Unit
Department of Neurology
Lund University Hospital
Lund S-221 85
Sweden

Bryan Kolb
Psychology Department
The University of Lethbridge
Lethbridge, Alberta T1K 3M4
Canada

Michael N. Lehman
Department of Cell Biology, Neurobiology, and
*   Anatomy*
University of Cincinnati College of Medicine
231 Bethesda Avenue
Cincinnati, Ohio 45267

Olle Lindvall
Restorative Neurology Unit
Department of Neurology
Lund University Hospital
Lund S-221 85
Sweden

Brian S. Meldrum
Department of Neurology
Institute of Psychiatry
De Crespigny Park, Denmark Hill
London SE5 8AF
United Kingdom

Guido Nikkhah
Department of Medical Cell Research
University of Lund
Biskopsgatan 5
Lund S-223 62
Sweden; and
Neurosurgical Clinic
Norstadt Hospital
Hanover D-3000
Germany

Martin R. Ralph
Department of Psychology
University of Toronto
100 St. George Street
Toronto, Ontario M5S 1A1
Canada

Michael Rasminsky
Department of Neurology
McGill University
Montreal General Hospital
1650 Cedar Avenue
Montreal, Quebec H3G 1A4
Canada

Paul J. Reading
Department of Experimental Psychology
University of Cambridge
Downing Street
Cambridge CB2 3EB
United Kingdom

Gal Richter-Levin
Department of Neurobiology
The Weizmann Institute
Rehovot 76100
Israel

Rosalind M. Ridley
Department of Psychiatry
Clinical Research Center
Watford Road
Harrow, Middlesex HA1 3UJ
United Kingdom

Hansjörg Sauer
Department of Medical Cell Research
University of Lund
Biskopsgatan 5
Lund S-223 62
Sweden

Menahem Segal
Department of Neurobiology
The Weizmann Institute
Rehovot 76100
Israel

John D. Sinden
Department of Psychology
Institute of Psychiatry
De Crespigny Park, Denmark Hill
London SE5 8AF
United Kingdom

Dalip Jaicaran Sirinathsinghji
Merck Sharp and Dohme Research
*   Laboratories*
Neuroscience Research Center
Terlings Park
Harlow, Essex CM20 2QR
United Kingdom

Matthew J. A. Wood
Department of Human Anatomy
University of Oxford
South Parks Road
Oxford OX1 3QX
United Kingdom

Zhiming Zhang
Department of Anatomy and Neurobiology
University of Kentucky Medical Center
800 Rose Street, MN224
Lexington, Kentucky 40536-0084

Acknowledgments

We wish to thank the authors for the energy and attention to detail with which they have assumed their task. Responsibility for the selectivity and biases of the resulting coverage must be laid at the door of the editors. We thank the editors of Raven Press who have provided continual patience, encouragement, and support in the prolonged process of bringing our initial ideas for this volume to fruition.

Preface

Within the neurosciences, the topic of neural transplantation has captured widespread interest over the last decade, from the general public as much as from biological scientists and medical practitioners. For the first time the techniques of neural transplantation in the adult brain appear to offer the possibility to alleviate and repair neurodegenerative disease in the brain—problems, such as Parkinson's disease and dementia or spinal cord injury, that have devastating consequences for the patients and their families and that have until now been completely untreatable. Yet, much of the debate about the potential applications of these new techniques is speculative and often based on fear and fantasy rather than on established scientific results.

Functional Neural Transplantation provides a critical assessment of the current status of biological research in the field of neural transplantation across the range of applications currently under consideration. We have restricted our focus to functional aspects of neural transplantation, since the basic biology of the techniques are already well reviewed in a number of previous volumes. Our goal has been to provide detailed reviews of the status of each main area of current research interest. In order to achieve an adequate breadth of coverage, we have not sought to represent each different and sometimes competing viewpoint. Rather, we have invited individual experts to provide a broad and detailed assessment of the current standing of research in their respective areas and to identify the key issues that are under experimental consideration. We believe that this strategy has provided a better coherent and detailed analysis of the fundamental issues under present investigation than would have been possible with a comprehensive, but piecemeal, account. We have sought to cover the major areas of active research in functional neural transplantation in the mammalian central nervous system, but we have considered the very different issues involved in transplantation within the peripheral nervous system and in non-mammalian species to be beyond the scope of the present volume.

Stephen B. Dunnett
Anders Björklund

Advances in Neuroscience

Volume 2

Functional Neural Transplantation

Functional Neural Transplantation,
edited by S. B. Dunnett and A. Björklund.
Raven Press, Ltd., New York © 1994.

1

Introduction

Stephen B. Dunnett and *Anders Björklund

*Department of Experimental Psychology, University of Cambridge, Cambridge CB2 3EB, United Kingdom; *Department of Medical Cell Research, University of Lund, S–223 62 Lund, Sweden*

THE HISTORY OF NEURAL TRANSPLANTATION

The field of neural transplantation has a long history, but only in recent years has it attracted widespread attention. It is now over a century since Thompson (43) reported on his first attempts at neural transplantation. In these studies, pieces of neocortex from adult dogs or cats were grafted into neocortical cavities in the brains of other adult dogs or cats. He reported "that brain tissue has sufficient vitality to survive seven weeks the operation of transplantation without wholly losing its identity," although, with the subsequent development of improved stains and the benefit of hindsight, it is likely that the remnants of the transplants that he saw represented the survival predominantly of glial and other nonneuronal elements rather than of neurons *per se*. Nevertheless, Thompson identified a series of critical questions that remain important issues to this day. What are the techniques necessary to yield good survival? What are the limitations in age and species for matching donor and host? Under what circumstances might the graft prove functional? Thompson considered that his first experiment suggested "an interesting field for further research, and I have no doubt that other experimenters will be rewarded by investigating it."

In fact, in the first half of the intervening century, rather few others took up Thompson's challenge. As shown in Table 1 and summarized in several more extended reviews (7,19), a number of alternative approaches were adopted with variable levels of success. Many of these early studies, for example by Forssman, Tello, and others, focused on the transplantability and regenerative capacity of peripheral nerves. By contrast, the first apparently successful grafting of CNS tissues into the brain was described by Elizabeth Dunn in 1917 (11). In a long series of experiments, she implanted wedges of neonatal cortical tissues into the cortex of littermate rat pups. In the best cases, even though the grafts were small, they retained features of cortical tissue, including a degree of lamination of their constituent neurons. Survival was poor, however, with only four viable grafts reported from a series of studies spanning over 10 years of attempts. Nevertheless, the successful cases provided important clues as to the likely factors necessary to promote good survival, including the use of donor tissues taken from developing rather than adult nervous systems, and the proximity of successful grafts to the choroid plexus of the lateral ventricles, suggesting the importance of establishing a good blood supply to the grafts.

Further studies in subsequent decades, for example by LeGros Clark (29) and Glees (21) confirmed the viability of transplanting developing cortical tissues into the mammalian brain, and they found that using em-

TABLE 1. *A brief chronologic history of neural transplantation*

Year	Author(s)	Reference	First published report(s) of . . . .
1890	W. G. Thompson	43	Attempt to graft adult CNS tissues to adult brain
1900	J. Forssman	17	Neurotropic effects of grafted CNS tissues
1907	G. Del Conte	10	Grafting embryonic CNS tissues to brain
1909	W. Ranson	38	Grafting spinal ganglia to brain
1911	F. Tello	42	Successful grafting of peripheral nerve to brain
1917	E. Dunn	11	Successful grafting of neonatal CNS to neonatal brain
1940	W. E. LeGros Clark	29	Successful grafting of foetal CNS to neonatal brain
1957	B. Flerko and J. Szentagothai	16	Successful grafting of neuroendocrine tissue i.c.v.
1962–1963	K. M. Knigge	27	Compensation of endocrine deficits with i.c.v. grafts of pituitary
	B. Halasz et al.	23	
1971–1972	L. Olson and Å. Seiger	34	Application of ³H-thymidine labeling and transmitter histochemistry for the study of CNS tissue grafts
	G. D. Das and J. Altman	9	
1976	U. Stenevi and A. Björklund	4	Characterization of the conditions for reliable fetal neural graft survival in the adult mammalian CNS
1979	M. J. Perlow et al.	5	Compensation of motor deficits with nigral grafts in rats
	A. Björklund and U. Stenevi	35	
1982	D. Krieger et al.	28	Compensation of neuroendocrine deficits with i.c.v. grafts of fetal hypothalamus
1982	S. B. Dunnett et al.	14	Compensation of cognitive deficits with cholinergic grafts in rats
1985	E.-O. Backlund et al.	2	Adrenal transplantation in Parkinson's disease
1988	O. Lindvall et al.	32	Fetal nigral transplantation in Parkinson's disease
	I. Madrazo et al.	33	
	E. G. Hitchcock et al.	26	

bryonic rather than neonatal donors produced better results than those described in Dunn's original report. These authors demonstrated clear growth, neuronal differentiation, and the maintenance of a laminar organization within the grafts, but provided little evidence of the growth of fibers between the graft and the host brain, which left the impression of graft tissues developing independently, in isolation from the normal connections of the host brain.

In light of the successful survival of the grafts in these and other studies in the middle decades of the present century, it is perhaps remarkable that so little attention was paid to them at the time. One factor was certainly the relative variability and unpredictability of the transplantation techniques then used. (In fact, most of the investigators studying transplants of neural tissues to the mammalian CNS in the first half of this century were completely unsuccessful, and considerable frustration can be noted in several of these reports.) Another is that when the grafts did survive, they appeared rather isolated when studied with the silver staining techniques then available. The realization of the rich cellular differentiation within neuronal grafts and their capacity to establish extensive connections both to and from the host brain has depended on the advent of modern neuroanatomic tract tracing and selective neurochemical staining techniques.

However, perhaps the most important factor was that these earlier studies on plasticity and regrowth in the brain ran counter to the prevailing *Zeitgeist,* that the adult mammalian brain is fixed and immutable. This view of the central nervous system as so inflexible is often attributed to Cajal (8), and his classic description that all attempts at regeneration after nerve injury in the adult brain are abortive—"everything may die, nothing may be regenerated." However, this does him discredit. Cajal himself used transplants of ganglia and pieces of peripheral nerve in a series of important experiments that were influential in establishing the neuron doctrine, including the key concepts of chemical and mechanical guidance, trophism and tropism, and neuron–glia interactions. Whereas his pessimistic conclusion in later years may represent many of his frustrations with the unreliability of the techniques available to him, he is nowhere near as dogmatic about the limited regenerative capacity of the mature nervous system as can be seen in the positions adopted by many of his followers. These prejudices, however, began to relax only with the advent of new and more sensitive techniques, such as the electron microscope, which allowed the first clear demonstration in 1969 that collateral sprouting and reorganization of damaged axons is possible in the adult mammalian brain after nerve injury (37). This was closely followed in the early 1970s by the development of new transplantation techniques and the characterization of the conditions necessary to yield more reliable graft survival than was hitherto possible (4,9,34,41), which opened up the present era in which neural transplantation provides a widely used tool in many different areas of neurobiology.

THE HISTORY OF FUNCTIONAL NEURAL TRANSPLANTATION

In those early years, the predominant interest in neural transplantation was its util-ity for the study of developmental and regenerative processes in the CNS. Thus, for example, the ability to transplant neural tissues (in developing urodeles and amphibians in particular) has allowed the independent manipulation of cellular origin, substrates for growth, and targets, and provided much of our present understanding on the establishment and guidance of axonal connections in the developing nervous system (36). By contrast, the interest in the functional capacity of neural tissues within the context of damage and repair of the nervous system is considerably more recent.

A few early studies speculate on the potential functional significance of neural grafts. For example, in their studies involving transplantation of human embryonic brain tissue into the guinea pig brain, Greene and Arnold (22) considered whether this might result in the transfer of human characteristics. When they observed the transplanted animals, however, the only change they could detect in the animals' behavior was an enhanced libido. In these studies, such considerations were tangential to the primary goals of the research, and the consideration of functional factors was essentially philosophical rather than analytical in nature. The first experimental consideration of the functional effects of intracerebral transplantation came with the neuroendocrine studies of Knigge (27) and Halasz and colleagues, (23,24) in which pituitary tissues implanted into the third ventricle and basal hypothalamus were shown to restore body growth and reproductive function in hypophysectomized rats. As described in more detail in Chapter 18, these early studies were important in the establishment of the concept of the hypophysiotropic area of the basal hypothalamus, and this line of research continues to contribute to our present understanding of hypothalamic–pituitary interactions in neuroendocrine regulation.

The second main area in which transplantation studies developed a central functional perspective was the development in the late 1970s of the nigral graft model of experimental parkinsonism. In 1979, two reports by Perlow et al. (35) and Björklund and Stenevi (5) appeared in close succession that showed that motor deficits induced by neurotoxic lesions of the nigrostriatal dopamine system were dramatically reduced after transplants of embryonic dopamine cells back into the denervated areas in the neostriatum. These were not the first studies to show measurable function of grafted catecholamine neurons—electrophysiologic techniques had already been used to show functional connections of grafted noradrenaline neurons in the hippocampus, for example (3)—but the studies in the dopamine system attracted particular interest. The reasons for this are not hard to identify: not only did the rats with nigral grafts show clear alleviation of a dramatic and easily observable motor impairment (whole-body rotation when activated with stimulant drugs), but the neuronal and neurochemical losses produced by nigrostriatal lesions in rats are widely used as a simple model of human Parkinson's disease. Even in the first reports, Perlow, Freed, and colleagues speculated that nigral cell transplantation might provide a radically new strategy to treat human neurodegenerative disease (35). Indeed, in the intervening 14 years, it is in the context of Parkinson's disease that the greatest advances have been made toward the development of neural transplantation as a viable clinical therapy (see Chapter 5).

The last decade has seen an almost exponential explosion in the number of studies involving neural transplantation, the issues being addressed, and the different experimental models under investigation. Some of these studies have principally a therapeutic focus, oriented directly toward identifying potential strategies for treatment of traumatic injury or neurodegenerative disease in the brain. At the other extreme, others are concerned with biologic issues, using neural transplantation as an additional experimental tool for the analy-

sis of the basic organization and function of the CNS. In between are studies oriented toward analysis of the extent and limits of plasticity within the developing and adult mammalian brain itself.

CURRENT ISSUES IN FUNCTIONAL NEURAL TRANSPLANTATION

The focus on functional aspects of neural transplantation starts with the basic question "Do transplants work?" Thus, the fact that the grafts are seen to survive, and possibly also establish axonal connections into and from the host brain, does not necessarily imply that they have any relevance to the host animal. The implanted tissues could simply be isolated and independent from the functional circuits of the host brain or, even worse, might create detrimental effects through the occupation of space and displacement of healthy tissues. The topic of functionality in many different systems has been addressed frequently, first by using physiologic and biochemical techniques to explore the restitution of spontaneous and evoked cellular activity within the graft and the host, the transmission of axon potentials between graft and host, the release of neurotransmitters in the host brain from graft-derived cells, changes in postsynaptic receptor sensitivity, and so on. The alternative approach has been to observe and measure changes in the functional capacities of the host animal after transplantation, whether in terms of neuroendocrine changes regulating physiologic processes such as body growth, sexual development, and water balance, or overt behavioral changes, from simple motor behaviors to more complex cognitive and learning-related processes. In such studies, a major concern has to be whether graft-induced changes are truly mediated by the grafted tissues or nonspecific effects of the surgery, and the use of appropriate control procedures becomes critical (see Chapter 21).

If there is good evidence that the transplants are functional, a second question is "How?"—that is, by what mechanisms do the grafts exert their functional effects? Thus, just because anatomic connections are seen to become reformed, it may be that the grafts exert their functional influences through more tonic or diffuse processes such as diffuse release of neurotransmitters, neurohormones, or growth factors (see Chapters 6 and 18). Conversely, such a pharmacologic mode of action is less plausible in interpreting functional recovery in other behavioral functions that are believed to be dependent on the relay of information in connected systems, such as in the retinotectal or corticostriatal pathways. Although this issue is considered explicitly in the final chapter (Chapter 21), it is an underlying theme that runs through all the chapters.

Other studies have investigated the functional consequences of neural transplantation to understand better the functional organization of the brain itself. Just as tissue transplantation can permit the independent manipulation of sources, substrates, and targets of axon growth in a developmental context, so also in functional studies neural grafts can provide a powerful tool to complement traditional lesion techniques in identifying the necessary and sufficient contributions of individual populations of cells in sustaining particular aspects of behavior. This can be illustrated with two simple examples from our own work. First, it has proved extremely difficult to manipulate cholinergic inputs to the hippocampus without causing extensive collateral damage to other ascending and descending subcortical connections of the hippocampus. The observation that, in rats with rather generalized, nonspecific lesions of the fimbria–fornix pathways, implants of cholinergic cells can provide alleviation of simple maze-learning functions but not of the animals' hyperactivity, whereas implants of noradrenergic neurons produced the converse profile of recovery, providing important clues about the relative contribution of

each set of inputs to integrated function of the hippocampus (13). Second, there has been a long discussion about the involvement of dopamine systems in the mediation of reward processes of the brain. Although lesions of ascending dopamine systems disrupt rats' performance of reward-related tasks, such as lever-pressing to self-administer electric stimulation in the brain (so called intracerebral self-stimulation), it might be that the lesions disrupt the animals' motor abilities to perform the task rather than affecting any underlying change in the rewarding value of the stimulation (25). The observation that electrodes positioned within a graft of nigral tissue can provide an efficient site for maintaining self-stimulation indicates that activation of nigral cells is sufficient to transduce the reinforcing properties of the stimulation (18). Thus, the role of dopamine inputs is more than that of simply providing the motor activation necessary to perform a response that is rewarded by activation of other independent systems of the forebrain.

Of course, it still remains the case that a large proportion of the interest in functional neural transplantation relates to the novel possibilities that are suggested for functional repair in traumatic brain damage and neurodegenerative disease. Consequently, in parallel with the basic experimental studies in particular anatomic systems of the brain, we are seeing an increasing number of transplantation research programs built on animal models of functional processes of disease—such as ischemia or epilepsy (see Chapters 14 and 15, respectively)—or the development of primate models of particular human diseases (see Chapters 4 and 13). Although clinical trials are well advanced only in the case of Parkinson's disease (see Chapter 5), applications to other types of damage such as spinal cord injury (see Chapter 20) and other diseases such as Huntington's and Alzheimer's diseases, motor neuron disease, and multiple sclerosis are the subject of current speculation and active research (30). Although many of these experimental programs are beginning to yield impressive results in experimental animals, it is too early to predict the extent of functional efficacy and practical difficulties that will be encountered in such diverse clinical applications.

ORGANIZATION OF THE PRESENT VOLUME

The present volume seeks to provide a critical assessment of the status of neural transplantation across the range of applications currently under consideration. We have restricted our focus to functional aspects of neural transplantation, because the basic biology of the techniques of neural transplantation in the central nervous system are already well reviewed in a number of previous volumes (1,6,7,12,15,20,31).

The underlying organization of the chapters is based on the neuroanatomic and functional systems of the central nervous system. The sequence of topics in part reflects the historical development of the field (for example, starting with the role of nigral grafts in experimental and clinical parkinsonism) and a progression from more basic to higher levels of functional complexity and difficulties of the problems to be solved (via striatal, hippocampal, and cortical circuitries), to conclude with an overview of the problems confronting repair of long-distance sensory and motor systems in the spinal cord. The selection of topics also reflects our own particular interests and desire to group together problems with a similar approach. The chapters that focus on particular systems are interleaved with chapters on distinctive conceptual approaches (such as the role of neurotrophic mechanisms of graft action, Chapter 6), or particular methodologic approaches (such as the use of electrophysiologic techniques or the study of peripheral nerves as substrates for growth, Chapters 12 and 17, respectively), which have been placed in the contexts where they fit most appropriately.

There are, however, two areas that are less well represented than we would like. First, we were sorry not to have been able to incorporate a separate chapter on the impressive functional studies by Ray Lund and colleagues on the restoration of pupillary reflexes and the transduction of visual information to sustain basic visual discrimination function in rats with retinal implants in the brain, but a brief overview of these studies has been provided in Chapters 17 and 21. Second, techniques for the implantation of adrenal chromaffin cells in the spinal cord for the treatment of intractable pain (39), and the efficient encapsulation of such cells for xenotransplantation (40), have progressed significantly since the present chapters were invited, and are referred to only briefly in Chapters 20 and 21.

Finally, we thank the editors of Raven Press who have provided continual patience, encouragement, and support in the prolonged process of bringing our initial ideas for this volume to fruition.

REFERENCES

1. Azmitia EC, Björklund A. *Cell and tissue transplantation into the adult brain.* New York: The New York Academy of Sciences; 1987.
2. Backlund EO, Granberg PO, Hamberger B, et al. Transplantation of adrenal medullary tissue to striatum in parkinsonism. *J Neurosurg* 1985;62:169–173.
3. Björklund A, Segal M, Stenevi U. Functional reinnervation of rat hippocampus by locus coeruleus implants. *Brain Res* 1979;170:409–426.
4. Björklund A, Stenevi U. Growth of central catecholamine neurones into smooth muscle grafts in the rat mesencephalon. *Brain Res* 1971;31:1–20.
5. Björklund A, Stenevi U. Reconstruction of the nigrostriatal dopamine pathway by intracerebral transplants. *Brain Res* 1979;177:555–560.
6. Björklund A, Stenevi U. *Neural grafting in the mammalian CNS.* Amsterdam: Elsevier; 1985.
7. Björklund A, Stenevi U. Intracerebral neural grafting: a historical perspective. In: Björklund A, Stenevi U, eds. *Neural grafting in the mammalian CNS.* Amsterdam: Elsevier; 1985:3–14.
8. Cajal S Ramon y. *Degeneration and regeneration of the nervous system.* Oxford: Oxford University Press; 1928.
9. Das GD, Altman J. Transplanted precursors of nerve cells: their fate in the cerebellums of young rats. *Science* 1971;173:637–638.

10. Del Conte G. Einpflanzungen von embryohalem Gewebe ins Gehirn. *Zieg Beit Patol Anat* 1907; 42:193–202.

11. Dunn EH. Primary and secondary findings in a series of attempts to transplant cerebral cortex in the albino rat. *J Comp Neurol* 1917;27:565–582.

12. Dunnett SB, Björklund A. *Neural transplantation: a practical approach.* Oxford: IRL Press; 1992.

13. Dunnett SB, Gage FH, Björklund A, Stenevi U, Low WC, Iversen SD. Hippocampal deafferentation: transplant-derived reinnervation and functional recovery. *Scand J Psychol* 1982; (Suppl 1):104–111.

14. Dunnett SB, Low WC, Iversen SD, Stenevi U, Björklund A. Septal transplants restore maze learning in rats with fornix–fimbria lesions. *Brain Res* 1982;251:335–348.

15. Dunnett SB, Richards SJ. *Neural transplantation: from molecular basis to clinical application.* Amsterdam: Elsevier; 1990.

16. Flerkó B, Szentágothai J. Oestrogen sensitive nervous structures in the hypothalamus. *Acta Endocrinol* 1957;26:121–127.

17. Forssman J. Zur Kenntniss des Neurotropismus. *Zieg Beit Patol Anat* 1900;27:407–430.

18. Fray PJ, Dunnett SB, Iversen SD, Björklund A, Stenevi U. Nigral transplants reinnervating the dopamine-depleted neostriatum can sustain intracranial self stimulation. *Science* 1983;219: 416–419.

19. Gash DM. Neural transplants in mammals: a historical overview. In: Sladek JR, Gash DM, eds. *Neural transplants: development and function.* New York: Plenum Press; 1984:1–12.

20. Gash DM, Sladek JR. *Transplantation into the mammalian CNS.* Amsterdam: Elsevier; 1988.

21. Glees P. Studies of cortical regeneration with special reference to cerebral implants. In: Windle WE, ed. *Regeneration in the central nervous system.* Springfield, IL: Charles C Thomas; 1955;94–111.

22. Greene HSN, Arnold H. The homologous and heterologous transplantation of brain and brain tumors. *J Neurosurg* 1945;2:315–331.

23. Halasz B, Pupp L, Uhlarik S, Tima L. Growth of hypophysectomised rats bearing pituitary transplants in the hypothalamus. *Acta Physiol Acad Sci Hung* 1963;23:287–292.

24. Halasz B, Pupp L, Uhlarik S, Tima L. Further studies on the hormone secretion of the anterior pituitary transplanted into the hypophysiotrophic areas of the rat hypothalamus. *Endocrinology* 1965;77:343–355.

25. Hall RD, Bloom FE, Olds J. Neuronal and neurochemical substrates of reinforcement. *Neurosci Res Prog Bull* 1977;15:133–314.

26. Hitchcock ER, Clough CG, Hughes RC, Kenny RG. Embryos and Parkinson's disease. *Lancet* 1988;1:1274.

27. Knigge KM. Gonadotrophic action of neonatal pituitary glands implanted in the rat brain. *Am J Physiol* 1962;202:387–391.

28. Krieger DT, Perlow MJ, Gibson MJ, et al. Brain grafts reverse hypogonadism of gonadotropin releasing hormone deficiency. *Nature* 1982;298: 468–471.

29. LeGros Clark WE. Neuronal differentiation in implanted foetal cortical tissue. *J Neurol Psychiatr* 1940;3:263–284.

30. Lindvall O. Prospects of transplantation in human neurodegenerative diseases. *Trends Neurosci* 1991;14:376–384.

31. Lindvall O, Björklund A, Widner H. *Intracerebral transplantation in movement disorders.* Amsterdam: Elsevier; 1991.

32. Lindvall O, Rehncrona S, Gustavii B. Fetal dopamine-rich mesencephalic grafts in Parkinson's disease. *Lancet* 1988;2:1483–1484.

33. Madrazo I, Leon V, Torres C, et al. Transplantation of fetal substantia nigra and adrenal medulla to the caudate nucleus in two patients with Parkinson's disease. *N Engl J Med* 1988;318:51.

34. Olson L, Seiger Å. Brain tissue transplanted to the anterior chamber of the eye: I. fluorescence histochemistry of immature catecholamine and 5-hydroxytryptamine neurons innervating the iris. *Z Zellforsch* 1972;195:175–194.

35. Perlow MJ, Freed WJ, Hoffer BJ, Seiger Å, Olson L, Wyatt RJ. Brain grafts reduce motor abnormalities produced by destruction of nigrostriatal dopamine system. *Science* 1979;204: 643–647.

36. Purves D, Lichtman JW. *Principles of neural development.* Sunderland, MA: Sinauer Associates; 1985.

37. Raisman G. Neuronal plasticity in the septal nuclei of the adult brain. *Brain Res* 1969;14:25–48.

38. Ranson SW. Transplantation of the spinal ganglion into the brain. *Quarterly Bulletin of N W University Medical School* 1909;11:176–178.

39. Sagen J, Pappas GD, Winnie AP. Alleviation of pain in cancer patients by adrenal medullary transplants in the spinal subarachnoid space. *Cell Transplant* 1993;2:259–266.

40. Sagen J, Wang H, Tresco PA, Aebischer P. Transplants of immunologically isolated xenogeneic chromaffin cells provide a long-term source of pain-reducing neuroactive substances. *J Neurosci* 1993;13:2415–2423.

41. Stenevi U, Björklund A, Svendgaard N-Aa. Transplantation of central and peripheral monoamine neurons to the adult rat brain: techniques and conditions for survival. *Brain Res* 1976; 114:1–20.

42. Tello F. La influencia del neurotropismo en la regeneracion de los contros nerviosos. *Trab Lab Invest Biol Univ Madr* 1911;9:123–159.

43. Thompson WG. Successful brain grafting. *New York Medical Journal* 1890;51:701–702.

Functional Neural Transplantation,
edited by S. B. Dunnett and A. Björklund.
Raven Press, Ltd., New York © 1994.

2

Functional Effects of Mesencephalic Dopamine Neurons and Adrenal Chromaffin Cells Grafted to the Rodent Striatum

Patrik Brundin, Wei-Ming Duan, and *Hansjörg Sauer

*Restorative Neurology Unit, Department of Neurology, University Hospital,
S–221 85 Lund, Sweden; *Department of Medical Cell Research, University of Lund,
S–223 62 Lund, Sweden*

The first trials with tissue implants in the human brain involved adrenal medulla autografts (8) and transplants of embryonic mesencephalic tissue (98,100) in patients with Parkinson's disease. Those initial trials have led to a large series of operations that, in the case of embryonic mesencephalic grafts, still are being extended [see chapter by Lindvall *(this volume)*] and it is likely that we have yet to experience the full potential of this approach to clinical brain repair. Animal experiments have played a very important role in guiding this clinical research, and particularly studies performed in rodents have provided crucial information of relevance both to the trials in Parkinson's disease and our understanding of nervous system plasticity.

The objectives of this review are, first, to describe briefly some of the rodent models of Parkinson's disease relevant to functional neural transplantation research, second, to give a short overview of the survival and morphological characteristics of grafted embryonic dopamine (DA) neurons and grafts of adrenal medulla cells; third, to describe the behavioral consequences of grafting embryonic mesencephalic tissue or adrenal chromaffin cells to the striatum of rodents (Table 1); and fourth, to discuss the

endogenous physiologic properties of such grafts. The direct physiologic effects of the transplanted catecholaminergic cells on the host brain are also reviewed.

Throughout this review, experiments concerning grafts of embryonic DA neurons will be treated first and at more length than those concerning transplants of adrenal medulla, since there is more information available on the functional characteristics of the former type of graft in rodents. In some cases, the particular functional features being discussed have not been explored for adrenal medullary grafts, and hence there is no mention of this type of graft in certain sections of the review.

RODENT MODELS OF PARKINSON'S DISEASE RELEVANT TO FUNCTIONAL TRANSPLANT RESEARCH

Most studies with intracerebral grafts of catecholamine-rich cells have been conducted in rodents with lesions of the DA system. There are several ways in which such lesions can be created, and in this section the lesion models that have been most important for grafting research in the DA system are briefly reviewed.

TABLE 1. *Behavioral effects of catecholamine-rich transplants in the dopamine-depleted striatum*

	Nigral dopamine neurons	Adrenal chromaffin cells
Apomorphine-induced rotation	+	+, But often transient
Amphetamine-induced rotation	+	Conflicting results
Spontaneous rotation	+	+, Only acutely
General motor function	+	Not reported
Sensory neglect	+	−
Disengage behavior	Conflicting results	Not reported
Paw-reaching	Conflicting results	Not reported
Aphagia and adipsia	+ In neonates	+ In neonates
Duration of effects	Long-term	Often transient

+, Well established effect; −, no effect.

6-Hydroxydopamine Lesion

Intracerebral injection of the neurotoxin 6-hydroxydopamine (6-OHDA) causes a rapid and selective degeneration of catecholaminergic neurons. If the neurotoxin is injected into the mesencephalic DA cell groups or their axons, one can achieve an almost complete depletion of forebrain DA in rats (173). Rats with extensive bilateral lesions of this kind manifest a severe motor symptomatology with akinesia reminiscent of that seen in advanced Parkinson's disease (176). Unfortunately, the extensive bilateral lesion also causes aphagia and adipsia in the rats (176), requiring them to be tube-fed, which has somewhat limited the use of the bilateral 6-OHDA lesion model in neural transplantation research.

The animal model of Parkinson's disease that undoubtedly has contributed the most to our understanding of DA-rich grafts is the rat with a unilateral 6-OHDA lesion of the mesostriatal pathway (169,173). Such rats display a marked asymmetry in their motor behavior. Thus, they tend to walk round in circles toward the side of the lesion, and when challenged with drugs acting on the DA system they will display active rotational behavior (173,175). For example the DA-releasing agent amphetamine (usually at doses of 1.5–5 mg/kg) will amplify the spontaneous ipsilateral circling whereas administration of the DA receptor agonist apomorphine (at a low dose, e.g., 0.05–0.25 mg/kg) will cause rotation con-

tralateral to the lesion by stimulating supersensitive receptors on the 6-OHDA denervated side (105,175). Drug-induced rotational behavior is easy to quantify (174) and does not disappear spontaneously in rats with very extensive lesions of the DA system. It is important to use only rats with complete or near-complete 6-OHDA lesions for behavioral studies of grafts. Schmidt et al. (140,141) found that it is possible to preselect rats with extensive lesions from a larger group of operated rats by testing their rotational response to 5 mg/kg amphetamine. Rats that performed an average of 7 or more full turns/min (over 90 min) ipsilateral to the lesion (after subtraction of any contralateral turns) were found to have 99% or greater depletions of striatal DA and never displayed spontaneous recovery of motor asymmetry. More recently, we have used rats with an initial mean net rotational asymmetry of 5.5 turns/min without observing spontaneous recovery; instead, there is often a small increase of asymmetry following repeated testing (refs. 6, 28, and unpublished observations). Because the lesion-induced behavioral changes are stable, amphetamine-induced rotation is eminently suited as a functional parameter to assess the effects of grafts. One slight disadvantage with amphetamine-induced rotation is that we have observed a significant mortality rate when repeatedly testing grafted rats with a dose of 5 mg/kg d-amphetamine or methamphetamine. In our experience, grafted rats are more likely to die than controls with 6-OHDA lesions only. Death typically occurs 60 to 120 minutes after drug injection, and we are not aware of the exact cause of death, although it seems to involve a gradual exhaustion of the rat. In recent years we have routinely opted for a lower dose (2.5 mg/kg) of d-amphetamine, and we believe that this has resulted in a lower mortality without significantly reducing the turning rate (55).

In addition to exhibiting rotational asymmetry, rats with unilateral mesostriatal lesions display deficits in sensorimotor integration on the side of the body contralateral to the lesion (107) and are also impaired in skilled forepaw use on that side (63,112,113).

The alterations in striatal physiology that occur after a 6-OHDA lesion of the mesostriatal pathway, including changes in the levels of striatal neurotransmitters, receptor densities, and neuronal firing patterns have all been characterized also. A brief overview of these changes is given later in this chapter, adjacent to the discussion of graft-induced effects on these physiologic parameters.

Injections of 6-OHDA can also be made into the pathways of the mesolimbocortical DA system. These lesions affect the locomotor behavior of the rats, which, in cases when the lesion is extensive, become spontaneously hypoactive, hyporesponsive to amphetamine challenge, and hyperresponsive to low doses of apomorphine (114). These rats also display deficits in more complex tasks such as food hoarding (84) and learning in a water maze (43). The effects of transplanting cells to the nucleus accumbens are dealt with in a chapter by Rogers *(this volume),* and will not be discussed further here.

Genetically Determined Degeneration of the Dopamine System

Weaver mutant mice are characterized by progressive degeneration in two systems associated with motor function: the cerebellar cortex (126) and the mesotelencephalic DA system (139). In the homozygote mutant, there is approximately a 70% loss of substantia nigra DA neurons (170) and a 75% reduction in striatal DA levels (139) at 3 months of age. These mice exhibit several behavioral deficits in locomotor, spatial orientation, and memory tasks (92–94). The young adult Weaver mouse presents with an unstable gait, impaired limb coordination, and a rapid, fine tremor of the trunk and limbs (150). The mice are unable to walk in a straight line and repeatedly topple over to the sides. The precise contribution of the neuropathology occurring in the substantia nigra as opposed to that in the cerebellum to the different parts of the symptomatology is not clear. Nevertheless, Weaver mice provide a unique opportunity to study DA-rich grafts in an environment with *ongoing* degeneration of the endogenous DA system, which thus mimics the situation in Parkinson's disease.

Lesions Induced by 1-Methyl-4-phenyl-1,2,3,6-tetrahydropyridine and its Metabolites

1-Methyl-4-phenyl-1,2,3,6-tetrahydropyridine (MPTP), which is known to cause DA depletion and a Parkinson-like state in humans (95) and other primates (33), does not affect the DA system of rodents quite as severely (22,125). In rats, systemic administration of MPTP does not give rise to a permanent depletion of DA (22), and the model has therefore not contributed in a major way to intracerebral transplant research. However, chronic (7-day) infusions of MPP+, which is the neurotoxic metabolite of MPTP, into the mesencephalon of rats causes degeneration of the nigrostriatal DA system (153) not unlike that seen after 6-OHDA administration, and has been used in a few experiments. Aside from the obvious practical disadvantage (the method requires chronic infusion via a minipump), its advocates point to the fact that, unlike with 6-OHDA, all the non-DA neuronal systems and the mesolimbic DA system are spared by MPP+ (153).

In contrast to the modest effects attained in rats, systemic treatment with MPTP can cause severe and long-term bilateral depletion of DA in mice (163,184). Because the lesion usually is not absolutely complete, the behavioral consequences are less marked and the model has therefore only been of limited use in functional intracerebral grafting research.

SURVIVAL AND MORPHOLOGY OF CATECHOLAMINE-RICH GRAFTS IN THE STRIATUM—A BRIEF OVERVIEW

Grafts of Embryonic Dopamine Neurons

Embryonic DA neurons do not only survive the intracerebral grafting procedure in rodents, but they develop extensive axonal projections that integrate with their normal target region, that is, the neostriatum (Fig. 1), and tend to avoid nontarget areas of the host brain (e.g., 18). Several studies have focused on basic conditions that govern the survival of the grafts. It is possible to graft DA neurons in solid blocks of mesencephalic tissue that are placed either in the lateral ventricle or a premade cortical cavity adjacent to the neostriatum. Alternatively, the tissue can be mechanically dissociated into a "cell suspension" and then injected stereotaxically into the parenchyma of virtually any brain region. To obtain large numbers of surviving DA neurons, the donor tissue must not be too mature at the time of grafting. In the case of solid grafts, the upper donor age limit is around embryonic day 17 (151), and for dissociated "cell suspension" grafts it is embryonic days 15 to 16 (24,29). When the donor mesencephalic tissue is prepared and grafted according to the dissociated "cell suspen-

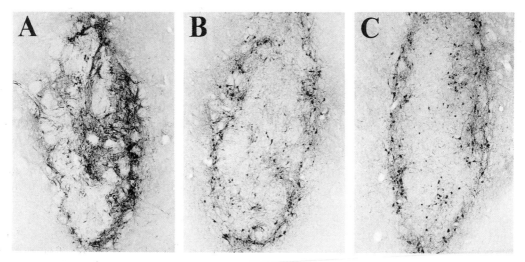

FIG. 1. Three photomicrographs each depicting a section through a nigral graft in a 6-OHDA denervated neostriatum. The sections are stained with an antibody against tyrosine hydroxylase. The rats were sacrificed at 4 days (**A**); 2 weeks (**B**); and 6 weeks (**C**) after transplantation surgery. The photographs show several darkly stained tyrosine hydroxylase-immunopositive cell bodies that extend fibers. At the earliest time point (**A**), relatively few fibers are seen to leave the graft tissue mass. At 2 (**B**) and 6 (**C**) weeks after grafting, there is a gradual increase in the amount of reinnervation of the denervated host striatum. In addition, as the grafts develop, there is a tendency for the tyrosine hydroxylase-immunopositive cells to arrange themselves around the perimeter of the grafts. × 120.

sion" technique, approximately 10% to 20% of the dissected DA neurons survive the grafting procedure (134,184), and they constitute in the order of 1 in 500 of the total number of surviving neurons (27). The grafted DA neurons have been identified using various techniques such as catecholamine histofluorescence (14), tyrosine hydroxylase immunohistochemistry (134), and *in situ* hybridization for tyrosine hydroxylase mRNA (155). In addition to containing DA neurons, it has been shown that mesencephalic grafts harbor CCK- (143), substance P-, enkephalin-, γ-aminobutyric acid (GABA)-, and serotonin-containing neurons (102). These grafts can give rise to a DA terminal network with a mean density just over 50% of normal adjacent to the graft, which drops to around 20% of normal about 1.0 mm from the graft border (54). The DA terminals have been found to synapse primarily on the dendritic spines and shafts of host striatal neurons (44,74,101), although "abnormal" synaptic contacts with giant striatal cell perikarya have also been described (74), which are not seen in the normal striatum. The grafts receive afferents from the host brain and, in a study using anterograde tracing and immunohistochemistry, have been shown to receive direct input from the neocortex and raphe nuclei (serotonergic fibers) and from a few striatal afferents (DARPP-32 positive) close to the graft host border (42,53).

Grafts of Adrenal Chromaffin Cells

Regarding transplants of adrenal medulla, there are few studies devoted to systematically investigating in which intracerebral sites and under which basic conditions the transplants survive best. In the initial experiments with intracerebral adrenal medulla grafts, the endocrine medulla from young rats (68) or cows (123) was dissected free of the cortex and injected into the lateral ventricle of adult rats. Freed and coworkers (68) counted between 66 and 4,080 surviving histofluorescent chromaffin cells derived from 4 to 6 dissected adrenal glands 2 months after grafting; however, the cells were confined to the ventricle and had formed almost no neurite-like extensions. In a recent study from the same laboratory, the proportions of graft recipients that contained surviving chromaffin cells in the ventricle were 67% and 44% at 5 and 10 months after surgery, respectively (166).

In general, it seems that adrenal grafts placed directly into the striatal parenchyma survive relatively poorly. This holds true both when the grafts are prepared as solid pieces of chromaffin tissue (72,88,160) and when they are implanted as dissociated chromaffin cells (13,23,121). Most grafted adrenal medullary cells die within a few hours after implantation in the striatum (88,160), and average numbers of cells that survive per host have been reported to range between 25 to 100 (13), 800 (72), and approximately 5,000 cells (121) (in the latter case estimated at 5% of the number of injected cells). An exception to the rule of small intrastriatal grafts comes from Decombe et al. (51) who injected bovine adrenal medulla into immunosuppressed rats and occasionally recovered relatively large grafts in which the cells were so tightly clustered that it precluded cell counting. However, the grafts always exhibited areas of necrosis, particularly in central regions, and only rarely was a process seen to extend from a grafted cell into the host brain.

An interesting approach to improving the survival of intrastriatal adrenal grafts has been to supplement the transplants with nerve growth factor (NGF), delivered either via minipumps (161) or in a "biologic" form through genetically engineered NGF-producing cells (46) or cografted peripheral nerve (48). When supplied for 4 weeks via minipumps, the NGF clearly increased the number of surviving chromaffin cells three- to fourfold at a 3-month analysis time point, and induced the extension of neurite-like fibers from the grafted cells into the surrounding host brain (161). Similar effects have been observed when dissociated chromaffin cells have been co-grafted intrastriatally together with genetically altered astrocytes that secrete NGF (46). Specifically, when the adrenal cells were taken from postnatal day 12 rat donors, the NGF-producing astrocytes increased graft cell survival three- to sixfold and induced a change into a neuronal-like morphology in the chromaffin cells. If the donor tissue was taken at postnatal day 90, the graft survival-enhancing effect was maintained, but there was no alteration in cellular phenotype (46). Since Schwann cells from transected peripheral nerve are known to produce NGF, Date and collaborators (48) cografted sciatic nerve with adrenal medulla from 30-day-old mice to the striatum of MPTP-treated mice. The survival of the chromaffin cells was increased two- to threefold by the sciatic nerve cografts, and several cells developed long neuronal processes (48).

Without the stimulus of NGF there is virtually no fiber outgrowth from grafted adrenal cells that are harvested from *adult* donors. When implanted into the striatum, they are usually round in shape with no (80,161) or very short neurite-like processes (13,72). If chromaffin cells from *newborn* rats are transplanted into the adult striatum, it has been suggested that they can undergo partial transdifferentiation into tyrosine hydroxylase (TH)-positive neurons and will adopt a morphology with multiple, elongated neurites bearing varicosities, and even make synaptic contacts with host striatal neurons (118), although these observations await further confirmation.

In summary, it seems that the survival of grafted adrenal medulla is rather inconsistent between different studies, and that conditions that may favor graft survival and development include the use of neonatal as opposed to adult donor tissue, placement of the implants in the lateral ventricle instead of the brain parenchyma, and the administration of NGF to the grafted cells.

BEHAVIORAL EFFECTS OF GRAFTS IN THE DOPAMINE-DENERVATED STRIATUM

Drug-Induced Rotational Behavior

Several studies have demonstrated that unilateral grafts of catecholamine-rich tissue can reverse drug-induced motor asymmetry in rodents with unilateral lesions of the mesostriatal DA system, and can induce an asymmetry in animals with bilateral lesions. Two categories of drugs that act on the DA system through principally different mechanisms have been tested. First are drugs that stimulate DA receptors directly and thereby reveal receptor supersensitivity by eliciting rotational behaviour away from the lesioned side. The prototype for these drugs is apomorphine, which stimulates both D1 and D2 receptors. Second, drugs such as amphetamine release DA from terminals on the side of the intact mesostriatal system and thereby cause turning in a direction ipsilateral to the lesion. Results obtained using these two categories of drugs are described separately below.

Rotation Induced by Dopamine Receptor Agonists

Grafts of Embryonic Dopamine Neurons Affect Rotation Elicited by Dopamine Receptor Agonists

It is possible to reverse apomorphine-induced asymmetry in rats with unilateral lesions of the mesostriatal DA system to approximately 10% to 60% of pretransplantation levels using grafts of rat (3,23,56, 60,63,67,122,127,128,155) or human (30,163, 177) mesencephalic DA neurons. The dose of apomorphine seems to play a crucial role. There are a few examples in the literature where, although there have been surviving transplants, there has been only a minor or no detectable graft effect using

0.25 to 0.5 mg/kg apomorphine (12,15,19) because all the rats became engaged in non-rotational stereotypic behavior, whereas at a dose of 0.05 mg/kg the graft effects have been clear (56). With intraparenchymal grafts of dissociated rat DA neurons, the functional recovery in the apomorphine rotation test gradually develops over the first 12 to 15 weeks after transplantation (23,63). Similar results of a reduction in drug-induced motor asymmetry have been obtained using other directly acting DA receptor agonists such as the D1 receptor selective agonists SKF 38393 (87,117,137), SKF 82958 (12), and CY 208243 (128); and the D2 receptor-selective agonists quinpirole (117) and LY171555 (12,87,128,137). In a study where L-dopa was given repeatedly to rats with unilateral 6-OHDA lesions, an augmentation of the contralateral rotational response (L-dopa here mimicking the action of a directly acting DA agonist), believed to be due to drug sensitization, was prevented by DA neuron grafts (78).

There is one problem inherent to the interpretation of graft-evoked effects on apomorphine-induced rotation that is related to the test being dependent on the integrity of striatal DA receptors on the side that undergoes transplantation surgery. Thus, any form of nonspecific damage (106) to the grafted striatum will cause a reduction in apomorphine-induced rotation and mimic a specific graft-induced effect. For example, we observed that the effect of a human nigral xenograft on apomorphine-induced rotation in an immunosuppressed rat was maintained, whereas the effect on amphetamine-induced rotation disappeared, when the grafted striatum showed cerebral pathology, presumably secondary to an infection (30).

Grafts of Adrenal Medulla Can Affect Apomorphine-Induced Rotation

With grafts of adrenal medulla, the observed functional effects have been less consistent. Freed and coworkers (68) initially described how intraventricular grafts of adrenal medulla from young donors could reduce apomorphine-induced rotation 2 months after surgery by approximately 40% compared to pretransplantation values. Similar grafts taken from older rat donors, aged 1 to 2 years, had no effect (69,73), and intrastriatal implants of adrenal tissue also were found by the same group to be ineffective at significantly reducing apomorphine-induced motor asymmetry 7 to 9 weeks after implantation (72). Similarly, Strömberg and coworkers (161) found that the effects of intrastriatal implants of adrenal tissue on apomorphine-induced rotation were relatively small (around 20%–30% reduction) and did not seem permanent, because they were apparent at 3 months after surgery but had disappeared by 6 months. However, they also found that after a 28-day intrastriatal infusion of NGF via a minipump, the effect of the adrenal graft on apomorphine-induced rotation was more prominent (70%–75% reduction after 2–4 weeks) and seemed to last longer, but perhaps not permanently because after 3 to 12 months the mean reduction had fallen to 44% to 48%. Control infusions of NGF into 6-OHDA-denervated striatum had no effect on apomorphine-induced motor asymmetry. An attractive explanation for the enhanced behavioral effects of the adrenal grafts is simply that, as mentioned previously, they survive better and develop more extensions when supplemented with NGF. Indeed, 3 months after surgery there was a mean of 449 histofluorescent cells in the NGF-treated rats as opposed to 127 in non-treated rats (161). Moreover, the NGF-treated grafts also contained several cells with a more neuronal phenotype and possessed several fibers extending into the host striatum, unlike the control transplants, which exhibited almost no fibers. However, the interpretation that the enhanced behavioral effect is due to improved survival and altered graft morphology is challenged by the findings of Pezzoli et al. (124). They also found that when NGF is infused into a brain containing a "sham" intraventricular implant of sciatic nerve or adipose tissue, there was a nearly 70% decrease in apomorphine-induced rotation, which was equivalent to the effect of NGF infusion in combination with an adrenal medullary transplant. The effect was not apparent with NGF alone, and thus the combination of nonspecific brain trauma and NGF seems to reduce behavioral manifestations of DA receptor supersensitivity in the denervated striatum.

In an important study, Brown and Dunnett (23) directly compared the effects of nigral grafts and different types of adrenal grafts (intrastriatal implants of dissociated chromaffin cells and intraventricular solid adrenal grafts taken from postnatal day 22–25 donors) on drug-induced rotation. The nigral transplants gradually induced a significant 40% reduction in apomorphine-induced rotation lasting until the end of the 14-week observation period. In contrast, the *intraventricular* adrenal grafts had no effect on apomorphine-induced rotation, and the dissociated *intrastriatal* implants of adrenal cells gave rise to 30% to 50% reductions in turning rates that were clearly apparent only during the first few weeks of testing, and then gradually disappeared. At sacrifice, most adrenal grafts were found to have died, and only a few rats in the intraventricular group contained a very low number of surviving chromaffin cells. This study supports the notion that when no trophic factors are added, the behavioral effects of adrenal grafts in rats are relatively minor, only temporary, and correlate with a poor survival of the grafts. However, because the adrenal grafts survived so poorly, the study does not resolve what the functional capacity of adrenal grafts would be if they could survive for longer periods. In a recent study, a subgroup of 11 rats with intraventricular adrenal grafts exhibited a mean 20% to 25%, statistically significant recovery in the apomorphine-induced rotation test, and this extent of recovery did not change between 1 and 9 months after trans-

plantation surgery (166). Less than half of the rats contained surviving chromaffin grafts, but nonetheless the authors do not report a correlation between survival of chromaffin cells and an effect in the apomorphine test.

In a study where bovine adrenal medulla was immunoisolated by polyelectrolyte microencapsulation and grafted to the denervated rat striatum, Aebischer et al. (1) observed a 60% reduction in apomorphine-induced rotational asymmetry. The effect was apparent already 1 week after transplantation and remained stable over the 4-week observation period. Although this different approach to grafting adrenal cells shows promise, its long-term efficacy remains to be established.

Rotation Induced by Dopamine-Releasing Agents

Grafts of Embryonic Dopamine Neurons Affect Amphetamine-Induced Rotation

As initially demonstrated by Björklund and Stenevi (14), grafts of mesencephalic DA neurons can completely reverse the amphetamine-induced rotation asymmetry in rats with unilateral 6-OHDA lesions. In a similar vein, unilateral transplants in rats with bilateral 6-OHDA lesions can induce a rotational asymmetry away from the grafted side after amphetamine administration (17,58,61,157). The effects of these grafts on rotation in the rat seem permanent in that there are reports of persistent recovery 2 years after surgery (ref. 119 and own unpublished observations). It also has been found that ipsiversive motor asymmetry induced by the DA reuptake blockers cocaine and nomifensine also can be reversed by DA neuron grafts in rats (110).

Amphetamine-induced rotation has also proven a useful tool to detect surviving DA neuron grafts in mice. Surviving grafts can reverse motor asymmetry in mice with unilateral intrastriatal 6-OHDA lesions (25), and are able to induce a motor asymmetry (contralateral rotation) in unilaterally implanted Weaver mice after amphetamine administration (52,99,171). Unilateral implants also have been found to support amphetamine-induced motor asymmetry in mice with bilateral lesions after systemic MPTP (184).

Time Course of Development of Effects on Amphetamine-Induced Rotation

The first signs of functional compensation of amphetamine-induced rotation can appear relatively early after transplantation. In rats with intraparenchymal implants of dissociated rat DA neurons, the first signs of a reduced rotational asymmetry typically appear as early as 2 to 3 weeks after surgery (16,23,157), whereas after solid grafts of rat tissue in cortical cavities overlying the striatum, the effects usually first appear as late as 2 to 3 months after transplantation surgery (15,56). After intraparenchymal implantation of cell suspension grafts, the reduction in turning asymmetry progressively develops to reach a stable level after 4 to 8 weeks (23). The speed with which graft-induced recovery appears seems to correlate to the rate of development of the grafted neurons. Thus, grafted human embryonic DA neurons, which normally exhibit a more protracted development compared to their rodent counterparts, do not give rise to functional effects in the amphetamine-induced rotation test until after 10 to 13 weeks, and the effects are not fully developed until 15 to 20 weeks after transplantation surgery (26,44). Interestingly, when dissociated rat nigral DA neurons are unilaterally implanted into the striatum of neonates that, 2 months later as adults, are subjected to an ipsilateral 6-OHDA lesion, the graft-induced reversal of amphetamine-induced rotation takes between 3 and 7 months to develop (4). Thus, it may be that the grafted DA neurons do not develop ex-

tensive axonal outgrowth until the host striatum is denervated, and when this occurs after the grafted neurons have been left to mature for 2 months, their rate of reinnervation of the host striatum is relatively retarded, explaining the latency of onset of functional effects.

Relationship between Nigral Graft Survival and Effects on Amphetamine-Induced Rotation

There seems to be a correlation between the number of surviving grafted DA neurons (24,29,127), their DA production (128,141), their fiber outgrowth into the host striatum (15), and the extent of the graft-induced changes in amphetamine-induced rotation. When postmortem tissue levels of DA were assessed, it was found that as little as 2% to 6% of the levels present in the normal striatum is sufficient to affect amphetamine-induced rotation (128, 141,142). With intraparenchymal grafts of dissociated DA neurons, it has been shown that as few as 120 to 400 (depending on the histologic technique used to detect the cells) surviving DA neurons are sufficient to elicit a 50% reduction in amphetamine-induced rotational asymmetry in the rat (24,29,134). This represents approximately 2% to 4% of the number of DA neurons that normally innervate the striatum, and a similar critical proportion seems to exist in the mouse with a unilateral 6-OHDA lesion, which needs a graft containing only 80 DA neurons before an effect on the rotation test is evident (25). One explanation for why so few grafted DA neurons are necessary to exert a significant effect on amphetamine-induced rotation is that they innervate only the small subregion of the striatum that is crucial for rotational behavior (i.e., the central and dorsal striatum) and which normally would receive afferents from only a minority of nigral DA neurons. The high sensitivity of the amphetamine-induced rotation test makes it an excellent assay to monitor survival of grafted DA neurons. One drawback is that, because the test is so sensitive, it does not distinguish rats with moderately sized grafts from those with large ones, because they all display complete reversal of the amphetamine-induced asymmetry.

"Overcompensation" of Amphetamine-Induced Rotation

Repeated studies have shown that intraparenchymal implants of dissociated DA neurons can give rise to an "overcompensation" of amphetamine-induced rotation, that is, the rats exhibit more turns *away* from the 6-OHDA-lesioned side, in contrast to before grafting, when they circle only *toward* the side of the lesion (60,83, 88,127,128). In contrast, rats with solid transplants placed in cavities overlying the caudate–putamen do not display overcompensation but exhibit at most 90% to 100% reductions in rotation (15). The reason why rats with intraparenchymal grafts show this overcompensation is unclear, and it sometimes also appears in rats with relatively small grafts that include only 5% (29,134) of the number of DA neurons that normally innervate the striatum, or produce around 5% of the normal total DA content of the striatum (128,142). When grafts in rats contain over 1,000 TH immunoreactive (134) or 300 histofluorescent (29) DA neurons, the rats are often "overcompensated," and there is usually a saturation effect, which means that additional DA neurons in the graft (29,134) or graft-derived DA fiber outgrowth (15) do not increase the extent of recovery in the amphetamine-induced rotation test.

The Importance of "Contralateral Turning"

The performance of a few turns contralateral to the lesion in response to amphet-amine is probably the most sensitive and specific indicator of a surviving nigral graft in the unilaterally 6-OHDA-lesioned rat. The contralateral turning is usually most marked in the first 20 minutes after amphetamine administration, and will in some rats gradually subside and revert to a net ipsilateral rotation over the ensuing 60 minutes (19,83,87,127,128) (Fig. 2A). Rioux et al. (128) have observed that when the grafts are relatively small, the contraversive turning is limited to the first 15 to 20 minutes (Fig. 2A), whereas in rats with larger grafts the contralateral rotation continues over the full 90-minute test period (Fig. 2B). Herman and coworkers (87) extended their observation period beyond 90 minutes and described the typical pattern of contralateral turning to be biphasic, with an early peak around 15 to 20 minutes after injection of 5 mg/kg amphetamine, and a second peak at 2 to 4 hours, before the active turning subsides. In contrast, ipsilateral turning in rats with 6-OHDA lesions only, or carrying nonfunctional grafts (Fig. 2C), typically peaks after 45 to 60 minutes and decreases linearly to reach baseline after around 4 hours (87). Herman and coworkers (83) have also noted that 0.4 mg/kg d-amphetamine sulfate, which, as opposed to doses of 1 to 5 mg/kg, did not give rise to marked ipsilateral rotational behavior in a 6-OHDA control group, nevertheless elicited very marked contralateral turning in rats with nigral grafts. This suggests that grafted DA neurons are hyperresponsive to amphetamine, and may be consistent with observations of transient contralateral rotation occurring shortly after drug injection when plasma levels of amphetamine presumably are low. However, the idea of hyperresponsiveness to amphetamine has been challenged (87,127), because with the *in vivo* microdialysis technique there is no evidence of an excessive (in comparison to the intact side) release of DA from grafts in response to amphetamine. It has also been speculated that the DA released from the grafts is acting on supersensitive receptors

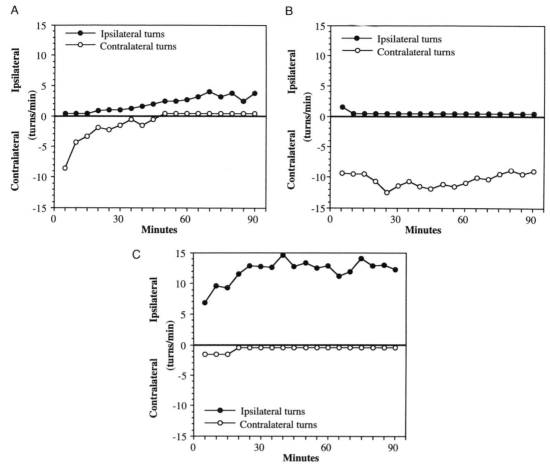

FIG. 2. Three diagrams illustrating the rotational behavior of three different unilaterally 6-OHDA-injected rats that received nigral grafts in the denervated striatum. The rats were given 5 mg/kg amphetamine at the start of the rotation test (minutes = 0). Before transplantation, all the rats exhibited a mean ipsilateral rotational bias of at least 7 full turns/minute. Grafting took place 22 weeks before the tests illustrated. The diagrams show the number of full turns per 5-minute bin ipsilateral and contralateral to the side of the lesion and graft over the full 90-minute test period. Three types of outcomes that can follow on nigral transplantation are illustrated: **A**: The results from a "compensated rat" in which the graft has eliminated the rotational bias. **B**: The results from an overcompensated rat in which the implant has induced a rotational bias in the direction contralateral to the graft. **C**: A "noncompensated" rat in which the graft has had no effect. Data modified from Duan et al. (55).

and therefore acts more efficiently than when released in an intact striatum. As will be discussed later in this chapter, there are several reports that grafts reduce receptor supersensitivity, but it is still conceivable that incomplete reversal of this phenomenon could be a contributing factor to behavioral "overcompensation." At least one ob-servation speaks against this interpretation. Herman et al. (83) studied apomorphine-induced turning, which is an index of receptor supersensitivity, and amphetamine-induced contralateral turning in the same grafted rats. They found no correlation between the two parameters, indicating that a grafted rat that performs several contralateral turns does not necessarily have a high level of residual receptor supersensitivity.

Removal of a Nigral Graft Reinstates Lesion-Induced Motor Asymmetry

In principle, it can be claimed that a surviving mesencephalic graft is a prerequisite for a greater than 50% reduction in amphetamine-induced rotation in a healthy rat that before grafting showed marked (> 6 turns/min) circling. The only exception to this rule seems to be that immunosuppressed rats that have exhibited functional effects of xenografted mouse DA neurons can continue to do so for some weeks after cessation of immunosuppression, even when the graft is undergoing rejection and no viable graft with DA cell bodies (but still some fibers) can be detected using catecholamine histofluorescence (31). Otherwise, it is noteworthy that when unilateral mesencephalic grafts that first have been shown to affect amphetamine-induced rotation are removed surgically by suction (15) or local injection of 6-OHDA (64), or are allowed to undergo complete immunologic rejection (31,35), the graft-induced effects on the rotational behavior disappear. Thus, rats with unilateral 6-OHDA lesions return to the rotational bias ipsilateral to the lesion that they displayed before grafting (Fig. 3). These observations demonstrate that the continued presence of the grafts is necessary for the functional effects to persist, and that the graft-induced behavioral changes are unlikely to be due to a trophic effect on the host brain requiring only a temporary exposure to the grafts.

No Strict Correlation between Nigral Graft Effects on Apomorphine- and Amphetamine-Induced Rotation

There is usually no strong correlation between the degree of recovery in the amphetamine-induced rotation tests and the

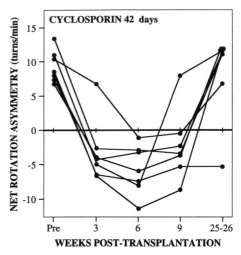

FIG. 3. Amphetamine-induced (5 mg/kg) rotational behavior of seven different unilaterally 6-OHDA-injected rats that received nigral xenografts from mouse donors in the denervated striatum. The rats were immunosuppressed with cyclosporin A for 42 days (6 weeks), after which the treatment was stopped. The rats were tested before grafting and at 3, 6, 9, and 25 to 26 weeks after transplantation surgery. All the rats exhibited "overcompensation" (contralateral turning) due to the grafts at 6 weeks. After cessation of immunosuppression, all the rats except one rejected their grafts and exhibited once again marked ipsilateral rotational behavior. Data modified from Brundin et al. (31).

extent of recovery in tests with directly acting DA receptor agonists. For example, Björklund and coworkers (15) noted, in an early study on solid nigral grafts placed in cortical cavities, that a complete reversal of amphetamine-induced rotation was not associated with an effect on apomorphine-induced circling, when the dose of apomorphine was 0.25 mg/kg. Subsequently, they tried a lower dose (0.05 mg/kg) and observed a 60% reduction in turning in a similar group of grafted rats (56), indicating that the dose of apomorphine is crucial when studying behavior related to DA receptor supersensitivity. However, using the low 0.05 mg/kg dose, Herman et al. (83) did not see any correlation between changes in apomorphine-induced rotation and amphetamine-induced contralateral turning in a group of rats with functional grafts. In a more recent study, Becker and Ariano (12) found a significant decrease of approximately 40% in amphetamine-induced asymmetry in a group of grafted rats that displayed unchanged apomorphine-induced (0.25 mg/kg) rotation after intraparenchymal grafting. No quantification of graft sizes was reported, but the relatively minor graft-induced effect in the amphetamine test suggests that the grafts were very small. Rioux and coworkers (127) have confirmed that small grafts, which cause only a little contralateral turning in the amphetamine test, do not significantly reduce apomorphine-induced turning. However, larger grafts, which completely reverse amphetamine-induced rotation, also reduce apomorphine-induced motor asymmetry (127). Thus, it seems that a change in amphetamine-induced turning, in particular the appearance of contralateral rotation in rats with complete 6-OHDA lesions of the mesostriatal DA system, is indeed a very sensitive and specific indicator of nigral graft function. These changes do not always correlate with alterations in apomorphine-induced motor asymmetry, which, as discussed previously, seem to be less specific and can be related to factors other than restored DA neurotransmission in the striatum. In cases when the reduction in apomorphine-induced asymmetry is due to a nigral transplant reinnervating the striatum, the transplant tends to be at least moderately large, exceeding the small sizes that are sufficient to affect amphetamine-induced rotation.

Testing for Apomorphine- before Amphetamine-Induced Rotation Can Give Confounding Results

When testing grafted rats for both apomorphine- and amphetamine-induced turning, it is important to be aware of the risk that rats can display spontaneous contralat-

eral turning when placed in the test apparatus even several days after an apomorphine test. This spontaneous contralateral turning can last for several minutes (unpublished observations), and can be misinterpreted as a graft effect if it appears in the early part of an amphetamine test, just before the amphetamine effect sets in. The phenomenon may be caused by a conditioning effect where the rats associate the "stimulus" of being inside the rotation test apparatus and performing contralateral turns, which they experienced during the prior session, with the "reward" of being given apomorphine. Indeed, in a well designed study, Annett and coworkers (6) have obtained evidence that grafted rats that are rotation tested with amphetamine develop a conditioned association between the test environment and the drug and rotate contralaterally (if the grafts are functional) when exposed to the test environment later under drug-free conditions.

Effects of Adrenal Medulla Grafts on Amphetamine-Induced Rotation Are Less Clear

In stark contrast to the effects of DA neuron grafts, it seems that grafts of adrenal medulla do not reliably reduce amphetamine-induced rotational asymmetry (10,23, 47,73,133,166). One study purports that amphetamine-induced motor asymmetry is reduced by intraventricular adrenal grafts; however, the evidence is not convincing. The authors report that the grafted rats exhibit a small, 27% reduction in circling compared to pretransplantation values (10). The results are difficult to evaluate because before transplantation surgery the rats were selected based on a criterion requiring a mean turning rate greater than only 0.83 full turns/minute in response to a relatively low dose (0.85–1.25 mg/kg) of amphetamine. Previous work indicates that this guarantees only a 90% depletion of striatal DA (81), and therefore does not exclude spontaneous behavioral recovery. A subsequent report, using the same paradigm, describes that 6 of 32 rats show a decrease in rotation, and that even when this subgroup is extracted from the whole transplant group, the mean reduction is only around 30% of baseline values (47). Another group of investigators (133) reports that the *increase* in amphetamine-induced rotation, which follows repeated tests, is marginally less in rats with intrastriatal implants of bovine adrenal medulla. However, the results are further confounded by the use of rats with only partial 6-OHDA lesions (58% reductions in DA in the lesion control group), and the authors also reallocated grafted rats with biochemical evidence of poor transplant survival to the control group when analyzing the behavioral data. In contrast, Bing et al. (13) report of an approximate 60% *reduction* in amphetamine-induced rotation 10 and 24 days after intrastriatal implantation of dissociated adrenal medulla. Thus, they did not provide evidence of long-term function of the grafts and, moreover, the results were somewhat unexpected in view of the fact that they observed only 25 to 100 surviving grafted chromaffin cells per rat.

In a singular report, Nishino and coworkers (118) observed a mean of 80% reduction in amphetamine-induced rotational asymmetry in 15 rats with intrastriatal grafts prepared from dissociated adrenal medulla of neonatal donors. The graft-induced effect developed gradually 2 to 8 weeks after surgery and remained over the 40-week observation period. The rats exhibited a recovery of motor asymmetry primarily in the later parts (more than 20 minutes after amphetamine injection) of each test session, which is quite unlike the findings in rats with embryonic mesencephalic grafts, which display the most marked reversal of asymmetry in the first part of each test session. Another subgroup of 20 rats in the same study that had received identical adrenal grafts exhibited no change in rotational asymmetry. Interestingly, the 15 rats that showed behavioral recovery contained

50 to 600 (mean, 120) TH-positive cells, whereas in the nonrecovered group there were virtually no surviving grafted cells. Moreover, the surviving TH-positive cells were (as mentioned in a previous section) often multipolar with a neuron-like morphology, including neurites that extended into the host striatum, and thus quite unlike the typical endocrine cell morphology of adrenal chromaffin cells are observed in most other transplantation experiments. In summary, the study by Nishino et al. (118) indicates that when chromaffin cells are taken from neonatal donors, they can still exhibit sufficient plasticity to adopt a neuronal-like morphology and are able to affect striatal-mediated behavior after amphetamine stimulation. Unfortunately, there are no published studies that directly follow up these original observations.

Nicotine-Induced Rotation in Rats with Chromaffin Grafts

In an original experiment involving intrastriatal grafts of bovine adrenal medulla to immunosuppressed rats, Decombe et al. (51) monitored no graft-evoked changes in amphetamine-induced rotation. However, interesting results were obtained when nicotine, which stimulates catecholamine release from normal adrenal medulla, was administered to the same rats. Those rats that on subsequent histologic examination were found to contain surviving transplants exhibited contralateral rotation, which was not blocked by the opiate receptor antagonist naloxone or the DA receptor antagonist pimozide, suggesting the effect was neither opiate nor DA receptor mediated. This study suggests that amphetamine is not the drug of choice for attempting to release transmitters from grafted adrenal medulla, and that nicotine provides an interesting alternative that warrants further study when assessing the functional capacity of adrenal grafts in the striatum. Recently, however, Takashima and coworkers (166) did not see any significant contralateral rotation after nicotine administration to rats with intraventricular grafts of rat chromaffin tissue.

Spontaneous Rotation

Nigral Grafts Affect Spontaneous Rotation

Spontaneous rotation in the unilateral 6-OHDA lesion rat model also is reduced by grafted DA neurons, both of rat (17,56,117) and human (30) origin. Similarly, rats with bilateral 6-OHDA lesions and unilateral nigral grafts will display preferred spontaneous turning contralateral to the grafted side (17,58,61,157). In general, the rate of spontaneous turning is quite low, around 15 net ipsilateral turns per hour for rats with unilateral 6-OHDA lesions during the active nocturnal period. The turning can be increased by tail-pinch activation (e.g., attaching a paper clip to the rat's tail), and under these conditions mesencephalic grafts also have been shown to increase the number of turns away from the transplanted side, both in unilaterally and bilaterally denervated rats (17,56,58,157). A different test of spontaneous behavior, where rats are trained to circle in response to a sugar-water reward (without drug administration), is called the conditioned rotation test (59). In this paradigm, rats with unilateral 6-OHDA lesions are unable to learn to turn away from the side of the lesion, whereas lesioned rats with grafts have been found to be able to perform the task, albeit not to control levels (62). Moreover, somewhat surprisingly, the grafted rats became partially impaired in their ability to perform conditioned turning ipsilaterally to the lesion, an impairment that was not apparent in rats with 6-OHDA lesions only.

No Evidence for Long-Term Effects of Chromaffin Grafts on Spontaneous Rotation

There are no reports indicating that grafts of adrenal chromaffin cells can induce long-term recovery in tests of spontaneous rotational behavior in rats with unilateral 6-OHDA lesions. The only published adrenal graft study dealing with spontaneous motor asymmetry is focused on the immediate postoperative effects of intrastriatal implantation of adrenal medulla, and shows that as the rats wake up from the anesthesia they can spontaneously rotate away from the grafted side (88). The rotational behavior was most intense around 100 minutes after grafting, and lasted approximately 400 minutes. It was most marked in rats grafted with large quantities of adrenal tissue in central parts of the striatum, and was interpreted as being secondary to a massive catecholamine release occurring when most of the implanted cells died and underwent lysis.

Tests of "Nonrotational" Spontaneous Behaviors Involving Motor and Sensory Asymmetry

Sensorimotor Integration

Nigral Grafts Reduce Deficits in Sensorimotor Integration

The impaired ability to respond to stimuli that appear contralateral to a unilateral 6-OHDA lesion of the mesostriatal pathway can be reversed by grafts of embryonic mesencephalic tissue. This has been achieved both with solid grafts (57) and implants of dissociated nigral tissue (60,103,117). The grafts must innervate the ventrolateral part of the striatum for the effects to appear (57,60,103). In rats with bilateral 6-OHDA lesions, a unilateral graft will support an increased sensorimotor responsiveness on the side opposite to the transplant (17, 58,61). T-maze bias, which can be taken as a measure of the rat's sensory attention on the two sides of the body, also is improved by mesencephalic transplants. Rats with unilateral lesions will make significantly more choices in the direction contralateral to the lesion after grafting (17,56,58,

60), and rats with bilateral lesions and unilateral implants show a marked preference for the maze arm contralateral to the graft (17,58).

Chromaffin Grafts Have Not Yet Been Shown to Reduce Deficits in Sensorimotor Integration

In a study on chromaffin grafts, Freed et al. (72) reported that intrastriatal implants of multiple small pieces of adrenal medullary tissue do not ameliorate sensory neglect compared to pretransplantation performance.

Disengage Behavior: Conflicting Results Concerning the Effects of Nigral Grafts

In the disengage behavior test, the rats are presented with a perioral sensory stimulus (e.g., poking with a pen) while engaged in eating. Normal rats are able to "disengage" from the ongoing activity (eating) and turn their heads toward the sensory stimulus, whereas rats with unilateral 6-OHDA lesions display reduced responsiveness on the side contralateral to the lesion (138). The deficit also has been found to remain in 6-OHDA-treated rats that exhibit spontaneous recovery in the conventional sensory neglect test (138). An initial transplantation study failed to detect any significant effects on disengage behavior by mesencephalic implants innervating only the ventrolateral part of the striatum, even though the same rats showed recovery in the sensory neglect test (103). In a more recent study (117), grafts innervating both the ventrolateral and central striatum displayed a partial, but significant, recovery of disengage behavior (40% reduction in response latency compared to controls). All the transplants were relatively large in this study and there were no significant differences in the size of the

grafts in rats that displayed functional compensation and those that did not.

Paw-Reaching/Forelimb Use: Conflicting Results Concerning the Effects of Nigral Grafts

In this test, the rats are presented with a skilled motor task in which they have to reach for a food reward using fine, controlled movements of the forepaw. Rats with unilateral 6-OHDA lesions are impaired contralateral to the lesion, and earlier work has failed to demonstrate a significant effect on paw-reaching performance by mesencephalic implants in such rats (63,112). A recent report (117) suggests that grafts in some cases can improve paw-reaching performance. Forty percent of the rats exhibited no improvement in paw-reaching even though the recovered in rotation tests with amphetamine and DA receptor agonists, whereas the remaining 60% showed a gradual improvement in paw function approaching control levels after 6 days of training. Notably, there were no differences in graft size between animals with improved paw function and those without. In contrast, in two other recent reports, Abrous and colleagues (3,4) have not observed any recovery of forepaw function secondary to mesencephalic implants placed in the neostriatum or the nucleus accumbens, although the same rats exhibited graft-related recovery in drug-induced rotation and activity tests. Pretreating the grafted rats with amphetamine before testing paw-reaching ability did not significantly improve their performance (3). Nor was there any effect on forelimb function when the nigral grafts were implanted into neonatal hosts (hypothetically, an environment that should favor anatomic graft–host interaction) that underwent unilateral 6-OHDA lesion surgery later as adults (4). The reason for the discrepancy in results between the aforementioned studies is not clear, but it does not seem to be related simply to differences in graft sizes or placement.

Behavioral Tests in Animals with Bilateral Functional Impairments

General Motor Function

Studies of the effects of grafts on locomotor activity have often involved lesions and grafts in the mesolimbic DA system, which fall outside the scope of this chapter and are dealt with in the chapter by Rogers et al. *(this volume)*. However, there are studies that focus on the locomotor effects of grafts placed in the caudate–putamen.

Nigral Grafts Affect Locomotor Activity

It has been possible to reverse akinesia in rats with bilateral lesions of the nigrostriatal pathways by solid nigral grafts placed in a cavity overlying the neostriatum (58) or by multiple implants of dissociated tissue into several striatal sites (61). In the study with multiple intrastriatal implants (61), both spontaneous and amphetamine-induced locomotor activity was increased by the grafts in some cases, whereas in the study with only one intracortical solid transplant (58), only amphetamine-induced locomotor activity was restored. Although it can be speculated that the responses were mediated by graft-derived DA fibers innervating the nucleus accumbens in the case of the multiple cell suspension grafts (61), it seems that reinnervation of the caudate–putamen proper must have mediated the behavioral recovery in the solid graft study, because in this case no graft fibers reached as far as the nucleus accumbens (58).

Effects of Nigral Grafts on Age-Related Motor Deficits Await Confirmation

Aged rats also have exhibited improvement in general motor function after grafts of mesencephalic tissue. Normally, most female Sprague-Dawley rats aged 21 to 23 months become motorically impaired and exhibit a deteriorating sensorimotor coordination. Eight such rats improved their motor performance compared to nine age-matched controls on tests of balance and limb coordination 12 weeks after bilateral implantation of nigral DA neurons into the head of the caudate–putamen (75). There were no beneficial graft-induced effects on general motor activity or swimming ability. Notably, there have been no published reports since 1983 demonstrating functional effects of nigral grafts on age-related motor impairments. This may reflect either that the studies are arduous to perform because the graft recipients often die of age-related causes, or simply that the graft-induced effects that were observed in this initial study are not very robust.

Nigral Grafts May Affect General Motor Function in Weaver Mutant Mice

Weaver mutant mice, which normally develop several motor impairments probably related both to their nigral and cerebellar pathologies (see section on genetically determined degeneration of the dopamine system), also can improve their general motor function after grafting. Thus, Weaver mice with bilateral nigral grafts have been reported to topple over to the side less often and perform better in tests of motor equilibrium (172).

Aphagia and Adipsia: Effects of Catecholamine-Rich Grafts on Ingestive Behaviors Depend on the Age of the Recipient

As mentioned previously, rats with extensive bilateral 6-OHDA lesions of the mesotelencephalic DA system exhibit aphagia and adipsia (176). Repeated, concerted efforts to reverse these deficits by grafting embryonic DA neurons to *adult* hosts have failed, and, at best, large grafts that reinnervate large regions of the forebrain DA target areas will induce very minor improvements in feeding and drinking behavior (17,58,61). However, if the graft surgery is performed on *neonatal* rats, and the bilateral 6-OHDA lesions created later when the rats are adult, a significant proportion of the grafted rats will not develop aphagia and adipsia (129,144). The difference between adult and neonatal recipients may be related to a greater neuronal plasticity present in the neonate, which may allow for a greater exchange of afferents and efferent connections between host and graft. Three recent independent studies (4,42,86) have reported that grafted DA neurons tend to migrate more into the host brain when implanted in neonates than when grafted to adult rats. However, when the host striatal projections into the graft tissue proper were labeled using DARPP-32 immunohistochemistry and their abundance compared in adult and neonate recipients, there was no indication that the neonatal striatal neurons had formed more extensive connections with the graft than those observed in the adult rats (42).

Using the same model, with grafts in neonatal hosts, Simonds et al. (152) have reported that bilateral intraventricular implants of adrenal medulla can induce an increase in eating and drinking behavior, although not to the same extent as seen after grafting embryonic DA neurons.

Functional Heterogeneity of the Striatum

Nigral Grafts Placed in Different Parts of the Striatal Complex Affect Different Types of Behavior

The different behavioral effects of DA neuron grafts described in the previous sections all depend on the grafts reinnervating a precise, crucial striatal region. The striatal region which is crucial varies according to the different types of behavior studied. For example, drug-induced rotation is primarily affected by grafts that reinnervate the central and dorsal striatum (56), whereas sensory neglect is reversed by grafts that reinnervate the ventrolateral striatum (57,60,103). The functional subdivision of the striatum seems strict, and also determines that nigral grafts innervating only the dorsal-central striatum do not diminish sensory neglect, and grafts that extend fibers just into the ventrolateral striatum do not reduce drug-induced rotational asymmetry. The sharpness of the anatomic borders that confine the behavioral effects of grafted DA neurons to those areas of the host striatum they reinnervate is clearly illustrated by an experiment involving mesencephalic implants into the nucleus accumbens and a behavioral test of caudate–putamen function (28). In this study, the hosts first received unilateral lesions of the mesostriatal DA pathway followed by bilateral local injections of 6-OHDA into the nucleus accumbens. The lesions of the mesolimbic DA fibers innervating the nucleus accumbens caused a decrease in the magnitude of the turning response after amphetamine administration, which was expected because DA neurotransmission in the accumbens/ventral striatum is believed to be crucial in regulating the magnitude of locomotion, without affecting direction. When the rats were given implants of DA neurons in the accumbens ipsilateral to the side of the unilateral mesostriatal lesion (i.e., in proximity to the denervated caudate–putamen), they increased their rotational asymmetry again (28). Intriguingly, a graft placed less than a millimeter away in the caudate–putamen would have according to the studies described previously, given the diametrically opposite effect, that is, a decrease or reversal of the motor asymmetry. Recently, Abrous and coworkers (3) obtained results of a similar kind in an analogous model consisting of a 6-OHDA denervation of both the neostriatum and nucleus accumbens on one side of the brain. They found that unilateral nigral grafts placed in the denervated nucleus accumbens did not affect amphetamine-induced rotation, whereas intrastriatal grafts did. Conversely, apomorphine-induced locomotor hyperactivity was attenuated by intraaccumbens grafts (because the nucleus accumbens is involved in locomotion), but remained significantly elevated in rats with grafts placed in the neostriatum. In summary, the results mentioned here suggest that the behavioral effects of mesencephalic grafts are strictly limited to the functions subserved by the regions that they innervate. Interestingly, as will be discussed later, there is evidence that nigral transplants can affect parameters of host striatal neuron physiology in areas beyond those actually reinnervated by the grafted DA neurons. The exact meaning of these distant effects remains enigmatic in view of the behavioral studies discussed above.

ENDOGENOUS PROPERTIES OF THE GRAFTED DOPAMINE NEURONS OR ADRENAL CELLS

Electrophysiologic Activity of Grafts

Grafted Embryonic Dopamine Neurons Exhibit Spontaneous Firing Activity

Regardless of whether implanted as an intrastriatal *cell suspension* (65) or, alternatively, as a *tissue fragment* into the lateral ventricle (181), a cortical cavity overlying the denervated host striatum (7), or directly into the striatal parenchyma (177), grafted mesencephalic DA neurons have been shown to display spontaneous firing activity. Most electrophysiologic characteristics of both DAergic and non-DAergic graft neurons have been reported to be strongly reminiscent of their mature *in situ* counterparts, although they can display some features normally encountered only during development. For example, Fisher and colleagues (65), in a study of the electrophysiologic characteristics of intrastria-

tal nigral suspension grafts, distinguished different classes of graft neurons on the basis of their physiologic characteristics and their morphology after intracellular dye injections and immunocytochemical staining. Although certain types of cells were reminiscent of non-DAergic neurons of the substantia nigra parts reticulata, and of neurons found in the mesencephalic reticular formation, respectively, another category of neurons displayed a physiologic activity pattern similar to that of nigral DA neurons. The authors noted that in grafts that were left to mature for 4 to 5 months, the firing rate tended to be lower and the action potentials wider than normally observed in the adult substantia nigra. Both these features are associated with developing neurons in the immature brain and, furthermore, they tended to be less prominent in recordings made 8 to 9 months after transplantation surgery.

From the early experiments of Wuerthele (181) on intraventricular nigral grafts, there is evidence that the grafted DA neurons possess some autoregulatory properties because local application of DA agonists decreased the firing of the neurons, whereas application of DA antagonists increased the neuronal activity. Subsequently, evidence suggesting that nigral grafts may be under some form of control from the host brain has emerged. Arbuthnott and colleagues (7) performed electrophysiologic recordings from solid mesencephalic grafts implanted into a cavity overlying the denervated host striatum and found that neurons in the graft could respond to stimulation of the host frontal cortex and the lower brain stem. More recently, the report by Fisher and coworkers (65) demonstrated that when the graft is implanted intrastriatally as a cell suspension, a large proportion of the grafted neurons are responsive to cortical or striatal stimulation if they have been given enough time to mature and, possibly, receive afferent connections from the host.

Because adrenal chromaffin cells are non-neuronal endocrine cells, there are no published accounts of the electrophysiologic properties of adrenal medulla transplants.

Graft Catecholamine Content and Release

Nigral Grafts Partially Restore Striatal Dopamine Levels

Even in rats with large mesencephalic grafts, the recovery of overall striatal DA levels and DA synthesis remains lower than normal. Schmidt et al. (140) revealed a mean recovery of 13% to 14% of normal striatal DA levels after placing the nigral graft into a cortical cavity overlying the denervated striatum. In subsequent studies on intrastriatal nigral suspension grafts, the DA levels in the grafted striatum have been reported to reach a similar recovery of 6% to 18% of normal (76,82,128,141). When taking punch samples of striatal tissue at various distances from an intraventricular nigral graft, Freed and colleagues (67) found that the recovery of tissue DA levels was highest in the tissue adjacent to the transplant (in the range of 30% of normal), and dropped to 5% to 15% in samples taken at a greater distance from the transplant. This indicates that the striatal region sampled is crucial when biochemically assessing the success of the grafts. More recently, Nikkhah et al. (117), using a novel transplantation method for distributing the graft suspension over 18 sites in the caudate–putamen, found a recovery of striatal DA levels, when including the multiple grafts in the dissection, to 30% of normal DA levels (see Björklund, Dunnett, and Nikkhah [*this volume*]).

Nigral Grafts Exhibit Increased Transmitter Turnover

The degree of functional recovery in the amphetamine-induced rotation test has been found to correlate with the amount of graft-derived DA in the lesioned striatum. Marked functional graft effects have been observed when DA levels in the grafted striatum exceeded 10% of normal control values, whereas grafts that exhibited only minor functional effects restored striatal DA only to about 6% (128,140,141). Although the modest recovery of striatal DA levels brought about by nigral grafts may at first seem disappointing, the fact that net reductions in total amphetamine-induced turning behavior can be seen with grafts that restore as little as 10% of total striatal DA content (128,140,141) points both to the grafts' remarkable functional efficiency and the high sensitivity of the amphetamine rotation test. There are indications that the grafted DA neurons have an increased transmitter turnover because grafted striata exhibit 3,4-dihydroxyphenylacetic acid (DOPAC):DA ratios that are 50% to 200% higher than normal (82,109,128, 140,141). However, the increase in turnover is less marked in rats with grafts that are large enough to reduce amphetamine-induced rotation significantly (141). A similar increase in DOPAC:DA ratio can be observed in the striatum after partial lesions of the mesostriatal pathway (132). Although the grafted nigral neurons normally synthesize DA at an increased rate, they still can increase their transmitter synthesis. Thus, when grafted rats are given the DA receptor blocker haloperidol (which is known to increase DA metabolism through a decreased negative feedback), the DOPAC:DA ratio is increased approximately twofold compared to saline-injected, grafted rats (82,109).

Nigral Grafts Spontaneously Release Dopamine

The spontaneous electrophysiologic activity of grafted mesencephalic neurons discussed in the previous section is paralleled by a tonic release of DA from the transplant. In intracerebral microdialysis studies, grafts of embryonic DA neurons have been found to restore the baseline levels of

DA partly (87,183), or wholly to normal control values (30,119,127,159). A comparison between the estimated striatal DA innervation density derived from the grafts and DA levels recovered in dialysis perfusates from the same rats suggests that grafted DA neurons release DA at a higher rate than normal rats (159,183).

Experiments made using the *in vivo* voltammetry technique also support the concept that grafted DA neurons are spontaneously active (66) or release DA in the denervated striatum in response to potassium application (131,164). The study by Forni and coworkers (66) used surface-treated multifiber carbon electrodes that were chronically implanted soon after transplantation surgery. The study demonstrated a very sudden recovery of voltammetric signal, usually occurring 6 to 8 weeks after grafting in rats with large transplants. There has been debate as to whether these electrodes actually monitor DA *in vivo*, rather than DA metabolites and ascorbate. However, assuming the validity of the claim that the electrodes monitor DA, the results suggest that there is little diffusion of DA from the graft-derived terminals and that the voltammetric signal therefore appears first when the graft-derived axons have grown far enough to reach the probe area and release DA from terminals immediately adjacent to the probe. Taking into consideration the distance between graft and probe and the time it took before a significant voltammetric signal appeared, the maximal speed of fiber outgrowth was estimated to be 0.1 mm per week (66).

Grafted Embryonic Dopamine Neurons Respond to Drugs and Possess Dopamine Reuptake Sites

In vivo dialysis studies have repeatedly demonstrated that grafted neurons release several-fold increased amounts of DA when the hosts are challenged with amphetamine (30,87,119,127,183). When nomifensine, a blocker of DA reuptake sites, is administered, the levels of extracellular DA derived from grafted human or rat DA neurons are increased threefold to tenfold (30,159). These *in vivo* findings are supported by *in vitro* studies on striatal slice preparations. Slices prepared from 6-OHDA-denervated striatum containing mesencephalic transplants show enhanced basal overflow of tritiated DA in response to amphetamine or nomifensine (89). More evidence for the existence of DA reuptake sites on graft-derived terminals comes from findings of a partial restoration in the binding of the DA reuptake site ligands [^{3}H]-mazindol (20), [^{3}H]-BTCP (50), and [^{3}H]-GBR 12935 (39, 41) in the 6-OHDA-denervated striatum that has been reinnervated by nigral grafts. In cases when careful quantification has been performed, the levels of DA reuptake sites have reached 60% to 70% of control (20,50). Using quantitative [^{3}H]-dopamine autoradiography, it has been possible to demonstrate that the DA uptake sites on the grafted neurons are functionally efficient both when grafted to the 6-OHDA-denervated rat striatum (54) and the partially denervated Weaver mutant mouse striatum (52).

As previously mentioned, it seems that the high baseline levels of DA are achieved by both a higher than normal DA turnover rate in the grafted neurons and a higher than normal release of DA relative to the density of terminals (140,183). However, this does not necessarily imply that the grafted neurons release DA in an unregulated manner because, first, as mentioned, they exhibit a functional DA reuptake system and, second, they seem to be subject to negative feedback through inhibitory DA autoreceptors, both of which may aid in maintaining a stable tonic level of DA release (159). When the DA receptor agonist apomorphine was administered, Strecker et al. (159) found that the graft-derived DA release dropped as much as 40%, suggesting that DA autoreceptor stimulation, just as in the electrophysiologic experiments of Wuerthele et al. (181), inhibited the grafted DA neurons.

Chromaffin Cells Release Catecholamines Acutely after Transplantation

The literature is relatively sparse with regard to transmitter content and transmitter release from grafted adrenal chromaffin cells. Evidence for poor survival of intraparenchymal grafts of adult chromaffin tissue has been obtained using a combined biochemical and morphologic approach. Strömberg et al. (169) measured the catecholamine levels between 2 and 400 minutes after intrastriatal implantation of one adult adrenal medulla. They found large amounts of adrenaline and noradrenaline and low levels of DA 2 minutes after implantation surgery. Over the following 400 minutes, the catecholamine levels decreased considerably. These findings were paralleled by microscopic observations of an intense catecholamine histofluorescence in and around the grafts at the 2-minute time point, and a drastic diminution of fluorescence by 400 minutes. Thus the results indicate that the major catecholamines present in the adrenal grafts are adrenaline and noradrenaline, and that they can be released at high concentrations immediately after implantation surgery, when a large proportion of the transplanted cells die. Five months after being implanted into the lateral ventricle, adrenal medullary grafts have been reported to harbor very variable levels of DA, which sometimes are in the range of those in normal, intact caudate–putamen (70). However, the total catecholamine concentration in analyzed pieces of graft tissue was still on average only 1% to 2% of that in normal adrenal medulla (70). The large variability of the data in this study, with catecholamine concentrations varying five orders of magnitude between grafts, and the absence of a systematic follow-up study make it difficult to evaluate

the true catecholamine-producing capacity of rat chromaffin tissue grafted to the brain. A more recent study on intrastriatal xenografts of bovine chromaffin tissue to rats suggests that the grafts will survive without immunosuppression for 8 weeks in less than half of the recipients, and that they then can produce large quantities of adrenaline and noradrenaline, but no DA (133).

Long-Term Chromaffin Grafts Do Not Release Large Quantities of Catecholamines

In a series of intracerebral microdialysis experiments, Becker and Freed (10) addressed the issue of catecholamine release from intraventricular adrenal medulla transplants in rats with unilateral 6-OHDA lesions. In a first experiment, a dialysis probe was placed in the lateral ventricle on the side of the transplant. Dialysate from the cerebrospinal fluid of chromaffin-grafted rats did not contain detectable levels of DA, but levels of DOPAC were slightly elevated compared to controls (10). In a second series of experiments, in which the dialysis probe was implanted into the striatum on the grafted side, there also was no increase in baseline DA levels in the chromaffin-grafted rats. In a subgroup of grafted rats that had displayed some reduction in amphetamine-induced rotation, the authors point out that there was a significantly greater percentage increase (around 550% versus 300%) in recovered DA after systemic amphetamine stimulation in comparison to control rats (10). However, although the baseline DA levels did not significantly differ between the two groups, the numerical mean for the baseline DA in the grafted group was half that of the controls. Hence, the absolute values for extracellular DA after amphetamine administration must have been approximately the same in the two groups. Thus, the significance of the apparent difference between the chromaffin-grafted and control groups is not clear and does not provide strong evidence for a DA-releasing capacity in adrenal medulla grafts. The interpretation of the results is hampered further by the inclusion of rats with relatively low turning rates in response to amphetamine, which means that some of the rats may have had as much as 10% of striatal DA remaining before transplantation surgery (81), and could have exhibited spontaneous biochemical and behavioral recovery (see discussion of the same experiment in section on rotation induced by dopamine-releasing agents).

In the study by Nishino et al., (118) who observed survival of intrastriatally grafted adrenal medullary cells with a neuron-like morphology and an effect of the grafts on amphetamine-induced rotation, five of the grafted rats were also subjected to an *in vivo* microdialysis experiment, 4 to 7 months after surgery. In the three rats that had exhibited behavioral recovery, it was possible to detect low levels of DA and DOPAC in the perfusates, whereas the two rats with no behavioral recovery exhibited undetectable levels of DA and trace levels of DOPAC. Because the number of rats analyzed is so low, it is difficult to draw any definite conclusions from this experiment, but it should be borne in mind that the study by Nishino et al. (118) differs from most other studies of adrenal grafts with regard to the survival, morphology, and behavioral capacity of the implants. Curran and Becker (47) used intrastriatal dialysis probes in a study of the DA-releasing capacity of intraventricular chromaffin transplants. Five of 25 studied rats with grafts were analyzed separately on the basis of having shown a 30% reduction in amphetamine-induced rotation during prior behavioral testing. These particular rats exhibited increased extracellular baseline levels of DOPAC and raised DA levels in the perfusates compared to nonrecovered and control rats. However, the DOPAC and DA levels were only on the order of four to six times greater than those recovered in

the 6-OHDA-denervated control striata. In other, similar studies (30,87,127,183), the DA and DOPAC levels in lesioned rats are extremely low. Although the presentation of the study does not permit direct comparison with release data from intact striatum, it would seem that the amounts of transmitter released from the intraventricular adrenal grafts are at best very small indeed. Decombe and coworkers (51) came to a similar conclusion when studying intrastriatal xenografts of bovine adrenal medulla using *in vivo* electrochemical detection. They found that the grafted chromaffin cells gave rise to no DOPAC signal under baseline conditions and produced low, if any, levels of catecholamines after systemic administration of a monoamine oxidase inhibitor. Because the authors also found no effect on apomorphine-induced rotation, they concluded that there was no functionally meaningful release of catecholamine from the bovine xenografts in their study, even though surviving grafts were subsequently found in 40% of recipients (51).

Somewhat surprisingly, it has been possible to detect increased DA concentrations in peripheral blood in rats with intraventricular adrenal medulla implants, and these changes have correlated to the behavioral efficacy of the grafts (10,11). Moreover, there are findings of increased penetration of peripherally administered DA into the brain and increased leakage of horseradish peroxidase into the brain in grafted rats (47). These findings led Freed, Becker, and coworkers to postulate that catecholamine secreted into blood vessels in the grafts is transported via the circulation into the host brain over a leaking blood–brain barrier (11,47). However, after a recent experiment, the same investigators refuted this hypothesis because they found that plasma catecholamine also was increased in control groups receiving sciatic grafts or sham surgery, even though these rats did not exhibit a marked reduction in apomorphine-induced rotation (166).

EFFECTS OF GRAFTS ON HOST STRIATAL NEURONS

The Effects of a Nigrostriatal Lesion on Striatal Physiology

Changes in Striatal Transmitters and Related Enzymes

Disruption of DA neurotransmission in the striatum by nigral lesions or DA receptor blockade is believed to cause a functional imbalance between the two different populations of striatal projection neurons, resulting in an increased activity in the GABA/enkephalinergic cells that project to the pallidum (the rodent analogue to the external pallidal segment), and a decreased activity in the GABA/dynorphin/substance P-ergic cells that project to the substantia nigra and the entopenduncular nucleus (the rodent analogue to the internal pallidal segment) (for review, see ref. 5). At the protein level, this imbalance is reflected in altered expression of striatal neuropeptides, namely increased levels of striatal and pallidal enkephalin-like immunoreactivity (104) and a decreased striatal and nigral immunoreactivity for substance P (180). These changes are accompanied by a pronounced upregulation of preproenkephalin (ppE)-mRNA and a more moderate downregulation of preprotachykinin (ppT) mRNA (the precursor molecule for substance P), and, according to some investigators, prodynorphin-mRNA as well (79,120,130,167,178,182). Both the enkephalinergic and dynorphin/substance-Pergic striatal cell populations coexpress GABA, and the net effects of a DA denervation on striatal GABAergic parameters are (1) an increased glutamic acid decarboxylase (GAD) activity, indicating increased GABA production (77,145,179) and release (168), and (2) elevated GAD mRNA levels (147,178). These findings are consistent with previous electrophysiologic studies demonstrating an increased firing rate of striatal neurons after 6-OHDA denervation of the striatum (142,149).

Changes in striatal interneuron physiology also have been observed after DA denervation, with an increase in the number of neurons immunostaining for neuropeptide Y (91) and an increased inhibition of acetylcholine release by DA receptor agonists acting on supersensitive D2 DA receptors located presynaptically on cholinergic interneurons (40).

Changes in Receptors in Striatal Neurons

In addition to the changes in transmitter levels, transmitter-related enzymes, and spike activity described above, supersensitivity of postsynaptic D1 and D2 DA receptors also has been described in response to a 6-OHDA-lesion. For the D2 receptor subtype, the literature unequivocally points to a marked upregulation of receptor binding after 6-OHDA denervation of the striatum (45,116,135,136). Although behavioral supersensitivity to D1 dopamine receptor agonists in 6-OHDA-lesioned rats is a well established phenomenon (158), D1 receptor binding in the 6-OHDA-lesioned striatum has been reported to be either increased (32,50,76,128), decreased (21,108), or unchanged (136).

As will be discussed below, the possibility of reversing all of the aforementioned lesion-induced changes has been addressed in intracerebral grafting studies (Fig. 4).

Effects of Grafts on Striatal Cell Activity, Protein Synthesis, and Receptor Expression

In agreement with the previously described behavioral results, intrastriatal nigral grafts have been found to compensate the lesion-induced changes completely in certain physiologic measures of striatal function, whereas other consequences of DA denervation are not or only partially counteracted.

Among the phenomena most effectively counteracted by nigral grafts are the "disinhibition" effects observed after disrup-

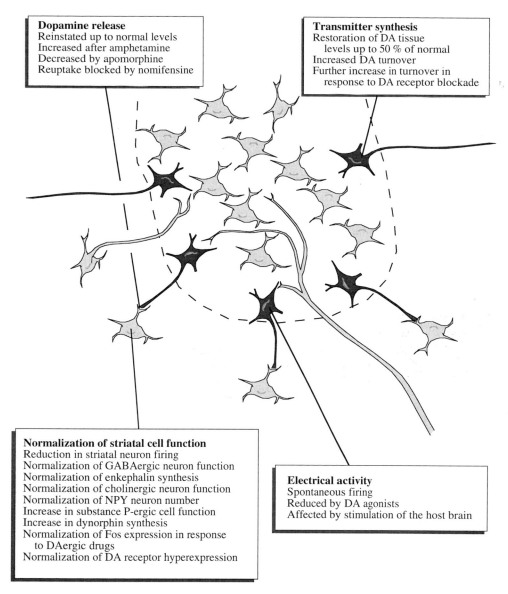

Dopamine release
Reinstated up to normal levels
Increased after amphetamine
Decreased by apomorphine
Reuptake blocked by nomifensine

Transmitter synthesis
Restoration of DA tissue
  levels up to 50 % of normal
Increased DA turnover
Further increase in turnover in
  response to DA receptor blockade

Normalization of striatal cell function
Reduction in striatal neuron firing
Normalization of GABAergic neuron function
Normalization of enkephalin synthesis
Normalization of cholinergic neuron function
Normalization of NPY neuron number
Increase in substance P-ergic cell function
Increase in dynorphin synthesis
Normalization of Fos expression in response
  to DAergic drugs
Normalization of DA receptor hyperexpression

Electrical activity
Spontaneous firing
Reduced by DA agonists
Affected by stimulation of the host brain

FIG. 4. Schematic diagram of a nigral graft in the striatum with darkly shaded dopamine neurons. The inset boxes list several properties of the grafted dopamine neurons and the effects the grafts have on the host striatal neurons. For details, see text. DA, dopamine; GABA, γ-aminobutyric acid; NPY, neuropeptide Y.

tion of striatal DAergic neurotransmission, namely, increases in striatal neuron firing rates, GAD mRNA expression, GAD enzymatic activity, ppE mRNA expression, and enkephalin immunoreactivity.

Firing Properties of Reinnervated Striatal Neurons

In a study that focused on the electrophysiologic effects of nigral grafts on the denervated host striatum, Strömberg and colleagues (162) implanted mesencephalic tissue fragments into a cortical cavity overlying the denervated striatum. Catecholamine histofluorescence showed that the zone of DA reinnervation extended approximately 1 to 1.5 mm from the transplant cavity into the denervated striatum. In electrophysiologic recordings performed in similar rats, the authors found that the spontaneous firing activity of striatal neurons located within the reinnervated area was only about one half to one third that of the rates recorded from areas that lay beyond this zone, and on the basis of these data suggested that the graft-derived fibers reestablished some degree of DAergic inhibitory control over the 6-OHDA-denervated striatum. The same group of investigators subsequently confirmed these findings in rats carrying xenografted human mesencephalic tissue (177).

Effects of Grafts on Striatal GABAergic Function

Since the vast majority of striatal neurons are GABAergic, graft-derived inhibitory control over these cells—as suggested by the experiments of Stromberg and coworkers (162,177)—should be reflected in parameters of GABAergic function. Segovia and colleagues (146), using a transplant paradigm quite similar to that of Strömberg et al. (162), measured GAD activity in DA-denervated and graft-reinnervated striata.

They found that the lesion-induced increase in GAD activity—most probably reflecting the disinhibition of these cells—was counteracted by the graft only to a minor degree, although the animals showed a nearly complete recovery of amphetamine-induced turning. Because ventral mesencephalic graft tissue inevitably contains large numbers of GABAergic cells derived from the developing pars reticulata of the substantia nigra, it is possible that fiber outgrowth from grafted GABAergic neurons could have increased the GAD levels in the host striatum and thus partly masked the DA-dependent downregulation of this enzyme in host striatal neurons. In a subsequent northern blot analysis for quantification of striatal GAD mRNA (excluding the grafted nigral tissue fragment) (148), the grafts were indeed found to be much more effective in attenuating the lesion-induced increases. In fact, they downregulated the expression of GAD mRNA to levels lower than normally encountered in an unlesioned striatum. Because GAD mRNA is believed to be confined to the soma of neurons, there probably was no contribution to the measured GAD mRNA levels from GABAergic neurons located in the graft tissue in this latter study.

It should be borne in mind that the striatal GABAergic projection neurons are not a homogeneous cell population, but can be divided into two categories that are distinguishable with respect to their primary projection area, and the neuropeptides and types of DA receptors they predominantly express. This distinct peptide expression offers an opportunity to study the differential effects a nigral graft may exert on these two striatal neuronal populations.

Effects of Nigral Grafts on Striatopallidal Neurons

In a quantitative immunocytochemical study, Manier and colleagues (104) focused on methionin enkephalin (metENK)-immunoreactive striatal neurons. They reported that the increased immunoreactivity for metENK observed after a 6-OHDA lesion of the nigrostriatal pathway can be effectively reversed by an intraparenchymal graft of DA neurons. Because the enkephalinergic striatal cells project mainly to the globus pallidus, both the lesion-induced increases of metENK immunoreactivity and the decreases caused by the graft also were observed in the stained pallidal terminals of these cells. As in the case for GAD mRNA (148), the grafts did not merely restore the metENK immunoreactivity to baseline levels but "overcompensated" the lesion-induced upregulation to below normal levels in areas close to, and reinnervated by, the grafts. Interestingly, a downregulation of metENK immunoreactivity also was noticeable in regions of the grafted striatum distant to the reinnervated zone, suggesting that the functional effects of the nigral grafts extended further than would be expected from their reinnervation patterns (104). There is further support that embryonic mesencephalic DA neurons can downregulate lesion-induced increases in enkephalin neuron activity from *in situ* hybridization histochemistry studies that have shown that there is significant attenuation of proenkephalin mRNA levels after intrastriatal implantation of such cells (9, 34,39,111,156). In a detailed analysis at the cellular level, Cenci et al. (39) noted that the levels of ppE mRNA per striatal cell were in fact decreased to below the levels encountered in the contralateral striatum, and also were significantly downregulated in nonreinnervated striatal areas, far caudal to the implantation sites. These detailed observations gave support to earlier preliminary findings by Sirinathsinghji and Dunnett (156), who noted an "overcompensation" of the DA denervation-induced ppE mRNA increase in the immediate vicinity of mesencephalic grafts and a generalized normalization of the ppE mRNA signal in areas distal to those actually reinnervated.

There is also evidence that nigral grafts can normalize DA denervation-induced changes in the opiate receptors associated with enkephalinergic neurotransmission. Normally, the striatum contains dense patches of μ-opiate receptors which correspond to striatal areas originally denoted "striosomes". Following DA-denervation there is complete disappearance of the μ-opiate receptor patches. Sirinathsinghji and Dunnett (154) observed a substantial restoration of these patches close to intrastriatal cell suspension nigral grafts, coinciding with the area graft-derived DA fibers would be able to reach. It remains unclear whether the μ-opiate receptors are located on the reinnervating DA terminals themselves or on their target neurons.

Because the enkephalinergic neurons in the striatum have been shown predominantly to express DA receptors of the D2 type (96,97) the pattern of lesion-induced changes and graft-induced restoration of D2 DA receptors would be likely to reflect the pattern of changes observed in enkephalinergic neurons. Several groups (21,41,50, 71,76,128,137,155) have studied DA D2 receptor binding in the 6-OHDA-denervated and grafted rat striatum, and have found that the receptor binding increases significantly in response to denervation; the increase is counteracted by intrastriatal grafts of embryonic DA neurons and shows a tendency to be overcompensated by the nigral grafts. Mesencephalic grafts also can affect D2 receptor binding in Weaver mice, which exhibit a partial DA denervation of the striatum, in that the implants can partially prevent an expected receptor upregulation that occurs as the DA system progressively degenerates (90). The reported transplant-induced changes in DA D2 receptor binding are further supported by a recent *in situ* hybridization histochemistry study demonstrating a reduced mRNA expression for this receptor subtype after grafting in the 6-OHDA-denervated rat striatum (41). In this study (41), both D2 mRNA levels and D2 receptor binding were analyzed on adjacent sections, revealing that normalization of D2 receptor-related changes, in analogy to previous findings on changes in enkephalinergic neuron function (93,104,156), in some cases extended to regions of the striatum beyond the area reinnervated by DAergic fibers from the graft.

Thus, in summary, the enkephalin/GABAergic population of striatal projection neurons, projecting mainly to the globus pallidus and expressing predominantly D2 DA receptors, seems to respond to DA denervation and subsequent transplantation of nigral DA cells in a consistent manner. The striking features in this response pattern are (1) a robust upregulation of the D2 DA receptor and the coexpressed neuropeptide enkephalin and its mRNA after the lesion; (2) these changes are readily responsive to intrastriatally grafted DA neurons and (3) show a tendency to be overcompensated by the graft; and (4) the graft-induced downregulation of the increases provoked by the lesion seems to extend further anatomically than the reinnervation of the striatum by the grafted cells.

Effects of Nigral Grafts on Striatonigral Neurons

Information on the responses of the second class of striatal projection neurons, which contains substance P/dynorphin/GABA, projects mainly to the substantia nigra, and predominantly expresses D1 DA receptors, is less consistent. As mentioned previously, behavioral supersensitivity to D1 receptors usually is clearly evident after 6-OHDA denervation, whereas the expected increases in D1 receptor binding—if they are detected at all—are small and difficult to quantify. Striatal postsynaptic D1 receptor supersensitivity has been reported to be partly (128) or wholly (50,76) normalized after intrastriatal nigral grafting. Dawson et al. (50) also described a significant unilateral increase in the number of D1 receptors in the substantia nigra ipsilateral to a 6-OHDA lesion, and found that it

was fully reversed by intrastriatal nigral grafts.

Other lesion-induced physiologic changes in the striatonigral projection neurons also have been reported to respond readily to intrastriatal nigral grafts. Thus, administration of direct or indirect dopaminergic agonists, which induces supranormal expression of the protooncogene c-*fos* in the 6-OHDA-denervated striatum, elicits only a normal expression of Fos immunoreactivity in rats bearing functional nigral grafts (2,38). Abrous and coworkers (2) noted that the nigral grafts induced an "overcompensation" by reducing the number of Fos-positive neurons in the anterolateral striatum to levels lower than control. Moreover, they found that there was a strong correlation between the degree of contralateral rotation in response to amphetamine in the graft host and extent of hyperexpression of Fos-positive nuclei. Interestingly, the normalization of DA agonist-induced Fos expression in the grafted striatum also has been found to extend beyond the immunocytochemically detectable zone of graft-derived dopaminergic reinnervation (2,38). This seems to correspond well to the results discussed earlier concerning striatopallidal neurons (39,41,104,156), which indicate that the activity of enkephalinergic neurons and levels of DA D2 receptors are normalized in areas beyond the reinnervated zone. However, Cenci and colleagues (37) have combined Fos immunohistochemistry with neuroanatomic tracing techniques to demonstrate that Fos is preferentially expressed not in the enkephalinergic, D2 receptor-bearing striatopallidal neurons, but rather in the substance P-ergic, D1 receptor-bearing striatonigral cell population.

Notably, the expression of ppT mRNA, which constitutes the precursor molecule for substance P and is downregulated after striatal DA denervation, also has been found to be normalized in the striata of animals bearing functional nigral grafts (39,111). In the detailed analysis on the cellular level performed by Cenci and colleagues (39), this normalization was found to be partial, and to be restricted to the portion of the striatum reinnervated by the graft-derived DAergic fibers. In addition, the grafts were able widely to prevent the upregulation of prodynorphin mRNA that could be induced by intermittent treatment of the 6-OHDA-denervated rats with apomorphine. Thus, it would seem that the graft-induced effects on the 6-OHDA-denervated host *striatonigral* cell population are heterogeneous: The nigral grafts give rise to a widespread normalization of DA agonist-induced upregulation of both the Fos protein and the prodynorphin mRNA, but the graft-induced restoration of ppT (substance P) mRNA expression in the same cell population is only partial and restricted to areas adjacent to the graft.

Effects of Nigral Grafts on Striatal Interneurons

In addition to the aforementioned studies that focused on striatal projection neurons, the effects of nigral transplants on striatal interneurons also have been studied. Unilateral intranigral injections of 6-OHDA give rise to an ipsilateral 30% increase in the number of neuropeptide Y-immunoreactive neurons in the striatum (91). These cells are medium-sized, spiny neurons that project within the striatum. After nigral grafting, the number of neuropeptide Y-immunoreactive neurons is normalized in the DA-denervated striatum, as well as in areas apparently beyond those reached by the DAergic fibers originating in the implant (115).

Further physiologic evidence for a normalization of interneuron function after grafting of DA neurons to the 6-OHDA-denervated striatum comes from a series of studies on *in vitro* superfused striatal slice preparations focusing on transmitter release from striatal cholinergic interneurons (36,85,89). Electrically evoked acetylcholine release from striatal slices was reduced

by the addition of apomorphine to the superfusion medium, and cholinergic interneurons in 6-OHDA-denervated striata exhibited a hypersensitivity to this apomorphine effect. Interestingly, striata carrying nigral grafts displayed a reduced sensitivity to apomorphine, that is, the acetylcholine release was less affected (85,89). Moreover, increasing the amounts of DA released in striatal slices by the addition of amphetamine or the reuptake blocker nomifensine was found to reduce acetylcholine release markedly from intact and grafted slices, but not 6-OHDA-treated preparations (36,85,89). Further support for the idea that grafted DA neurons can restore inhibitory control over striatal cholinergic interneurons comes from a study on muscarinic receptor binding in rats with 6-OHDA lesions (49). Long-term DA denervation causes a 25% downregulation of striatal muscarinic receptors, which can be interpreted as a consequence of excessive acetylcholine release due to a disinhibition of cholinergic neurons, secondary to a loss of DAergic presynaptic inhibition (49). Nigral implants that give rise to behavioral compensation in the amphetamine-induced rotation test also normalize striatal muscarinic receptor density (49).

Possible Mechanisms Underlying Effects of Nigral Grafts on Striatal Neuronal Populations outside the Reinnervated Zone

As discussed above, there are several indications that grafted DA neurons affect host neuron physiology in striatal regions beyond those they actually reinnervate. The precise importance of these "distant effects" is unclear because several studies of drug-induced behaviors support exactly the contrary notion (see section on functional heterogeneity of the striatum), that is, the functional effects of the grafts are limited to the areas they actually reinnervate. Nevertheless, since there now are many robust observations of distant effects of grafts, the mechanisms underlying these effects are worthy of speculation.

On the basis of their finding that normalization of ppE mRNA expression is complete and widespread in the grafted striatum, whereas substance P mRNA expression is only partially restored and restricted to the area reinnervated by the graft, Cenci and colleagues (39) have formulated the hypothesis that striatonigral neurons require synaptic interaction with the graft DA neurons for normalization of their function, whereas striatopallidal neurons can normalize their neuropeptide mRNA expression in response to lower concentrations of DA diffused over some distance in the striatum. An alternative attractive explanation for the graft-induced effects that extend beyond the striatal regions innervated by graft-derived DAergic fibers has been proposed by Manier et al. (104). They hypothesize that these effects are mediated by some of the medium-sized, spiny neurons that are inside the DA-reinnervated zone and in turn extend axon collaterals over several hundred micrometers to other striatal regions. According to this hypothesis, cholinergic interneurons, whose function has been shown to be affected by grafted DA neurons (85,89), may directly or via other medium-sized spiny neurons (e.g., neuropeptide Y-containing (115)) influence transmitter, receptor, and protooncogene expression in striatal neurons that are not reached directly by the graft-derived fibers or diffusing DA. Because grafted DA neurons possess an efficient DA reuptake system and exhibit autoregulatory mechanisms (see section on graft catecholamine content and release), it is an appealing idea that the distant effects of the grafts are primarily mediated via interneurons rather than diffusing DA.

Effects of Adrenal Grafts on Striatal Neuron Physiology

Regarding grafts of adrenal chromaffin cells, there are no published systematic investigations on their effects on host striatal neuron physiology. However, several studies have focused on the possible trophic effects of adrenal grafts directly on the host DAergic system. This topic lies outside the focus of this review, and is dealt with extensively in the chapter by Gash and coworkers *(this volume)*.

CONCLUDING REMARKS

The field of neural transplantation research is still, if not in its infancy, at least in its adolescence. Throughout its brief history, studies of transplants to the DA-denervated striatum have played a pioneering role. In this paradigm, the first behavioral effects of neural grafts were observed; the biologic parameters that govern graft survival and growth were carefully established; the first clinical trials were conducted in the DA-depleted striatum of patients with Parkinson's disease; and now, the first detailed description of neurobiologic mechanisms that govern the function of neural grafts is emerging from research into catecholamine-rich transplants to the striatum.

The past 4 to 5 years have witnessed a large number of experiments that, by using more refined experimental designs and novel behavioral tests, have further characterized the functional limitations of implants in the DA-denervated striatum and have begun to challenge these limitations using alternative transplantation strategies. Moreover, the application of modern techniques from the rapidly developing field of molecular neurobiology has shed light on the extent to which the grafts can normalize the physiologic changes that occur in the DA-depleted striatum. These recent studies indicate that grafted embryonic DA neurons possess a remarkable capacity to mimic the functions that nigral neurons normally exert in the striatum (see Fig. 4). The functional effects of transplanted adrenal chromaffin cells seem less consistent and, when they occur, tend to be more subtle.

This should by no means preclude further research into adrenal transplants, because in the future it is possible that genetic engineering or the supply of specific neurotrophic factors could furnish the chromaffin cells with properties that would make them suitable as donor tissue even in a clinical setting.

ACKNOWLEDGMENTS

During part of the preparation of this chapter, W-M Duan was supported by the Thorsten and Elsa Segerfalk foundation. Our own work cited in the text was supported in part by grants from the Medical Faculty at the University of Lund, the Swedish MRC, the Neurologically Handicapped Society (NHR), and the Crafoord foundation, which are all gratefully acknowledged. We are also very grateful to Bengt Mattson for his excellent help with the illustrations.

REFERENCES

1. Aebischer P, Tresco PA, Sagen J, Winn SR. Transplantation of microencapsulated bovine chromaffin cells reduces lesion-induced rotational asymmetry in rats. *Brain Res* 1991; 560:43–49.
2. Abrous DN, Torres EM, Annett LE, Reading PJ, Dunnett SB. Intrastriatal dopamine-rich grafts induce a hyperexpression of Fos protein when challenged with amphetamine. *Exp Brain Res* 1992;91:181–190.
3. Abrous DN, Shaltot AR, Torres EM, Dunnett SB. Dopamine-rich grafts in the neostriatum and/or nucleus accumbens: effects on drug-induced behaviours and skilled paw-reaching. *Neuroscience* 1993;53:187–197.
4. Abrous DN, Torres EM, Dunnett SB. Dopaminergic grafts implanted into the neonatal or adult striatum: comparative effects on rotation and paw reaching deficits induced by subsequent unilateral nigrostriatal lesions in adulthood. *Neuroscience* 1993;54:657–668.
5. Albin RL, Young AB, Penney JB. The functional anatomy of basal ganglia disorders. *Trends Neurosci* 1989;12:366–375.
6. Annett LE, Reading PJ, Tharumaratnam D, Abrous DN, Torres EM, Dunnett SB. Conditioning versus priming of dopaminergic grafts by amphetamine. *Exp Brain Res* 1993;93: 46–54.
7. Arbuthnott G, Dunnett SB, MacLeod N. Electrophysiological properties of single units in mesencephalic transplants in rat brain. *Neurosci Lett* 1985;57:205–210.
8. Backlund EO, Granberg PO, Hamberger B, et al. Transplantation of adrenal medullary tissue to striatum in parkinsonism: first clinical trials. *J Neurosurg* 1985;62:169–173.
9. Bal A, Savasta M, Chritin M, Mennicken F, et al. Transplantation of fetal nigral cells reverses the increase of preproenkephalin mRNA levels in the rat striatum caused by 6-OHDA lesion of the dopaminergic nigrostriatal pathway: a quantitative in situ hybridization study. *Mol Brain Res* 1993;18:221–227.
10. Becker JB, Freed WJ. Adrenal medulla grafts enhance functional activity of the striatal dopamine system following substantia nigra lesions. *Brain Res* 1988;462:401–406.
11. Becker JB, Curran EJ, Freed WJ, Poltorak M. Mechanisms of action of adrenal medulla grafts: the possible role of peripheral and central dopamine systems. *Prog Brain Res* 1990; 82:499–507.
12. Becker JB, Ariano MA. Behavioral effects of fetal substantia nigra tissue grafted into the dopamine-denervated striatum: responses to selective D_1 and D_2 dopamine receptor agonists. *Rest Neurol Neurosci* 1991;3:187–195.
13. Bing G, Notter MFD, Hansen JT, Gash DM. Comparison of adrenal medullary, carotid body and PC12 cell grafts in 6-OHDA lesioned rats. *Brain Res Bull* 1988;20:399–406.
14. Björklund A, Stenevi U. Reconstruction of the nigrostriatal pathway by intracerebral nigral transplants. *Brain Res* 1979;177:555–560.
15. Björklund A, Dunnett SB, Stenevi U, Lewis ME, Iversen SD. Reinnervation of the denervated striatum by substantia nigra transplants: functional consequences as revealed by pharmacological and sensorimotor testing. *Brain Res* 1980;199:307–333.
16. Björklund A, Schmidt RH, Stenevi U. Functional reinnervation of the neostriatum in the adult rat by use of intraparenchymal grafting of dissociated cell suspensions from the substantia nigra. *Cell Tissue Res* 1980;212:39–45.
17. Björklund A, Stenevi U, Dunnett SB, Iversen SD. Functional reactivation of the deafferented neostriatum by nigral transplants. *Nature* 1981; 289:497–499.
18. Björklund A, Stenevi U, Schmidt RH, Dunnett SB, Gage FH. Intracerebral grafting of neuronal cell suspensions: II. survival and growth of nigral cell suspensions implanted in different brain sites. *Acta Physiol Scand (Suppl)* 1983; 522:9–18.
19. Blunt SB, Jenner P, Marsden CD. The effect of chronic L-dopa treatment on the recovery of motor function in 6-hydroxydopamine-lesioned rats receiving ventral mesencephalic grafts. *Neuroscience* 1991;40:453–464.
20. Blunt SB, Jenner P, Marsden CD. The effect of L-DOPA and carbidopa treatment on the survival of rat fetal dopamine grafts assessed by tyrosine hydroxylase immunohistochemis-

try and [³H] mazindol autoradiography. *Neuroscience* 1991;43:95–110.

21. Blunt SB, Jenner P, Marsden CD. Autoradiographic study of striatal D_1 and D_2 dopamine receptors in 6-OHDA-lesioned rats receiving foetal ventral mesencephalic grafts and chronic treatment with L-DOPA and carbidopa. *Brain Res* 1992;582:299–311.

22. Boyce S, Kelly E, Reavill C, Jenner P, Marsden CD. Repeated administration of N-methyl-4-phenyl-1, 2, 3, 6-tetrahydropyridine to rats is not toxic to striatal dopamine neurons. *Biochem Pharmacol* 1984;33:1747–1752.

23. Brown VJ, Dunnett SB. Comparison of adrenal and foetal nigral grafts on drug-induced rotation in rats with 6-OHDA lesions. *Exp Brain Res* 1989;78:214–218.

24. Brundin P, Isacson O, Björklund A. Monitoring of cell viability in suspensions of embryonic CNS tissue and its use as a criterion for intracerebral graft survival. *Brain Res* 1985; 331:251–259.

25. Brundin P, Isacson O, Gage FH, Prochiantz A, Björklund A. The rotating 6-hydroxydopamine lesioned mouse as a model for assessing functional effects of neuronal grafting. *Brain Res* 1986;366:346–349.

26. Brundin P, Nilsson OG, Strecker RE, Lindvall O, Åstedt B, Björklund A. Behavioural effects of human fetal dopamine neurons grafted in a rat model of Parkinson's disease. *Exp Brain Res* 1986;65:235–240.

27. Brundin P, Björklund A. Survival, growth and function of dopaminergic neurons grafted to the brain. *Prog Brain Res* 1987;71:293–308.

28. Brundin P, Strecker RE, Londos E, Björklund A. Dopamine neurons grafted unilaterally to the nucleus accumbens affect drug-induced circling and locomotion. *Exp Brain Res* 1987; 69:183–194.

29. Brundin P, Barbin G, Strecker RE, Isacson O, Prochiantz A, Björklund A. Survival and function of dissociated dopamine neurons grafted at different developmental stages or after being cultured in vitro. *Dev Brain Res* 1988;39:233–243.

30. Brundin P, Strecker RE, Widner H, et al. Human fetal dopamine neurons grafted in a rat model of Parkinson's disease: immunological aspects, spontaneous and drug-induced behaviour, and dopamine release. *Exp Brain Res* 1988;70:192–208.

31. Brundin P, Widner H, Strecker RE, Nilsson OG, Björklund A. Intracerebral xenografts of dopamine neurons: the role of immunosuppression and the blood-brain barrier. *Exp Brain Res* 1989;75:195–207.

32. Buonamici M, Caccia M, Carpentieri M, Pegrassi L, Rossi AC, Di Chiara G. D-1 receptor supersensitivity in the rat striatum after unilateral 6-hydroxydopamine lesions. *Eur J Pharmacol* 1986;126:347–348.

33. Burns BS, Chiueh CC, Markey SP, Ebert MH, Jacobowitz DM, Kopin IJ. A primate model of parkinsonism: selective destruction of dopaminergic neurons in the pars compacta of the substantia nigra by N-methyl-4-phenyl-1,2,3,6-tetrahydropyridine. *Proc Natl Acad Sci USA* 1983;80:4546–4550.

34. Cadet JL, Zhu SM, Angulo JA. Intrastriatal implants of fetal mesencephalic cells attenuate the increases in striatal proenkephalin mRNA observed after unilateral 6-hydroxydopamine-induced lesions of the striatum. *Brain Res Bull* 1991;27:707–711.

35. Carder RK, Snyder Keller AM, Lund RD. Behavioral and anatomical correlates of immunologically induced rejection of nigral xenografts. *J Comp Neurol* 1988;277:391–402.

36. Carder RK, Jackson D, Morris HJ, Lund RD, Zigmond MJ. Dopamine released from mesencephalic transplants restores modulation of striatal acetylcholine release after neonatal 6-hydroxydopamine: an in vitro analysis. *Exp Neurol* 1989;105:251–259.

37. Cenci MA, Campbell K, Wictorin K, Björklund A. Striatal c-fos induction by cocaine or apomorphine occurs preferentially in output neurons projecting to the substantia nigra in the rat. *Eur J Neurosci* 1992;4:376–380.

38. Cenci MA, Kalén P, Mandel RJ, Wictorin K, Björklund A. Dopaminergic transplants normalize amphetamine- and apomorphine-induced Fos expression in the 6-hydroxydopamine lesioned striatum. *Neuroscience* 1992;46:943–957.

39. Cenci MA, Campbell K, Björklund A. Neuropeptide-messenger RNA expression in the 6-hydroxydopamine-lesioned striatum reinnervated by fetal dopaminergic transplants: differential effects of the grafts on preproenkephalin-, preprotachykinin- and prodynorphin messenger RNA levels. *Neuroscience* 1993;57:275–296.

40. Chesselet MF. Presynaptic regulation of neurotransmitter release in the brain: facts and hypothesis. *Neuroscience* 1984;12:347–375.

41. Chritin M, Savasta M, Mennicken F, et al. Intrastriatal dopamine-rich implants reverse the increase of dopamine D_2 receptor mRNA levels caused by lesion of the nigrostriatal pathway: a quantitative *in situ* hybridization study. *Eur J Neurosci* 1992;4:663–672.

42. Chkirate M, Vallée A, Doucet G. Host striatal projections into fetal ventral mesencephalic tissue grafted to the striatum of immature or adult rat. *Exp Brain Res* 1993;94:357–362.

43. Choulli K, Herman JP, Abrous N, Le Moal M. Behavioral effects of intraaccumbens transplants in rats with lesions of the mesocorticolimbic dopamine system. *Ann NY Acad Sci* 1987;495:497–509.

44. Clarke DJ, Brundin P, Nilsson OG, Strecker RE, Björklund A, Lindvall O. Human fetal dopamine neurons grafted in a rat model of Parkinson's disease: ultrastructural evidence for synapse formation using tyrosine hydroxylase immunocytochemistry. *Exp Brain Res* 1988;73: 115–126.

45. Creese I, Burt DR, Snyder SH. Dopamine receptor binding enhancement accompanies le-

sion-induced behavioural supersensitivity. *Science* 1977;197:596–598.

46. Cunningham LA, Hansen JT, Short MP, Bohn MC. The use of genetically altered astrocytes to provide nerve growth factor to adrenal chromaffin cells grafted into the striatum. *Brain Res* 1991;561:192–202.

47. Curran EJ, Becker JB. Changes in blood–brain barrier permeability are associated with behavioral and neurochemical indices of recovery following intraventricular adrenal medulla grafts in an animal model of Parkinson's disease. *Exp Neurol* 1991;114:184–192.

48. Date I, Felten SY, Felten DL. Cografts of adrenal medulla with peripheral nerve enhance the survivability of transplanted adrenal chromaffin cells and recovery of the host nigrostriatal dopaminergic system in MPTP-treated young adult mice. *Brain Res* 1990;537:33–39.

49. Dawson TM, Dawson VL, Gage FH, Fisher LJ, Hunt MA, Wamsley JK. Downregulation of muscarinic receptors in the rat caudate–putamen after lesioning of the ipsilateral nigrostriatal dopamine pathway with 6-hydroxydopamine (6-OHDA): normalization by fetal mesencephalic transplants. *Brain Res* 1991;540:145–152.

50. Dawson TM, Dawson VL, Gage FH, Fisher LJ, Hunt MA, Wamsley JK. Functional recovery of supersensitive dopamine receptors after intrastriatal grafts of fetal substantia nigra. *Exp Neurol* 1991;111:282–292.

51. Decombe R, Rivot JP, Aunis D, Abrous N, Peschanski M, Herman JP. Importance of catecholamine release for the functional action of intrastriatal implants of adrenal medullary cells: pharmacological analysis and in vivo electrochemistry. *Exp Neurol* 1990;107:143–153.

52. Doucet G, Brundin P, Seth S, et al. Degeneration and graft-induced restoration of dopamine innervation in the weaver mouse neostriatum: a quantitative radioautographic study of [^{3}H] dopamine uptake. *Exp Brain Res* 1989;77:552–568.

53. Doucet G, Murata Y, Brundin P, et al. Host afferents into intrastriatal transplants of fetal ventral mesencephalon. *Exp Neurol* 1989;106:1–19.

54. Doucet G, Brundin P, Descarries L, Björklund A. Effect of prior dopamine denervation on survival and fiber outgrowth from intrastriatal fetal mesencephalic grafts. *Eur J Neurosci* 1990;2:279–290.

55. Duan W-M, Widner H, Björklund A, Brundin P. Sequential intrastriatal grafting of allogeneic embryonic dopamine-rich neuronal tissue in adult rats: will the second graft be rejected? *Neuroscience* 1993;57:261–274.

56. Dunnett SB, Björklund A, Stenevi U, Iversen SD. Behavioural recovery following transplantation of substantia nigra in rats subjected to 6-OHDA lesions of the nigrostriatal pathway: I. unilateral lesions. *Brain Res* 1981;215:147–161.

57. Dunnett SB, Björklund A, Stenevi U, Iversen SD. Grafts of embryonic substantia nigra reinnervating the ventrolateral striatum ameliorate sensorimotor impairments and akinesia in rats with 6-OHDA lesions of the nigrostriatal pathway. *Brain Res* 1981;229:209–217.

58. Dunnett SB, Björklund A, Stenevi U, Iversen SD. Behavioural recovery following transplantation of substantia nigra in rats subjected to 6-OHDA lesions of the nigrostriatal pathway: II. bilateral lesions. *Brain Res* 1981;229:457–470.

59. Dunnett SB, Björklund A. Conditioned turning in rats: dopaminergic involvement in the initiation of movement rather than the movement itself. *Neurosci Lett* 1983;41:173–178.

60. Dunnett SB, Björklund A, Schmidt RH, Stenevi U, Iversen SD. Intracerebral grafting of neuronal cell suspensions: IV. behavioural recovery in rats with unilateral 6-OHDA lesions following implantation of nigral cell suspensions in different brain sites. *Acta Physiol Scand (Suppl)* 1983;522:29–37.

61. Dunnett SB, Björklund A, Schmidt RH, Stenevi U, Iversen SD. Intracerebral grafting of neuronal cell suspensions: V. behavioural recovery in rats with bilateral 6-OHDA lesions following implantation of nigral cell suspensions. *Acta Physiol Scand (Suppl)* 1983;522:39–47.

62. Dunnett SB, Whishaw IQ, Jones GH, Isacson O. Effects of dopamine-rich grafts on conditioned rotation in rats with unilateral 6-OHDA lesions. *Neurosci Lett* 1986;68:127–133.

63. Dunnett SB, Whishaw IQ, Rogers DC, Jones GH. Dopamine-rich grafts ameliorate whole body motor asymmetry and sensory neglect but not independent limb use in rats with 6-hydroxydopamine lesions. *Brain Res* 1987;415:63–78.

64. Dunnett SB, Hernandez TD, Summerfield A, Jones GH, Arbuthnott G. Graft-derived recovery from 6-OHDA lesions: specificity of ventral mesencephalic graft tissues. *Exp Brain Res* 1988;71:411–424.

65. Fisher LJ, Young SJ, Tepper JM, Groves PM, Gage FH. Electrophysiological characteristics of cells within mesencephalon suspension grafts. *Neuroscience* 1991;40:109–122.

66. Forni C, Brundin P, Strecker RE, El Ganouni S, Björklund A, Nieoullon A. Time-course of recovery of dopamine neuron activity during reinnervation of the denervated striatum by fetal mesencephalic grafts as assessed by in vivo voltammetry. *Exp Brain Res* 1989;76:75–87.

67. Freed WJ, Perlow MJ, Karoum F, et al. Restoration of dopaminergic function by grafting of fetal substantia nigra to the caudate nucleus: long-term behavioural, biochemical and histochemical studies. *Ann Neurol* 1980;8:510–519.

68. Freed WJ, Morihisa J, Spoor E, et al. Transplanted adrenal chromaffin cells in rat brain reduce lesion-induced rotational behavior. *Nature* 1981;292:351–352.

69. Freed WJ. Functional brain tissue transplantation: reversal of lesion-induced rotation by intraventricular substantia nigra and adrenal me-

dulla grafts, with a note on intracranial retinal grafts. *Biol Psychiatry* 1983;18:1205–1267.

70. Freed WJ, Karoum F, Spoor HE, Morihisa JM, Olson L, Wyatt RJ. Catecholamine content of intracerebral adrenal medulla grafts. *Brain Res* 1983;269:184–189.

71. Freed WJ, Ko GN, Niehoff D, et al. Normalization of spiroperidol binding in the denervated rat striatum by homologous grafts of substantia nigra. *Science* 1983;222:937–939.

72. Freed WJ, Cannon-Spoor HE, Krauthamcr E. Intrastriatal adrenal medulla grafts in rats: long-term survival and behavioral effects. *J Neurosurg* 1986;65:664–670.

73. Freed WJ, Poltorak M, Becker JB. Intracerebral adrenal medulla grafts: a review. *Exp Neurol* 1990;110:139–166.

74. Freund TF, Bolam JP, Björklund A, et al. Efferent synaptic connections of grafted dopaminergic neurons reinnervating the host neostriatum: a tyrosine hydroxylase immunocytochemical study. *J Neurosci* 1985;5:603–616.

75. Gage FH, Dunnett SB, Stenevi U, Björklund A. Aged rats: recovery of motor impairments by intrastriatal nigral grafts. *Science* 1983;221:966–969.

76. Gagnon C, Bédard PJ, Rioux L, Gaudin D, Martinoli MG, Pelletier G, DiPaolo T. Regional changes of striatal dopamine receptors following denervation by 6-hydroxydopamine and fetal mesencephalic grafts in the rat. *Brain Res* 1991;558:251–263.

77. Gale K, Casu M. Dynamic utilization of GABA in substantia nigra: regulation by dopamine and GABA in the striatum and its clinical and behavioral implications. *Mol Cell Biochem* 1981;39:369–405.

78. Gaudin DP, Rioux L, Bédard PJ. Fetal dopamine neuron transplants prevent behavioral supersensitivity induced by repeated administration of L-dopa in the rat. *Brain Res* 1990;506:166–168.

79. Gerfen CR, McGinty JF, Young WS III. Dopamine differentially regulates dynorphin, substance P and enkephalin expression in striatal neurons: in situ hybridization histochemical analysis. *J Neurosci* 1991;11:1016–1031.

80. Hansen JT, Bing G, Notter MFD, Gash DM. Paraneuronal grafts in unilateral 6-hydroxydopamine-lesioned rats: morphological aspects of adrenal chromaffin and carotid body glomus cell implants. *Prog Brain Res* 1988;78:507–511.

81. Hefti F, Melamed E, Sahakian BJ, Wurtman RJ. Circling behavior in rats with partial, unilateral nigro-striatal lesions: effect of amphetamine, apomorphine, and DOPA. *Pharmacol Biochem Behav* 1979;12:185–188.

82. Herman JP, Choulli K, Le Moal M. Activation of striatal dopaminergic grafts by haloperidol. *Brain Res Bull* 1985;15:543–546.

83. Herman JP, Choulli K, Le Moal M. Hyperreactivity to amphetamine in rats with dopaminergic grafts. *Exp Brain Res* 1985;60:521–526.

84. Herman JP, Choulli K, Geffard M, Nadaud D, Taghzouti K, Le Moal M. Reinnervation of the nucleus accumbens and frontal cortex of the rat by dopaminergic grafts and effects on hoarding behavior. *Brain Res* 1986;372:210–216.

85. Herman JP, Lupp F, Abrous DN, Le Moal M, Hertting G, Jackisch R. Intrastriatal dopaminergic grafts restore inhibitory control over striatal cholinergic neurons. *Exp Brain Res* 1988;73:236–248.

86. Herman JP, Abrous DN, Le Moal M. Anatomical and behavioral comparison of unilateral dopamine-rich grafts implanted into the striatum of neonatal and adult rats. *Neuroscience* 1991;40:465–475.

87. Herman JP, Rouge-Pont F, Le Moal M, Abrous DN. Mechanisms of amphetamine-induced rotation in rats with unilateral intrastriatal grafts of embryonic dopaminergic neurons: a pharmacological and biochemical analysis. *Neuroscience* 1993;53:1083–1095.

88. Herrera-Marschitz M, Strömberg I, Olsson D, Ungerstedt U, Olson L. Adrenal medullary implants in the dopamine-denervated rat striatum: II. acute behavior as a function of graft amount and location and its modulation by neuroleptics. *Brain Res* 1984;297:53–61.

89. Jackisch R, Duschek M, Neufang B, Rensing H, Hertting G, Herman JP. Long-term survival of intrastriatal dopaminergic grafts: modulation of acetylcholine release by graft-derived dopamine. *J Neurochem* 1991;57:267–276.

90. Kaseda Y, Ghetti B, Low WC, et al. Age-related changes in striatal dopamine D2 receptor binding in weaver mice and effects of ventral mesencephalic grafts. *Exp Brain Res* 1990;83:1–8.

91. Kerkerian L, Bosler O, Pelletier G, Nieoullon A. Striatal neuropeptide Y neurons are under the influence of the nigrostriatal dopaminergic pathway: immunohistochemical evidence. *Neurosci Lett* 1986;66:106–112.

92. Lalonde R. Delayed spontaneous alternation in weaver mutant mice. *Brain Res* 1986;398:178–180.

93. Lalonde R, Botez MI. Navigational deficits in weaver mutant mice. *Brain Res* 1986;398:175–177.

94. Lalonde R. Motor abnormalities in weaver mutant mice. *Exp Brain Res* 1987;65:479–481.

95. Langston JW, Ballard P, Tetrud JW, Irwin I. Chronic parkinsonism in humans due to a product of meperidine-analog synthesis. *Science* 1983;219:979–980.

96. Le Moine C, Normand E, Guitteny AF, Fouque B, Teoule R, Bloch B. Dopamine receptor gene expression by enkephalin neurons in the rat forebrain. *Proc Natl Acad Sci USA* 1990;87:230–234.

97. Le Moine C, Normand E, Bloch B. Phenotypical characterization of the rat striatal neurons expressing the D-1 dopamine receptor gene. *Proc Natl Acad Sci USA* 1991;88:4205–4209.

98. Lindvall O, Rehncrona S, Brundin P, et al. Human fetal dopamine neurons grafted into the

striatum in two patients with severe Parkinson's disease. *Arch Neurol* 1989;46:615–631.

99. Low WC, Triarhou LC, Kaseda Y, Norton J, Ghetti B. Functional innervation of the striatum by ventral mesencephalic grafts in mice with inherited nigrostriatal dopamine deficiency. *Brain Res* 1987;435:315–321.

100. Madrazo I, Franco-Bourland R, Ostrosky-Solis F, et al. Fetal homotransplants (ventral mesencephalon and adrenal tissue) to the striatum of parkinsonian subjects. *Arch Neurol* 1990; 47:1281–1285.

101. Mahalik TJ, Finger TE, Strömberg I, Olson L. Substantia nigra transplants into denervated striatum of the rat: ultrastructure of graft and host interconnections. *J Comp Neurol* 1985; 240:60–70.

102. Mahalik TJ, Clayton GH. Specific outgrowth from neurons of ventral mesencephalic grafts to the catecholamine-depleted striatum of adult hosts. *Exp Neurol* 1991;113:18–27.

103. Mandel RJ, Brundin P, Björklund A. The importance of graft placement and task complexity for transplant-induced recovery of simple and complex sensorimotor deficits in dopamine denervated rats. *Eur J Neurosci* 1990;2:888–894.

104. Manier M, Abrous DN, Feuerstein C, Le Moal M, Herman JP. Increase of striatal methionin enkephalin content following lesion of the nigrostriatal dopaminergic pathway in adult rats and reversal following the implantation of embryonic dopaminergic neurons: a quantitative immunohistochemical analysis. *Neuroscience* 1991;42:427–439.

105. Marshall JF, Ungerstedt U. Supersensitivity to apomorphine following destruction of the ascending dopamine neurons: quantification using the rotational model. *Eur J Pharmacol* 1977;41:361–367.

106. Marshall JF, Ungerstedt U. Striatal efferents play a role in maintaining rotational behaviour in the rat. *Science* 1977;198:62–64.

107. Marshall JF, Berrios N, Sawyer S. Neostriatal dopamine and sensory inattention. *J Comp Physiol Psychol* 1980;94:833–846.

108. Marshall JF, Navarette R, Joyce JN. Decreased striatal D-1 binding following mesotelencephalic 6-OHDA injections: an autoradiographic analysis. *Brain Res* 1989;493:247–257.

109. Meloni R, Childs J, Gerogan F, Yurkifsky S, Gale K. Effect of haloperidol on transplants of fetal substantia nigra: evidence for feedback regulation of dopamine turnover in the graft and its projections. *Prog Brain Res* 1988; 78:457–461.

110. Meloni R, Gale K. Cocaine-induced turning behavior in rats with 6-hydroxydopamine lesions: effect of transplants of fetal substantia nigra. *Eur J Pharmacol* 1991;209:113–117.

111. Mendez IM, Naus CCG, Elisevich K, Flumerfelt BA. Normalization of striatal proenkephalin and preprotachykinin mRNA expression by fetal substantia nigra grafts. *Exp Neurol* 1993;119:1–10.

112. Montoya CP, Astell S, Dunnett SB. Effects of nigral and striatal grafts on skilled forelimb use in the rat. *Prog Brain Res* 1990;82:459–466.

113. Montoya CP, Campbell-Hope LJ, Pemberton KD, Dunnett SB. The "staircase" test: a measure of independent forelimb reaching and grasping abilities in rats. *J Neurosci Methods* 1991;36:219–228.

114. Moore KE, Kelly PH. Biochemical pharmacology of mesolimbic and mesocortical dopaminergic neurons. In: Lipton MA, Di Mascio A, Killam KF, eds. *Psychopharmacology: a generation of progress.* New York: Raven Press; 1978:221–234.

115. Moukhles H, Nieoullon A, Daszuta A. Early and widespread normalization of dopamine–neuropeptide Y interactions in the rat striatum after transplantation of fetal mesencephalon cells. *Neuroscience* 1992;47:781–792.

116. Neve KA, Altar CA, Wong CA, Marshall JF. Quantitative analysis of ^{3}H-spiroperidol binding to rat forebrain sections: plasticity of neostriatal dopamine receptors after nigrostriatal injury. *Brain Res* 1984;302:9–18.

117. Nikkhah G, Duan W-M, Knappe U, Björklund A. Restoration of complex sensorimotor behavior and skilled forelimb use by a modified nigral cell suspension transplantation approach in the rat Parkinson model. *Neuroscience* 1993;56:33–43.

118. Nishino H, Ono T, Shibata R, et al. Adrenal medullary cells transmute into dopaminergic neurons in dopamine-depleted rat caudate and ameliorate motor disturbances. *Brain Res* 1988;445:325–337.

119. Nishino H, Hashitani T, Kumazaki M, et al. Long-term survival of grafted cells, dopamine synthesis/release, synaptic connections, and functional recovery after transplantation of fetal nigral cells in rats with unilateral 6-OHDA lesions in the nigrostriatal dopamine pathway. *Brain Res* 1990;534:83–93.

120. Normand E, Popovici T, Onteniente B, et al. Dopaminergic neurons of the substantia nigra modulate proenkephalin A gene expression in rat striatal neurons. *Brain Res* 1988;439:39–46.

121. Patel-Vaidya U, Wells MR, Freed WJ. Survival of dissociated adrenal chromaffin cells of rat and monkey transplanted into rat brain. *Cell Tissue Res* 1985;240:281–285.

122. Perlow MJ, Freed WJ, Hoffer B, Seiger Å, Olson L, Wyatt RJ. Brain grafts reduce motor abnormalities produced by destruction of nigrostriatal dopamine system. *Science* 1979;204:643–647.

123. Perlow MJ, Kukkura K, Guidotti A. Prolonged survival of bovine adrenal chromaffin cells in rat cerebral ventricles. *Proc Natl Acad Sci USA* 1980;77:5278–5281.

124. Pezzoli G, Fahn S, Dwork A, et al. Non-chromaffin tissue plus nerve growth factor reduces experimental parkinsonism in aged rats. *Brain Res* 1988;459:398–403.

125. Pileblad E, Fornstedt B, Clark D, Carlsson A. Acute effects of 1-methyl-4-phenyl-1,2,3,6-tet-

rahydropyridine on dopamine metabolism in mouse and rat striatum. *J Pharm Pharmacol* 1985;7:707–711.

126. Rakic P, Sidman RL. Sequence of developmental abnormalities leading to granule cell deficit in cerebellar cortex of Weaver mutant mice. *J Comp Neurol* 1973;152:103–132.

127. Rioux L, Gaudin DP, Bui LK, Grégoire L, DiPaolo T, Bédard PJ. Correlation of functional recovery after a 6-hydroxydopamine lesion with survival of grafted fetal neurons and release of dopamine in the striatum of the rat. *Neuroscience* 1991;40:123–131.

128. Rioux L, Gaudin DP, Gagnon C, DiPaolo T, Bédard PJ. Decrease of behavioral and biochemical denervation supersensitivity of rat striatum by nigral transplants. *Neuroscience* 1991;44:75–83.

129. Rogers DC, Martel FL, Dunnett SB. Nigral grafts in neonatal rats protect from aphagia induced by subsequent adult 6-OHDA lesions: the importance of striatal location. *Exp Brain Res* 1990;80:172–176.

130. Romano GJ, Shivers BD, Harlan RE, Howells RD, Pfaff DW. Haloperidol increases proenkephalin mRNA levels in the caudate–putamen of the rat: a quantitative study at the cellular level using in situ hybridisation. *Mol Brain Res* 1987;2:33–41.

131. Rose G, Gerhardt G, Strömberg I, Olson L, Hoffer B. Monoamine release from dopamine-depleted rat caudate nucleus reinnervated by substantia nigra transplants: an *in vivo* electrochemical study. *Brain Res* 1985;341:92–100.

132. Roth RH, Murrin C, Walters JR. Central dopaminergic neurons: effects of alterations in impulse flow on the accumulation of dihydroxyphenylacetic acid. *Eur J Pharmacol* 1976;36:163–171.

133. Rydelek-Fitzgerald L, Glick SD, Schneider AS. Effect of striatal implantation of bovine adrenal chromaffin cells. *Brain Res* 1989;481:373–377.

134. Sauer H, Brundin P. Effects of cool storage on survival and function of intrastriatal ventral mesencephalic grafts. *Rest Neurol Neurosci* 1991;2:123–135.

135. Savasta M, Dubois A, Feuerstein C, Manier M, Scatton B. Denervation supersensitivity of striatal D-2 dopamine receptors is restricted to the ventro- and dorsolateral regions of the striatum. *Neurosci Lett* 1987;74:180–186.

136. Savasta M, Dubois A, Benavides J, Scatton B. Different plasticity changes in D-1 and D-2 receptors in rat striatal subregions following impairment of dopaminergic transmission. *Neurosci Lett* 1988;85:119–124.

137. Savasta M, Mennicken F, Chritin M, et al. Intrastriatal dopamine-rich implants reverse the changes in dopamine-D2 receptor densities caused by 6-hydroxydopamine lesion of the nigrostriatal pathway in rats: an autoradiographic study. *Neuroscience* 1992;46:729–738.

138. Schallert T, Hall S. "Disengage" sensorimotor deficit following apparent recovery from unilat-

eral dopamine depletion *Behav Brain Res* 1988; 30:15–24.

139. Schmidt MJ, Sawyer BD, Perry KW, Fuller RW, Foreman MM, Ghetti B. Dopamine deficiency in the Weaver mutant mouse. *J Neurosci* 1982;2:376–380.

140. Schmidt RH, Ingvar M, Lindvall O, Stenevi U, Björklund A. Functional activity of substantia nigra grafts reinnervating the striatum: neurotransmitter metabolism and [^{14}C] 2-deoxy-D-glucose autoradiography. *J Neurochem* 1982; 38:737–748.

141. Schmidt RH, Björklund A, Stenevi U, Dunnett SB, Gage FH. Intracerebral grafting of neuronal cell suspensions: III. activity of intrastriatal nigral suspension implants as assessed by measurements of dopamine synthesis and metabolism. *Acta Physiol Scand [Suppl]* 1983; 522:19–28.

142. Schultz W, Ungerstedt U. Short-term increase and long-term reversion of striatal cell activity after degeneration of the nigrostriatal dopamine system. *Exp Brain Res* 1978;33:159–171.

143. Schultzberg M, Dunnett SB, Björklund A, et al. Dopamine and cholecystokinin immunoreactive neuronses in mesencephalic grafts reinnervating the neostriatum: evidence for selective growth regulation. *Neuroscience* 1984; 12:17–32.

144. Schwarz S, Freed WJ. Brain tissue transplantation in neonatal rats prevents a lesion-induced syndrome of adipsia, aphagia, and akinesia. *Exp Brain Res* 1987;65:449–454.

145. Segovia J, Garcia-Munoz M. Changes in the activity of GAD in the basal ganglia of the rat after striatal dopaminergic denervation. *Neuropharmacology* 1987;26:1449–1451.

146. Segovia J, Meloni R, Gale K. Effect of dopaminergic denervation and transplant-derived reinnervation on a marker of striatal GABAergic function. *Brain Res* 1989;493:185–189.

147. Segovia J, Tillakaratne NJK, Whelan K, Tobin AJ, Gale K. Parallel increases in striatal glutamic acid decarboxylase activity and mRNA levels in rats with lesions of the nigrostriatal pathway. *Brain Res* 1990;529:345–348.

148. Segovia J, Castro R, Notario V, Gale K. Transplants of fetal substantia nigral regulate glutamic acid decarboxylase gene expression in host striatal neurons. *Mol Brain Res* 1991; 10:359–362.

149. Siggins G, Hoffer B, Ungerstedt U. Electrophysiological evidence for the involvement of cyclic adenosine monophosphate in dopamine responses of caudate neurons. *Life Sci* 1974;15:779–792.

150. Sidman RL, Green MC, Appel SH. Catalog of the Neurological Mutants of the Mouse. Cambridge, MA: Harvard University Press; 1965:66–67.

151. Simonds GR, Freed WJ. Effects of intraventricular substantia nigra allografts as a function of donor age. *Brain Res* 1990;530:12–19.

152. Simonds GR, Schwarz S, Krauthamer E, Freed WJ. Effects of adrenal medulla grafts in neo-

natal rat hosts on subsequent bilateral substantia nigra lesions. *Rest Neurol Neurosci* 1990; 1:315–322.

153. Sirinathsinghji DJS, Heavens RP, Richards SJ, Beresford IJM, Hall MD. Experimental hemiparkinsonism in the rat following chronic unilateral infusion of MPP$^+$ into the nigrostriatal dopamine pathway: I. behavioural, neurochemical and histological characterization of the lesion. *Neuroscience* 1988;27:117–128.

154. Sirinathsinghji DJS, Dunnett SB. Disappearance of the μ-opiate receptor patches in the rat neostriatum following lesioning of the ipsilateral nigrostriatal dopamine pathway with, 1-methyl-4-phenylpyridinium ion (MPP$^+$): restoration by embryonic nigral dopamine grafts. *Brain Res* 1989;504:115–120.

155. Sirinathsinghji DJS, Dunnett SB, Northrop AJ, Morris BJ. Experimental hemiparkinsonism in the rat following chronic unilateral infusion of MPP$^+$ into the nigrostriatal dopamine pathway: III. reversal by embryonic nigral dopamine grafts. *Neuroscience* 1990;37:757–766.

156. Sirinathsinghji DJS, Dunnett SB. Increased proenkephalin mRNA levels in the rat neostriatum following lesion of the ipsilateral nigrostriatal dopamine pathway with 1-methyl-4-phenylpyridinium ion (MPP$^+$): reversal by embryonic nigral dopamine grafts. *Mol Brain Res* 1991;9:263–269.

157. Snyder-Keller AM, Carder RK, Lund RD. Development of dopamine innervation and turning behavior in dopamine-depleted infant rats receiving unilateral nigral transplants. *Neuroscience* 1989;30:779–794.

158. Sonsalla PK, Manzino L, Heikkila RE. Interactions of D1 and D2 receptors on the ipsilateral vs contralateral side in rats with unilateral lesions of the dopaminergic nigrostriatal pathway. *J Pharmacol Exp Ther* 1988;247:180–185.

159. Strecker RE, Sharp T, Brundin P, Zetterström T, Ungerstedt U, Björklund A. Autoregulation of dopamine release and metabolism by intrastriatal nigral grafts as revealed by intracerebral microdialysis. *Neuroscience* 1987;22:169–178.

160. Strömberg I, Herrera-Marschitz M, Hultgren L, Ungerstedt U, Olson L. Adrenal medullary implants in the dopamine-denervated rat striatum: I. acute catecholamine levels in grafts and host caudate as determined by HPLC-electrochemistry and fluorescence histochemical image analysis. *Brain Res* 1984;297:41–51.

161. Strömberg I, Herrera-Marschitz M, Ungerstedt U, Ebendal T, Olson L. Chronic implants of chromaffin tissue into the dopamine-denervated rat striatum: effects of NGF on graft survival, fiber growth and rotational behavior. *Exp Brain Res* 1985;60:335–349.

162. Strömberg I, Johnson S, Hoffer B, Olson L. Reinnervation of the dopamine-denervated striatum by substantia nigra transplants: immunohistochemical and electrophysiological correlates. *Neuroscience* 1985;14:981–990.

163. Strömberg I, Bygdeman M, Goldstein M, Seiger Å, Olson L. Human fetal substantia nigra grafted to the dopamine-denervated striatum of immunosuppressed rats: evidence for functional reinnervation. *Neurosci Lett* 1986; 71:271–276.

164. Strömberg I, Almquist, P, Bygdeman M, et al. Human fetal mesencephalic tissue grafted to dopamine-denervated striatum of athymic rats: light- and electron-microscopical histochemistry and in vivo chronoamperometric studies. *J Neurosci* 1989;9:614–624.

165. Sundström E, Strömberg I, Tsutsumi T, Olson L, Jonsson G. Studies on the effects of 1-methyl-4-phenyl-1,2,3,6-tetrahydropyridine (MPTP) on central catecholamine neurons in C57BL/6 mice: comparison with three other strains of mice. *Brain Res* 1987;405:26–38.

166. Takashima H, Poltorak M, Becker JB, Freed WJ. Effects of adrenal medulla grafts on plasma catecholamines and rotational behavior. *Exp Neurol* 1992;118:24–34.

167. Tang F, Costa E, Schwartz JP. Increase of proenkephalin mRNA and enkephalin content of rat striatum after daily injection of haloperidol for 2 to 3 weeks, *Proc Natl Acad Sci USA* 1983;80:3841–3844.

168. Tossman U, Segovia J. Ungerstedt U. Extracellular levels of amino acids in striatum and globus pallidus of 6-hydroxydopamine lesioned rats measured with microdialysis. *Acta Physiol Scand* 1986;127,547–551.

169. Trantzer JP, Thoenen H. Ultramorphologische Veränderungen der sympatischen Nervenendigungen der Katze nach Vorbehandlung mit 5- und 6-hydroxy-dopamin. *Naunyn Schmiedebergs Arch Exp Pathol Pharmakol* 1967;257: 343–344.

170. Triarhou LC, Norton J, Ghetti B. Mesencephalic dopamine cell deficit involves areas A8, A9 and A10 in Weaver mutant mice. *Exp Brain Res* 1988;70:256–265.

171. Triarhou LC, Brundin P, Doucet G, Norton J, Björklund A, Ghetti B. Intrastriatal implants of mesencephalic cell suspension in Weaver mutant mice: ultrastructural relationships of dopaminergic dendrites and axons issued from the graft. *Exp Brain Res* 1990;79:3–17.

172. Triarhou LC, Low W, Ghetti B. Dopamine neuron grafting to the Weaver mouse striatum. *Prog Brain Res* 1990;82:187–195.

173. Ungerstedt U. 6-hydroxydopamine induced degerneration of central monoamine neurons. *Eur J Pharmacol* 1968;5:107–110.

174. Ungerstedt U, Arbuthnott GW. Quantitative recording of rotational behavior in rats after 6-hydroxy-dopamine lesions of the nigrostriatal dopamine system. *Brain Res* 1970;24:485–493.

175. Ungerstedt U. Post-synaptic supersensitivity after 6-hydroxydopamine induced degeneration of the nigro-striatal dopamine system. *Acta Physiol Scand (Suppl)* 1971;367:49–68.

176. Ungerstedt U, Aphagia and adipsia after 6-hydroxydopamine induced degeneration of the nigro-striatal dopamine system. *Acta Physiol Scand (Suppl)* 1971;367:95–122.

177. van Horne CG, Mahalik T, Hoffer B, et al. Be-

havioral and electrophysiological correlates of human mesencephalic dopaminergic xenograft function in the rat striatum. *Brain Res Bull* 1990;25:325–334.

178. Vernier P, Julien JF, Rataboul P, Fourier O, Feuerstein C, Mallett J. Similar time course changes in striatal levels of glutamic acid decarboxylase and proenkephalin mRNA following dopaminergic deafferentation in the rat. *J Neurochem* 1988;51:1375–1380.

179. Vincent SR, Nagy JI, Fibiger HC. Increased striatal glutamate decarboxylase after lesions of the nigrostriatal pathway. *Brain Res* 1978; 143:168–173.

180. Voorn P, Roest G, Groenewegen HJ. Increase of enkephalin and decrease of substance P immunoreactivity in the dorsal and ventral striatum of the rat after midbrain 6-hydroxydopamine lesions. *Brain Res* 1987;412:391–396.

181. Wuerthele SM, Freed WJ, Olson L, et al. Effect of dopamine agonists and antagonists on the electrical activity of substantia nigra neurons transplanted into the lateral ventricle of the rat. *Exp Brain Res* 1981;44:1–10.

182. Young WS III, Bonner TI, Brann MR. Mesencephalic dopamine neurons regulate the expression of neuropeptide mRNAs in the rat forebrain. *Proc Natl Acad Sci USA* 1986; 83:9827–9831.

183. Zetterström T, Brundin P, Gage FH, et al. In vivo measurement of spontaneous release and metabolism of dopamine from intrastriatal nigral grafts using intracerebral microdialysis. *Brain Res* 1986;362:344–349.

184. Zuddas A, Corsini GU, Barker JL, Kopin IJ, di Porzio U. Specific reinnervation of lesioned mouse striatum by grafted mesencephalic dopaminergic neurons. *Eur J Neurosci* 1991;3:72–85.

Functional Neural Transplantation,
edited by S. B. Dunnett and A. Björklund.
Raven Press, Ltd., New York © 1994.

3

Nigral Transplants in the Rat Parkinson Model

Functional Limitations and Strategies to Enhance Nigrostriatal Reconstruction

*Anders Björklund, †Stephen B. Dunnett, and *‡Guido Nikkhah

*Department of Medical Cell Research, University of Lund, S–223 62 Lund, Sweden;
†Department of Experimental Psychology, University of Cambridge, Cambridge CB2 3EB,
United Kingdom; ‡Neurosurgical Clinic, Nordstadt Hospital, Hanover D-3000, Germany*

EXTENT AND LIMITS OF NIGRAL GRAFT RECOVERY

The two preceding chapters amply illustrate the extent of functional recovery that can be obtained after transplantation of dopamine-rich (usually fetal nigral) tissues in the striatum in adult rats and monkeys. The animal experimental work has been the subject of many reviews [see Brundin, Annett (this volume)], and has provided the basis for the progress to clinical trials of adrenal and nigral cell transplantation in human Parkinson's disease (PD) [see Lindvall (this volume)]. Nevertheless, in spite of the dramatic and relatively complete functional recovery observed on some tests, such as drug-induced rotation or akinesia in rats with forebrain dopamine lesions, it has always been apparent that the transplanted animals show less recovery on other tests.

This issue was first apparent in early studies of solid grafts of fetal ventral mesencephalon implanted into a cavity in the frontoparietal cortex overlying the dorsal neostriatum of rats with unilateral or bilateral 6-hydroxydopamine (6-OHDA) lesions of the nigrostriatal dopamine pathway.

Whereas rats with unilateral lesions showed good graft-induced recovery on spontaneous and drug-induced rotation, they remained impaired on tests of sensorimotor neglect (11,23). Similarly, rats with bilateral lesions and unilateral transplants showed good recovery on tests of locomotor akinesia, but they never recovered from their life-threatening disturbances in food and water intake (aphagia and adipsia, respectively) (11,25). It soon became apparent that this heterogeneity of response was in part due to the placement of the nigral transplants. The neostriatum is topographically organized, such that it is necessary to place the grafts into the relevant sites if one was to elicit a functional response on a particular test. Such functional heterogeneity could account for some of the early results: Whereas placement of grafts into the dorsal site is capable of reversing whole-body rotation asymmetry, it is necessary to place the grafts in or adjacent to the lateral striatum to alleviate the rats' sensorimotor deficits (24,26). Conversely, topographic heterogeneity alone was unable to account for the failure of recovery in other functional impairments, such as the aphagia and adipsia after bilateral nigrostriatal lesions. Profound eating and drinking deficits remained whether the grafts were placed in single or multiple striatal or extrastriatal sites (11, 25,27).

Subsequently, a number of other classes of behavioral deficit have been identified in 6-OHDA-lesioned rats that are relatively resistant to functional alleviation by grafts implanted into the deafferented neostriatum and ventral striatum. In our own laboratories, these include deficits in the rats' abilities to use the forepaws for skilled manipulation, as assessed in tests of reaching for food (2,31,50), and deficits in the rats' ability to orient toward distracting sensory stimuli while engaged in eating ("disengage" behavior) (46). Along similar lines, Herman and colleagues (41–43) have seen little recovery in more complex behaviors, such as hoarding, after dopamine cell implants in either neostriatum or nucleus accumbens.

The problem, then, is to understand why nigral grafts produce recovery on some tests but not on others. This has led us first to develop new tests to analyze the functional deficits in greater detail. Next, we consider alternative explanations for the cases in which recovery is not seen and in particular whether some of the limits to recovery are due to the ectopic placement of conventional nigral grafts into the host neostriatum. Finally, we evaluate the functional efficacy of alternative graft strategies oriented toward enhancing nigrostriatal reconstruction.

LIMITATIONS OF ECTOPIC NIGRAL GRAFTS

Paw-Reaching Tests

Of these various tests of nigrostriatal deficits resistant to recovery, the deficits in paw-reaching and response initiation offer the most obvious parallels with the motor impairments in PD. These kinds of tests thus are particularly relevant for understanding the extent and limitations of repair in the rat Parkinson model.

The first type of paw-reaching test we adopted was one in which the rats had to reach through the cage bars to collect and retrieve small pellets of food. The forelimbs can be bandaged or restricted one at a time to test the reaching capacity and extent of deficit in each paw separately (70). Unilateral nigrostriatal lesions induce marked deficits in this reaching task: if given a free choice of which paw they may use, the rats not surprisingly manifest a relatively complete bias toward preferred use of the paw ipsilateral to the lesion. However, if use of the unaffected paw is restricted, the rats will attempt to use the affected paw but with a very low level of success. In particular, they make uncoordinated flailing movements in contrast to the accurate, directed reaching observed in an intact rat. They frequently contact the food pellets with the open palm, but they appear unable to make a coordinated grasp in response to the somatosensory feedback from contact with the food, and their attempts are generally without success (70). In this test, the "hit rate" (successful reaches divided by total attempts) was about 50% to 60% for a normal rat, whereas a rat with a nigrostriatal lesion generally scored under 10% with the contralateral limb (70). In a first transplant study, nigral cell suspension implants in the denervated caudate–putamen were completely without effect on the host animals' paw-reaching deficits, even though the same animals showed complete recovery on tests of rotation asymmetry and contralateral sensorimotor neglect (31).

To assess residual capacity and recovery in the affected contralateral limb (i.e., contralateral to the lesioned side), these first tests of skilled paw-reaching relied on binding or otherwise restricting use of the "good" paw (contralateral to the intact side), a process that can induce a degree of postural imbalance. We have therefore developed an alternative test of paw-reaching deficits in which use of the two limbs is constrained by the structure of the test apparatus rather than by any direct curtailment of the animals' movements. Known as the "staircase" test, the apparatus permits the rat to reach down on either side of a central platform to retrieve pellets located in a deep, narrow trough on either side (51). The base of each trough comprises a staircase with steps down from the level of the platform to a depth well beyond an animal's reach. Two food pellets are placed on each step of the staircase, and the rats are then free to collect and consume all food pellets within their reach and within a certain time. The apparatus is designed so that a rat can reach down only into the left-hand trough with its left forepaw and into the right trough with its right forepaw, so that the number of steps from which the pellets are displaced on each side provides a direct measure of how far the rat can reach with the paw on that side.

Unilateral nigrostriatal 6-OHDA lesions induce a marked deficit in the number of pellets retrieved with the contralateral paw, with a small deficit also in ipsilateral forelimb use. As in the previous paw-reaching study, whereas nigral grafts, placed into the head of the caudate–putamen, were functional in restoration of the rats' rotation asymmetries, the grafted rats showed improved paw-reaching on the ipsilateral side but no detectable recovery with the paw contralateral to the graft (50) (Fig. 1). An additional group of animals received unilateral ibotenic acid lesions of the lateral striatum that produced a similar marked reaching deficit. Interestingly, grafts of fetal striatal tissue implanted into the lesioned striatal area produced significant improvement in both ipsilateral and contralateral paw-reaching (Fig. 1). This demonstrates that the paw-reaching task is not intrinsically resistant to graft-derived recovery, even though the nigral grafts used in this experiment were largely ineffective.

Sensorimotor Tests

In the "disengage" behavior test, as introduced by Schallert and Hall (60), the rat's ability to initiate orienting movements is applied similarly to the standard test for sensorimotor neglect, except that the latency for responding is evaluated while the rat is engaged in eating. This switching from one behavior (eating) to another (orientation toward a tactile stimulus applied to the perioral region) depends on an intact mesostriatal dopamine system. In unilateral 6-OHDA-lesioned rats, the animals continue to respond promptly toward the side ipsilateral to the lesion, whereas response toward the side contralateral to the lesion is severely impaired. Interestingly, in the study by Schallert and Hall (60), rats that showed spontaneous recovery of simple sensorimotor orienting responses on the contralateral side remained severely impaired in the disengage test. This suggests that disengage behavior may be a more rigorous test of dopamine-dependent integrative sensorimotor behavior in the rat Parkinson model than the simple sensorimotor orienting tests used in the earlier studies.

In a first experiment using this test, Mandel et al. (46) studied the effect of standard nigral cell suspension grafts implanted into the central or lateral subfields of the head of the caudate–putamen. Consistent with previous findings, lateral, but not centrally placed grafts restored virtually completely simple sensorimotor orienting responses, whereas the impaired responding during eating remained unaffected.

Mesolimbic Deficits

While replicating the restoration of basic motor responses in activity and rotation tests, Herman and colleagues (42,43) have reported on other behavioral measures of dopamine system damage that are resistant to alleviation by nigral grafts. In their studies, they have focused on motivational be-

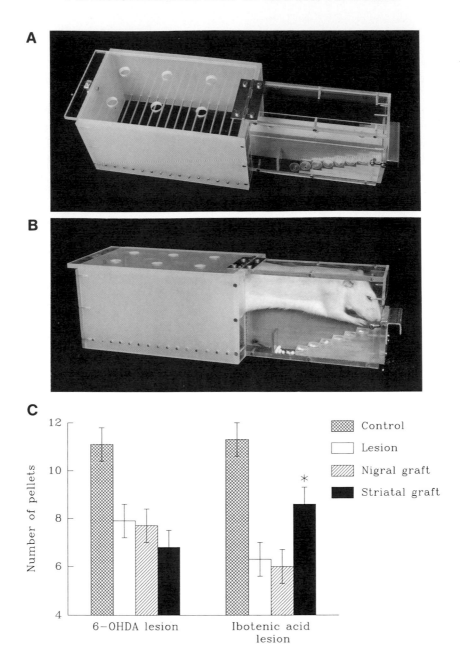

FIG. 1. Effects of lesions and transplants on skilled paw-reaching in the "staircase test." **A, B**: Two views of the box used in the Montoya et al. (51) test. At the start of the test, the steps of the staircase are baited with pellets on both sides. The number of pellets remaining after the 15-min test session is counted in each of the five test days. **C**: Numbers of pellets successfully retrieved by the paw contralateral to a 6-OHDA lesion of the nigrostriatal bundle (*left*) or an ibotenic acid lesion of the striatum (*right*). The striped bars represent lesioned rats receiving intrastriatal grafts of E14 fetal nigral tissue; the filled bars represent lesioned rats receiving grafts of E14 fetal striatal tissue. Three months postlesion; means of 5 tests. Asterisk indicates significant graft-induced improvement. Data from Montoya et al. (50).

haviors subserved by mesocorticolimbic dopamine projections to the ventral striatum–nucleus accumbens area. Animals with mesolimbic dopamine depletions induced by injection of 6-OHDA into the nucleus accumbens show marked deficits in hoarding behavior (the natural tendency of hungry rats to collect food and store it in a corner of their home cages), which is not restored by nigral grafts unless, interestingly, the grafts are stimulated with a low dose of amphetamine. The situation was found to be more complicated in rats with more extensive mesocorticolimbic lesions induced by injections of 6-OHDA into the area of the cell bodies in the ventral tegmental area (43). This lesion produced a more widespread dopamine depletion throughout the limbic forebrain and resulted in stable deficits in locomotor activity, and a decline in both exploratory activity and hoarding. Dopamine-rich grafts placed in the nucleus accumbens again alleviated the animals' deficits in drug-induced locomotor activity, but in this case had no effect on the exploratory and hoarding deficits, even when the grafts were stimulated with a low dose of amphetamine (43). These authors therefore suggest an interpretation based on cooperativity between different forebrain areas receiving mesolimbic dopamine projections (including the nucleus accumbens, septum, and amygdala) in the maintenance of normal performance on these more complex and subtle tests of the animals' motivational status.

INTERPRETATIONS OF RESIDUAL DEFICITS

Hypothesis I: Recovery in More Complex Integrative Tasks Requires More Extensive Reinnervation of Denervated Striatal (or Extrastriatal) Forebrain Areas

An obvious limitation of the standard type of intrastriatal nigral transplant is that the associated dopamine fiber outgrowth reaches only a limited subregion of the various striatal and extrastriatal structures that are denervated by the 6-OHDA lesion. This is well illustrated by the biochemical data of Schmidt et al (61). In this study, the 6-OHDA lesion reduced the total forebrain dopamine content by 94% to 97% (from 640 to about 30 ng). The nigral cell suspension grafts, implanted as three 3-μl deposits in the head of the caudate–putamen, restored the total forebrain dopamine content by 35 to 80 ng, which is equivalent to 5% to 13% of the dopamine content lost by the lesion. The parallel microscopic analysis (12) showed that reinnervation was dense in an area of about 1 to 1.5 mm around the graft, but that large areas of the neostriatum remained denervated (see also ref. 20).

There is quite convincing evidence that dopamine released from intrastriatal nigral grafts can act over a wider area than that reached by the outgrowing axons. Thus, Savasta et al. (59) and Chritin et al. (18) have observed that normalization of dopamine receptor supersensitivity (D1 and D2 receptor binding and D2 mRNA expression) around single graft deposits extends well beyond the immediate area reinnervated by the graft. This has been shown to be the case also for the graft-induced normalization of dopamine receptor-mediated Fos expression (15) and enkephalin expression (16,47,65) in striatal projection neurons. However, other aspects of nigral graft function are likely to depend on dopamine release at specialized synaptic sites. In a recent *in situ* hybridization study, Cenci et al. (16) have shown that behaviorally functional nigral grafts (as assessed by the rotation test) normalize enkephalin synthesis in the striatal projection neurons throughout the denervated striatum, whereas normalization of substance P synthesis (which is a property of the striatonigral neurons) is restricted to the area densely reinnervated by the grafted dopamine neurons.

These data strongly suggest that both quantitative and region-specific effects are important for the pattern and extent of functional recovery induced by nigral grafts in the rat PD model. In general support of this idea are our previous data on multiple striatal nigral grafts, showing that a full range of effects on turning bias, sensorimotor orientation, sensorimotor limb use, and drug-induced locomotion is obtained only with transplants innervating several striatal subfields (i.e., lateral, dorsal, anteromedial, and ventral striatum, including the nucleus accumbens) (26).

In a recent study, (54,55) we made an attempt to obtain more extensive reinnervation of the entire head of the caudate–putamen in unilaterally 6-OHDA-lesioned rats. A modified cell suspension approach was used, which allowed distribution of the graft tissue over multiple sites with minimal trauma. A total of 450,000 cells (equivalent to about one fetal mesencephalon) was distributed over 18 deposits along 6 needle penetrations in the head of the caudate–putamen. As compared to our standard type of grafts (same numbers of cells implanted as two deposits), the distributed "micro" grafts resulted in a nearly threefold increase

in dopamine neuron survival, a 2.5-fold increase in the recovery of striatal dopamine (to 30% of normal levels), and a more substantial reinnervation throughout the head of the grafted caudate–putamen (54). In these animals it was for the first time possible to obtain a significant recovery in paw-reaching on the contralateral lesioned and grafted side (Fig. 2). Although the overall improvement was partial, it is notable that about half of the rats (six of ten) achieved a performance level similar to that of normal controls. Although the rats with single large-sized graft deposits (same number of cells implanted at two sites) showed a similar trend, their improvement in the paw-reaching task did not reach significance (55).

These rats also were tested for sensorimotor orientation and disengage behavior. Consistent with previous studies, simple sensorimotor orientation was markedly improved in all rats with the single large as well as multiple small deposits. In addition, the distributed "micro" grafts produced an approximately 45% reduction in response latency in the disengage test (55). However,

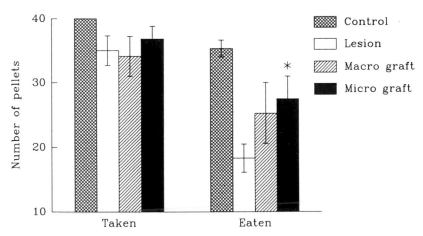

FIG. 2. Recovery of skilled paw-reaching in the staircase test (see Fig. 1) seen 3 months after transplantation of single large E14 fetal nigral cellsuspension grafts ("macro" graft) or multiple distributed small graft deposits ("micro" grafts) into the 6-OHDA lesioned striatum. The diagram shows the performance of the paw contralateral to the lesion and graft side on the last day of the test, when only the contralateral staircase was baited. Asterisk indicates significant graft-induced recovery in the micro graft group. Data from Nikkhah et al. (55).

most of the grafted animals remained impaired relative to the nonlesioned side.

These data are in good agreement with those obtained in marmosets. As described by Annett (*this volume*), single grafts in the caudate nucleus can reverse drug-induced turning but have no or only marginal effects on forelimb use. However, after multiple grafts involving both caudate nucleus, putamen, and nucleus accumbens, there was a significant improvement in forelimb reaching, although certain aspects of limb use, as well as neglect, remained impaired.

Taken together, these data support the idea that nigral transplants that reinnervate limited striatal subfields may be sufficient to restore basic parameters of dopamine-dependent motor behaviors, such as simple sensorimotor orientation and turning bias, whereas more extensive reinnervation is required to influence deficits in more complex sensorimotor tasks.

Hypothesis II: Ectopic Grafts Cannot Reconstruct the Full Nigrostriatal Circuitry

Resolution of the question of why ectopic nigral grafts yield good, and sometimes complete, recovery on some behavioral measures but no or only partial recovery on other behavioral tests requires a clear formulation of the alternative mechanisms of how neural grafts can mediate their functional effects. These issues, which have been the topic of several earlier reviews (13,21,22), will be discussed in more general terms in the final chapter of this volume [see Dunnett and Björklund (*this volume*)]. However, in the present context, the essential issue involves the extent, limitations, and precise patterning of efferent and afferent of graft connectivity with the host brain.

The first clue about the level of anatomic reconstruction required of nigral grafts comes from an analysis of alternative pharmacologic treatments of human PD. It is clear that in the early stages of the disease,

patients receive substantial relief from many of their symptoms with drugs, such as L-dopa, that promote central dopamine function. This suggests that direct activation of striatal dopamine receptors may be sufficient to restore the normal cellular activity of striatal neurons. If so, then simple dopamine replacement in the striatum could provide an effective therapeutic strategy for central dopamine depletion in experimental animals or specifically for parkinsonism in humans. Thus, creating a transplant that can secrete dopamine at stable physiologic levels into circumscribed brain targets may be all that is required of a therapeutically effective transplant. Such a rationale underlies the development of dopamine-secreting polymers and the encapsulation of stable dopamine-secreting cell lines (7,76).

Nevertheless, several lines of evidence suggest that the "pharmacologic minipump" strategy of neural transplantation may prove insufficient, particularly in later stages of the disease. Thus, L-dopa itself produces an increasing number of side effects and has declining efficacy in more advanced cases of PD. It is likely that L-dopa requires presynaptic regulation to be effective, and that this drug exerts its effects in part by promoting the functional capacity of residual neurons spared by the disease, rather than by replacing them. Similarly, L-dopa or direct dopaminergic agonists can be effective in experimental animals with partial lesions but provide minimal benefit in animals with relatively complete bilateral lesions (44,48). Perhaps most critically, whereas dopamine-secreting polymers, encapsulated cells, or nonneuronal tissues (such as adrenal medulla) can alleviate drug-induced locomotor and rotational asymmetries, improvement in spontaneous sensorimotor behaviors, such as contralateral sensory neglect, has not been achieved so far in animals with relatively complete lesions (36). Moreover, in the few situations where they have been compared directly, nigral grafts have been found to yield more extensive functional recovery than adrenal grafts (14).

Taken together, these results suggest that biologic minipumps, which provide a non-regulated tonic activation of dopamine receptors in the striatum, may not provide a sufficient level of repair for full restoration of function in the Parkinson model. It is a reasonable assumption, therefore, that regulated synaptic or nonsynaptic dopamine release, achieved through dopaminergic reinnervation and formation of synaptic connections with their striatal targets, contributes importantly to the pattern of functional recovery obtained with intrastriatal nigral transplants. In the intact brain, the nigral dopamine neurons are likely to exert their striatal function not only through tonic dopamine release (which is largely independent of changes in axonal impulse flow) but also through phasic changes in neuronal impulse activity (17,39,52). Of particular importance in this regard is the burst firing properties of the nigral dopamine neurons, which depend on afferent inputs to the nigral neurons, above all on the glutamatergic afferents (see ref. 39 for a recent review). Consequently, we can hypothesize that normal function of the nigrostriatal dopamine system depends on afferent regulation; whereas certain aspects of striatal function can be subserved by tonic dopamine release, full functional recovery may be obtained only when the dynamic flow of information that is normally relayed by the nigrostriatal connections is restored. In other words, simple striatal reinnervation without the graft itself receiving and transducing information afferent to the substantia nigra in the intact brain may not be sufficient to restore full function.

Of course, ectopic nigral transplants implanted into the caudate–putamen are not entirely devoid of regulatory afferent inputs (6,34). In a recent electrophysiologic study, Fisher et al. (34) have shown that over 50% of the grafted nigral neurons respond to stimulation of the host prefrontal cortex or striatum (which are normal sources of af-ferents to the nigra). Burst firing was indeed present in some of the putative dopaminergic graft neurons, but it developed slowly and retained immature features. Thus, functional afferents are likely to be established in ectopic nigral grafts, but they may be insufficient to normalize the phasic aspect of dopamine neuron function.

The failure to achieve full reconstruction of the nigrostriatal circuitry may provide an explanation for the failure to alleviate some deficits such as the aphagia and adipsia after bilateral lesions (21). A clue as to the basis of this disorder comes from observation of the similarities between nigrostriatal bundle damage on the one hand and the classic lateral hypothalamic syndrome on the other (28,49,68,69). In particular, the aphagia and adipsia that follows both types of lesions is most plausibly interpreted in terms of the two lesions producing serial damage at different levels of a connected system, specifically that involving the relay of hypothalamic information on the animal's homeostatic status via the substantia nigra to striatal centers involved in the selection and initiation of appropriate regulatory behaviors (29,77). Although the homeostatic afferents to the substantia nigra may remain after nigrostriatal lesion, that information will not reach ectopic nigral grafts located in the neostriatum itself.

ALTERNATIVE TRANSPLANTATION STRATEGIES

These various considerations raise the question whether it may be possible to modify or improve the transplantation approach to obtain more complete reconstruction of the nigrostriatal circuitry in the rat PD model. Several alternative strategies are being explored with this goal in mind. These include the use of (1) neonatal hosts to provide an environment that may promote more extensive graft–host interactions and be more permissive of long-distance axon growth and connectivity; (2)

homotopic transplantation into the substantia nigra itself; (3) co-grafts to provide a growth-promoting bridge between a nigral graft and its remote striatal targets; and (4) xenograft donor tissues with a greater growth capacity than embryonic rat neurons.

Grafting in Neonatal Hosts

One alternative approach to promoting functional integration of nigral grafts was suggested by Schwarz and Freed (64) in the context of further attempts to achieve recovery from the regulatory eating and drinking deficits induced by bilateral nigrostriatal lesions. A variety of anatomic studies have suggested that embryonic tissues implanted into the developing brain survive better and yield improved graft–host connectivity than when implanted into mature hosts (35,40,45,66,80). Schwarz and Freed, therefore, implanted nigral grafts not into the lesioned adult brain, but into the brain of neonatal rat pups. In this environment,

the grafts do indeed survive well, but they develop a more diffuse organization and the grafted dopamine cells are typically seen to migrate and become scattered within the host neostriatum rather than being restricted to a discrete graft cluster (1,57). The neonatal grafted animals are then subsequently given bilateral 6-OHDA lesions when they reach maturity; Schwarz and Freed (64) reported that 30% to 40% of the animals did not manifest the full aphagia/adipsia syndrome, but spontaneously resumed eating and maintained themselves without special care. We have replicated the protection provided by neonatal implantation of nigral grafts (Fig. 3), and demonstrated that the recovery of the neonatally grafted animals is not secondary to any protection provided by disturbance of the developing intrinsic dopamine system of the host brain (57).

Schwarz and Freed (64) interpreted these data as suggesting that fetal nigral grafts implanted at an early stage of development may become more fully incorporated into the host neostriatal circuitry than when the

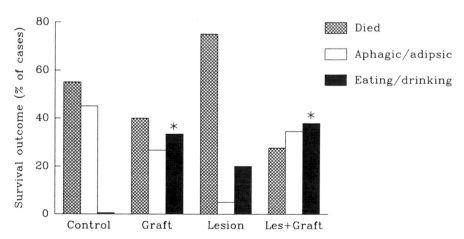

FIG. 3. Nigral grafts implanted into neonatal animals provide partial protection from the severe regulatory deficits induced by bilateral 6-OHDA lesions in adulthood. During the first week of life, the four groups of animals received either bilateral intracerebroventricular injections, nigrostriatal lesions, and/or bilateral nigral grafts. Whereas most neonatal lesion and control rats were either profoundly aphagic and adipsic or died after the adult lesion, approximately one third of the rats with neonatal grafts showed good recovery (whether or not they had also received neonatal lesions) and were able to eat and drink spontaneously. Data from Rogers and Dunnett (57).

grafts are implanted into the mature neostriatum. In consideration of the circuitries involved in the maintenance of food and water intake (see above), it seems possible that those cases in which the neonatal nigral grafts were successful in protecting from the regulatory effects of adult bilateral 6-OHDA lesions were the ones where the grafts had received hypothalamic afferents. In fact, the neonatal grafts were seen to be effective only when placed in the posterior ventral neostriatum, that is, in a site close to the lateral hypothalamus (58). More direct evidence, comparing the patterns of afferent connections of grafts in neonatal and adult hosts, is under investigation using neuroanatomic tracing techniques.

Studies to attempt reversal of the paw-reaching deficits have been less successful. Following a similar experimental design to the Schwarz and Freed study, nigral grafts were implanted unilaterally into the neostriatum of neonatal rats and the animals were allowed to grow to maturity before a subsequent ipsilateral nigrostriatal lesion made in adulthood. The grafted rats showed as great an impairment in accurate reaching with the contralateral paw as rats receiving implants in the conventional sequence into the lesioned adult striatum (3,4). Consequently, it is not yet established whether the functional benefit conferred by the neonatal implantation of nigral grafts observed in the protection from aphagia and adipsia is a general feature of neonatal grafts or is a phenomenon restricted to the particular anatomic organization and prophylactic response involved in specific regulatory functions.

Transplantation into the Substantia Nigra in Adult and Neonatal Hosts

The substantia nigra itself may be a most interesting transplantation site for two reasons: First, nigral neurons implanted in their normal location may be able to interact with regulatory afferent inputs not available to them in other ectopic locations. Second, experimental pharmacologic studies in rats have provided evidence that dopamine released (probably from dendrites) within the substantia nigra plays an important role in the regulation of striatal motor functions (see ref. 56, for a recent review).

In a first attempt to transplant nigral cell suspensions to the substantia nigra region in 6-OHDA-lesioned rats (12,26), we observed that the dopamine neurons survived but that they did not grow any axons toward the denervated striatum, and no functional effects were observed on either amphetamine-induced turning or sensorimotor orientation. We have made a more detailed study of nigra-to-nigra transplants in both adult and neonatal 6-OHDA-lesioned rats using the microtransplantation approach (ref. 53, and Nikkhah et al., in preparation). Multiple small grafts (about 25,000 cells in 0.2 μl each) were implanted in adult 6-OHDA-lesioned rats at four to eight sites within the lesioned nigra using a microcapillary to minimize tissue damage. Tyrosine hydroxylase (TH) immunohistochemistry has shown that the implanted dopamine neurons survive and become well integrated with the surrounding host tissue (particularly within the pars reticulata) (Fig. 4). The survival rate of the implanted neurons, however, was clearly much lower (in the order of 10%–20%) compared to grafts placed within the caudate–putamen, and no directed TH-positive axonal outgrowth could be detected, either locally or along the nigrostriatal pathway. The TH-positive dopamine neurons occurred in two locations: clustered within the small, circumscribed graft deposits, and scattered within the pars reticulata of the host substantia nigra. Tyrosine hydroxylase-positive fibers with a dendritic morphology were seen to extend to form patches of TH-positive terminal networks in the adjacent parts of the pars reticulata.

The functional analysis revealed a marked graft-induced effect on dopamine receptor agonist-induced turning, both after apomor-

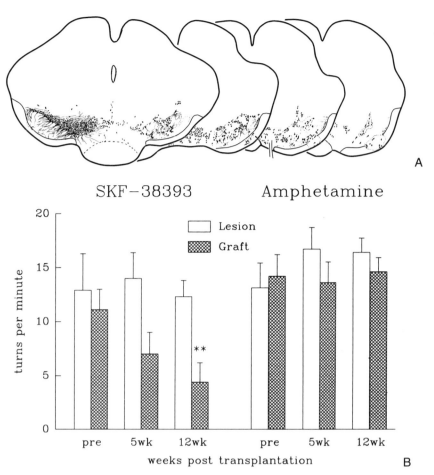

FIG. 4. E14 fetal nigral suspension grafts implanted with a microtransplantation procedure into the substantia nigra region of adult 6-OHDA-lesioned rats. **A**: Distribution of tyrosine hydroxylase-positive grafted neurons illustrated in camera lucida drawings of four coronal sections through the lesioned substantia nigra. Eight 200-nl graft deposits were made with a 50-μm glass capillary into the rostral and caudal substantia nigra. **B**: Effect of 6-OHDA lesion and grafts on D1 receptor agonist (SKF 38393; 2 mg/kg)-induced rotation (*left*) and on amphetamine (5 mg/kg)-induced rotation (*right*). Asterisks indicate significant reduction of D1 agonist-induced rotation. Data from Nikkhah et al. (53).

phine and after selective, D1 and D2 agonists (Fig. 4). The turning behavior induced by amphetamine (which is substantially reduced by intrastriatal nigral grafts) was unaffected. Likewise, there was no clear-cut effect on paw-reaching in these rats.

In the studies in neonatal rats, two 0.3-μl deposits of nigral cell suspension were implanted unilaterally into the substantia nigra in 3-day-old rat pups that had received a bilateral 6-OHDA lesion 2 days earlier

(110 μg into the lateral ventricle, bilaterally). The survival and growth of the implanted nigral neurons was strikingly different from that seen in the adult substantia nigra. Substantial numbers of TH-positive neurons survived, and they gave rise to a TH-positive terminal network that extended throughout large areas of the ipsilateral caudate–putamen. The transplant origin of this newly formed TH innervation was confirmed by backlabeling with a ret-

rograde tracer (Fluoro-Gold) from the striatum.

The functional effects of the neonatal nigra-to-nigra transplants were clearly more extensive than those seen after grafting to the nigra in adult recipients (Fig. 5). Marked effects were seen on both spontaneous and stress-induced rotation, as well as on amphetamine- and apomorphine-induced rotation. These rats also displayed a significant spontaneous locomotor hyperactivity compared to both the intact and 6-OHDA-lesioned controls. These effects resemble those seen after grafting to the striatum in neonatal rats (1,3), which suggests that the behavioral changes are likely to be mediated by dopamine release from the axons innervating the striatum. However, in contrast to previous neonatal graft studies using ectopic intrastriatal graft placements (see above), an improvement also was obtained in contralateral forelimb

use. This effect, however, seemed to be less pronounced than that obtained with extensive intrastriatal nigral grafts in adult rats in the study of Nikkhah et al. (55) (see above), and it was evident only in the final part of the paw-reaching test when only one side of the staircase was baited.

Long-Distance Axon Growth Using Tissue Bridges as Conduits

Previous studies have established that the Schwann cells of peripheral nerves, unlike the glia in the CNS, can provide a good milieu for the growth of regenerating central as well as peripheral axons over relatively long distances. This is well demonstrated in the studies of Aguayo and colleagues using pieces of sciatic nerve to promote axon growth, such as from axotomized retinal ganglion neurons or across

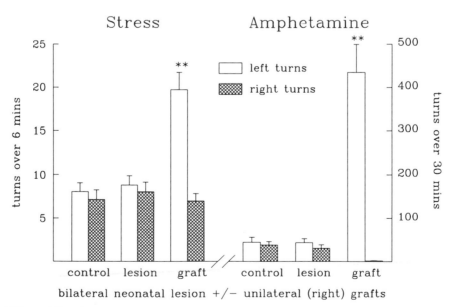

FIG. 5. Effect of E14 fetal nigral grafts implanted into the right substantia nigra region on postnatal day 3 in rats that had received bilateral intraventricular injections of 6-OHDA (110 μg total) on day 1. Stress-induced rotation (tail-pinch) and amphetamine-induced rotation (2 mg/kg, i.p.). The grafted rats turn actively in the direction contralateral (left turns) to the grafted side. Asterisks indicate significant graft-induced effects (p <0.001) . Unpublished data from Nikkhah et al.

a lesion in the spinal cord (8,19; see also chapter by Rasminsky et al. [*this volume*]). The peripheral nerve implant provides a channel (or "bridge") that will stimulate and direct growth of CNS axons to span the lesioned area and reconnect with the denervated target. This strategy provided the basis for a first attempt to induce long-distance growth from nigral graft axons to reconnect to their distant targets. In these experiments, a nigral graft was implanted over the dorsal tectum, and a 2- to 3-cm piece of autologous sciatic nerve was used as a bridge to connect the nigral graft via a track overlying the cortex to the neostriatum in the forebrain (5,37) (Fig. 6A). In this configuration, the peripheral nerve graft can stimulate dopaminergic fibers to grow from the nigral graft all the way along the full length of the bridge co-graft to reach the distant neostriatum. On reaching the far end of the bridge graft, the dopaminergic axons were seen to sprout short distances into the denervated host striatum. Inside the CNS environment, however, further growth was quite limited. Nevertheless, this level of structural reconnection was sufficient to yield some functional effects, at least in the alleviation of the sensitive amphetamine-induced rotation response (37).

This co-graft model provides a first demonstration of the feasibility of the bridge approach, but it is not ideal for practical purposes. First, it involves laying a piece of peripheral nerve over the surface of the brain with one end joined to the fetal nigral graft, so that the required distance for regeneration is relatively great. Second, the nigral graft is placed on the superficial surface of the brain stem, rather than in its natural location, in the depth of the mesencephalon, which would be more appropriate for the reformation of reciprocal host–graft connections. We have therefore used an alternative approach to attempt nigrostriatal reconstruction using a direct intracerebral bridge graft (32). Animals with unilateral 6-OHDA lesions first received nigral graft suspensions implanted conven-

tionally into the substantia nigra. These grafts survived well, but (as previously) by themselves had no influence on the amphetamine-induced rotation of the host animals. Then, tissue meant to serve as intracerebral bridges was implanted via an oblique approach through the frontal pole to lay a straight track between the substantia nigra and the neostriatum of the host brain (Fig. 6B). Of the alternative tissues that were tested in this experiment, only one (fetal striatal tissue) provided an efficient substrate for growth of dopamine axons from the nigral grafts toward the striatal targets (32). A dopaminergic reinnervation of the striatum sufficient to reduce amphetamine-induced rotation was achieved in approximately half of the nigral graft/striatal bridge group, but took a full 6 months to develop, which was four to six times longer than the time required for a similar degree of recovery after direct striatal implantation.

These bridge graft experiments demonstrate that long-distance growth of nigrostriatal connections is a feasible goal. Nevertheless, with the present techniques the procedure is still unreliable and inefficient, so that none of these models have yet been tested on any of the more complex behavioral tests. The co-graft approach clearly needs further improvement and refinement if it is going to be useful. In particular, fetal striatal cells are probably not the best substrate because most dopaminergic axons terminated on striatal neurons within the co-grafts rather than extending through that receptive environment to reinnervate the target striatum. The peripheral nerve grafts appear to be more efficient at sustaining long-distance axon growth. It would therefore be natural to expect that oblique nigrostriatal injection of Schwann cell suspensions might be a better choice. However, preliminary experiments along this line indicate that grafted Schwann cells migrate from the injection track and no longer provide an effective bridge for nigral graft axon elongation (Fawcett and Dun-

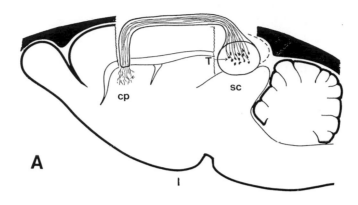

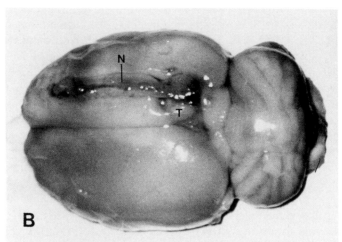

FIG. 6. A: Schematic illustration of the bridge experiment, when a piece of sciatic nerve is placed to connect a solid fetal nigral graft (*T*), placed on the dorsal surface of the superior colliculus (*sc*), over the cortex into the denervated caudate–putamen (*cp*) in a 6-OHDA-lesioned rat. Tyrosine hydroxylase-positive axons could be traced along the nerve graft into the host striatum. **B**: Dorsal view of a grafted brain, showing the fetal nigral transplant, (*T*) connected to the nerve bridge (*N*), which extends over the cortical surface. Rostrally, the nerve turns ventrally through the cortex and the corpus callosum into the caudate–putamen as indicated in B. **C**: In some of the grafted rats there was a significant reduction in amphetamine-induced rotation, which was partially abolished after cutting the nerve graft. Data from Gage et al. (38).

nett, unpublished observations). An active search is underway for potential sources of neurons, glia, nonneural cells, or other growth substrates, that can provide effective conduits for directing and stimulating long-distance growth of developing axons from nigral and other tissue grafts within the CNS environment.

Long-Distance Axon Growth from Intranigral Xenografts

With CNS tissue obtained from rat (or mouse) embryos, extensive reinnervation of a previously denervated region requires that the transplant is placed within, or very close to, the target area (11,12,66,78,79).

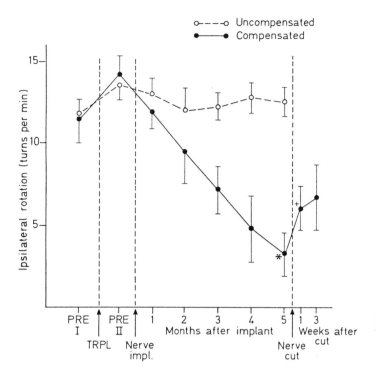

As discussed earlier, fetal rat dopamine neurons can exhibit directed axonal growth toward the denervated caudate–putamen if they are placed less than 1 mm from the striatal border (11,12). Implants placed along the trajectory of the nigrostriatal pathway, or close to the substantia nigra itself, have failed to show any long, directed axon growth toward the striatum.

Neuroblasts taken from the developing brain of early (6–9 weeks old) human embryos have a considerably greater growth capacity when implanted into the lesioned rat brain. This most probably reflects the fact that the human CNS neurons have a much more protracted developmental growth period, and that they have the capacity to grow over much greater distances. For example, the nigrostriatal pathway in humans is about 3 to 4 cm, compared to about 4 to 6 mm in the rat. In a first series of experiments (71), cell suspensions of dissociated striatal primordia from 6- to 8-week old embryos were implanted into the ibotenic acid-lesioned caudate–putamen of immunosuppressed adult rats. Immunohistochemistry, performed 12 to 25 weeks after implantation, showed that the graft-derived axons (visualized with a species-specific antibody specifically recognizing human, but not rat, intermediary neurofilaments) had grown along the internal capsule and the cerebral peduncle to reach the globus pallidus, substantia nigra, and the pontine nuclei (8–10 mm from the graft), and some fibers had extended as far as the cervical spinal cord (about 20 mm from the graft). Graft-derived axons also extended within the corpus callosum to reach large areas of the cerebral cortex on both sides.

As a follow-up of this work, Wictorin et al. (72) implanted human mesencephalic neuroblasts from donors of similar age (containing the developing dopaminergic neurons of the substantia nigra and the ventral tegmental area) at different points along the trajectory of the nigrostriatal dopamine system. As illustrated in Figure 7, the graft-

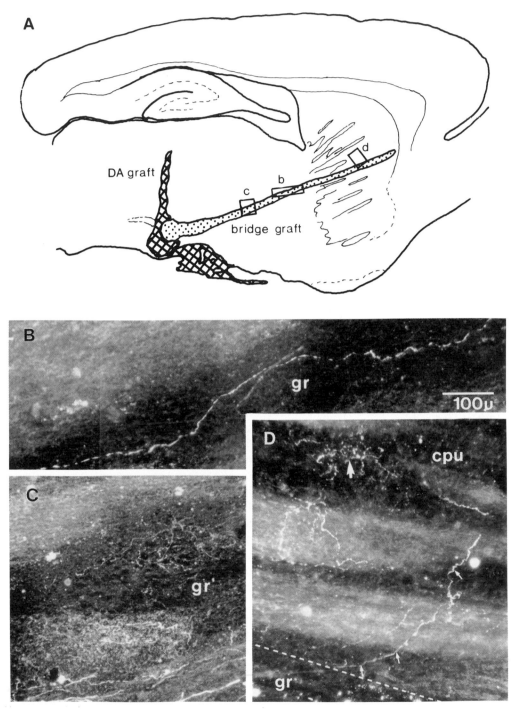

FIG. 7. Camera lucida drawing (**A**) of the intracerebral nigrostriatal bridge experiments, in which a nigral suspension graft (*cross hatch*) is implanted in the substantia nigra in combination with a nigrostriatal bridge graft of striatal tissue (*dotted*). Tyrosine hydroxylase staining showed long fibers derived from the nigral graft running through the bridge graft (**B**), and forming terminal fiber clusters both within the bridge (**C**) and within the host neostriatum (*arrow*) (**D**). gr, bridge graft; cpu, host caudate–putamen. Data from Dunnett et al. (32).

derived axons (visualized with human neurofilament (HNF)-specific antibodies) were seen to extend in large numbers rostrally along the medial forebrain bundle and the internal capsule and ramify within the caudate–putamen, the ventral striatum, and the amygdaloid nuclei (a distance of about 5–6 mm), and more sparsely in the frontal cortex and the olfactory bulb (a distance of about 10 mm). Tyrosine hydroxylase immunohistochemistry revealed that the vast majority of the rostrally projecting HNF-positive axons were also TH positive, and that the graft-derived axons gave rise to dense TH-positive terminal networks in, for example, large areas of the previously denervated caudate–putamen. The outgrowth pattern of the human nigral neuroblasts was remarkable in several ways: The axons grew over large distances (up to about 10 mm); they elongated along major myelinated fiber tracts to form prominent ascending fiber pathways; they followed to a large extent those pathways (i.e., the medial forebrain bundle and the internal capsule) that are the normal trajectories of the nigrostriatal and mesolimbocortical pathways; they exhibited a remarkable directional specificity in that they grew preferentially in the rostral direction along the fiber bundles; and their areas of termination were largely confined to those regions of the forebrain that normally are densely innervated from the ventral mesencephalon.

In intracerebral transplantation studies, a capacity to extend axons over longer distances along myelinated fiber tracts has been observed previously only in neonatal rats, that is, during the time when the intrinsic systems are still developing their axonal projections and the pathways are not yet fully myelinated (see above, and also refs. 35,40,45,67). In adult recipients, outgrowing axons from grafted rat neurons extend primarily or exclusively within the gray matter of the target territory (e.g., within the hippocampus or spinal cord) to reach more distant sites of termination. These outgrowth patterns, therefore, seem consistent with the idea that the white matter substrate is inhibitory to axonal growth in the adult CNS (33,62,63). These data also are in good agreement with other observations of axonal regeneration in the adult rat CNS, such as the extensive axonal regrowth that can occur in the serotonergic and noradrenergic projection systems after neurotoxin-induced axotomy. Also in such cases, where the lesioned axons can regrow over long distances (up to at least 10–20 mm in the spinal cord), the growth occurs exclusively within the gray matter of the target territory (9,10,75). The only instance where axons (of rat or mouse origin) have been seen to grow in large numbers along a myelinated fiber tract in the adult mammalian CNS is in the case of embryonic rat or mouse striatal grafts, implanted into the excitotoxin-lesioned striatum of adult rats (73,74). In this case, fascicles of axons have been seen to grow within and along the myelinated fiber bundles of the internal capsule to innervate synaptically the host globus pallidus neurons, a distance of about 1.5 to 2 mm, and these outgrowing axons become themselves myelinated (73).

Axonal elongation across foreign territory, along major myelinated fiber pathways, thus appears to constitute a major obstacle for successful axonal regeneration in the adult mammalian CNS. The observations of Wictorin et al. (71,72) indicate that growing human neuroblasts can escape or neutralize the nonpermissive nature of the mammalian CNS tissue environment, which normally acts to inhibit the elongation of regenerating axons along myelinated fiber tracts (62,63). Indeed, the long-distance directed axon growth exhibited by the human mesencephalic and striatal neuroblasts implies, first, that the guidance and growth-promoting mechanisms necessary for pathway formation and successful regrowth of axons toward their targets are present not only during development but also in the adult lesioned brain, and, second, that the growing human neurons possess the necessary properties to respond to these growth-promoting influences.

Functional studies on rats with human

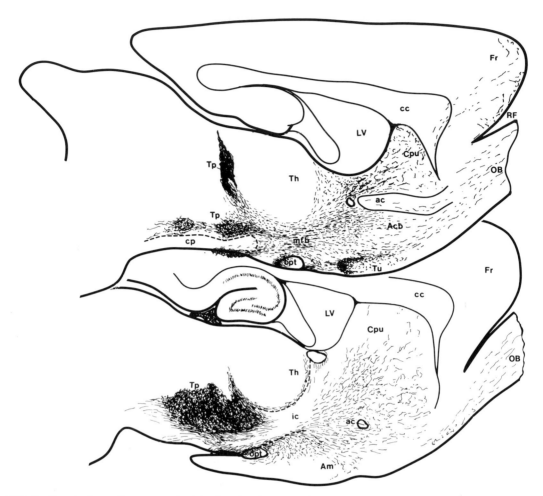

FIG. 8. Semischematic camera lucida drawing from a 6-OHDA-lesioned rat that had received a graft of human fetal ventral mesencephalic tissue into the substantia nigra region. Axonal outgrowth was revealed by immunohistochemistry using an antibody detecting human (but not rat) neurofilaments. Abundant axonal outgrowth (which was to a large extent also tyrosine hydroxylase positive) was seen along the medial forebrain bundle (*mfb*) and the internal capsule (*ic*) into striatal and limbic forebrain areas, including the caudate–putamen (*Cpu*), nc accumbens (*Acb*), amygdala (*Am*), olfactory tubercle (*Tu*), olfactory bulb (*OB*), and frontal cortex (*Fr*). *Tp,* neurofilament-positive graft tissue. From Wictorin et al. (72).

and primate nigra-to-nigra xenografts are in progress. The main problem so far has been related to the relatively poor survival of the human fetal mesencephalic cells when they are implanted into the nigral region. Indeed, in the study by Wictorin et al. (72), good graft survival was obtained only when the implantation site was prelesioned with an injection of ibotenic acid (which apparently creates a more favorable environment for the implanted cells). Nevertheless, the xenograft model may provide entirely new possibilities for the reconstruction of the nigrostriatal dopamine pathway in the rat PD model. If our assumptions are correct, human nigral grafts placed in their natural position within the substantia nigra region may be able to establish more accurate afferent and efferent functional connections with the host basal ganglia circuitry than the standard type of rat nigral transplants, which are placed within, or adjacent to, the striatal target areas. If so, the xenograft approach may offer new strategies to overcome the functional limitations inherent in the use of ectopically placed transplants.

CONCLUDING REMARKS

The initial results obtained in the clinical trials so far performed in patients with PD show that it is possible to achieve marked and sustained improvement in sensorimotor function after transplantation of dopamine-rich fetal nigral tissue into the dopamine-depleted striatum. There now seem to be sufficient data to conclude that the fetal nigra transplantation paradigm is effective in dopamine-depleted brains of affected patients also [see Lindvall (*this volume*)], but that the symptomatic improvement is only partial. In principle, these results are consistent with the experimental studies in the rat and primate PD models. In tests of more complex integrative sensorimotor behaviors, the graft-induced recovery obtained in rats and monkeys has been incomplete or on some tasks entirely absent. It is clear that there can be complete recovery on some basic functional parameters, such as drug-induced turning and simple sensorimotor orienting responses, while the animals remain impaired on other more complex measures. The reasons for these shortcomings of current transplantation procedures so far have been insufficiently explored. As discussed earlier, there are several alternative (although not necessarily mutually exclusive) explanations.

One possibility is that the functional properties of ectopically placed nigral grafts (i.e., grafts implanted into the denervated forebrain target regions) are fully sufficient, but that recovery of function will not be complete unless dopamine transmission is restored throughout the entire striatum as well as in affected nonstriatal regions, including the substantia nigra itself. It is clear that all experimental studies performed so far have resorted to partial engraftment covering parts of the caudate–putamen, or selected limbic or cortical areas. Moreover, even within the grafted area, the graft-induced recovery of dopamine levels and dopamine innervation density (typically in the range of 10%–30% in the rat experiments) is far from complete. Similarly, not even the most extensive transplantations attempted so far in patients with PD (using combined placements in caudate and putamen) have been able to restore total striatal ^{18}F-fluorodopa uptake (as assessed by positron emission tomography) back to the range seen in nonsymptomatic individuals. It remains a valid hypothesis, therefore, that more complete functional recovery will require more complete dopamine replacement. To achieve this, it will be necessary to increase the efficacy of the nigral transplants, by increasing the number of grafted neurons and by increasing their growth capacity, or by grafting into multiple striatal and nonstriatal target sites.

Alternatively, it is quite possible that ectopically placed grafts do not possess the full range of functional properties necessary for the recovery of complex integrative functions in the basal ganglia. In particular, certain critical regulatory afferent inputs may not be available to dopamine neurons located within the striatum. If so, dopamine neuron replacement may require that the grafted neurons be placed in their normal location, that is, within the substantia nigra itself, to restore both afferent and efferent connectivity. It is a challenge for future experimental studies to find ways to achieve this. The initial studies reviewed in this chapter suggest some promising lines that deserve to be pursued much more systemically in the future.

Issues raised by the ongoing clinical trials in patients with PD highlight the need for more refined analysis of nigral graft function in the rat PD model. Such studies are needed both to clarify the mechanisms underlying recovery of different components of the dopamine deficiency syndrome, as well as to define the limitations of current transplantation procedures. Used to its full capacity, the rat PD model will be a highly useful tool for this purpose.

REFERENCES

1. Abrous DN, Choulli K, Simon H, Le Moal M, Herman JP. Behavioral effects of intracerebral dopaminergic grafts after neonatal destruction of the mesencephalic dopaminergic system. *Prog Brain Res* 1990;82:481–487.
2. Abrous DN, Shaltot A, Torres EM, Dunnett SB. Dopamine-rich grafts in the neostriatum and/or nucleus accumbens: effects on drug-induced behaviours and skilled paw reaching. *Neuroscience* 1993;53:187–198.
3. Abrous DN, Wareham AT, Torres EM, Dunnett SB. Unilateral dopamine lesions in neonatal, weanling and adult rats: comparison of rotation and reaching deficits. *Behav Brain Res* 1992;51:67–75.
4. Abrous DN, Torres EM, Dunnett SB. Dopaminergic grafts implanted into the neonatal or adult striatum: comparative effects on rotation and paw reaching deficits induced by subsequent unilateral nigrostriatal lesions in adulthood. *Neuroscience* 1993;54:657–668.
5. Aguayo AJ, Björklund A, Stenevi U, Carlstedt T. Fetal mesencephalic neurones survive and extend long axons across PNS grafts inserted into the adult rat neostriatum. *Neurosci Lett* 1984;45:53–58.
6. Arbuthnott G, Dunnett SB, MacLeod N. The electrophysiological properties of single units in mesencephalic transplants in rat brain. *Neurosci Lett* 1985;57:205–210.
7. Becker JB, Robinson TE, Barton P, Sintov A, Siden R, Levy RJ. Sustained behavior recovery from unilateral nigrostriatal damage produced by the controlled release of dopamine from a silicone polymer pellet placed into the denervated striatum. *Brain Res* 1990;508:60–64.
8. Benfey M, Aguayo AJ. Extensive elongation of axons from rat brain into peripheral nerve grafts. *Nature* 1982;296:150–153.
9. Björklund A, Lindvall O. Regeneration of normal terminal innervation patterns by central noradrenergic neurons after 5,7-dihydroxytryptamine-induced axotomy in the adult rat. *Brain Res* 1979;171:271–293.
10. Björklund A, Wiklund L. Mechanisms of regrowth of the bulbospinal serotonin system following 5,6-dihydroxytryptamine induced axotomy: I. biochemical correlates. *Brain Res* 1980;191:109–127.
11. Björklund A, Dunnett SB, Stenevi U, Lewis ME, Iversen SD. Reinnervation of the denervated striatum by substantia nigra transplants: functional consequences as revealed by pharmacological and sensorimotor testing. *Brain Res* 1980;199:307–333.
12. Björklund A, Stenevi U, Schmidt RH, Dunnett SB, Gage FH. Intracerebral grafting of neuronal cell suspensions: II. survival and growth of nigral cell suspensions. *Acta Physiol Scand* 1983;(Suppl 522):9–18.
13. Björklund A, Lindvall O, Isacson O, Brundin P, Strecker RE, Dunnett SB. Mechanisms of action of intracerebral neural implants. *Trends Neurosci* 1987;10:509–516.
14. Brown V, Dunnett SB. Comparison of adrenal and foetal nigral grafts on drug-induced rotation in rats with 6-OHDA lesions. *Exp Brain Res* 1989;78:214–218.
15. Cenci MA, Kalén P, Mandel RJ, Wictorin K, Björklund A. Dopaminergic transplants normalize amphetamine- and apomorphine-induced Fos expression in the 6-hydroxydopamine-lesioned striatum. *Neuroscience* 1992;46:943–957.
16. Cenci MA, Campbell K, Björklund A. Neuropeptide-mRNA expression in the 6-hydroxydopamine-lesioned rat striatum reinnervated by fetal dopaminergic transplants: differential effects of the grafts on preproenkephalin-, preprotachychinin- and prodynorphin-mRNA levels. *Neuroscience* 1993;57:275–296.
17. Chiodo LA, Antelman SM, Caggiula AR, Lineberry CG. Sensory stimuli alter the discharge rate of dopamine (DA) neurons: evidence for two functional types of DA cells in the substantia nigra. *Brain Res* 1980;189:544–549.
18. Chritin M, Savasta M, Mennicken F, et al. Intrastriatal dopamine-rich implants reverse the increase of dopamine D_2 receptor mRNA levels caused by lesion of the nigrostriatal pathway: a quantitative in situ hybridization study. *Eur J Neurosci* 1992;4:663–672.
19. David S, Aguayo AJ. Axonal elongation into peripheral nervous system "bridges" after central nervous system injury in adult rats. *Science* 1981;214:931–933.
20. Doucet G, Brundin P, Descarries L, Björklund A. Effect of prior denervation on survival and fiber outgrowth from intrastriatal fetal mesencephalic grafts. *Eur J Neurosci* 1990;2:279–290.
21. Dunnett SB. Functional analysis of neural grafts in the neostriatum. In: Björklund A, Aguayo AJ, Ottoson D, eds. *Brain repair.* London: Macmillan; 1990:355–373.
22. Dunnett SB, Björklund A. Mechanisms of function of neural grafts in the adult mammalian brain. *J Exp Biol* 1987:132:263–289.
23. Dunnett SB, Björklund A, Stenevi U, Iversen SD. Behavioural recovery following transplantation of substantia nigra in rats subjected to 6-OHDA lesions of the nigrostriatal pathway: I. unilateral lesions. *Brain Res* 1981;215:147–161.
24. Dunnett SB, Björklund A, Stenevi U, Iversen SD. Grafts of embryonic substantia nigra reinnervating the ventrolateral striatum ameliorate sensorimotor impairments and akinesia in rats with 6-OHDA lesions of the nigrostriatal pathway. *Brain Res* 1981;229:209–217.
25. Dunnett SB, Björklund A, Stenevi U, Iversen

SD. Behavioural recovery following transplantation of substantia nigra in rats subjected to 6-OHDA lesions of the nigrostriatal pathway: II. bilateral lesions. *Brain Res* 1981;229:457–470.

26. Dunnett SB, Björklund A, Schmidt RH, Stenevi U, Iversen SD. Intracerebral grafting of neuronal cell suspensions: IV. behavioural recovery in rats with unilateral implants of nigral cell suspensions in different forebrain sites. *Acta Physiol Scand* 1983;(Suppl 522):29–37.

27. Dunnett SB, Björklund A, Schmidt RH, Stenevi U, Iversen SD. Intracerebral grafting of neuronal cell suspensions: V. behavioural recovery in rats with bilateral 6-OHDA lesions following implantation of nigral cell suspensions. *Acta Physiol Scand* 1983;(Suppl 522):39–46.

28. Dunnett SB, Lane D, Winn P. Ibotenic acid lesions of the lateral hypothalamus: comparison with 6-hydroxydopamine-induced sensorimotor deficits. *Neuroscience* 1985;14:509–518.

29. Dunnett SB, Robbins TW. The functional role of mesotelencephalic dopamine systems. *Biol Rev* 1992;67:419–518.

30. Dunnett SB, Whishaw IQ, Jones GH, Isacson O. Effects of dopamine-rich grafts on conditioned rotation in rats with unilateral 6-OHDA lesions. *Neurosci Lett* 1986;68:127–133.

31. Dunnett SB, Whishaw IQ, Rogers DC, Jones GH. Dopamine-rich grafts ameliorate whole body motor asymmetry and sensory neglect but not independent skilled limb use in rats with 6-hydroxydopamine lesions. *Brain Res* 1987;415:63–78.

32. Dunnett SB, Rogers DC, Richards SJ. Reconstruction of the nigrostriatal pathway after 6-OHDA lesions by combination of dopamine-rich nigral grafts and nigrostriatal "bridge" grafts. *Exp Brain Res* 1989;75:523–535.

33. Fawcett JW. Factors responsible for the failure of structural repair in the central nervous system. In: Hunter AJ, Clark M, eds. *Neurodegeneration*. London: Academic Press; 1992:81–96.

34. Fisher LJ, Young SJ, Tepper JM, Groves PM, Gage FH. Electrophysiological characteristics of cells within mesencephalon suspension grafts. *Neuroscience* 1991;40:109–122.

35. Floeter MK, Jones EJ. Connections made by transplants to the cerebral cortex of rat brains damaged in utero. *J Neurosci* 4:141–150.

36. Freed WJ. Functional brain tissue transplantation: reversal of lesion-induced rotation by intraventricular substantia nigra and adrenal medulla grafts, with a note on intracranial retinal grafts. *Biol Psychiatry* 1983;18:1205–1267.

37. Gage FH, Stenevi U, Carlstedt T, Foster G, Björklund A, Aguayo AJ. Anatomical and functional consequences of grafting mesencephalic neurons into a peripheral nerve "bridge" connected to the denervated striatum. *Exp Brain Res* 1985;60:584–589.

38. Gage FH, Stenevi U, Carlstedt T, Foster G, Björklund A, Aguayo AJ. Anatomical and functional consequences of grafting mesencephalic neurons into a peripheral nerve 'bridge' connected to the denervated striatum. *Exp Brain Res* 1985;60:584–589.

39. Grace AA. Phasic versus tonic dopamine release and the modulation of dopamine system responsitivity: a hypothesis for the etiology of schizophrenia. *Neuroscience* 1991;41:1–24.

40. Hankin MH, Lund RD. Role of the target in directing the outgrowth of retinal axons: transplants reveal surface-related and surface-independent cues. *J Comp Neurol* 1987;263:455–466.

41. Herman JP, Abrous N, Le Moal M. Anatomical and behavioral comparison of unilateral dopamine-rich grafts implanted into the striatum of neonatal and adult rats. *Neuroscience* 1991;40:465–475.

42. Herman JP, Choulli K, Geffard D, Nadaud D, Taghzouti K, Le Moal M. Reinnervation of the nucleus accumbens and frontal cortex of the rat by dopaminergic grafts and effects on hoarding behavior. *Brain Res* 1986;372:210–216.

43. Herman JP, Choulli K, Abrous N, Dullac J, Le Moal M. Effects of intra-accumbens dopaminergic grafts on behavioral deficits induced by 6-OHDA lesions of the nucleus accumbens or A10 dopaminergic neurons: a comparison. *Behav Brain Res* 1988;29:73–83.

44. Ljungberg T, Ungerstedt U. Reinstatement of eating by dopamine agonists in aphagic dopamine denervated rats. *Physiol Behav* 1976;16:277–283.

45. Lund RD, Radel JD, Hankin MH, Klassen H, Coffey PJ, Rawlins JNP. Developmental and functional integrations of retinal transplants with host rat brains. In: Björklund A, Aguayo AJ, Ottoson D, eds. *Brain repair*. London: Mcmillan; 1990:327–340.

46. Mandel R, Brundin P, Björklund A. The importance of graft placement and task complexity for transplant-induced recovery of simple and complex sensorimotor deficits in dopamine denervated rats. *Eur J Neurosci* 1990;2:888–894.

47. Marier M, Abrous DN, Feuerstein C, Le Moal M, Herman JP. Lesion of the nigrostriatal dopaminergic pathway in adult rats and reversal following the implantation of embryonic dopaminergic neurons: a quantitative immunohistochemistry analysis. *Neuroscience* 1991;42:427–439.

48. Marshall JF, Gotthelf T. Sensory inattention in rats with 6-hydroxydopamine-induced lesions of ascending dopaminergic neurons: apomorphine-induced reversal of deficits. *Exp Neurol* 1979;65:389–411.

49. Marshall JF, Richardson JS, Teitelbaum P. Nigrostriatal bundle damage and the lateral hypothalamic syndrome. *J Comp Physiol Psychol* 1974;87:808–830.

50. Montoya CP, Astell S, Dunnett SB. Effects of nigral and striatal grafts on skilled forelimb use in the rat. *Prog Brain Res* 1990;82:459–466.

51. Montoya CP, Campbell-Hope LJ, Pemberton KD, Dunnett SB. The "staircase" test: a measure of independent forelimb reaching and

grasping abilities in rats. *J Neurosci Methods* 1991;36:219–228.

52. Nieoullon A, Cheramy A, Glowinski J. Nigral and striatal dopamine release under sensory stimuli. *Nature* 1977;269:340–342.
53. Nikkhah G, Bentlage C, Cunningham MG, Björklund A. Intranigral fetal dopamine grafts induce behavioral compensation in the rat Parkinson model. *J Neuro Sci* 1994 (*in press*).
54. Nikkhah G, Cunningham MG, Jödicke A, Knappe U, Björklund A. Improved graft survival and striatal reinnervation by microtransplantation of fetal nigral cell suspensions in the rat Parkinson model. *Brain Res* 1994;633: 133–143.
55. Nikkhah G, Duan WM, Knappe U, Jödicke A, Björklund A. Restoration of complex sensorimotor behavior and skilled forelimb use by a modified nigral cell suspension transplantation approach in the rat Parkinson model. *Neuroscience* 1993;56:33–43.
56. Robertson HA. Dopamine receptor interactions: some implications for the treatment of Parkinson's disease. *Trends Neurosci* 1992;15:201–206.
57. Rogers DC, Dunnett SB. Neonatal dopamine-rich grafts and 6-OHDA lesions independently provide partial protection from the adult nigrostriatal lesion syndrome. *Behav Brain Res* 1989;34:131–146.
58. Rogers DC, Martel FL, Dunnett SB. Nigral grafts in neonatal rats protect from aphagia induced by subsequent adult 6-OHDA lesions: the importance of striatal location. *Exp Brain Res* 1990;80:172–176.
59. Savasta M, Mennicken F, Chritin M, et al. Intrastriatal dopamine-rich implants reverse the changes in dopamine D_2 receptor densities caused by 6-hydroxydopamine lesion of the nigrostriatal pathway in rats: an autoradiographic study. *Neuroscience* 1992;46:729–738.
60. Schallert T, Hall S. 'Disengage' sensorimotor deficit following apparent recovery from unilateral dopamine depletion. *Behav Brain Res* 1988;30:15–24.
61. Schmidt RH, Björklund A, Stenevi U, Dunnett SB, Gage FH. Intracerebral grafting of neuronal cell suspensions: III. activity of intrastriatal nigral suspension implants as assessed by measurements of dopamine synthesis and metabolism. *Acta Physiol Scand* 1983;(Suppl 522): 19–28.
62. Schnell L, Schwab ME. Axonal regeneration in the rat spinal cord produced an antibody against myelin-associated neurite growth inhibitors. *Nature* 1990;343:269–272.
63. Schwab ME. Myelin-associated inhibitors of neurite growth and regeneration in the CNS. *Trends Neurosci* 1990;13:452–455.
64. Schwarz SS, Freed WJ. Brain tissue transplantation in neonatal rats prevents a lesion-induced syndrome of adipsia, aphagia and akinesia. *Exp Brain Res* 1987;65:449–454.
65. Sirinathsinghji DJS, Dunnett SB. Increased proenkephalin mRNA levels in the rat neostriatum following lesion of the ipsilateral nigrostriatal dopamine pathway with 1-methyl-4-phenylpyridinum ion (MMP$^+$): reversal by embryonic nigral dopamine grafts. *Mol Brain Res* 1991; 9:263–269.
66. Sotelo C, Alvarado-Mallart RM. Reconstruction of the defective cerebellar circuitry in adult purkinje cell degeneration mutant mice by purkinje cell replacement through transplantation of solid embryonic implants. *Neuroscience* 1987;20:1–22.
67. Stanfield BB, O'Leary DDM. Fetal occipital cortical neurones transplanted to the rostral cortex can extend and maintain a pyramidal tract axon. *Nature* 1985;313:135–136.
68. Teitelbaum P, Epstein AN. The lateral hypothalamic syndrome: recovery of feeding and drinking after lateral hypothalamic lesions. *Psychol Rev* 1962;69:74–80.
69. Ungerstedt U. Adipsia and aphagia after 6-hydroxydopamine induced degeneration of the nigrostriatal dopamine system. *Acta Physiol Scand* (Suppl)1971;367:95–122.
70. Whishaw IQ, O'Connor WT, Dunnett SB. The contributions of motor cortex, nigrostriatal dopamine and caudate–putamen to skilled forelimb use in the rat. *Brain* 1986;109:805–843.
71. Wictorin K, Brundin P, Gustavii B, Lindvall O, Björklund O. Reformation of long axon pathways in adult rat central nervous system by human forebrain neuroblasts. *Nature* 1990;347: 556–558.
72. Wictorin K, Brundin P, Sauer H, Lindvall O, Björklund A. Long distance directed axonal growth from human dopaminergic mesencephalic neuroblasts implanted along the nigrostriatal pathway in 6-hydroxydopamine lesioned adult rats. *J Comp Neurol* 1992;323:475–494
73. Wictorin K, Clarke DJ, Bolam JP, Björklund A. Fetal striatal neurons grafted into the ibotenate lesioned adult striatum: efferent projections and synaptic contacts in the host globus pallidus. *Neuroscience* 1990;37:301–315.
74. Wictorin K, Lagenauer CF, Lund RD, Björklund A. Efferent projections to the host brain from intrastriatal striatal mouse-to-rat grafts: time course and tissue-type specificity as revealed by a mouse specific neuronal marker. *Eur J Neurosci* 1991;3:86–101.
75. Wiklund L, Björklund A. Mechanisms of regrowth in the bulbospinal serotonin system following 5,6-dihydroxytryptamine induced axotomy: II. fluorescence histochemical observations. *Brain Res* 1980;191:129–160.
76. Winn SR, Wahlberg L, Tresco P, Aebischer P. An encapsulated dopamine-releasing polymer alleviates experimental parkinsonism in rats. *Exp Neurol* 1989;105:244–250.
77. Wright AK, Tulloch IF, Arbuthnott GW. Possible links between hypothalamus and substantia nigra in the rat. *Appetite* 1980;1:43–51.
78. Zhou C-F, Raisman G, Morris RJ. Specific pat-

terns of fibre outgrowth from transplants to host mice hippocampi, shown immunohistochemically by the use of allelic forms of thy-1. *Neuroscience* 1985;16:819–833.

79. Zhou C-F, Li Y, Raisman G. Embryonic entorhinal transplants project selectively to the deafferented entorhinal zone of adult mouse hippocampi, as demonstrated by the use of thy-1 allelic immunohistochemistry: effect of timing of transplantation in relation to deafferentation. *Neuroscience* 1989;32:349–362.

80. Zimmer J, Finsen B, Sörensen T, Sunde N. Hippocampal transplants: synaptic organization, their use in repair of neuronal circuits and mouse to rat xenografting. In: Althaus H, Seifert W, eds. *Glial–neuronal communication in development and regeneration.* Heidelberg: Springer-Verlag; 1987:545–563.

Functional Neural Transplantation
edited by S. B. Dunnett and A. Björklund.
Raven Press, Ltd., New York © 1994.

4

Functional Studies of Neural Grafts in Parkinsonian Primates

Lucy E. Annett

Department of Experimental Psychology, University of Cambridge, Cambridge CB2 3EB, United Kingdom

The distinct clinical improvements reported recently in patients with idiopathic (44,54, 75) and 1-methyl-4-phenyl-1,2,3,6-tetrahydropyridine (MPTP)-induced parkinsonism (87) after transplantation of embryonic dopaminergic tissue into the striatum provide considerable support for the view that neural transplantation may eventually become an option in the treatment of Parkinson's disease. At present, however, neural transplantation in the clinic is an experimental procedure. The optimal procedures for grafting have not yet been established and the degree of improvement in motor symptoms in the large number of patients worldwide who have received neural grafts has been extremely variable (ref. 53, and Lindvall [*this volume*]). Further work in animals is needed to determine which procedural factors are critical for a successful outcome. Rodent studies have been, and will continue to be, central to the development of neural transplantation techniques (Björklund et al., and Brundin [*this volume*]). The role of primate studies is to resolve those issues relevant to the clinical application of neural transplantation that cannot be addressed easily in rodents—for example, because the monkey and the human (but not the rat) neostriatum is differentiated into discrete caudate nucleus and putamen, whether grafts located at sites in one or the other of these structures alone

are sufficient to ameliorate parkinsonian symptoms (see Dunnett and Annett (32)). A particularly important reason for using primates in neural transplantion studies is to extend the range of tests used to assess the behavioral effects of grafts. Ultimately, the decision to use neural transplants therapeutically depends on evidence from animal studies that grafts produce behavioral changes that are likely to benefit patients. The complex behavioral repertoire of monkeys provides greater scope for determining the extent of the functional recovery produced by grafts.

The purpose of this chapter is to review functional studies of neural grafts in parkinsonian primates and, in particular, to focus on the nature and extent of any reported graft effects on behavior. Each section of the chapter deals with evidence relevant to one particular type of behavior or behavioral test. Thus, a single study may be discussed in several different sections if more than one method was used to assess the behavior of the monkeys in that study. This organization facilitates analysis of the quality and quantity of the evidence relating to each type of behavior. Studies of neural transplantation in parkinsonian primates have not been numerous, and those that have reported quantitative behavioral data from monkeys with grafts have been even fewer in number. Thus, it is possible to review in some detail the numbers of monkeys examined on each type of behavioral test. Indeed, such an analysis is essential because inadequate subject numbers may seriously limit the conclusions that may be drawn. By focusing on behavior in this way, this chapter complements and extends an earlier review of neural grafts in parkinsonian primates (32).

The behavioral tests used in primate neural transplantation studies have necessarily depended on the lesion model employed and, in particular, on whether the lesion was bilateral or unilateral. The preferred method of producing bilateral dopaminergic lesions has been the systemic administration of MPTP either by intravenous or intramuscular injection. The principal advantage of this type of lesion is that the associated behavioral syndrome closely resembles the symptoms experienced by patients with Parkinson's disease (21). The capacity of neural grafts to ameliorate the syndrome, and by analogy parkinsonian symptoms, can therefore be assessed directly. The disadvantages of using bilateral MPTP-induced lesions have been discussed in Dunnett and Annett (32). In brief, if the dopamine depletion is not extensive, considerable spontaneous recovery may occur, which confounds the interpretation of any recovery that may be observed in monkeys with grafts (37,51). On the other hand, if the dopamine depletion is relatively complete, the monkeys may die or be profoundly debilitated. The inability or lack of motivation of monkeys with bilateral MPTP lesions to perform tasks on which they were trained before the lesion has been a problem in some neural transplantation studies (45,78). Tasks designed to reveal residual deficits in otherwise asymptomatic monkeys may avoid this problem, but as yet such tasks have not been widely used (78). The principal methods used to assess the behavior of monkeys with bilateral MPTP lesions and neural grafts have therefore been observer evaluation of parkinsonian symptoms by rating scales or scoring of sponta-

neous behaviors or activity levels in the home cage.

An alternative method of using MPTP to produce dopaminergic lesions, which was developed by Bankiewicz and colleagues (11) and has been used in a number of neural graft studies (14–17,62), is infusion of the toxin unilaterally into one internal carotid artery. Because the half-life of MPTP is short, the lesion is restricted to the hemisphere on the side of the infusion and the motor impairments appear primarily on the contralateral side of the body. Unilateral injections of MPTP directly into the substantia nigra also have been used to induce hemiparkinsonian in one primate neural graft study (31). A major advantage of these unilateral models is that the monkeys remain healthy and are able to feed and maintain themselves. The behavioral tests that are possible with hemiparkinsonian monkeys differ from those used in the case of monkeys with bilateral lesions. Thus, side biases and rotation can be quantified and performance with the affected contralateral limb compared to that of the ipsilateral limb. However, just as with bilateral MPTP lesions, some spontaneous recovery may occur over a period of several weeks (51). Although some degree of hemiparkinsonism is common in patients with Parkinson's disease, unilateral neurotoxic lesions in monkeys do not closely model this condition because the imbalance in dopamine function between the two sides is far greater than is ever likely to be the case in patients. A recent study has described a two-stage lesion approach in which an initial infusion of MPTP into one carotid artery to induce hemiparkinsonism was followed several months later by a second infusion of MPTP into the other carotid artery to induce bilateral parkinsonism (74). This approach combines the advantages of the carotid route of administration, which is less debilitating for the monkeys than the systemic route, and the bilateral lesion model, which more closely resembles Parkinson's disease. The behavioral deficits produced by the two-stage lesion appeared to be relatively stable, but the technique has not yet been used in neural graft studies.

A third method of producing dopaminergic lesions that has been used in functional studies of neural transplantation in parkinsonian primates is the stereotaxic injection of 6-hydroxydopamine (6-OHDA) unilaterally into the substantia nigra or ascending nigrostriatal pathway (2,4,27,28,32). Because spontaneous behavioral recovery is apparently less of a problem in rats with 6-OHDA lesions than in monkeys with MPTP lesions, we decided to examine the stability of the behavioral deficits in marmosets with unilateral 6-OHDA lesions to see whether this type of lesion might provide a suitable model for assessing dopaminergic graft function in primates (7). Deficits were observed that persisted for at least 6 months in a group of lesioned marmosets compared with sham lesioned controls; however, the extent of the deficits varied considerably between individual animals in different behavioral tests. The extent of the dopamine depletion rather than the type of toxin (MPTP or 6-OHDA) used to produce the lesion may be the most important factor determining the probability of spontaneous recovery (7). Behavioral variability between monkeys therefore needs to be taken into account in neural graft studies using either toxin. Ideally, all studies should include adequate numbers of subjects to allow for behavioral variability and should compare the behavior of monkeys with grafts with that of lesion controls matched with respect to behavioral scores before grafting. A period of at least 2 months between lesion and graft is also desirable to allow sufficient time for most of the spontaneous recovery to occur (51). Unfortunately, very few primate neural transplantation studies have implemented these controls, no doubt because of the difficulty and expense of working with monkeys.

The donor tissue used in most neural transplantation studies in parkinsonian primates has been either ventral mesencephalon derived from embryos/fetuses of the same species as the host, or adrenal medulla derived either from the host (autograft) or from another adult of the same species (allograft). Survival of catecholamine-rich chromaffin cells in grafts of adrenal medulla in monkeys generally has been poor, and survival of embryonic/fetal dopaminergic neurons in grafts of ventral mesencephalon variable, possibly because of factors such as the exact age of the donor tissue used (see Dunnett and Annett (32)). Comparison of the behavioral effects of different types of tissue grafts (i.e., dopaminergic and nondopaminergic) in monkeys has stimulated debate about the mechanisms of graft action in animal models of Parkinson's disease. The question of mechanisms is therefore considered in a separate section of this review. However, comparisons between different types of grafts have rarely been made within a single study, or even within a paradigm. Many technical differences complicate comparisons between studies—for example, whether the tissue was transplanted using stereotaxic or open cavitation surgery, the location of the grafts in the striatum, and the lesion model and hence the behavioral tests used. Nevertheless, this chapter aims to determine whether any general principles emerge from a review of this somewhat disparate literature.

OBSERVER EVALUATION OF PARKINSONIAN SYMPTOMS

Transplantation of adrenal medulla and fetal nigral tissue into the striatum of monkeys was first reported in 1984 (59). No behavioral tests were conducted in this first study, and although some adrenal tissue survived, dopamine cells in the nigral grafts did not. This report was soon followed by studies in which the behavior of monkeys with more successful neural grafts was assessed. The obvious starting point for these initial behavioral studies was the parkinsonian syndrome produced by the systemic administration of MPTP.

Nigral Grafts

Among the earliest studies of nigral graft function in primates were those of Bakay and colleagues in which three rhesus monkeys, previously treated systemically with MPTP, received cell suspension grafts placed bilaterally at three sites in the caudate nucleus (8,9,41). The cell suspension was prepared from the ventral mesencephalon of 35- to 37-day, 15- to 16-mm crown–rump length (CRL) embryos. The functional measures used to assess these monkeys were described in most detail in Bakay et al (8). A scale from 0 to 4 was used to rate the parkinsonian symptoms "hypokinesia," "rigidity," "flexed posture," and "tremor," whereas the occurrence of, or time spent in, behaviors such as "up in cage," "crossover," and "active behavior" were scored from 6-hour videotapes of spontaneous behavior in the home cage. All three monkeys were described as showing functional improvement during the 2 months after transplantation and before sacrifice. The parkinsonian symptoms, which had been scored at level 2 or 3 after MPTP treatment (except for tremor, which was observed only for a short period in one animal), were reduced to 1 or 0 in two of the monkeys. However, in the third case, flexed posture remained at level 3, whereas hypokinesia and rigidity were reduced to level 2 only. The changes in spontaneous behaviors scored from the videotapes were harder to interpret because in several instances the MPTP treatment did not produce clear deficits. In one monkey, "active behavior" was substantially reduced by MPTP; however, this behavior was not restored to pre-MPTP baseline levels by the grafts. The numbers of catecholaminergic cells that survived transplantation were estimated at between 300 and 600 cells in the two monkeys whose clinical rating scales improved. In addition, dopamine and L-dopa levels in the CSF of these two animals increased posttransplantation. It is not possible to draw any firm conclusions about the functional capacities of these grafts from such a limited number of animals, especially without data from lesion-alone animals for comparison. Although additional monkeys were treated with MPTP that did not receive grafts, and one monkey that was not treated with MPTP did receive grafts, quantitative behavioral data for these animals were not presented. A further problem with this study, acknowledged by the authors, is the relatively short time period of only 2 months allowed for the behavioral observations. In several subsequent studies reviewed later, the behavioral changes produced by nigral grafts did not become fully apparent until at least 3 months after transplantation surgery.

An initial report of another early study of nigral grafts in primates by Redmond, Sladek, and colleagues, described three African green monkeys made parkinsonian with MPTP (63). Two of these monkeys received grafts of fetal nigra into the caudate nucleus, whereas the third received control grafts of inappropriate tissue (hypothalamus and locus coeruleus) into the striatum/ventricle and grafts of mesencephalon into an inappropriate site (cingulate cortex). The transplants comprised stereotaxic implants of minced (1 mm³) tissue at multiple sites. The tissue used for the appropriate grafts into the first two monkeys was taken from a single late gestational fetus (17 cm CRL), whereas the tissue for the inappropriate grafts was from a much younger donor (1.3 cm CRL). Details of the implantation procedures and of the graft morphology were given in three further papers (70,71,73). Parkinsonian symptoms were rated before, during, and after MPTP treatment, during the 18 days immediately after grafting, and between 18 and 69 days after grafting and before sacrifice. Reduced parkinsonian summary scores were recorded during the 18- to 69-day period for the two monkeys that received the appropriate grafts of nigral tissue into the caudate nucleus. In one of these animals (A in ref. 63; S092 in refs. 70,73) the improvements were noted as early as 1 to 2 days after surgery. In contrast, the monkey that received the inappropriate grafts did not recover and died at 56 days postgraft.

Histologic examination of the striatum revealed large numbers of tyrosine hydroxylase (TH)-positive cells in the two monkeys that received nigral grafts, approximately 60,000 cells in one case (S092) and 15,000 in the other (S054) (70,71,73). However, the distribution of these cells was extensive and not limited to the immediate vicinity of the implantation sites. The authors suggested that catecholaminergic cells may have migrated from the transplanted tissue as far as the boundaries of the caudate nucleus and putamen. An alternative explanation is that the neurons that stained positive for TH may have been intrinsic rather than graft derived. Endogenous TH neurons within or immediately adjacent to the striatum have been observed in both long-tailed macaques (30) and marmosets (40,82, 88). A later report gives the number of TH-positive cells located within the transplant of monkey S054 as 30 (79). Also in this later report, monkey S092 was excluded from the functional analysis because it was only mildly affected by MPTP and thus might have recovered spontaneously even if it had not received a graft (N.B.—this was the monkey that showed signs of recovery 1 to 2 days after surgery). Overall, then, the initial reports on these three monkeys alone do not provide sufficient evidence on which to judge the functional efficacy of nigral grafts.

Subsequent reports from Redmond, Sladek, and colleagues included data from additional monkeys with grafts and considerably more detail on the methodology and outcome of the behavioral tests. The most comprehensive and quantitative behavioral account of this expanded series was given by Taylor et al (79). Histologic descriptions of some of these additional cases also were

given in Sladek et al. (72), and biochemical evidence of increased DA levels in punches of tissue adjacent to nigral graft sites in two monkeys in Elsworth et al (39). A preliminary account of some of the behavioral data appeared in Taylor et al. (78), which included a cognitive object retrieval task reviewed in the section on cognitive tasks in this chapter.

In all, ten monkeys with grafts of fetal neural tissue (including S054 and S114 from the initial reports) were described in the 1991 paper (79): Four of these received grafts of nigral tissue into the caudate nucleus approximately 1 month after systemic MPTP treatment; three received inappropriate grafts of either substantia nigra into the cortex (n = 2) or cerebellum into the caudate nucleus (n = 1), again after prior MPTP treatment; three that had not been treated with MPTP received multiple grafts of various tissues, including cerebellum, olfactory bulb, locus coeruleus, and substantia nigra, into the caudate nucleus. For two subjects in this no-MPTP control group, the tissue was cryopreserved, whereas in all other cases the implanted tissue pieces were fresh. The size of the donor embryos ranged considerably from 1.3 to 21 cm, and neonatal tissue was implanted into one of the no-MPTP control monkeys.

Grafts containing TH-positive cells were seen at histology in each of the four monkeys that received grafts of fetal nigral tissue into the caudate nucleus, although the numbers of cells that survived were small (+ 28, 30, 42, 506). Despite the limited number of cells, networks of TH-positive fibers were observed that sometimes were dense and often extended into the ventricle. All four of these monkeys showed behavioral improvements before they were sacrificed between 2 and 7.5 months after grafting, whereas none of the three monkeys with inappropriate grafts improved. Indeed, these monkeys either died at 2 months or were sacrificed for humane reasons 5 to 6 months after surgery because of the severe consequences of the MPTP treatment.

Quantification of the behavioral changes was achieved by rating a range of behaviors as normal or abnormal on a scale from 0 to 5 and by scoring other behaviors as present or absent during 5-sec intervals in 5-min observation periods. In general, parkinsonian signs such as "delayed movement," "poverty of movement," and "tremor" were rated, whereas normal behaviors, including "bipedal lookout," "self-groom," and "vertical climb," were scored as present or absent. A parkinsonian summary score and a healthy behavior score were derived from the data. On both measures the groups differed significantly at a number of time points after treatment. After an initial decline during the first month after transplantation surgery, the nigral graft group gradually improved so that by months 7 to 8 the parkinsonian summary score was at pre-MPTP baseline levels and did not differ significantly from the score of the no-MPTP control group. The healthy behavior score of the nigral graft group also improved, and at 5 to 6 months was not significantly different from the score of the no-MPTP controls, although it remained lower than pre-MPTP baseline levels. In contrast, the MPTP-treated group with inappropriate grafts did not improve on either measure, whereas the scores of the no-MPTP control graft group were unchanged during the course of the experiment, apart from a slight decline in the healthly behavior score that may have been a result of surgery. Anxiety and arousal summary scores also improved in the nigral compared with the inappropriate graft group, although the arousal score did not return to baseline levels and remained considerably depressed even 7 to 8 months after transplantation surgery.

As well as the summary scores, group data for some of the individual behaviors were presented. The most dramatic of these was the "facedown" score, which illustrated the severe nature of the syndrome produced by the MPTP treatment, so that the monkeys that received the inappropriate grafts spent most of the observation periods lying face down on the floor of the cage. The improvement in the nigral graft group on this measure mirrored the changes in the parkinsonian summary score. Because of the predominance of "facedown" behavior, data for some of the other individual behaviors are hard to interpret. For example, "delayed movement" was reduced in the nigral graft group and, from the quantitative data presented, also appeared to be reduced in the inappropriate graft group. However, this group initiated so little movement that it was difficult to judge whether movement was delayed. Similar problems are apparent with the attempts to measure "freeze" and "intention tremor" in these severely affected monkeys. In effect, for each of these individual behaviors, there is no control group with MPTP-produced deficits against which to compare the changes in the nigral graft group. Nevertheless, in spite of this difficulty with the detailed analysis of the functional changes, this study is important because it provided the first clear demonstration, with sufficient subjects to allow statistical comparisons between groups, of the amelioration of parkinsonian symptoms and general improvements in the health of the monkeys with fetal nigral grafts in the striatum. Tremor was a notable exception in that, although reduced during periods of quiescence, it was still evident, and indeed increased with the intention to respond, 7 to 8 months after implantation of the nigral tissue in the caudate nucleus.

One caveat with regard to this study is that all the monkeys received grafts, albeit of different tissue types placed in various locations. There were no subjects that had been treated with MPTP alone and were not subjected to transplantation surgery. Might the inappropriate grafts have contributed to the functional decline of this important control group? The question cannot be answered without explicit behavioral comparisons between MPTP-treated monkeys with inappropriate grafts and with no grafts at all.

An important question arising from the

study by Taylor et al. (79) concerns the mechanism of the observed functional recovery. Relatively few TH-positive cells were found at the graft sites in the caudate nucleus. Were these few cells sufficient to produce the considerable functional improvements, or might some other mechanism, such as damage to the striatum during implantation, account for the behavioral changes? The gradual improvement over a period of months, indeed the initial decline during the first month after transplantation, suggests that the recovery was not an immediate consequence of the surgical procedures. Nevertheless, Fiandaca and colleagues (42) and Bankiewicz et al. (14) have proposed that injury-induced regeneration of host dopaminergic neurons may underlie functional recovery produced by tissue implants in the striatum (see section on mechanisms of graft action). Monkeys with grafts of inappropriate tissue in the striatum are of crucial importance in this debate. However, only one of the inappropriate graft controls in the study by Taylor et al. received implants of inappropriate tissue in the caudate nucleus. The size and placement of the inappropriate graft were comparable with the nigral grafts in other monkeys, except that the graft was devoid of TH-positive neurons (39,72). There was no evidence of regeneration of the host dopaminergic neurons (79). The monkey did not recover, which is against the regeneration hypothesis, but, clearly, functional assessments of more subjects with inappropriate tissue grafts located in the striatum are needed to answer this question.

Adrenal and Other Tissue Grafts

To date, no study designed specifically to assess the parkinsonian symptoms of monkeys with bilateral dopaminergic lesions and grafts of adrenal medulla implanted in the striatum has been published in full. One monkey with a bilateral lesion produced by systemically administered MPTP received a unilateral graft of fetal cerebellum into the caudate nucleus in the study of Bankiewicz et al. (14) (see "Adrenal and other tissue grafts" in the sections on rotation and hand and arm movements). Recovery from bradykinesia and tremor was described as dramatic during the months after transplantation and was maintained over the next 6 months; however, no quantitative assessment of the behavioral changes was made. In the study by Nakai et al. (60), in which the primary behavioral measure was activity (see section on locomotion—adrenal and other tissue grafts), two monkeys with bilateral MPTP lesions were described as showing reduced bradykinesia and muscular rigidity 5 to 6 days after autologous bilateral transplantation of the superior cervical ganglion (SCG) into the caudate nucleus, whereas recovery was incomplete in a third animal also with a SCG graft. A fourth parkinsonian monkey that did not receive a graft did not recover.

Most studies that have attempted to examine functional changes in monkeys with grafts of tissue other than embryonic nigra have used subjects with unilateral lesions and measured either rotation or hand and arm use rather than parkinsonian symptoms. Watts et al. (86) commented that there was some clinical improvement in their hemiparkinsonian monkeys that received adrenal medulla grafts, although the improvement lagged behind the changes in apomorphine-induced rotation (see section on rotation—adrenal and other tissue grafts) and was not quantified. Thus, there are very few data on which to judge the efficacy of adrenal or other tissue grafts in reducing clinically rated parkinsonian symptoms in primates.

LOCOMOTION

Nigral Grafts

Surprisingly few studies have recorded activity levels in monkeys with nigral grafts. In the observer evaluation studies reviewed under "Nigral Grafts" in the previous section, behaviors that involved whole-body movements were among the list of items scored. For example, in the study by Bakay et al., (8) "crossover," "active," and "acrobatic" behaviors were quantified, although, as we have seen, too few monkeys were studied to draw any definite conclusions. In the study by Taylor et al., (79) "shift" and "vertical climb" were components of the arousal summary score, which, although improved slightly in the nigral graft group, did not recover to baseline levels. Only two studies have used automated systems to quantify locomotion in monkeys with nigral grafts, and only one of these (43) has looked at the effects of grafts placed bilaterally in the striatum.

In the study by Fine and colleagues (43), the locomotor activity of marmosets rendered parkinsonian by the systemic administration of MPTP was measured in cages fitted with photodetectors once before, and at several time points after transplantation of marmoset embryonic (10–15 mm CRL) tissue into the putamen. Two monkeys received bilateral "dopaminergic" grafts of ventral mesencephalon, two received bilateral "control nondopaminergic" grafts of striatal eminence, and two remained without transplants. Stereotaxic injections of dissociated cell suspensions were made into one of the "dopaminergic" and one of the "control nondopaminergic" monkeys, whereas the injections were of undissociated tissue fragments in the other two cases. The number of TH-positive cells in the striatum of the monkey that received the undissociated "dopaminergic" graft was estimated at more than 40,000, and in the monkey that received the dissociated "dopaminergic" graft at approximately 3,000. In both monkeys, spontaneous locomotion was reported as markedly increased at 3 months, and amphetamine-induced locomotion when tested at 9 to 10 months after transplantation surgery, although quantitative data from only one of the two animals were presented. In contrast, the marmosets with the "control nondopaminergic" grafts

remained as inactive as the MPTP-treated controls, which did not receive grafts. This latter comparison is of importance with regard to the debate about the mechanisms of functional recovery because it provides two more cases, in addition to the one described by Taylor et al (79), of monkeys with implants of inappropriate tissue in the striatum that did not show any functional benefit. Unfortunately, the size and location of the "control nondopaminergic" grafts in these two cases were not described.

A photocell cage also was used in the study by Annett et al. (4) to measure locomotion by marmosets with nigral grafts, although in this experiment the lesions and grafts were unilateral rather than bilateral (see the section on rotation—nigral grafts, for details of the grafts). Individual locomotor counts were extremely variable and there were no group differences between monkeys with nigral grafts and lesion-alone controls. The study is of note, however, because the graft placements included a site in the nucleus accumbens, the location at which nigral grafts have been found to be most effective for influencing levels of locomotion in rats (50), and where injections of amphetamine induce locomotion in marmosets (6). Most primate neural graft studies have focused on the caudate nucleus and/or putamen, and none has specifically examined the functional effects of nigral grafts placed in the nucleus accumbens alone. In summary, although individual cases have been described in which locomotion increased after transplantation, statistically confirmed differences between groups of monkeys with and without nigral grafts have not been reported to date, and most studies have not included graft placements at potentially the most appropriate striatal site.

Adrenal and Other Tissue Grafts

Even fewer studies have evaluated locomotion by monkeys with adrenal or other tissue grafts than is the case with nigral grafts. A telemetric method in which electrical signals generated by the monkey's movements were transmitted to a receiver outside the cage was used by Nakai et al. (60) to quantify the spontaneous activity of four *Macaca fuscata* monkeys before and after systemic MPTP treatment. Three of these monkeys went on to receive autologous grafts of SCG into the caudate nucleus bilaterally, whereas the fourth served as a lesion-alone control. Five to 6 days after surgery, the activity of the grafted monkeys started to increase, and by 4 to 5 weeks had returned to pre-MPTP baseline levels in two cases, although the activity of the third grafted monkey remained considerably depressed. The lesion-alone control monkey did not recover. However, the period between the final dose of MPTP and grafting of the SCG tissue was very short (less than 1 week in the two monkeys in which recovery was most complete), and considerable spontaneous recovery from the effects of MPTP treatment commonly occurs during this period (51). Watts et al. (86) used a computerized tracking system to analyze monkeys' movements in the home cage. The hypokinesia of a hemiparkinsonian compared to an intact rhesus monkey was illustrated dramatically by records produced by the system. A small increase in the mobility of monkeys with adrenal medulla grafts was reported, but quantitative records for these monkeys were not presented. The total number of 90° turns in either direction was used by Dubach (28) as a measure of activity in hemiparkinsonian long-tailed macaques with adrenal medulla grafts (see the section on rotation—adrenal and other tissue grafts, for details of the grafts). Activity levels were unaffected by the transplants.

ROTATION

The most widely used behavioral measure of graft function in rats with unilateral dopaminergic lesions is undoubtedly the rotation induced by the stimulant drugs amphetamine and apomorphine. The well defined effect of the lesion combined with the simplicity of quantification in bowls based on the design of Ungerstedt and Arbuthnott (83) make rotation a particularly useful behavioral measure. Like rats, monkeys with unilateral dopaminergic lesions rotate toward the side of the lesion, both spontaneously and after an injection of amphetamine, whereas the rotation induced by apomorphine and other direct dopamine agonists is away from the side of the lesion (7,11,24). Although rotation bowls are not practical for use with primates, a number of methods of quantifying rotation have been devised that involve, for example, a flexible cable tether in the home cage (28), a system of infrared phototransmitters in a jacket worn by the monkey and detectors around the home cage (15), or simply counting the number of complete turns from video records of behavior as the film is replayed on fast-forward (2,7). Although absolute levels of rotation may vary considerably between monkeys, individual scores are generally stable over periods of several months (7,11), an important requisite for graft studies. Indeed, most primate neural graft studies that have used unilateral dopaminergic lesions have included some measure of rotation. A few cases of rotation by monkeys with bilateral lesions and unilateral grafts also have been described.

Nigral Grafts

In an early study by Dubach and colleagues (31), one long-tailed macaque received injections of a suspension of embryonic mesencephalic cells into sites in the caudate nucleus and putamen 5 months after a unilateral lesion had been produced by direct injection of MPTP into the substantia nigra. Rotation was measured by a potentiometer mounted on top of the cage to which a nylon jacket worn by the monkey was attached via a flexible cable. The potentiometer registered any turn greater than 6° (the procedure is described in detail in ref. 28). Before transplantation surgery, only about 4% of all turns made by this animal were toward the contralateral side. Ten days after the transplant, this doubled to about 8%. Turning toward the contralateral side averaged 8% for the next 3 weeks before returning to baseline levels. Thus, the extent and duration of the change in turning were extremely limited compared to most other reports of nigral graft effects on rotation, described later. Few TH-positive cells were found at the injection sites in the striatum, although there were such cells some 3 to 4 mm medial to the transplant sites adjacent to the ventricle, which may have been intrinsic rather than graft derived because intrinsic TH-positive neurons have been described in the intact primate neostriatum (30). Thus, it is not clear whether the reported change in rotation was related to the transplant.

In contrast, the marmoset (S1) described by Fine et al. (43), which rotated spontaneously 10 weeks after receiving a unilateral graft, had a large number of surviving TH-positive cells at the graft site in the putamen, and reinnervation that extended from the putamen, through the internal capsule, into the caudate nucleus. The spontaneous rotation was away from the grafted side, whereas apomorphine-induced rotation was toward the grafted side. This monkey was one of four that had been treated systemically with MPTP before receiving unilateral grafts of a nigral cell suspension prepared from 10- or 14-mm CRL marmoset embryos. The three other marmosets that received unilateral grafts did not rotate. This may have been because the tissue used for their grafts was from the older embryo, and graft survival was not as good. It is of interest that a graft site in the putamen should produce rotation because we have reported that only grafts in the caudate nucleus, and not in the putamen, affect rotation (3,32). However, because the reinner-

vation in this monkey extended into the caudate nucleus, the putamen site may not have been crucial for producing the rotation.

Another monkey with bilateral MPTP-induced parkinsonian and a unilateral nigral graft that rotated spontaneously has been described by Bankiewicz and colleagues (15). A unilateral transplant of 1- to 2-mm pieces of 35- to 42-day embryonic ventral mesencephalic tissue was made into the precavitated caudate nucleus of this rhesus monkey. Infrared photodetectors around the cage and a transmitter in a jacket worn by the monkey were used to record turns (angle not given). Five months after transplantation, the monkey started to turn spontaneously away from the transplanted side. Amphetamine increased turning away from the transplant, whereas after apomorphine administration the monkey turned toward the transplanted side. The rotation by this monkey is of particular interest for two reasons. First, although rotation was first seen 5 months after transplantation surgery, parkinsonian symptoms were reported to improve during the first week after surgery. Thus, the rotation did not parallel other functional changes. Second, the caudate nucleus was precavitated bilaterally, even though the transplant was unilateral. The damage caused by such a procedure has been reported to induce sprouting of surviving intrinsic dopaminergic fibers, which may promote functional recovery (14,16,42, 62) (see section on mechanisms of graft action). The rotation by this monkey with the unilateral transplant suggests that the embryonic mesencephalic tissue produced a greater functional effect on the transplanted side than the cavity alone on the nontransplanted side.

In the same study by Bankiewicz and colleagues (15), three hemiparkinsonian monkeys also received transplants of embryonic ventral mesencephalon. In these cases, the transplants were made bilaterally, again into the precavitated caudate nucleus. In all three monkeys, apomorphine-induced rotation decreased during the first 3 weeks after implantation. The extent of the decrease was not reported quantitatively in the original paper, but in a subsequent paper in which transplants of different types were compared, decreases of about 80% were reported in tests at 3 and 6 months after transplantation (14). Although the decrease was sustained for 6 months in two of the monkeys, rotation by the third monkey increased again after 6 weeks because of rejection of the implant, which had been derived from two fetuses. Despite the decrease in apomorphine-induced rotation in the two monkeys with successful grafts, spontaneous turning toward the MPTP-treated side was unaffected by the transplants.

Among the battery of behavioral tests used by Annett et al. (2,4) to make a functional assessment of embryonic nigral grafts in marmosets, the most striking effects of the grafts were observed in rotation tests. Six marmosets with unilateral 6-OHDA lesions of the nigrostriatal pathway and subsequent grafts of embryonic nigra in the striatum were compared with four marmosets with the lesion alone and five unlesioned controls. The grafts comprised injections of cell suspensions prepared from the ventral mesencephalon of 74-day marmoset embryos (Carnegie stage 18–19, equivalent developmentally to E14–15 rat embryos, see ref. 32) into four sites in the caudate nucleus, three in the putamen, and one in the nucleus accumbens on the same side as the initial lesion. The monkeys were filmed for 30 or 60 min while in transparent Perspex boxes, and then complete 360° turns in either direction were counted when the videotape was replayed on fast-forward. Both amphetamine-induced and spontaneous rotation toward the side of the lesion were significantly reduced in the monkeys with grafts compared to the lesion-alone controls from the third month onward after transplantation surgery. Apomorphine-induced rotation away from the lesioned side, assessed at 10 to 12 months postgraft, also

was significantly reduced by the grafts. Rotation was not only reduced in the amphetamine and spontaneous tests, but in the three marmosets with the largest grafts (>1,500 TH-positive cells in the striatum), the direction of rotation was reversed so that the monkeys turned away from the side of the lesion and graft (i.e., contralaterally). A similar phenomenon of overcompensation by grafts on amphetamine rotation tests has been observed in many studies of embryonic nigral grafts in rats (1,5,23, 34,35). The mechanisms underlying this overcompensation are not yet fully understood. However, abnormally high c-*fos* activity has been reported in the striatum of rats with nigral grafts after amphetamine treatment, which suggests that neurons postsynaptic to the grafts may become functionally overactive while under the influence of drug (1,23).

Reduced spontaneous rotation in the study by Annett et al. (2,4) contrasts with the report by Bankiewicz et al. (15) that spontaneous turning toward the side of the lesion remained at about the same level for 7 months after transplantation surgery. Methodologic differences between the two studies may account for the apparent anomaly. In the study by Bankiewicz et al. (15), the monkeys wore primate jackets fitted with an infrared phototransmitter so that turns could be counted by infrared detectors while the monkeys remained in the home cage. In the study by Annett et al. (2,4), the monkeys were removed from the home cage and taken to another room where, on different days, both spontaneous and drug-induced rotation were assessed. Therefore, rotation during the spontaneous tests may have been influenced by previous experience of rotation during amphetamine tests; that is, rotation recorded during the spontaneous tests may have been conditioned. The marmosets with grafts that rotated contralaterally during the spontaneous tests did so only after they had previously rotated contralaterally during an amphetamine test. Overcompensation is not normally seen in no-drug tests of nigral graft function in rats (5,34,36). However, rats with nigral grafts did exhibit conditioned contralateral rotation during a no-drug test when placed again in an environment in which they had previously rotated contralaterally while under the influence of amphetamine (5). Thus, in the marmoset graft study, the decrease in spontaneous rotation may have been specific to the formal test situation. Indeed, in the home cage, the same monkeys occasionally rotated ipsilaterally. They also tended to sit in the home cage looking over their ipsilateral shoulder, and rarely looked contralaterally. This ipsilateral bias, quantified by recording the position of the head with respect to the rest of the body every second during 1-min intervals, was not reduced by the grafts. Further examples of ipsilateral biases that persisted, despite the graft effects on rotation, included hand preference and neglect of visual and somatosensory stimuli (see "Nigral Grafts" in the sections on hand and arm movements and neglect). Overall, the results of the study by Annett et al. (2,4) were interpreted as partial recovery of function: although sufficient to reduce drug-induced rotation and produce some improvements in a reaching task (see section on hand and arm movements—nigral grafts), function on the grafted side was not restored to prelesion levels, and hence ipsilateral biases remained.

The location of grafts in the striatum determines the profile of behavioral changes in rats, with dorsal or central placements being more effective than ventrolateral sites for reducing amphetamine-induced rotation (35,57). In monkeys, the importance of graft location has been examined in a second study by Annett et al. (3,32). Embryonic nigral grafts were prepared exactly as in the previous study, except that in four marmosets the implants were made only into the caudate nucleus, whereas in another five marmosets the grafts were made only into the putamen. The behavior of these monkeys with transplants was com-

pared to that of six monkeys with the unilateral 6-OHDA lesion alone and with five unoperated controls. The ipsilateral rotation induced by amphetamine was reduced, and in three cases reversed, in the monkeys with grafts in the caudate nucleus. The magnitude and time course of the effect were very similar to those observed in the previous study in which grafts were placed at multiple striatal sites, including sites in the caudate nucleus. In contrast, grafts in the putamen alone did not affect rotation. However, these putamen grafts did produce functional improvements in a reaching task (see section on hand and arm movements—nigral grafts). The absence of rotation effects in the putamen graft group provides another example of rotation not necessarily predicting functional changes in other behavioral tests.

In our most recent study, rotation has been used as a behavioral measure of graft viability in an experiment comparing donor tissue taken from embryos of different ages. In rats, the success of neural transplants depends critically on the age of the donor embryos (61). For nigral grafts the optimal age is E14 to 15, which corresponds to 10- to 14-mm CRL and Carnegie developmental stages 18 to 21 (33). Many primate studies have used tissue derived from donors at equivalent developmental stages (see Table 6 in ref. 32). However, in the early studies of Redmond and Sladek, relatively old (fetal rather than embryonic) monkey nigral tissue was reported to survive transplantation and produce functional effects (63,79). Thus, the critical time window during which nigral tissue could be taken for transplantation might be considerably broader in primates than in rats. Conversely, studies of human embryonic xenografts in rats suggest that there is an optimal age for transplantation of human donor tissue, the upper limit for suspension grafts being about 8 weeks postconception, which is equivalent to Carnegie stage 22 (20,46). For solid implants, the upper limit may be extended slightly by about 9 days

(46). Histologic evidence of graft survival is described by Freed et al. in three bonnet monkeys that received grafts of nigral tissue derived from 18-, 45-, or 150-mm embryos/fetuses (45). Only the grafts from the youngest donor survived well and produced behavioral improvements, whereas a few transplanted nigral cells survived in the middle case, and there was essentially no graft survival or behavioral improvement in the last monkey, which received tissue from the oldest donor. In more recent studies, Sladek, Redmond, and colleagues have reported much greater dopamine cell survival in transplants from E44 compared to E49 embryos in vervet monkeys (69).

The numbers of monkeys that have received grafts from donors of different ages and have been compared both histologically and functionally are therefore very small. We decided to use the marmoset unilateral 6-OHDA lesion model to make a systematic comparison of nigral grafts from donors of different ages. In our previous studies described earlier, all donor embryos were taken at 74 days postconception (Carnegie stages 18–19 in the marmoset; see ref. 32). In the new study, grafts of nigral tissue taken from 83- or 84-day marmoset embryos (Carnegie stages 20+) were placed at sites in the caudate nucleus of six marmosets with the unilateral 6-OHDA lesion. A further six lesioned marmosets received nigral grafts into the caudate nucleus of tissue derived from 92- or 93-day donors (by which stage they are more appropriately categorized as fetal rather than embryonic). Attempts to dissect the ventral mesencephalon from younger (E64 and E68) embryos proved unsuccessful because the brains were too small. Amphetamine-induced rotation was monitored before and after the lesion and once a month for 6 months after transplantion. In contrast to the significant effects on rotation with the E74 grafts observed in the two previous studies, monkeys in both the E83 to 84 and E92 to 93 groups continued to rotate ipsilaterally for the duration of the study (Fig. 1A). At his-

tology, graft sites with a few surviving TH-positive cells were found in most monkeys in both groups; however, the numbers of cells were very much smaller than in the previous two experiments (<10%; Fig. 1B). Thus, although a few dopaminergic cells survived, these were not sufficient to produce functional improvements in rotation tests. Therefore, there does seem to be a critical time window, which may be as short as a few days, for successful transplantion of nigral tissue in marmosets.

In summary, changes in rotation have been reported in a number of monkeys that have received transplants of embryonic nigra in the striatum, either decreased rotation in those cases in which the grafts were placed on the same side as a unilateral dopaminergic lesion, or increased rotation in cases with bilateral lesions and unilateral grafts (Table 1). The most convincing effects have been observed in amphetamine or apomorphine tests; it is not clear whether spontaneous rotation is also affected in monkeys with unilateral lesions and grafts, although the gradual appearance of rotation in the animals with bilateral lesions and unilateral grafts would appear to be spontaneous. Characteristics of nigral graft effects in rats that also have been observed in monkeys include overcompensation in amphetamine rotation tests, and the importance of graft location and the age of the donor tissue. However, it is important to note that graft-dependent changes in rotation do not always parallel, and therefore cannot be used to predict, other functional changes. Nevertheless, rotation would seem to a useful behavioral tool in monkeys as a sensitive and reliable *in vivo* indicator of nigral graft viability.

Adrenal and Other Tissue Grafts

Reductions in apomorphine-induced rotation have been described in several studies by Bankiewicz, Plunkett, and colleagues of hemiparkinsonian rhesus monkeys with

A.

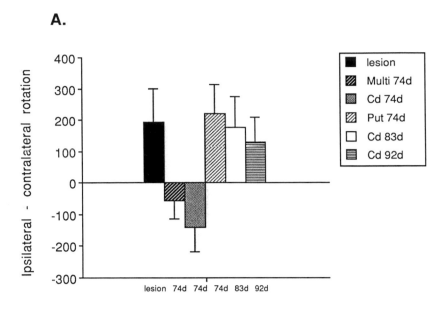

B.

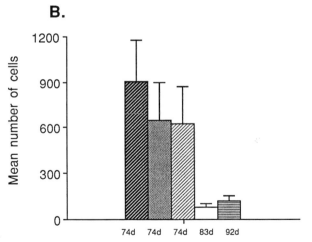

FIG. 1. A: Amphetamine-induced (0.5 mg/kg i.m.) rotation in marmosets with unilateral 6-OHDA lesions of the nigrostriatal bundle and, in some cases, with grafts of embryonic ventral mesencephalon of various ages in the striatum. The figure summarizes combined data from three experiments reported in the text (refs. 2–4,32 and unpublished observations). lesion, lesion-alone controls (n = 10); Multi 74d, graft tissue derived from 74-day embryos (Carnegie stages 18–19) placed at sites in the caudate nucleus, the putamen, and the nucleus accumbens (n = 6); Cd 74d, graft tissue derived from 74-day embryos placed in the caudate nucleus alone (n = 4); Put 74d, graft tissue derived from 74-day embryos placed in the putamen alone (n = 5); Cd 83d, graft tissue derived from 83–84-day embryos (Carnegie stages 20 +) placed in the caudate nucleus alone (n = 6); Cd 92d, graft tissue derived from 92–93-day embryos (fetal rather than embryonic) placed in the caudate nucleus alone (n = 6). Scores are total ipsilateral minus contralateral 360° turns made during 30-min rotation tests conducted at 4, 5, and 6 months after grafting. **B**: Number of TH-positive cells in the striatum of the same marmosets with grafts as in (A). Legend as for (A), except that n = 4 for the Put 74d group because cell counts were unavailable from one of the monkeys in this group. For the purpose of comparison, only cells in the caudate nucleus of the Multi 74d group are presented in this figure, although additional TH-positive cells were located in the putamen and in the nucleus accumbens of these monkeys.

bilateral grafts of adrenal medulla or various other types of tissue in the precavitated caudate nucleus, or, indeed, in monkeys in which cavities were made but no tissue was implanted (13,14,16,17). Rotation was reduced by about 70%, compared with pretransplant scores, in four monkeys tested 3 months after receiving adrenal medulla allografts. However, when the same animals were tested 6 months after surgery, the reduction was only about 40% (16). No TH-positive cells survived in the grafts of these animals, so although the initial reductions in rotation may have been due to dopamine released from chromaffin cells in the grafts, other mechanisms must account for the long-term behavioral effects (see section on mechanisms of graft action). In a second experiment, gradual but substantial reductions in rotation over a period of about 10 to 12 months were observed in two monkeys with bilateral autografts of adrenal medulla, but in a third case rotation increased over the same period (62). Again, survival of the graft tissue was poor. Four control monkeys in this experiment in which cavities were made in the caudate nucleus, but no tissue was implanted, also showed reductions in rotation, as did one other monkey with cavitation alone in the first experiment. Reductions of about 40% in rotation tested 3 and 6 months after surgery also were reported in one monkey that received grafts of adrenal cortex and in another monkey that received grafts of adult monkey fat tissue (16). Similarly, transplants of fetal nondopaminergic neural tissue (cerebellum in one monkey and spinal cord in another) also reduced rotation, the time course and magnitude of the effect being described as "similar to that reported for monkeys receiving a foetal mesencephalon implant" (14). A third monkey in this study with bilateral parkinsonism produced by systemic MPTP treatment that then received a unilateral graft of fetal cerebellum into the caudate nucleus did not rotate (cf. parkinsonian monkeys with unilateral grafts of fetal nigra; see section on rotation—ni-

gral grafts). Finally, decreases of 57% to 67% in apomorphine-induced rotation up to 6 months after surgery were reported in three of four monkeys that received transplants of fetal amnion in the caudate nucleus (13).

For all these studies, the conclusion that the transplants or cavities were primarily responsible for the reductions in rotation depends, of course, on absence of any spontaneous recovery in hemiparkinsonian, but otherwise intact, monkeys. Data from three such animals indicating stable rotation levels for at least 6 months were presented in the first study (16), but direct comparisons between implanted and surgically intact monkeys were not made in the other studies (13,14,62). Five hemiparkinsonian monkeys with stable levels of rotation over 10 or 40 months were described in one paper (14), but it is not clear whether these included the three animals previously described. Statisical comparisons between groups were not made in any of the studies. The presence, or absence, of graft effects on amphetamine-induced or spontaneous rotation was not reported.

Reductions in apomorphine-induced rotation in hemiparkinsonian monkeys with adrenal medulla grafts also have been reported by Watts et al (86). Four rhesus monkeys received grafts of adrenal medullary tissue fragments into the caudate nucleus ipsilateral to the unilateral MPTP lesion, two received cografts of adrenal medulla and sural nerve, also into the ipsilateral caudate, whereas in two further monkeys adrenal medulla was grafted to the contralateral unlesioned caudate. All of the monkeys that received grafts showed reductions in drug-induced rotation within 1 month of grafting, whereas rotation remained stable for periods of up to 1 year in three hemiparkinsonian, surgically intact controls. The reductions, ranging from 63% to 95%, were maintained for several months despite poor survival of chromaffin cells in the grafts. From the results presented, it is not clear whether the improvements were

TABLE 1. *Graft effects on rotation*

Reference	Species	Lesion	Graft tissue (or control procedure)	n	Target	Rotation		
						Spont.	Amphet.	Apom.
Dubach et al. (31)	Long-tailed macaque	MPTP u	Embryonic nigra	1	C+P	(+)	−	−
Fine et al. (43)	Marmoset	MPTP b	Embryonic nigra	1 (4)	Pu[a]	+	−	+
Bankiewicz et al. (15)	Rhesus, cynomolgus	MPTP b	Embryonic nigra (lesion alone)	1	Cu	+	+	+
				3		−	−	−
		MPTP u	Embryonic nigra (lesion alone)	3	Cb	0	−	+
				5		0	−	0
Annett et al. (2,4)	Marmoset	6-OHDA u	Embryonic nigra	6	C+P+A	+	+	+
			(lesion alone or saline injection)	4		0	0	0
Annett et al. (3) and Dunnett and Annett (34)	Marmoset	6-OHDA u	Embryonic nigra	4	C	−	+	−
				5	P	−	0	−
			Embryonic nigra (lesion alone)	6		−	0	−
Annett (*this chapter*)	Marmoset	6-OHDA u	Aged embryonic nigra	12	C	−	0	−
Bankiewicz et al. (16)	Rhesus	MPTP u	Adrenal medulla	4	C	−	−	+
			Adrenal cortex, fatty tissue	1	C	−	−	+
			(lesion plus cavitation)	1	C	−	−	+
			(lesion no cavitation)	3		−	−	0

Reference	Species	Lesion	Graft	n	Target	Rotation			Graft effect
						Spont.	Amphet.	Apom.	
Plunkett et al. (62)	Rhesus	MPTP u	Adrenal medulla (lesion plus cavitation)	2 (3)	C	—	—	—	+
				4		—	—	—	+
Bankiewicz et al. (14)	Rhesus	MPTP b	Embryonic cerebellum	1	Cu	0	—	—	—
		MPTP u	Embryonic spinal cord	1	Cb	—	—	—	+
		MPTP u	Embryonic cerebellum	1	Cb	—	—	—	+
Bankiewicz et al. (13)	Rhesus	MPTP u	Amnion	3 (4)	C	—	—	—	+
Watts et al. (86)	Rhesus	MPTP u	Adrenal medulla	4	C	0	—	—	+
		MPTP u	Adrenal medulla plus sural nerve	2	C	0	—	—	+
			(lesion alone)	3		0	—	—	0
Dubach (28)	Long-tailed macaques	6-OHDA u	Adrenal medulla "ribbon grafts"	4 (6)	C+P	+	—	—	0
			Adrenal medulla non-"ribbon grafts"	16	C+P	0	—	—	—

Species: donor and host species of monkey.

Lesions: u, unilateral; b, bilateral.

n: The total number of monkeys in the group is given in brackets if not all monkeys in the group were affected by the grafts.

Target: C, caudate; P, putamen; A, nucleus accumbens; u and b indicate that the grafts were placed unilaterally or bilaterally if this differed from the lesion.

Rotation: Spont., spontaneous rotation; Amphet., amphetamine-induced rotation; Apom., apomorphine-induced rotation.

+, Graft effect; (+), weak graft effect; 0, no graft effect; —, not reported.

aGraft was placed in the putamen but reinnervation extended into the caudate nucleus.

seen only in those animals in which the grafts were placed ipsilateral to the side of the lesion. Nor is it clear whether the improvements were greater in the animals with co-grafts, although this was one of the stated conclusions. Spontaneous rotation persisted despite the grafts; effects on amphetamine-induced rotation were not reported.

The largest series of monkeys with adrenal medulla grafts for which rotation data are available has been reported by Dubach. Histologic descriptions of the autografts, including evidence of surviving chromaffin cells in a number of cases, are presented in two papers (27,29), and a third paper gives details of the behavioral results (28). A range of techniques was used to prepare and transplant the tissue into four or more sites in the caudate nucleus and the putamen of 24 long-tailed macaques with unilateral 6-OHDA lesions of the substantia nigra. The most successful of the techniques, both in terms of numbers of surviving chromaffin cells and behavioral improvements, were the "ribbon" grafts, which were produced by slicing the medulla with an assembly of razors and then implanting the tissue stereotactically using an arrangement of inner and outer needles so that the "ribbon" shape of the tissue was maintained in the host striatum (26). Additional infusions of neuron growth factor were made into the ventricles of some monkeys, although this did not appear to be crucial because cell survival was good in one monkey that did not receive such an infusion. Four of the six monkeys that received ribbon grafts, and that had consistently shown low levels of spontaneous contralateral turning after the lesion, improved within 10 to 20 days of receiving the grafts, and the improvement was maintained until sacrifice at 4 to 8 weeks. In contrast, monkeys that received grafts of minced or cubed tissue, or earlier versions of the ribbon grafts, did not improve. Taking the nonribbon grafts as surgical controls, the improvement in turning preference with the ribbon grafts was statistically significant. The changes appeared to be related to the size of the implants rather than the number of viable grafted cells, although it is not clear why two of the monkeys with successful "ribbon" grafts did not improve. This series differs in two key respects from the other studies of adrenal medulla grafts reviewed earlier. First, 6-OHDA and not MPTP was used to produce the dopaminergic lesion, which, together with the stereotaxic rather than cavitation implantation technique, reduces the likelihood that the behavioral improvements were due to sprouting of host dopaminergic fibers. Indeed, no such sprouting was observed (28). Second, the behavioral measure was spontaneous rather than drug-induced rotation. No other previous study of adrenal grafts in primates has observed changes in spontaneous rotation, and only a few studies have reported such changes in monkeys with embryonic nigral grafts (see section on rotation—nigral grafts).

HAND AND ARM MOVEMENTS

Assessment of neural graft effects in clinically relevant situations becomes particularly important given that grafts may not produce equivalent functional recovery in all behavioral tests. The ability to use the hand and arm to reach out toward an object would seem to be an example of a behavioral skill that is clinically relevant and that can be usefully examined in monkeys with neural grafts. However, so far only a few studies have attempted to quantify motor performance in tasks involving reaches by monkeys to retrieve objects, or pull or release levers, in tests designed to measure reaction and movement times (Table 2).

Nigral Grafts

Freed et al. (45) used a lever-pull task to measure motor performance with each hand by bonnet monkeys that received cell

TABLE 2. *Graft effects on hand and arm movements*

Reference	Species	Lesion	Graft tissue (or control procedure)	n	Target	Graft effect
Freed et al. (45)	Bonnet	MPTP b	Embryonic nigra	1	C+P	+
Bankiewicz et al. (15)	Rhesus	MPTP u	Embryonic nigra	3	Cb	+
Annett et al. (2,4)	Marmoset	6-OHDA u	Embryonic nigra (lesion alone or saline injection)	6 4	C+P+A	+ 0
Annett et al. (3) and Dunnett and Annett (34)	Marmoset	6-OHDA u	Embryonic nigra Embryonic nigra (lesion alone)	4 5 6	C P	(+) + 0
Bankiewicz et al. (16)	Rhesus	MPTP u	Adrenal medulla Adrenal cortex, fatty tissue (lesion plus cavitation) (lesion no cavitation)	4 1 1 1 3	C C C	(+) 0 0 0 0
Plunkett et al. (62)	Rhesus	MPTP u	Adrenal medulla (lesion plus cavitation)	1 (3) 4	C	(+) 0
Bankiewicz et al. (14)	Rhesus	MPTP b MPTP u MPTP u	Embryonic cerebellum Embryonic spinal cord Embryonic cerebellum	1 1 1	Cu Cb Cb	0 (+) 0
Bankiewicz et al. (13)	Rhesus	MPTP u	Amnion	3 (4)	C	+
Watts et al. (86)	Rhesus	MPTP a	Adrenal medulla plus sural nerve	1	C	+
Ellis et al. (38)	Rhesus	MPTP u	Adrenal medulla plus sural nerve	1	C	+
Goddard et al. (48)	Long-tailed macaques	MPTP u	Encapsulated PC12 cells	4 (5)	?	+
			(control implants)	3	?	0

Species: donor and host species of monkey.

Lesions: u, unilateral; b, bilateral.

n: The total number of monkeys in the group is given in brackets if not all monkeys in the group were affected by the grafts.

Target: C, caudate; P, putamen; A, nucleus accumbens; u and b indicate that the grafts were placed unilaterally or bilaterally if this differed from the lesion.

+, Graft effect; (+), weak or transient graft effect; 0, no graft effect.

suspension grafts of fetal ventral mesencephalon unilaterally into the caudate nucleus and into the putamen some 6 months after systemic MPTP treatment. Although six monkeys were originally trained on the task, one was put down and two others were completely unable to perform the task as a result of the MPTP treatment, and were therefore tested on a simpler task involving reaching for pellets presented by the experimenter. Data were presented for only one monkey performing the lever-pull task before and after the transplant. The donor tissue in this case was derived from a 45-mm CRL embryo, and a few TH-positive neurons were seen in the vicinity of the injection tracks when the monkey was sacrificed 6 months later. A clear improvement in use of the hand contralateral to the side of the graft, measured as an increase in the number of lever pulls per second, was seen from about 6 weeks after surgery, together with a slight improvement at about 12 weeks in the use of ipsilateral hand. Although three other monkeys received grafts of embryonic or fetal monkey nigra into the striatum, and two of these were reported to show behavioral improvements, it is not clear on which tests these improvements were seen.

A simple, but ingenious, method of assessing the capacity of each hand to make volitional movements has been used by Bankiewicz and colleagues to evaluate motor function in monkeys with grafts of embryonic nigral tissue (15,17) and with a range of other tissue grafts discussed in this section under "Adrenal and Other Tissue Grafts" (14,17,62). The monkeys were presented with a piece of food that was held in one hand and taken to the mouth. A second piece of food was then presented. Monkeys without lesions normally used their other hand to take this second piece of food. However, hemiparkinsonian monkeys used the hand that had been used for the initial response again to take the second piece of food. Bankiewicz et al. (15) described six rhesus and two cynomolgus monkeys that did not use the hand contralateral to the side of a unilateral intracarotid infusion of MPTP to take the second piece of food. Three months after the administration of MPTP, three of these monkeys received grafts comprising transplants of $1 \times 1 \times 2$-mm pieces of ventral mesencephalic tissue obtained from 35- to 42-day (i.e., Carnegie stages 17–22) gestational monkey embryos into the precavitated caudate nucleus. Precavitation and transplantation was bilateral even though the lesion was unilateral. In the reaching test, all three monkeys were described as showing marked increases in use of the affected arm 1 month after transplantation, although quantitative data were not presented. The improvement persisted in two of the monkeys for at least 7 months, whereas in the third monkey performance regressed about 6 weeks after transplantation, which the authors proposed was due to rejection of the graft.

Two different tasks requiring reaches to retrieve food were used by Annett et al. (2,4) to assess performance with each hand by the six marmosets with embryonic nigral grafts placed at multiple striatal sites, described under "Nigral Grafts" in the section on rotation. In one task, pieces of apple were placed in a series of trials at various distances inside tubes constructed from 10-ml syringes. Monkeys with the lesion alone were impaired with respect to the maximum distance from which they successfully retrieved apple pieces from inside the tubes, either when they were forced, by means of a jacket with a sleeve set into only one arm hole, to use the hand contralateral to the lesion, or when a tube was positioned at an angle so as to encourage reaches with the contralateral hand. The impairment was abolished in the monkeys with grafts. However, in a second task in which the monkeys retrieved apple pieces moving on a conveyor belt, the nigral grafts did not influence the strong ipsilateral hand preference produced by the earlier 6-OHDA lesion. Persistant impairments in the accuracy of reaches by the monkeys with grafts also were observed at the conveyor belt when performance with each hand was assessed independently using the jacket with one sleeve. Taken together, these results suggested graft-dependent recovery that was partial rather than complete, so that the contralateral hand could be used to reach for food, but was still impaired for reaches toward moving targets and was not preferred to the ipsilateral hand. An important question for future studies is whether more complete recovery in these reaching tasks would have been produced by more extensive grafts.

The relationship between graft location in the striatum and functional outcome is clearly an important issue for clinical transplantation programs. The differential effects on amphetamine-induced rotation of nigral grafts placed either in the caudate nucleus alone or in the putamen alone of marmosets with unilateral 6-OHDA lesions has been described under "Nigral Grafts" in the section on rotation. In the same experiment, the ability of the monkeys to use each hand to reach for apple pieces placed inside tubes also was assessed (3). The marmosets with grafts in the putamen reached significantly further into a tube with their contralateral hand when the ipsilateral hand was constrained than did control marmosets with the lesion alone. The marmosets with grafts in the caudate nucleus improved slightly on this task and their scores fell in between, and were not significantly different from, the putamen graft group and the lesion-alone group. When the tube was placed at an angle so as to encourage reaches with the contralateral hand, both the putamen and the caudate graft groups reached significantly further than the lesion-alone group. These improvements were evident 3 months after grafting, and at 6 months the performance of both graft groups matched that of unlesioned controls. The contrast between the significant improvements in this reaching task for the marmosets with grafts in the putamen and the absence of graft effects in the amphet-

amine rotation tests for the same animals indicates that the profile of functional recovery produced by grafts may depend precisely on where the grafts are located in the striatum.

Adrenal and Other Tissue Grafts

The reaching test in which two pieces of food were presented sequentially has also been used by Bankiewicz, Plunkett, and colleagues to assess the hemiparkinsonian monkeys with grafts of adrenal medulla (16,62), adrenal cortex (16), fatty tissue (16), fetal nondopaminergic neural tissue (14), and fetal amnion (13,17) used in the apomorphine rotation tests described under "Adrenal and Other Tissue Grafts" in the section on rotation. In all these studies, the subjects were rhesus monkeys that received unilateral intracarotid infusions of MPTP followed by bilateral transplants of tissue into the precavitated caudate nucleus. The allografts of adrenal medulla (n = 4) were reported to produce a temporary increase, evident 3 but not 6 months after transplantation, in the number of occasions the affected arm was used to accept the second piece of food. Because no surviving TH-positive cells were found at histology, the behavioral changes were attributed to sprouting of residual host dopaminergic fibers. The monkeys with implants of adrenal cortex (n = 1), fat taken from an adult rhesus monkey (n = 1), precavitation of the caudate nucleus alone and no transplant (n = 1), or the MPTP infusion alone and no further surgery (n = 3), did not improve on this test (16). In the second study (62), autografts of adrenal medulla (n = 3) did not produce functional recovery, apart from one case in which the affected arm was used again 8 months after the transplant, although movement was not as fluent as in the unaffected arm, and tremor remained. Further controls with cavities but no transplants (n = 4) did not recover. The transplants of fetal cerebellum (n = 1) or fetal spinal cord (n = 1) also were ineffective in the reaching tests, apart from a transient improvement during the first 6 weeks in the monkey with the spinal cord transplant (14). Hand preference was unaffected in the monkey with bilateral parkinsonism that received a unilateral graft of fetal cerebellum into the caudate nucleus, despite recovery of bradykinesia and tremor (14). The most successful of the alternative tissue transplants performed by Bankiewicz and colleagues with regard to improved use of the affected arm would appear to be the grafts of fetal amnion, although the effects of these grafts have not been reported in full (13). Three of the four monkeys that received amnion grafts started to use the affected arm to take offered pieces of food from 2 to 6 weeks after transplantation. As with the other tissue grafts, the functional changes were attributed to sprouting of host dopaminergic fibers.

An alternative approach to the quantitative assessment of performance with each hand, used by Bakay, Watts, and colleagues, has been to train monkeys to hold and then release or move manipulanda in response to visual signals. Accurate measures of reaction and movement times were then gathered over many trials. In a preliminary report, Watts et al. described one hemiparkinsonian rhesus monkey that was trained to move a handle by making wrist flexion and extension movements (86). Response initiation and movement times with the affected hand were prolonged up to 10 months after MPTP treatment. After a cograft of adrenal medulla and sural nerve into the caudate nucleus, performance gradually improved so that 6 months after the transplant movement times were in the normal range, although response initiation times remained prolonged. Performance with the other hand and histologic details for this particular animal were not reported.

A more detailed account of a task in which a rhesus monkey with an adrenal medulla/sural nerve co-graft was required to depress two levers concurrently, one with each hand, until a signal was given to release one of the levers and touch an illuminated target on a touch-sensitive screen, has been given by Ellis et al (38). During the 18-week period between the unilateral intracarotid infusion of MPTP and the transplant into the caudate nucleus, the monkey was unable to complete any trials with the hand contralateral to the side of the MPTP infusion, whereas performance with the ipsilateral hand remained fairly stable. From about 4 weeks after the transplant, a few responses were completed with the contralateral hand, although these were slow and inaccurate. During subsequent weeks, performance with the contralateral hand gradually improved, until by the end of the study, 30 weeks after transplantation, it approached that with the ipsilateral hand. At histology, surviving chormaffin cells within the graft and sprouting of host TH-positive fibers were observed. Further hemiparkinsonian monkeys with or without cografts of adrenal medulla and sural nerve are being studied on this task (10).

Finally, a novel development in primates has been the use of polymer-encapsulated PC12 cells to provide a source of dopamine that avoids the use of embryonic tissue and the immunologic problems associated with cross-species grafts (48). Four of the five hemiparkinsonian long-tailed macaques that received implants of encapsulated PC12 cells in the striatum were reported to show significant improvements in their ability to use their impaired hand to pick food rewards from wells in a tray, whereas three monkeys that received implants of encapsulated chromaffin cells or the polymer envelopes alone remained impaired. Further details of this experiment, including the location in the striatum of the implants and a full description and time course of the behavioral effects, have yet to be published.

NEGLECT

Neglect of stimuli presented on the side contralateral to a unilateral 6-OHDA lesion is a well documented phenomenon in rats

(55,58,66,67). Hemiparkinsonian monkeys also may neglect stimuli presented on the side contralateral to a prior intracarotid infusion of MPTP (12) or 6-OHDA lesion of the substantia nigra (7). Visual neglect has been measured as a reduction in the angle in the contralateral visual field at which food treats were taken from a revolving arm (12), and as a decrease in the number of attempts to pick up apple pieces arriving from the contralateral side on a conveyor belt (7). A modified version of the adhesive label test designed by Schallert et al. (66,67) for rats has been used to quantify somatosensory neglect as an ipsilateral bias in the response to labels placed bilaterally around monkeys' feet (7). Although neglect may appear like a failure of sensory input, the origin of the deficit in the case of dopamine lesions is more likely to be an impairment in the intention to respond (i.e., a hemiakinesia) (7,12,22,85).

Nigral Grafts

Neglect of contralateral stimuli was assessed in the six marmosets with nigral grafts placed at sites in the caudate nucleus, putamen, and nucleus accumbens studied by Annett et al (2,4). Neglect of either visual or somatosensory stimuli was not abolished by the grafts. In the conveyor belt task, there was some improvement during the months after transplantation in the number of responses when apple pieces arrived from the contralateral side, but the rate of improvement was no greater in the monkeys with grafts than in the lesion-alone controls. In the adhesive label test, the strong lesion-induced bias to contact and remove the label on the ipsilateral foot before that on the contralateral foot persisted for the duration of the study. Long-term ipsilateral biases in the adhesive label test also were observed in the second study, in which marmosets with grafts placed either in the caudate nucleus or in the putamen were compared (3).

How might these negative results be rec-

onciled with a number of reports of graft-dependent recovery of neglect in rats (34–36,57)? Typically, positive graft effects have been observed in studies in which neglect has been measured as impaired response to a tactile probe presented on the side contralateral to the lesion and graft. However, in a more complex version of the test, rats with lesions and grafts ignored the probe if it was presented while they were eating a preferred food, unlike control rats with no lesion that "disengaged" from their current behavior to attend to the stimulus [Björklund et al. (*this volume*)] (57). Also, in the Schallert test (66,67) in which adhesive labels were placed on rats' paws, neglect was not abolished by nigral grafts. Thus, graft-dependent recovery of neglect in rats may be partial rather than complete. In the marmosets with grafts at multiple striatal sites, there may have been some diminution of neglect, although not sufficient to overcome the ipsilateral bias, because the latency to contact the label on the contralateral foot decreased during the months after transplantation (4). In the second study, the marmosets with grafts in the putamen tended to contact the label on the contralateral foot more quickly than the marmosets with grafts in the caudate nucleus or the lesion-alone controls, although the difference between the groups did not achieve statistical significance. This result would be of particular interest if confirmed in future studies, because it would suggest that graft placements that influence somatosensory neglect in monkeys (putamen) may be analogous to those that are known to be effective in rats (ventrolateral striatum) (3,34). Thus, although the data on neglect in monkeys with nigral grafts are extremely limited, they are not incompatible with graft effects on neglect in rats.

Neglect is not normally thought of as a symptom of Parkinson's disease, although it has been reported in some hemiparkinsonian patients (76,84). It is perhaps not surprising that neglect is not a more obvious feature of the disease because, even in cases of hemiparkinsonism, the imbalance in dopamine function between the two striata is unlikely to be as great in patients as it is in animals with unilateral neurotoxic lesions. Nevertheless, neglect is an exceedingly interesting phenomenon and, as a functional deficit that can be assessed quantitatively in monkeys, deserves further investigation in primate neural graft studies.

COGNITIVE TASKS

Cognitive impairments, including deficits in planning, temporal sequencing, and shifting between conceptual sets, have been described in a number of studies of parkinsonian subjects (18,25,52,64,77). The impairments resemble, in some respects, deficits produced by damage to the frontal lobe. Although most MPTP or 6-OHDA primate studies have focused on the motor disabilities produced by the lesion, a few studies have reported cognitive deficits in tasks sensitive to frontal damage in monkeys either with 6-OHDA lesions or dopamine receptor blockade in the frontal cortex (19,65) or after systemic treatment with MPTP (68,80,81). Only one study, by Taylor and colleagues, has attempted to use such a task to assess the cognitive abilities of monkeys with nigral grafts (78).

Nigral Grafts

The paradigm used by Taylor et al. (78) was an object retrieval task in which monkeys were required to reach into a transparent box, open on one side only, to retrieve a piece of banana. The position of the open side of the box, relative to the subject, varied from trial to trial, so on many trials the monkeys had to supress the tendency to reach directly in the line of sight and instead make a detour reach around the box into the open side. The position of the box on the test tray and the position of the banana reward within the box also varied from trial to trial. By manipulating these three vari-

ables, trials were generated that differed in the level of cognitive or motor difficulty required for the monkey to achieve a successful response. The task is described in detail in two papers that report acquisition and performance deficits, respectively, in otherwise asymptomatic MPTP-treated monkeys (without grafts) (80,81). Both cognitive and motor impairments were observed in the MPTP-treated subjects compared to sham controls. Deficits classified as cognitive included more barrier reaches, that is, reaches directed at a closed side of the box, and fewer rewards collected on trials classified as cognitively hard (e.g., when the position of the open side of the box was changed from a preceeding sequence of trials). Motor deficits included failures to retrieve the reward on the first reach into the box and increased initiation times, especially on motorically difficult trials.

The African green monkeys with nigral grafts tested on this complex motor/cognitive task were the same animals for which anatomic (63,70–73) and biochemical (39) descriptions of the grafts were presented in a preceding series of papers, and for which changes in overall motor function were described in a subsequent report (79) (see section on observer evaluation of parkinsonian symptoms—nigral grafts). After systemic pretreatment with MPTP, the monkeys received implants of approximately 1-mm^3 pieces of fetal tissue, either appropriate grafts of nigral tissue into the caudate nucleus (n = 3–4), or inappropriate tissue (cerebellum) into the caudate nucleus (n = 1), or nigral tissue into an inappropriate cortical site (n = 2). Control monkeys that had not been treated with MPTP also received grafts of fetal nigral tissue into the caudate nucleus (n = 3). Statistically significant improvements within subjects over time were reported for three of the monkeys with appropriate grafts on a number of parameters of the object retrieval task. Thus, the number of barrier reaches at the closed side of the box, which had increased after MPTP treatment, declined so that by the fourth month after transplantation performance had reached pretreatment levels and by months 7 to 8 was no different from that of the controls with grafts that had not been treated with MPTP. A similar profile of recovery was reported for impairments classified as motor rather than cognitive, such as the latency to initiate a reach, the percentage of first reaches that successfully retrieved reward, and the number of reaches into the open side of the box on each trial before the reward was retrieved. Crucially, however, no comparison could be made between the cognitive abilities of the monkeys with appropriate and inappropriate grafts because severe motor impairments developed in the subjects in the latter group as a result of the MPTP treatment, which prevented them from even attempting the object retrieval task. Without this comparison, the probability of spontaneous recovery of the cognitive/complex motor skills with practice on the task over the time period of this experiment is uncertain. On the other hand, the long-term performance deficits in otherwise asymptomatic MPTP-treated monkeys reported in a preceding paper suggest that spontaneous recovery of these skills is not inevitable (81).

MECHANISMS OF GRAFT ACTION

The range of mechanisms by which different types of neural grafts may come to produce functional effects is considered in other chapters in this book [Björklund et al., Dunnett and Björklund, and Gash et al. (*this volume*)]. However, the primate work has made an important contribution to the debate about mechanisms of graft action, in particular the processes that may underlie functional recovery in experimental models of parkinsonism. It has been proposed that dopamine released from grafted neurons may not be essential for recovery, but instead damage caused by transplantation procedures may indirectly produce functional benefits (15,16,62). A number of re-

ports have presented histologic evidence of host TH-immunoreactive fibers growing toward graft sites of embryonic nigra, adrenal medulla, or nondopaminergic tissue in the striatum of MPTP-treated monkeys in which cavities were made in the caudate nucleus before transplantation (14–16,42,47,49,62, 86). Sprouting or upregulation of host TH-positive fibers, possibly from mesolimbic dopamine neurons spared by the MPTP lesion, also has been reported in cases in which cavities were made, or a silver coil tissue carrier was embedded in the striatum, but no tissue was transplanted (42,62). Thus, changes in the host dopamine system, perhaps induced by neurotrophic factors released as a consequence of the damage, might conceivably account for behavioral improvements observed in primates with neural grafts. Before such a conclusion can be drawn, however, the evidence for functional recovery in the absence of viable dopaminergic grafts must be considered carefully, because only limited behavioral data are available from a small number of monkeys. Two key questions will be considered here: (1) what evidence is there that surgical damage or transplantation of nondopaminergic tissue into the striatum produce behavioral improvements beyond those that may occur spontaneously; and (2) what evidence is there that viable dopaminergic grafts produce behavioral improvements beyond those that might be accounted for by nonspecific mechanisms related to surgical damage or transplantation of nondopaminergic tissue?

Evidence that surgical damage or transplantation of nondopaminergic tissue in the striatum may reduce behavioral deficits produced by dopaminergic lesions comes primarily from the work of Bankiewicz, Plunkett, and colleagues—specifically, the reductions in apomorphine-induced rotation in the hemiparkinsonian monkeys in which the caudate nucleus was precavitated before tissue transplantation (13,14, 16,17,62). In all, some 18 monkeys have been described in which rotation decreased by 40% to 80% after cavitation alone, or cavitation plus grafts of nondopaminergic neuronal or nonneuronal tissue, including grafts of adrenal medulla in which chromaffin cell survival was poor (see section on rotation—adrenal and other tissue grafts). Crucially, there was no spontaneous recovery of apomorphine-induced rotation in three hemiparkinsonian, surgically intact controls (16). Only two hemiparkinsonian monkeys with cavities and grafts did not show reduced rotation (one adrenal medulla (62) and one fetal amnion graft (13)), the explanation offered in both cases being that there was no sprouting of host TH-positive fibers because the grafts were positioned caudally in the striatum at a site distant from the nucleus accumbens. The study by Watts et al. (86) provides further examples of decreases in apomorphine-induced rotation in monkeys with adrenal medulla grafts despite poor survival of chromaffin cells in the grafts. Again, rotation levels were stable in three hemiparkinsonian, surgically intact controls. Thus, although not confirmed by statistical comparisons between groups in any single report, the weight of available evidence favors the conclusion that transplantation procedures in the absence of viable dopaminergic grafts may affect apomorphine-induced rotation.

In contrast, the evidence that surgical damage or nondopaminergic grafts in the striatum promote recovery of behaviors other than apomorphine-induced rotation is extremely limited. Of the monkeys studied by Bankiewicz, Plunkett, and colleagues, only two with adrenal medulla and one with fetal spinal cord grafts improved in their ability to use the hand contralateral to the MPTP lesion, but the improvements were not sustained (14,16), whereas recovery was delayed and incomplete in a fourth monkey in which the caudate nucleus was cavitated but no tissue was implanted (62). Three of the four monkeys with grafts of fetal amnion were reported to improve in the test of contralateral hand use, but no quantitative data were presented for comparison

with hemiparkinsonian, surgically intact controls (13) (see section on hand and arm movements—adrenal and other tissue grafts). No reductions in amphetamine-induced or spontaneous rotation have been reported in any hemiparkinsonian monkeys in which the caudate nucleus has been cavitated or nondopaminergic tissue implanted. Evidence that transplantation of nondopaminergic tissue ameliorates bilateral parkinsonian symptoms is limited to a descriptive account of recovery in one monkey with a unilateral graft of fetal cerebellum (14) (see section on observer evaluation of parkinsonian symptoms—adrenal and other tissue grafts).

All reports of functional improvements in monkeys in which the striatum has been damaged or nondopaminergic tissue transplanted have been in animals in which MPTP was used to make the initial dopaminergic lesion, and any transplants were made using the open microsurgical approach, which necessarily destroys regions of the caudate nucleus adjacent to the lateral ventricle (56). The possibility that damage-related processes in other regions, for example in the putamen, might improve behaviors such as volitional use of the contralateral hand has not been explored. Nondopaminergic grafts placed stereotactically in the striatum did not promote recovery in two MPTP-treated monkeys reported by Fine et al. (43) and one reported by Taylor et al. (78,79) (see "Nigral Grafts" in sections on observer evaluation of parkinsonian symptoms, and locomotion). Because the mechanism of recovery proposed by Bankiewicz and colleagues (15,16) depends on residual host mesolimbic dopaminergic fibers spared by the MPTP lesion, it seems unlikely that striatal damage could lead to recovery in cases in which mesolimbic dopamine loss was more complete, for example after a 6-OHDA lesion (7). Unfortunately, there have been no behavioral comparisons of 6-OHDA-lesioned monkeys with and without damage or nondopaminergic grafts in the striatum. In our own work with 6-OHDA-lesioned marmosets, any damage to the striatum that may have been caused by injections of saline (4), rejection of cross-species grafts (unpublished observations), or grafts of relatively old embryonic ventral mesencephalon (see section on rotation—nigral grafts), did not reduce amphetamine-induced rotation. Recovery due to surgical damage or transplantation of nondopaminergic tissue in the striatum may therefore be limited to apomorphine-induced rotation, and also may occur only under certain conditions, namely if the dopamine lesion is incomplete and damage in the striatum is relatively severe (i.e., that caused by cavitation and not by stereotaxic surgery).

Evidence relevant to the second question comes mainly from studies of the behavior of monkeys with grafts of embryonic nigra. Again, no single report has compared, with statistically confirmed differences between groups, the behavior of monkeys with embryonic nigral grafts to that of controls with surgical damage or alternative tissue grafts in the striatum. However, although limited, there is evidence that suggests that viable dopaminergic grafts may have functional effects beyond those that might be accounted for by nonspecific, damage-related mechanisms. The absence of recovery in the monkeys with control grafts of nondopaminergic tissue reported by Fine et al. (43) and by Taylor et al. (78,79) contrasts with functional improvements in monkeys with embryonic nigral grafts in the same studies (see "Nigral Grafts" in sections on observer evaluation of parkinsonian symptoms, and locomotion). Bankiewicz, Plunkett, and colleagues commented that the degree and time course of recovery in their monkeys with nigral grafts were greater and faster than those observed in the monkeys with grafts of adrenal medulla, adrenal cortex or fat, or cavitation of the caudate nucleus. Most importantly, the nigral grafts restored volitional use of the hand contralateral to the MPTP lesion (15,16,62) (see section on hand and arm movements—ni-

gral grafts). Two further pieces of evidence from Bankiewicz's work suggest that the functional impact of nigral grafts was greater than that of cavitation alone: first, the spontaneous rotation by the parkinsonian monkey in which the caudate nucleus was cavitated bilaterally but the nigral graft placed unilaterally, and second, the temporary behavioral improvement in the hemiparkinsonian (bilaterally cavitated) monkey that was not sustained when the nigral graft was rejected (see section on rotation—nigral grafts).

Whereas the grafts of adult nondopaminergic tissue clearly were not as effective as the embryonic nigral grafts in the experiments of Bankiewicz, Plunkett, and colleagues, the recovery observed after transplantation of nondopaminergic tissue of embryonic/fetal origin did more closely resemble that observed after transplantation of embryonic nigra. Thus, the magnitude of the effect of the fetal cerebellar and spinal cord grafts on apomorphine-induced rotation was equal to that of embryonic nigral grafts (although volitional use of the contralateral hand was not restored) (14), whereas the amnion grafts reduced apomorphine-induced rotation and improved contralateral hand use (13). The amnion and embryonic nigra grafts were compared in a table in ref. 17: good recovery (behavioral measure not specified) was seen in two of the four monkeys with amnion grafts and three of the five with nigral grafts. On the other hand, evidence against transplantation of embryonic tissue *per se* promoting recovery is, of course, the absence of any behavioral change in the control monkeys with embryonic nondopaminergic grafts described by Fine et al. (43) and Taylor et al (78,79). Clearly, further behavioral comparisons between monkeys with grafts of embryonic dopaminergic and nondopaminergic tissue are needed to clarify this issue. At present, insufficient quantitative behavioral data are available to warrant any firm conclusions about the capacity of embryonic/fetal nondopaminergic grafts, compared to embryonic dopaminergic grafts, to ameliorate parkinsonian symptoms in primates.

CONCLUSIONS

Overall, the published reports of behavioral effects of neural grafts in parkinsonian primates have been disappointing in several respects. It remains the case, some 9 years after the first reports of neural tissue transplantion into monkeys, that in most studies the effects of neural grafts on behavior have either not been rigorously assessed or adequately reported. In particular, in many studies too few subjects have been used to permit statistical comparisons between groups of subjects in a controlled experimental design. Behavioral assessment of monkeys with grafts often has not been conducted in parallel with assessment of monkeys in lesion control groups. Whereas there is no doubt that neurotoxic dopaminergic lesions can produce stable, long-term behavioral deficits in individual monkeys, this cannot be assumed to be the case in every monkey that receives such a lesion. Thus, for each behavioral test, adequate lesion controls are essential to provide estimates of the probability of spontaneous recovery and the variability between animals against which potential graft effects can be judged. Although the main purpose of using primates in neural graft studies is to address questions directly relevant to the clinical application of neural transplantation, so far most studies have not advanced beyond a basic demonstration that neural grafts can have functional effects in parkinsonian primates. Those studies that have examined specific issues have done no more than confirm what was already known from rodent work. For example, the recent demonstration that the age of the donor embryo is important for successful transplantation of embryonic nigra in monkeys confirms previous findings with grafts of both rat and human nigral tissue in rats. Investigation of the functional importance of graft location

within the striatum has only just begun in monkeys, and this work must be extended to include further graft sites and behavioral tests to determine which sites, or combination of sites, are likely to bring the greatest functional benefits to patients.

On a more positive note, some of the most recent studies of neural grafts in parkinsonian primates have presented firm evidence of recovery of function after transplantation—for example, the improvements in the parkinsonian symptoms (with the possible exception of tremor) and general health of monkeys with bilateral MPTP lesions after transplantation of embryonic nigra into the striatum (79). Rotation tests also have provided definite evidence of functional graft effects in a number of monkeys (2,4,15,28). Unfortunately, although useful as a demonstration of graft viability *in vivo,* graft effects on rotation are not particularly useful for predicting other behavioral changes in the same animals, nor for anticipating how grafts might affect motor deficits in parkinsonian patients. Of more direct clinical relevance are the demonstrations of improved use of the hand and arm contralateral to the grafted striatum, principally in monkeys with grafts of embryonic nigra (2,4,15,45), but also in a few cases with co-grafts of adrenal medulla and sural nerve (38,86). Development of tasks such as these that quantify motor performance with the limb contralateral to a neural graft may prove especially worthwhile in future primate studies with the aim of defining more precisely the extent to which grafts can restore normal function.

With respect to the mechanisms of graft action in animal models of parkinsonism, the monkey neural graft literature has raised a number of questions that must be addressed in future studies. The behavioral evidence that viable dopaminergic cells in grafts are not essential for functional recovery in parkinsonian primates depends almost exclusively on one behavioral measure, apomorphine-induced rotation, and has been explored in only one type of lesion model, MPTP-induced hemiparkinsonism. That grafts of nondopaminergic tissue, or indeed surgical damage in the striatum, can produce reliable and substantial reductions in parkinsonian symptoms in monkeys remains unproven. From the evidence currently available, dopaminergic grafts appear to be behaviorally more effective than transplants of nondopaminergic tissue or surgical damage in the striatum, with the possible exception of transplants of nondopaminergic tissue of embryonic/fetal origin. The conclusion is only tentative, however, given the paucity of data directly comparing the behavioral effects of different types of grafts and surgical procedures. Experiments designed specifically to make such comparisons, using a range of behavioral measures, are needed to clarify mechanisms of graft action in parkinsonian primates.

ACKNOWLEDGMENTS

I thank S. B. Dunnett, E. M. Torres, R. M. Ridley, H. F. Baker, and D. J. Clarke for collaborating in experiments reviewed in this chapter, and Professor C. D. Marsden for his interest and encouragement in our research. Our work has been generously supported by the Parkinson's Disease Society of Great Britain and The Wellcome Trust.

REFERENCES

1. Abrous DN, Torres EM, Annett LE, Reading PJ, Dunnett SB. Intrastriatal dopamine-rich grafts induce a hyperexpression of Fos protein when challenged with amphetamine. *Exp Brain Res* 1992;91:181–190.
2. Annett LE, Dunnett SB, Martel FL, et al. A functional assessment of embryonic dopaminergic grafts in the marmoset. *Prog Brain Res* 1990;82:535–542.
3. Annett LE, Dunnett SB, Torres EM, Ridley RM, Baker HF, Marsden CD. Behavioural assessment of embryonic nigral grafts placed in the caudate nucleus and/or putamen of 6-OHDA lesioned marmosets. *Eur J Neurosci* 1991;(Suppl 4):248.
4. Annett LE, Martel FL, Rogers DC, Ridley RM, Baker HF, Dunnett SB. Behavioural assessment of the effects of embryonic nigral grafts in marmosets with unilateral 6-OHDA lesions of the nigrostriatal pathway. *Exp Neurol* 1994;125:228–246.
5. Annett LE, Reading PJ, Tharumaratnam D, Abrous DN, Torres EM, Dunnett SB. Conditioning versus priming of dopaminergic grafts by amphetamine. *Exp Brain Res* 1993;93:46–54.
6. Annett LE, Ridley RM, Gamble SJ, Baker HF. Behavioural effects of intracerebral amphetamine in the marmoset. *Psychopharmacology* 1983;81:18–23.
7. Annett LE, Rogers DC, Hernandez TD, Dunnett SB. Behavioural analysis of unilateral monoamine depletion in the marmoset. *Brain* 1992; 115:825–856.
8. Bakay RAE, Barrow DL, Fiandaca MS, Iuvone PM, Schiff A, Collins DC. Biochemical and behavioural correction of MPTP Parkinsonian-like syndrome by fetal cell transplantation. *Ann NY Acad Sci* 1987;495:623–640.
9. Bakay RAE, Fiandaca MS, Barrow DL, Schiff A, Collins DC. Preliminary report on the use of fetal tissue transplantation to correct MPTP-induced parkinsonian-like syndrome in primates. *Appl Neurophysiol* 1985;48:358–361.
10. Bakay RAE, Watts RL, Byrd LD, Mandir A. Quantifying the improvement following CNS transplantation in hemiparkinsonian monkeys using operant behavioural tasks. *Rest Neurol Neurosci* 1992;4:175.
11. Bankiewicz KS, Oldfield EH, Chiueh CC, Doppman JL, Jacobowitz DM, Kopin IJ. Hemiparkinsonism in monkeys after unilateral internal carotid artery infusion of 1-methyl-4-phenyl-1,2,3,6-tetrahydropyridine (MPTP). *Life Sci* 1986; 39:7–16.
12. Bankiewicz KS, Oldfield EH, Plunkett RJ, et al. Apparent unilateral visual neglect in MPTP-hemiparkinsonian monkeys is due to delayed initiation of motion. *Brain Res* 1991;541:98–102.
13. Bankiewicz KS, Plunkett RJ, Jacobowitz DM, Kopin IJ, Cummins AC, Oldfield EH. Behavioural recovery in MPTP-hemiparkinsonian monkeys after amnion implantation into the head of the caudate nucleus. *Rest Neurol Neurosci* 1990;1:110.
14. Bankiewicz KS, Plunkett RJ, Jacobowitz DM, Kopin IJ, Oldfield EH. Fetal nondopaminergic neural implants in parkinsonian primates. *J Neurosurg* 1991;74:97–104.
15. Bankiewicz KS, Plunkett RJ, Jacobowitz DM, et al. The effect of fetal mesencephalon implants on primate MPTP-induced parkinsonism. *J Neurosurg* 1990;72:231–244.
16. Bankiewicz KS, Plunkett RJ, Kopin IJ, Jacobowitz DM, London WT, Oldfield EH. Transient behavioural recovery in hemiparkinsonian primates after adrenal medullary allografts. *Prog Brain Res* 1988;78:543–549.
17. Bankiewicz KS, Plunkett RJ, Mefford I, Kopin IJ, Oldfield EH. Behavioural recovery from MPTP-induced parkinsonism in monkeys after intracerebral tissue implants is not related to

CSF concentrations of dopamine metabolites. *Prog Brain Res* 1990;82:561–571.

18. Brown RG, Marsden CD. Cognitive function in Parkinson's disease: from description to theory. *Trends Neurosci* 1990;13:21–29.

19. Brozoski TJ, Brown RM, Rosvold IIE, Goldman PS. Cognitive deficit caused by regional depletion of dopamine in prefrontal cortex of rhesus monkey. *Science* 1979;205:929–932.

20. Brundin P. Dissection, preparation, and implantation of human embryonic brain tissue. In: Dunnett SB, Björklund A, eds. *Neural transplantation: a practical approach*. Oxford: IRL Press; 1993:139–160.

21. Burns RS, Chiueh CC, Markey SP, Ebert MH, Jacobowitz DM, Kopin IJ. A primate model of parkinsonism: selective destruction of dopaminergic neurons in the pars compacta of the substantia nigra by N-methyl-4-phenyl-1,2,3,6-tetrahydropyridine. *Proc Natl Acad Sci USA* 1983; 80:4546–4550.

22. Carli M, Evenden JL, Robbins TW. Depletion of unilateral striatal dopamine impairs initiation of contralateral actions and not sensory attention. *Nature* 1985;313:679–682.

23. Cenci MA, Kalen P, Mandel RJ, Wictorin K, Björklund A. Dopaminergic transplants normalize amphetamine- and apomorphine-induced Fos expression in the 6-hydroxydopamine lesioned striatum. *Neuroscience* 1992;46:943–957.

24. Clarke CE, Boyce S, Robertson RG, Sambrook MA, Crossman AR. Drug-induced dyskinesia in primates rendered hemiparkinsonian by intracarotid administration of 1-methyl-4-phenyl-1, 2,3,6-tetrahydropyridine (MPTP). *J Neurol Sci* 1989;90:307–314.

25. Downes JJ, Roberts AC, Sahakian BJ, Evenden JL, Morris RG, Robbins TW. Impaired extra-dimensional shift performance in medicated and unmedicated Parkinson's disease: evidence for a specific attentional dysfunction. *Neuropsychologia* 1989;27:1329–1343.

26. Dubach M. Adrenal medullary "ribbon" grafts in non-human primates: transplant method. *J Neurosci Methods* 1991;39:19–28.

27. Dubach M. Viable adrenal medullary transplants in non-human primates: increasing the number of grafts. *J Neural Trans Plasticity* 1992;3:81–96.

28. Dubach M. Behavioural effects of adrenal medullary transplants in non-human primates. *J Neural Trans Plasticity* 1992;3:97–114.

29. Dubach M, German DC. Extensive survival of chromaffin cells in adrenal medulla "ribbon" grafts in the monkey neostriatum. *Exp Neurol* 1990;110:167–180.

30. Dubach M, Schmidt R, Kunkel D, Bowden DM, Martin R, German DC. Primate neostriatal neurons containing tyrosine hydroxylase: immunohistochemical evidence. *Neurosci Lett* 1987; 75:205–210.

31. Dubach M, Schmidt RH, Martin R, German DC, Bowden DM. Transplant improves hemiparkinsonian syndrome in nonhuman primate: intracerebral injection, rotometry, tyrosine hydroxy-lase immunohistochemistry. *Prog Brain Res* 1988;78:491–496.

32. Dunnett SB, Annett LE. Nigral transplants in primate models of parkinsonism. In: Lindvall O, Björklund A, Widner H, eds. *Intracerebral transplantation in movement disorders*. Amsterdam: Elsevier; 1991:27–51.

33. Dunnett SB, Björklund A. Staging and dissection of rat embryos. In: Dunnett SB, Björklund A, eds. *Neural transplantation: a practical approach*. Oxford: IRL Press; 1992:1–19.

34. Dunnett SB, Björklund A, Schmidt RH, Stenevi U, Iversen SD. Intracerebral grafting of neuronal cell suspensions: IV. behavioural recovery in rats with unilateral implants of nigral cell suspensions in different forebrain sites. *Acta Physiol Scand [Suppl]* 1983;522:29–37.

35. Dunnett SB, Björklund A, Stenevi U, Iversen SD. Behavioural recovery following transplantation of substantia nigra in rats subjected to unilateral 6-OHDA lesions of the nigrostriatal pathway. *Brain Res* 1981;215:147–161.

36. Dunnett SB, Whishaw IQ, Rogers DC, Jones GH. Dopamine-rich grafts ameliorate whole body motor asymmetry and sensory neglect but not independent limb use in rats with 6-hydroxydopamine lesions. *Brain Res* 1987;415:63–78.

37. Eidelberg E, Brooks BA, Morgan WW, Walden JG, Kokemoor RH. Variability and functional recovery in the N-methyl-4-phenyl-1,2,3,6-tetrahydropyridine model of parkinsonism in monkeys. *Neuroscience* 1986;18:817–822.

38. Ellis JE, Byrd LD, Bakay RAE. A method for quantitating motor deficits in a nonhuman primate following MPTP-induced hemiparkinsonism and co-grafting. *Exp Neurol* 1992;115:376–387.

39. Elsworth JD, Redmond DE, Sladek JR Jr, Deutch AY, Collier TJ, Roth RH. Reversal of MPTP-induced parkinsonism in primates by fetal dopamine cell transplants. In: Franks AJ, Ironside JW, Mindham RHS, Smith RJ, Spokes EGS, Winlow W, eds. *Function and dysfunction in the basal ganglia*. Manchester: Manchester University Press; 1990:161–180.

40. Everitt BJ, Sirkia TE, Roberts AC, Jones GH, Robbins TW. Distribution and some projections of cholinergic neurons in the brain of the common marmoset. *J Comp Neurol* 1988;271:533–558.

41. Fiandaca MS, Bakay RAE, Sweeney KM, Chan WC. Immunologic response to intracerebral fetal neural allografts in the rhesus monkey. *Prog Brain Res* 1988;78:287–296.

42. Fiandaca MS, Kordower JH, Hansen TJ, Jiao SS, Gash DM. Adrenal medullary autografts into the basal ganglia of cebus monkeys: injury-induced regeneration. *Exp Neurol* 1988;102: 76–91.

43. Fine A, Hunt SP, Oertel WH, et al. Transplantation of embryonic marmoset dopaminergic neurons to the corpus striatum of marmosets rendered parkinsonian by 1-methyl-4-phenyl-1,2,3,6-tetrahydropyridine. *Prog Brain Res* 1988; 78:479–489.

44. Freed CR, Breeze RE, Rosenberg NL, et al. Survival of implanted fetal dopamine cells and neurologic improvement 12 to 46 months after transplantation for Parkinson's disease. *N Engl J Med* 1992;327:1549–1555.

45. Freed CR, Richards JB, Sabol KE, Reite ML. Fetal substantia nigra transplants lead to dopamine cell replacement and behavioural improvement in bonnet monkeys with MPTP induced parkinsonism. In: Beart PM, Woodruff GN, Jackson DM, eds. *Pharmacology and functional regulation of dopaminergic neurons.* London: Macmillan; 1988:353–360.

46. Freeman TB, Nauert GM, Olanow CW, Kordower JH. Influence of donor age on the survival of human embryonic dopaminergic neural grafts. *Rest Neurol Neurosci* 1992;4:180.

47. Gash DM, Kordower JH, Fiandaca MS, Hansen JT. Adrenal medullary transplants in primates. In: Lindvall O, Björklund A, Widner H, eds. *Intracerebral transplantation in movement disorders.* Amsterdam: Elsevier; 1991:15–25.

48. Goddard M, Signore AP, Timpson RL, Aebischer P. Functional recovery in hemiparkinsonian primates transplanted with polymer encapsulated PC12 cells. *Rest Neurol Neurosci* 1992;4:169–170.

49. Hansen JT, Kordower JH, Fiandaca MS, Jiao SS, Notter MFD, Gash DM. Adrenal medullary autografts into the basal ganglia of cebus monkeys: graft viability and fine structure. *Exp Neurol* 1988;102:65–75.

50. Herman JP, Choulli K, LeMoal M. Hyper-reactivity to amphetamine in rats with dopaminergic grafts. *Exp Brain Res* 1985;60:521–526.

51. Kurlan R, Kim MH, Gash DM. The time course and magnitude of spontaneous recovery of parkinsonism produced by intracarotid administration of 1-methyl-4-phenyl-1,2,3,6-tetrahydropyridine to monkeys. *Ann Neurol* 1991;29:677–679.

52. Lees AJ, Smith E. Cognitive deficits in the early stages of Parkinson's disease. *Brain* 1983;106:257–270.

53. Lindvall O. Prospects of transplantation in human neurodegenerative diseases. *Trends Neurosci* 1991;14:376–384.

54. Lindvall O, Widner H, Rehncrona S, et al. Transplantation of fetal dopamine neurons in Parkinson's disease: one year clinical and neurophysiological observations in 2 patients with putaminal implants. *Ann Neurol* 1992;31:155–165.

55. Ljungbert T, Ungerstedt U. Sensory inattention produced by 6-hydroxydopamine-induced degeneration of ascending dopamine neurons in the brain. *Exp Neurol* 1976;53:585–600.

56. Madrazo I, Drucker-Colìn R, Dìaz V, Martìnez-Mata J, Torres C, Becerril JJ. Open microsurgical autograft of adrenal medulla to the right caudate nucleus in two patients with intractable Parkinson's disease. *N Engl J Med* 1987;316:831–834.

57. Mandel RJ, Brundin P, Björklund A. The importance of graft placement and task complexity for transplant-induced recovery of simple and complex sensorimotor deficits in dopamine denervated rats. *Eur J Neurosci* 1990;2:888–894.

58. Marshall JF, Teitelbaum P. Further analysis of sensory inattention following lateral hypothalamic damage in rats. *J Comp Physiol Psychol* 1974;86:375–395.

59. Morihisa JM, Nakamura RK, Freed WJ, Mishkin M, Wyatt RJ. Adrenal medulla grafts survive and exhibit catecholamine-specific fluorescence in the primate brain. *Exp Neurol* 1984;84:643–653.

60. Nakai M, Itakura T, Kamei I, et al. Autologous transplantation of the superior cervical ganglion into the brain of parkinsonian monkeys. *J Neurosurg* 1990;72:91–95.

61. Olson L, Seiger Å, Strömberg I. Intraocular transplantation in rodents: a detailed account of the procedure and examples of its use in neurobiology with special reference to brain tissue grafting. In: Fedoroff S, Hertz L, eds. *Advances in cellular neurobiology.* Vol 4. New York: Academic Press; 1983:407–422.

62. Plunkett RJ, Bankiewicz KS, Cummins AC, Miletich RS, Schwartz JP, Oldfield EH. Long-term evaluation of hemiparkinsonian monkeys after adrenal autografting or cavitation alone. *J Neurosurg* 1990;73:918–926.

63. Redmond DE, Sladek JR Jr, Roth RH, et al. Fetal neuronal grafts in monkeys given methylphenyltetrahydropyridine. *Lancet* 1986;1:1125–1127.

64. Sagar HJ, Sullivan EV, Gabrieli JDE, Corkin S, Growdon JH. Temporal ordering and short-term memory deficits in Parkinson's disease. *Brain* 1988;111:525–539.

65. Sawaguchi T, Goldman-Rakic PS. D1 dopamine receptors in prefrontal cortex: involvement in working memory. *Science* 1991;251:947–950.

66. Schallert T, Upchurch M, Lobaugh N, et al. Tactile extinction: distinguishing between sensorimotor and motor asymmetries in rats with unilateral nigrostriatal damage. *Pharmacol Biochem Behav* 1982;16:455–462.

67. Schallert T, Upchurch M, Wilcox RE, Vaughn DM. Posture-independent sensorimotor analysis of inter-hemispheric receptor asymmetries in neostriatum. *Pharmacol Biochem Behav* 1983;18:753–759.

68. Schneider JS, Kovelowski CJ. Chronic exposure to low doses of MPTP: I. cognitive deficits in motor asymptomatic monkeys. *Brain Res* 1990;519:122–128.

69. Sladek JR Jr, Collier TJ, Elsworth JD, Taylor JR, Roth RH, Redmond DE. Fetal dopamine neuronal grafts in parkinsonian non-human primates. *Rest Neurol Neurosci* 1992;4:185.

70. Sladek JR Jr, Collier TJ, Haber SN, et al. Reversal of parkinsonian by fetal nerve cell transplants in primate brain. *Ann NY Acad Sci* 1987;495:641–657.

71. Sladek JR Jr, Collier TJ, Haber SN, Roth RH, Redmond DE. Survival and growth of fetal catecholamine neurons transplanted into primate brain. *Brain Res Bull* 1986;17:809–818.

72. Sladek JR Jr, Redmond DE, Collier TJ, et al. Fetal dopamine neural grafts: extended reversal of methylphenyltetrahydropyridine-induced parkinsonism in monkeys. *Prog Brain Res* 1988;78:497–506.

73. Sladek JR Jr, Redmond DE, Collier TJ, Haber SN, et al. Transplantation of fetal dopamine neurons in primate brain reverses MPTP induced parkinsonism. *Prog Brain Res* 1987;71:309–323.

74. Smith RD, Zhang Z, Kurlan R, McDermott M, Gash DM. Developing a stable bilateral model of parkinsonism in rhesus monkeys. *Neuroscience* 1993;52:7–16.

75. Spencer DD, Robbins RJ, Naftolin F, et al. Unilateral transplantation of human fetal mesencephalic tissue into the caudate nucleus of patients with Parkinson's disease. *N Engl J Med* 1992;327:1541–1548.

76. Starkstein S, Leiguarda O, Gershanik O, Berthier M. Neuropsychological disturbances in hemiparkinson's disease. *Neurology* 1987;37:1762–1764.

77. Taylor AE, Saint-Cyr JA, Lang AE. Frontal lobe dysfunction in Parkinson's disease. *Brain* 1986;109:845–883.

78. Taylor JR, Elsworth JD, Roth RH, Collier TJ, Sladek JR Jr, Redmond DE. Improvements in MPTP-induced object retrieval deficits and behavioural deficits after fetal nigral grafting in monkeys. *Prog Brain Res* 1990;82:543–559.

79. Taylor JR, Elsworth JD, Roth RH, Sladek JR Jr, Collier TJ, Redmond DE. Grafting of fetal substantia nigra to striatum reverses behavioural deficits induced by MPTP in primates: a comparison with other types of grafts as controls. *Exp Brain Res* 1991;85:335–348.

80. Taylor JR, Elsworth JD, Roth RH, Sladek JR Jr, Redmond DE. Cognitive and motor deficits in the acquisition of an object retrieval/detour task in MPTP-treated monkeys. *Brain* 1990;113:617–637.

81. Taylor JR, Roth RH, Sladek JR Jr, Redmond DE. Cognitive and motor deficits in the performance of an object retrieval task with barrier/detour in monkeys treated with MPTP: long-term performance and effect of transparency of the barrier. *Behav Neurosci* 1990;104:564–576.

82. Torres EM, Rogers DC, Annett LE, Sirinathsinghji DJS, Dunnett SB. A novel population of tyrosine hydroxylase immunoreactive neurons in the basal forebrain of the common marmoset (*Callithrix jacchus*). *Neurosci Lett* 1993;150:29–32.

83. Ungerstedt U, Arbuthnott GW. Quantitative recording of rotational behaviour in rats after 6-hyrodroxydopamine lesions of the nigrostriatal dopamine system. *Brain Res* 1970;24:485–493.

84. Villardita C, Smirni P, Zappalà G. Visual neglect in Parkinson's disease. *Arch Neurol* 1983;40:737–739.

85. Watson RT, Heilman KM, Miller BD, King FA. Neglect after mesencephalic reticular formation lesions. *Neurology* 1974;24:294–298.

86. Watts RL, Bakay RAE, Herring CJ, et al. Preliminary report on adrenal medullary grafting and cografting with sural nerve in the treatment of hemiparkinsonian monkeys. *Prog Brain Res* 1990;82:581–591.

87. Widner H, Tetrud J, Rehncrona S, et al. Bilateral fetal mesencephalic grafting in two patients with parkinsonism induced by 1-methyl-4-phenyl-1,2,3,6-tetrahydropyridine (MPTP). *N Engl J Med* 1992;327:1556–1563.

88. Wisniowski L, Ridley RM, Baker HF, Fine A. Tyrosine hydroxylase-immunoreactive neurons in the nucleus basalis of the common marmoset (*Callithrix jacchus*). *J Comp Neurol* 1992;325:379–387.

Functional Neural Transplantation,
edited by S. B. Dunnett and A. Björklund.
Raven Press, Ltd., New York © 1994.

5

Neural Transplantation in Parkinson's Disease

Olle Lindvall

*Restorative Neurology Unit, Department of Neurology, University Hospital,
S–22 1 85 Lund, Sweden*

Idiopathic Parkinson's disease (PD) is a progressive neurodegenerative disorder of unknown etiology characterized by tremor, rigidity, hypokinesia, and postural instability (155). The disease usually begins between 40 and 60 years of age, with the peak of onset in the sixth decade. The prevalence of PD has been estimated to be between 85 to 187 per 100,000 population (155). The characteristic pathologic finding is a loss of dopaminergic neurons in the pars compacta of the substantia nigra, resulting in a degeneration of the mesostriatal pathway and a severe depletion of striatal dopamine (DA). This loss of dopaminergic input to the striatum is responsible for the major motor symptomatology of PD. L-dopa treatment initially provides a marked symptomatic relief in most cases, but within 5 to 10 years, most patients with PD show a progressive loss of efficacy of L-dopa associated with diurnal oscillations in motor performance ("on–off" phenomena) and dyskinesias. Although at this stage the patients often temporarily benefit from changes in medication, most patients become severely incapacitated. For this large group of patients, there is a need for new therapeutic approaches.

Cell transplantation as a possible new treatment for patients with PD was suggested in the late 1970s, when it was first reported that intrastriatal implants of DA-rich ventral mesencephalic tissue from rat embryos could reduce the symptoms of ex-

perimental parkinsonism in adult rats (14, 115). Since then, the bulk of experimental evidence from studies in rats with 6-hydroxydopamine (6-OHDA)-induced lesions of the mesostriatal DA system indicates that grafted embryonic DA neurons can reinnervate and form synaptic contacts with host striatal neurons, receive afferent inputs from the host, release DA spontaneously, restore striatal DA levels and lesion-induced deficits in gene expression in striatal neurons, and reverse some of the motor and sensorimotor behavioral abnormalities [see chapter by Brundin (*this volume*)]. Similar studies in monkeys with parkinsonism induced by 1-methyl-4-phenyl-1,2,3,6-tetrahydropyridine (MPTP) or 6-OHDA have indicated graft survival, fiber outgrowth, restoration of DA turnover, and reduction of parkinsonian symptoms [see chapter by Annett (*this volume*)]. Based on these data obtained in animal models, clinical trials with transplantation of embryonic, DA-rich mesencephalic tissue have been initiated in patients with PD. From the clinical point of view, the most attractive feature with neural grafts in PD is the possibility of reinstating a physiologic, at least partly regulated, synaptic release of DA in the striatum. Such a restoration of DA transmission, confined to the region deprived of its intrinsic dopaminergic input, cannot be achieved with any other therapeutic approach. It must be underscored, however, that the neural grafting proce-

TABLE 1. *Study design of clinical trials with grafting of human embryonic mesencephalic tissue into the striatum of patients with Parkinson's disease*

Authors	Number of patients	Tissue preparation[a]/ surgical technique[b]/ unilateral or bilateral	Location[d]/ number[e] of implantations	Number[f]/age[g] of fetal cadavers
Lindvall et al. (87,88)	2	Diss/ster/uni	Caud/1 + Put/2	4/8–10 w (m)
Lindvall et al. (86,89,90)	2	Diss/ster/uni	Put/3	4/8–10 w (m)
Madrazo et al. (97,99)	4	Fragm/open/uni	Caud/1	1/12–14 w (g)
Molina et al. (104)	30	Fragm/open/uni	Caud/1	1/6–12 w
Henderson et al. (61)	12	Diss/ster/uni	Caud/1	1/11–19 w (g)
Freed et al. (47,48)	7	Diss or strand/ster/ uni (2)[c] or bi (5)	Caud + Put uni (2)[c] or Put bi (5)/10–14	1 (6)[c] or 2 (1)/7–8 w (g)
Lopez-Lozano et al. (93)	7	Fragm/open/uni	Caud/1	1/8–17 w (m)
Widner et al. (162)	2	Diss/ster/bi	Caud/1 + Put/ 3 bi (1); Caud/0–1 + Put/3 bi (1)	6–8/6–8 w (pc)
Spencer et al. (140)	4	Fragm (cryo)/ster/uni	Caud/2–4	1/7–11 w (g)

[a]Diss, cell suspension or dissociated tissue; Fragm, tissue fragments; Strand, strand of tissue; Cryo, cryopreserved.

[b]Ster, stereotaxic implantation; open, open microsurgery with implantation into a cavity.

[c]Number of patients within parentheses.

[d]Caud, caudate nucleus; Put, putamen; uni, unilateral; bi, bilateral.

[e]Number of implantation sites.

[f]Number of fetal donors for tissue implanted in each patient.

[g]Age of fetal cadavers (weeks) as reported: m, menstrual; g, gestational; pc, postconception.

[h]Time period during which the patient is included in the transplantation program and subjected to regular clinical assessments: n.r., not reported.

[i]Defined as from start of preoperative assessment to 6 months postoperatively.

[j]PET, positron emission tomography; CSF, cerebrospinal fluid.

dures have not yet been optimized in animal experiments; even in animals, a complete reversal of parkinsonian symptoms cannot be effected by neural grafts. The major scientific question in the first studies in patients therefore has not been to clarify whether neural grafting is better than established drug treatments, but to explore if survival and function of such grafts are at all possible in patients with PD. The more general goal of the clinical trials carried out so far has been to explore if the basic principles of cell replacement, established in animal experiments, are valid in the diseased human brain as well.

The objective of this chapter is to summarize the evidence that surviving functional neural grafts can be obtained in the human parkinsonian brain, and, further-more, to discuss, from a clinical perspective, both the present status of neural grafting as a therapeutic strategy in PD, and the further developments to increase symptomatic relief as well as find DA-producing implants other than ventral mesencephalic tissue from aborted human embryos.

CLINICAL TRIALS IN PATIENTS WITH PARKINSON'S DISEASE

Transplantation of Embryonic Dopamine Neurons: Design and Results of Studies

An estimated 140 patients with PD have so far received implants of human embryonic mesencephalic tissue into the striatum.

Duration of pre/ postoperative assessment period[h]	Changes of antiparkinsonian medication during study period[i]	Immunosuppression	Attempts to show graft survival[j]
6 mo/20 mo	No	Yes	PET
6–11 mo/36 mo	No	Yes	PET
n.r./19–32 mo	Yes	Yes	No
30–45 d/ – 24 mo	Yes	Yes	CSF
1–6 w/12 mo	Yes	No	No
4–12 mo/12–46 mo	Yes	Yes (4)[c]; No (3)	PET
n.r./7 mo	Yes	Yes	No
18 mo/22–24 mo	No	Yes	PET
n.r./18 mo	Yes	Yes	PET

Tables 1 and 2 summarize the (often incomplete) data reported from clinical studies performed on 70 patients. Two major surgical approaches have been used: stereotaxic implantation of dissociated tissue directly into the striatum (Fig. 1), or placement of pieces or fragments of nigral tissue into a cavity in the head of the caudate nucleus. The grafts have been placed unilaterally and, in seven patients, bilaterally in the caudate nucleus or putamen. In most studies, tissue from only one embryo has been used in each patient, but Lindvall et al. (86–90) implanted tissue from four embryos, and the patients grafted bilaterally by Widner et al. (162) received mesencephalic tissue from six to eight embryonic cadavers. Embryonic ages have varied from 6 to 19 weeks. The preoperative assessment period ranges from 1 to 12 months, and in several cases has not been reported. In most studies, except in those of Lindvall et al. (86–90) and Widner et al. (162), doses of antiparkinsonian medication were changed at the time of transplantation or during the first 6 postoperative months. All patients were subjected to immunosup-

pressive treatment except those operated by Hitchcock and coworkers (61) and three of the patients of Freed et al. (47,48). Few attempts to show graft survival have been undertaken.

The reported results can be summarized as follows (see Table 2): (1) Some general improvement of motor symptoms has been observed in almost all patients after implantation of embryonic mesencephalic tissue. The degree of this functional change varies from minor to moderate, but in no case has there been a full reversal of symptomatology. (2) The improvement has been observed as a prolonged duration of L-dopa response (86,90), and by several groups as an increased percentage of time spent in the "on" phase and a reduction of the severity of symptoms, particularly during "off" (Figs. 2, 3) (3). Regarding individual symptoms, tremor has shown little change except in the patients of Molina et al. (104). The most consistent improvement has been observed for rigidity and hypokinesia/bradykinesia, but significant changes in gait and balance also have been reported by Madrazo et al. (97,99), Molina et al. (104),

TABLE 2. *Results from clinical trials with grafting of human embryonic mesencephalic tissue into the striatum of patients with Parkinson's disease*[a]

Authors	Number of patients[b]	Degree of reported improvement[d]				
		Overall motor performance	% On time[e]	Duration of L-dopa response[f]	Tremor	Rigidity
Lindvall et al. (87,88)	2	+	0	0	0	0
Lindvall et al. (86,89,90)	1	+ +	+ +	+ +	0	+ +
	1	+ + (+)	+ + +	+ +	0	+ + (+)
Madrazo et al. (97,99)	2	+ + (+)	+ +	n.r.	0	+ +
	2	+ +				
Molina et al. (104)	26	+ + (+)	+ + (+)	n.r.	+ +	+ +
	4	+ +				
Henderson et al. (61)[c]	1	+ +	+	n.r.	n.r.	n.r.
	2	+ (+)				
	6	0				
Freed et al. (47,48)	4	+ +	+ +	n.r.	n.r.	n.r.
	2	+				
	1	0				
Lopez-Lozano et al. (93)	7	+	n.r.	n.r.	n.r.	n.r.
Widner et al. (162)	2	+ + (+)	+ +	+	+	+ + (+)
Spencer et al. (140)	3	+	n.r.	n.r.	+	+
	1	0				

[a]The results summarized in Table 2 refer to the clinical trials in Table 1.

[b]The patients are grouped according to the reported changes in overall motor performance.

[c]Clinical data reported in 9 of 12 operated patients.

[d]The symptomatic relief has on basis of the data presented been scored as follows: 0, no improvement; +, small improvement of no or minor therapeutic value; + +, moderate improvement of clear therapeutic value; + + +, excellent, of major therapeutic value, complete reversal of symptoms, no medication.

[e]Percent of time awake spent in mobile phase; n.r., not reported.

[f]In specific tests of motor response after a single dose of L-dopa.

[g]n.o., Not observed.

[h]One patient died at 17 months of causes not related to grafting.

[i]Changes of fluorodopa uptake in grafted striatum as assessed by positron emission tomography were, on basis of data presented, scored as follows: 0, no change; +, small increase; + +, moderate increase, still pathologic uptake; + + +, major increase, uptake within the normal range.

Freed et al. (47), and Widner et al. (162). (4) Some studies have described therapeutically valuable reduction in the severity and duration of dyskinesias after transplantation. (5) The latency reported for the appearance of the first positive signs has varied considerably (from immediately after implantation, up to 3–6 months), and improvement has continued up to 24 months postgrafting. (6) No major adverse effects related to the implantation of embryonic tissue have been reported. One patient had a brain abscess (99), another partial motor seizures (140), and a third patient (89) showed increased blood pressure possibly secondary to immunosuppressive treatment with cyclosporine. All patients operated on by Molina et al. (104), using an open micro-surgical technique, showed a transient "postsurgical syndrome." Some clinical features of this syndrome, which came regularly up to 3 months after grafting, were anxiety, hyperthermia, flushing, arterial hypertension, tachycardia, and polyuria. Such symptoms have not been observed in any other clinical grafting studies. (7) Evidence for increased DA transmission in the grafted striatum has been provided for only five patients (47,86,132,162). Positron emission tomography (PET) has demonstrated a significant increase, compared to preoperative levels, of 6-L-(^{18}F) fluorodopa uptake confined to the grafted putamen in two patients with idiopathic PD who improved clinically (Figs. 2–4) (86,89,132). Similarly, two patients with MPTP-induced parkin-

Bradykinesia/ hypokinesia	Gait	Dyskinesia[g]	Balance	Latency to first signs/peak of improvement	Adverse effects	Evidence of graft survival[i]
+	+	n.o.	0	1–3 mo/5–6 mo	No	(+)[h]
+ +	0	n.o	0	6 w/5 mo	No	+ +
+ +	0	n.o	0	3 mo/24 mo	Minor	+ + +
+ +	+ +	n.r.	+ +	1–2 mo/8 mo	Brain abscess (1)	No
+ +	+ +	+ +	+ +	12 h/6 mo	"Postsurgical syndrome"	No
+	n.r.	+	n.r.	Immediate/3 mo	No[h]	No
+ +	+(+)	+ +	+ +	6 w/6 mo	No	(+) (1)
n.r.	n.r.	n.r.	n.r.	3 mo/7 mo	No	No
+ +(+)	+ +(+)	+ +	+ +	6 mo/24 mo	No	+ +
+	+	n.r.	n.r.	n.r/n.r.	Minor	No

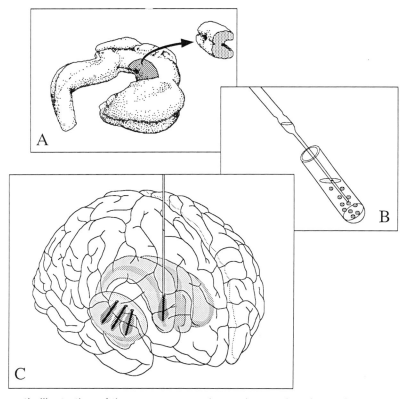

FIG. 1. Schematic illustration of the most commonly used procedure for grafting human embryonic dopaminergic neurons into the striatum in patients with PD. Ventral mesencephalic DA-rich tissue (**A**) from human embryos aged 6 to 9 weeks postconception is dissociated (**B**) and then implanted unilaterally or bilaterally using stereotaxic surgery into the caudate nucleus or the putamen, or both (**C**).

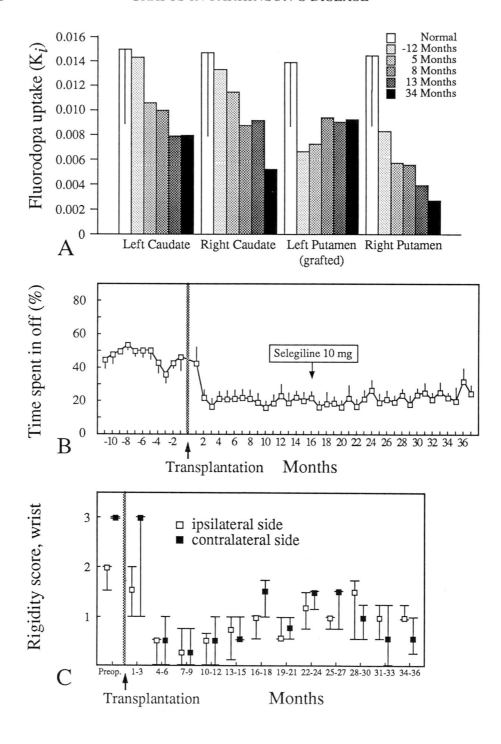

sonism, who were grafted bilaterally in the caudate nucleus and putamen, have exhibited a gradual and marked increase of striatal fluorodopa uptake on both sides (Fig. 5) (162). Freed et al. (47) described significant increase in fluorodopa uptake in the grafted putamen at 33 months compared to 9 months after surgery.

In conclusion, the clinical trials reported so far indicate that embryonic mesencephalic tissue can be implanted into the human brain without major risks. Improvements have been observed, but even in the best cases, no complete reversal of multiple or single parkinsonian symptoms has been obtained. The differences in the design of available studies with regard to duration of preoperative assessment period, drug regimens and methods of evaluation, and the lack of data on graft survival in most patients make the results from various groups difficult to compare. Variations in the design also mean that it is difficult to draw any conclusions about the relative importance for graft survival and function of, for example, surgical and tissue preparation techniques, number of implantation sites, number and age of embryos, and use of immunosuppression.

Transplantation of Embryonic Dopamine Neurons: Graft Survival and Mechanisms of Improvement

When analyzing the data obtained in the clinical studies performed so far, two scientific questions are particularly relevant: First, do the implanted DA neurons survive in the human parkinsonian brain and restore striatal DA synthesis and storage? Second, are the symptomatic improvements in patients caused by the action of functional dopaminergic grafts? Preliminary data from autopsies have indicated surviving DA neurons in three of five patients with embryonic mesencephalic implants in the striatum (Bankiewicz and Hitchcock, personal communication). The only *in vivo* evidence for graft survival comes from PET studies in five patients (47,86,89,132,162) showing increased fluorodopa uptake focally at the site of tissue implantation in the striatum. In PD, striatal fluorodopa uptake is reduced (83,84), and the uptake in putamen correlates with the severity of rigidity and akinesia (83,84). The level of fluorodopa uptake visualized by PET probably represents a combination of the number of dopaminergic terminals

FIG. 2. Parallel changes of motor performance and striatal fluorodopa uptake in a patient with PD who received implants of mesencephalic tissue from four human embryos at three sites in the left putamen. **A**: Sequential changes in regional fluorodopa uptake. Compared to before surgery, fluorodopa uptake increased in the grafted putamen during the first postoperative year, whereas there was a progressive fall of tracer uptake in nongrafted striatal regions. Between 1 and 3 years after grafting, fluorodopa uptake was stable in the left, grafted putamen, whereas there was a further reduction of the uptake in the right, nongrafted caudate nucleus and putamen. **B**: Mean monthly percentage of awake time spent in "off" phase (based on daily autoscoring by the patient). There was a marked reduction of the time spent in "off" phase during the second postoperative month with no major further change up to 3 years. Bars indicate 99% confidence limits. **C**: Limb rigidity (shown for the wrist). During the third and subsequent postoperative months, there was a clear reduction of rigidity, most marked on the right side, contralateral to the graft. From 1 year after grafting and onward, there was a slight bilateral increase of muscle tone in the arms. Consistent with the fluorodopa uptake data, rigidity continued to be markedly reduced on the side contralateral to the graft but increased on the ipsilateral side during the third postoperative year. 3, Severe rigidity; 2, moderate rigidity; 1, slight rigidity; 0, no rigidity. Median values with the lines representing quartiles. Data from Lindvall et al. (89) In (A), comparative data are given for a group of healthy volunteers ("normal"; error bar represents normal mean minus 2 standard deviations) (132).

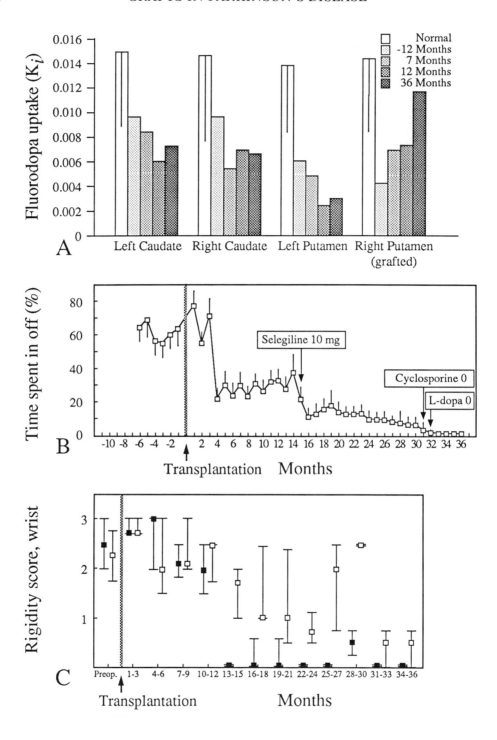

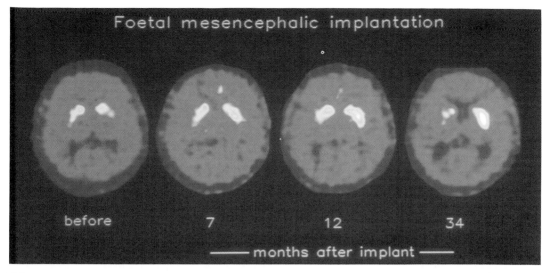

FIG. 4. Images of (^{18}F) fluorodopa uptake from four sequential studies in the patient whose motor performance and serial PET scan data are illustrated in Figure 3. The fluorodopa PET images show tracer uptake at the site of implantation in the right putamen, indicating the presence of a surviving dopaminergic graft. Each image has been scaled to the activity recorded in the occipital cortex such that sequential studies may be directly compared. The images are from a similar anatomic level. (Courtesy of Dr. Guy Sawle, Hammersmith Hospital, London, United Kingdom.)

and the concentration of L-aromatic amino acid decarboxylase (AAAD). Because there is no evidence from animal studies that transplanted embryonic mesencephalic tissue can change host AAAD activity, the most likely explanation for the progressive increase of fluorodopa uptake after transplantation (86,89,132,162) is a surviving dopaminergic graft reinnervating the striatum. A breach in the blood–brain barrier (BBB), leading to a more efficient tracer uptake, seems less likely because magnetic resonance imaging (MRI) performed after gadolinium-DTPA injection at 10 postoperative months in a patient with increased fluorodopa uptake (90), and at 5 months after grafting in another patient (48) showed no signal enhancement at the implant site. Furthermore, in animal experiments it has been shown that intracerebral neural grafts establish a well-developed physical BBB within 1 to 2 weeks after implantation

FIG. 3. Parallel changes of motor performance and striatal fluorodopa uptake in a patient with PD who received implants of mesencephalic tissue from four human embryos at three sites in the right putamen. **A:** During the first postoperative year, fluorodopa uptake increased in the grafted putamen, whereas tracer uptake fell in both caudate and in the nongrafted putamen. Between 1 and 3 years after transplantation, there was a further marked increase of fluorodopa uptake (to normal levels) in the grafted putamen, whereas uptake in other structures was unchanged. **B:** The patient exhibited a marked reduction of the time spent in "off" phase from the fourth postoperative month. During the second and third years after grafting, "off" phases became gradually shorter and were no longer observed from 32 months postsurgery, when L-dopa could be withdrawn. **C:** Rigidity showed no significant changes during the first postoperative year, but then almost completely disappeared on the left side (contralateral to the graft), whereas improvements were variable and less pronounced on the right side (ipsilateral to the graft). Note that cyclosporine was withdrawn at 31 months without any negative effects on motor function and fluorodopa uptake. For further explanations, see Figure 2. Data from Lindvall et al. (89)

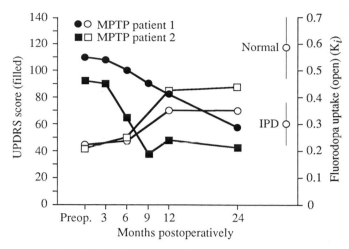

FIG. 5. Score according to the Unified Parkinson's Disease Rating Scale (UPDRS) and total striatal fluorodopa uptake in two patients with MPTP-induced parkinsonism before and at various time points after bilateral implantation of embryonic mesencephalic tissue in the caudate nucleus and putamen (tissue from three to four mesencephalons on each side). There is a close correlation between fluorodopa uptake and clinical scores; after a delay of 3 to 6 months there is from 9 to 12 months and onward both a major improvement and a marked increase of fluorodopa uptake. The circles and bars on the right side denote mean fluorodopa uptake ($\pm$SD) for a group of normal subjects and for another group of severely disabled patients with idiopathic PD (IPD) studied with the same scanner. Data from Widner et al. (162)

(17,24). Also, brain tissue from rat embryos placed in the anterior chamber of the rat eye is completely revascularized from the host 5 days after transplantation (149), and the newly formed vessels exhibit an enzymatic barrier toward L-dopa soon after they have been formed. Even if the endothelial cells in the graft vessels were donor derived in implanted patients, it seems likely that the enzymatic BBB had already developed at the time of the PET scans. Thus, the enzymatic barrier for L-dopa has been demonstrated as early as 20 to 22 weeks postgestation in human fetal cortical tissue (60). The progressive increase of striatal fluorodopa uptake up to 1 to 3 years after grafting in four patients (89,132,162), and especially the lack of changes at 6 months that were then observed at 12 and 24 months in the two patients with MPTP-induced parkinsonism, (162) also argue against a breach in the BBB.

On the basis of morphologic observations (8,16) suggesting plastic responses after transplantation procedures in MPTP-treated animals with partial lesions of the mesostriatal DA system, it may be argued that the increased fluorodopa uptake after grafting in patients was caused by sprouting of host dopaminergic neurons induced by the surgical trauma or the implanted embryonic tissue. However, two patients operated on stereotaxically using an implantation instrument with a 2.5-mm outer diameter (87) displayed nonsignificant changes on PET, whereas four patients subjected to grafting with a thinner (1.0-mm) instrument showed marked increased of fluorodopa uptake on PET (86,89,132,162). Trauma-induced sprouting thus seems unlikely, but trophic effects exerted by the graft cannot be excluded. However, whereas sprouting responses in experimental animals have been reported only after partial lesions of the DA system, major restoration of fluorodopa uptake to near-normal levels (89, 162) has been observed in patients with PD with severe (probably more than 95%) depletion of DA in striatal regions. In rats and monkeys with such complete lesions of the mesostriatal DA system, the functional improvements after transplantation are due to a graft-derived reinnervation of the denervated striatum [see chapter by Brundin (*this volume*)]. Furthermore, there is evidence in two grafted patients with idiopathic PD of a continuous degeneration of the intrinsic DA system caused by the disease (89). The increased fluorodopa uptake in the grafted putamen observed from 5 and 7 months after grafting, respectively, could hypothetically be attributed to sprouting of the patients' own remaining DA neurons. If that were so, the stability of the fluorodopa uptake in the grafted putamen up to at least 3 years after surgery, despite a progressive fall in tracer uptake in nongrafted striatal structures, would imply that implantation of embryonic, DA-rich mesencephalic tissue was able to prevent degeneration of the intrinsic DA system. However, there are no data from animal experiments suggesting that neural grafts can protect DA neurons from an ongoing degeneration.

Although the mechanisms of improvement are unknown in most patients subjected to neural transplantation, the most likely explanation for the therapeutically valuable improvement seen in four patients monitored both clinically and with repeated PET scans is restoration of striatal DA transmission by a surviving functional graft (86,89,132,162). In these patients, as well as in two patients with modest clinical changes, the degree of parkinsonian symptoms correlated well with fluorodopa uptake in grafted and nongrafted striatal regions. In two patients grafted unilaterally in the caudate and putamen and showing only modest clinical improvement, there were only minor changes of fluorodopa uptake (87). In contrast, the symptomatic relief and the increase in striatal fluorodopa uptake in four patients operated on with an improved technique were much more marked (86,89,90,132,162). In two of these, with MPTP-induced parkinsonism, and bilateral grafts in the caudate and putamen, the increase in fluorodopa uptake and clinical improvement occurred after a 3- to 6-month delay (Fig. 5). Two patients with idiopathic PD who were grafted unilaterally in the putamen improved on both sides, but mainly contralaterally, up to 1 year after surgery (90) (Figs. 2, 3). At the same time, fluorodopa uptake increased within the grafted putamen despite a progressive decrease in tracer uptake in the unoperated striatal structures (Figs. 2, 3). The long-term clinical course and changes on PET differed in these two patients, but there was still a good correlation between symptomatology and fluorodopa uptake. Between 1 and 3 years after surgery, one patient (Fig. 2) showed only minor changes in symptoms on the side contralateral to the graft, whereas there was a worsening on the ipsilateral side. Fluorodopa uptake was unchanged in the grafted putamen, but decreased in the nongrafted putamen. In the other patient, the reduction of parkinsonian symptoms on the side contralateral to the graft became even more pronounced from 1 year after surgery, whereas the ipsilateral side improved to a lesser extent. Fluorodopa uptake further increased in the grafted putamen, whereas no change was detected in the nongrafted putamen.

Spontaneous fluctuations and placebo effects, which are common in PD, seem unlikely because symptomatology was stable over the preoperative assessment period and improvement persisted up to 3 years. The gradual and marked improvement starting about 2 to 4 months after surgery had a time course consistent with the slow development of a growing graft. Furthermore, the major improvement occurred on the side contralateral to the transplant in unilaterally operated patients (89,90), and in one patient has remained stable up to 3 years despite a progressive worsening of parkinsonian symptoms on the ipsilateral side (89). Changes in medication can lead to clinical improvement, but the patients of Lindvall et al. (89,90) and Widner et al. (162) received the same doses of medication during the preoperative assessment period and up to 1 to 2 years after surgery, when major improvements occurred. A more efficient entry of L-dopa after grafting also seems a less likely explanation for increased motor function because improvements persisted after L-dopa withdrawal in one of the patients (Fig. 3) (89). Nonspecific effects of stereotactic surgery probably can be ruled out because two patients subjected to adrenal medulla autotransplantation in the putamen (85) and the two patients grafted with embryonic DA neurons unilaterally in the caudate and putamen (87) showed only very modest clinical changes despite the use of an implantation instrument that probably caused more tissue damage.

In patients receiving unilateral implants, clinical improvement has been most pronounced in the contralateral limbs, which agrees well with what could be expected for a functioning dopaminergic graft (e.g., on basis of previous data obtained in patients with hemiparkinsonism) (51,66). However, ipsilateral amelioration of parkinsonian symptoms as well as reduction of the duration and number of "off" periods (when the patients have bilateral symptoms) also have been observed. Could this ipsilateral effect also be graft induced? It seems highly unlikely that a unilateral graft, placed deeply in the striatal parenchyma, could influence function in the contralateral striatum through diffusion of DA. Several lines of evidence indicate, however, that manipulations of striatal function on one side can have bilateral effects. First, the two nigrostriatal DA systems are not functionally independent; rather, any modification in the activity of one pathway influences the activity of the contralateral pathway (107). Unilateral lesions of the DA input to the striatum lead to a marked increase in DA release in the contralateral striatum (166) and reduction of γ-aminobutyric acid (GABA) release in the contralateral globus pallidus (135). Second, electrical stimulation of the striatum has been reported to increase GABA release in both the ipsilateral and contralateral globus pallidus (12). Third, and perhaps most important, a major output from

the striatum is, via the pallidum and thalamus, directed to the supplementary motor area (SMA) (3,57), which has bilateral connections. Interestingly, administration of the DA agonist apomorphine, which alleviates akinesia, also reverses the impaired activation of the SMA in PD (72). It is tempting to speculate that unilateral DA grafts reduce motor symptoms bilaterally by restoring the functional integrity of the ipsilateral cortico-striato-thalamo-cortical loop (72) and thereby the activity of the SMA, which controls both sides of the body.

Transplantation of Adrenal Medulla

The first clinical trials with cell transplantation in PD were carried out using stereotaxic implantation of the patient's own adrenal medulla, mainly to avoid the ethical and immunologic problems linked to the use of human embryonic tissue. Only minor and transient improvements, lasting for a couple of months, were observed after unilateral grafting to either the caudate nucleus or the putamen in four patients (7,85). The major interest in this approach emerged from the study by Madrazo et al. (94), in which they reported successful adrenal medulla autotransplantation in two young patients with PD. Instead of a stereotaxic approach, Madrazo and coworkers used open microsurgical techniques and implanted pieces of adrenal medullary tissue through the cerebral cortex into a pre-made cavity in the head of the caudate nucleus on one side. Madrazo et al. (95,98) have summarized their findings up to 1 to 3 years after surgery in 42 consecutive cases. Four patients died, and four others could not be followed up. As assessed by different rating scales, 60% of the remaining 34 patients showed good response, 20% moderate improvement, and only 20% responded poorly. The quality of life improved clearly in 53% of the patients. The improvement developed gradually, was always bilateral, and affected primarily rigidity, bradykinesia, postural instability, and gait disturbances. The mean L-dopa dose could be reduced by 60%. Madrazo et al. (96) also have summarized briefly the clinical outcome in 106 patients after adrenal medulla autotransplantation performed in Mexico, Chile, Cuba, and Spain (so-called Hispanic Registry of Graft Procedures for Parkinson's Disease; see also ref. 92). Nine patients died (8%), and the others were followed for 6 months or more. Of these, 32% showed a good response (50%–90% improvement), 27% a moderate response (30%–50%), 15% had a poor response (5–30% improvement), and 9% showed no change. There were numerous complications.

Other groups, however, have not observed any dramatic improvements after adrenal medulla autotransplantation (4,53–56,70,76,109). In a series of 61 cases (54,55), comparable to those operated by Madrazo et al. (95,98), 2-year follow-up data were collected on 56 patients subjected to adrenal medulla autotransplantation using either stereotaxic surgery or open craniotomy. The patients showed a significant, though modest, reduction in the severity and duration of "off" periods. The mean percentage of "off" time during the day decreased from 50% before transplantation to 39% at both 1 and 2 years after surgery. Even if the patients were more independent during "off" periods and showed significant improvement of all measures of "off" function, the changes were small and the patients remained prominently affected by their disease. Motor fluctuations persisted in all patients. Moreover, the doses of antiparkinsonian medication could not be reduced after transplantation. There were numerous medical complications, including 11 deaths; half of these were judged as possibly related to the surgery. The morbidity involved several body systems, but was focused mostly on neurologic, psychiatric and respiratory dysfunction. At 2 years after surgery, only about 32% of survivors were improved, and 22% had persistent psychiatric morbidity.

There have been several attempts to reduce the morbidity and mortality after adrenal medulla autotransplantation: First, use a retroperitoneal approach instead of a frontal abdominal incision to take out the adrenal gland has been advocated (54,55). Second, patients have been operated on in two steps using stereotaxic surgery (119). The adrenal medullary tissue has then been implanted in a cavity in the caudate nucleus prepared some weeks earlier. Pezzoli et al. (119) have concluded from results in two patients that, in addition to increased safety, the precavitation technique also improves the functional outcome after adrenal medulla autotransplantation. Third, the neurosurgical technique has been changed to an even less traumatic one, namely, to stereotaxic implantation using specially designed cannulas (7,74,85,150). No significant adverse effects have been reported in patients operated on with this technique. The improvements have been described as very modest and transient (in four patients, two of whom were implanted in the caudate nucleus and two in the putamen) (7,85), and moderate, lasting for 6 months (in one patient with putaminal implants) (150); and, after implantation in the caudate nucleus, as permanent and slight (two patients), moderate (four patients), or significant (four patients) (74). It should be mentioned, however, that Tanner et al. (151), after examining some of these latter patients, reported that the improvements were, in fact, only moderate. After stereotaxic implantation of adrenal medullary tissue into or near the left caudate nucleus, Fazzini et al. (40) observed modest improvement in two patients and a "dramatic" increase in the percentage of "on" time and a decrease in the severity of the "off" phases in one patient. This patient died of glioblastoma 1 year after grafting; autopsy showed no surviving adrenal medulla cells. No improvement was observed in a fourth patient with the graft misplaced in the medial thalamus. In the series of Apuzzo et al. (6) (nine patients, five grafted unilaterally and four bilaterally in the caudate nucleus; one patient died of causes unrelated to transplantation), 50% of the cases showed modest improvement. No further enhancement of the clinical response was observed after bilateral compared to unilateral graft placement.

Most investigators agree that the development of intracerebral adrenal medulla transplantation into a useful treatment for PD should be pursued primarily in the laboratory. After all, using the open microsurgical procedure, only a modest improvement has been documented in about 30% to 50% of the patients, and the patients have continued to show motor fluctuations. Importantly, the morbidity and mortality have been considerable. The mechanisms of improvement are largely unknown, and no evidence has been obtained to support the hypothesis that the reduction of PD symptoms is due to catecholamine release from the implanted cells, as originally intended. In animal experiments, it also has not been possible to detect any spontaneous catecholamine release from intrastriatal implants of chromaffin cells (30). In the few patients that have been subjected to autopsy, either no surviving graft (31,45,62, 70,117) or a very limited number of presumed adrenal medulla cells (67,79) have been demonstrated. It should be pointed out, however, that most of the cases analyzed have shown very little clinical benefit from the operation (which agrees with a poor graft survival), and it therefore cannot be excluded that in the more successful cases there is also a higher yield of surviving chromaffin cells. Analyses of cerebrospinal fluid from patients with PD subjected to adrenal medulla autotransplantation have not demonstrated significant and consistent increases of catecholamines and their metabolites (46,70,120,154), which would support the presence of a surviving graft acting through catecholamine release. Finally, attempts to use PET to show graft survival and increases of striatal DA innervation have not been successful. In the study of Guttman et al., (59) three of five patients showed accumulation of fluorodopa at the site of the implant, but this was probably due to leakage of the BBB.

RESEARCH STRATEGIES FOR DEVELOPMENT OF A TRANSPLANTATION THERAPY IN PARKINSON'S DISEASE

Clinical trials have provided good evidence that grafts of human embryonic DA neurons can survive and exert functional effects in the parkinsonian brain. However, this advancement constitutes only a first step toward a transplantation therapy in PD. The symptomatic relief observed in operated patients is not of the magnitude that would justify the procedure in a large number of patients. Further work is necessary to optimize the transplantation procedures with respect to the yield of surviving DA neurons and the location and number of implantation sites necessary to achieve the largest possible symptomatic improvement. It also remains to be clarified how frequently graft survival and function can be obtained in patients, and whether nigral grafts survive permanently and have long-lasting functional effects. If the graft is destroyed (e.g., due to the disease process itself, immunologic mechanisms, or the lack of trophic factors), new treatment strategies must be developed to prevent this degeneration. It is necessary to agree on common principles for the design of clinical trials with embryonic DA neuron transplantation to make the results obtained by different investigators directly comparable. It is of critical importance to establish with a noninvasive technique such as PET to what extent the graft has survived and restored DA transmission in the striatum. Verification of graft survival is necessary to evaluate in detail different factors of possible importance for successful grafting in patients, such as embryonic age, number of embryos used, placement (caudate nucleus versus putamen versus both; unilateral versus bilateral grafts), time interval between abortion and implantation, whether antiparkinsonian drug treatment affects graft function and survival, and if immunosuppressive treatment is necessary.

Monitoring Graft Survival and Function

At present, PET seems to be the only imaging technique that can provide quantitative *in vivo* data regarding DA function within both the graft and the host brain. 6-L-(^{18}F) Fluorodopa is the tracer most commonly used to demonstrate the functional integrity of the human DA system (83,84). For clinical studies with DA neuron grafting in PD, the PET technique has several uses: First, it characterizes the pattern of DA denervation in each patient before transplantation, which in addition to providing a preoperative baseline, also is of importance for the selection of implantation sites; second, it can be used to monitor survival and possibly also growth of the graft, which is essential to elucidate mechanisms underlying functional improvements in transplanted patients with PD; and, third, it can be used to follow degeneration of intrinsic DA neurons in nongrafted regions. In fact, sequential fluorodopa PET scans in two patients with idiopathic PD have provided evidence not only for survival and growth of grafted DA neurons but also for disease progression, as suggested by reduced tracer uptake in parts of the striatum outside the graft (89,132).

The CAPIT (Core Assessment Program for Intracerebral Transplantations) contains guidelines for how clinical trials with transplantation in PD should be standardized, mainly with respect to inclusion criteria and methods of assessment (82). The main recommendations are the following: (1) The patient should have idiopathic PD and respond to L-dopa. (2) Antiparkinsonian medication should be kept unchanged (if possible) for a minimum of 3 months before and 12 months after surgery. (3) The patient

should be observed for at least 3 months before and 12 months after surgery. A minimum of three examinations before and four examinations after transplantation must be performed. (4) The clinical assessment protocol has to include autoscoring of time spent in the "on" and "off" phases, staging according to Hoehn and Yahr, scoring according to the Unified Parkinson's Disease Rating Scale (UPDRS) and the Dyskinesia Rating Scale, timed neurologic tests such as repeated pronation–supination, and tests of the response to a single dose of L-dopa after drug withdrawal overnight. (5) If possible, a fluorodopa PET scan should be performed before surgery and at 6 months after grafting. (6) The staging of the donor embryos must be defined exactly.

Yield of Surviving DA Neurons and their Volume of Reinnervation

Experimental data obtained with grafting of dissociated human embryonic mesencephalic tissue into the rat model of PD indicate that about 40,000 tyrosine hydroxylase (TH)-immunopositive, presumed dopaminergic neurons survive grafting from one embryo (aged 6–8 weeks postconception) (50). Each substantia nigra in the normal human brain contains 550,000 dopaminergic (identified as pigmented) neurons (113). Thus, less than 4% of human DA neurons survive grafting into rats, which is a lower survival rate than has been found in rat-to-rat grafting experiments. The survival after implantation into the human brain is unknown, but probably is not higher than 5% to 10%. The survival rate of DA neurons must be increased in future transplantations, in particular to allow for a significant DA reinnervation at multiple deposits despite the limited availability of human embryonic tissue. Currently, the low yield of surviving DA neurons after grafting is poorly understood. One important factor seems to be the degree of tissue damage at the implantation site (20), which suggests that the size of the implantation instrument may be of crucial importance for neuron survival. It also may be related to acute cell trauma during the dissection and tissue preparation, prolonged anoxia, or lack of trophic factors in the adult host brain. In this context, it should be pointed out that the age of the human donor is critical for the survival rate, and that very few or no DA neurons survive from grafts of dissociated embryonic tissue older than 9 weeks postconception.

Based on cell counting by Pakkenberg et al. (113), it may be estimated that about 250,000 DA neurons in the human substantia nigra innervate the putamen, and a similar number project to the caudate nucleus. If 40,000 DA neurons from each human embryo survive transplantation in patients, as in experimental animals (50), grafting of tissue from one mesencephalon into either the putamen or the caudate nucleus would be able to restore 16% of the number of neurons normally innervating this structure. In support of this occurring in the human brain, serial PET scans showed high fluorodopa uptake at implantation sites in two patients who received implants of dissociated tissue amounting to three complete mesencephalons into the putamen (89,132). In fact, in one of these patients, putaminal fluorodopa uptake at 3 years after implantation was close to normal (89). These and other findings in clinical trials indicate that, with the present survival rate of human embryonic DA neurons, tissue from more than one mesencephalon needs to be implanted in each striatal structure to obtain a significant increase of fluorodopa uptake detectable by PET. Thus, two patients who were grafted with tissue corresponding to 1.3 mesencephalons in both caudate and putamen displayed only minor changes of fluorodopa uptake on PET (87,88). One patient who received tissue from 0.5 mesencephalon in the putamen showed no change in fluorodopa uptake (47). In another patient, no focal increase in fluorodopa uptake in the grafted caudate nucleus was found after

implantation of tissue from one cryopreserved mesencephalon (140).

The volume of the striatum is about 200 times larger in the human than in the rat brain, and even with a large number of surviving DA neurons, the volume of graft-derived innervation in a patient with PD might be insufficient. To what extent the striatum will be reinnervated depends not only on the total number of surviving grafted DA neurons but on the number and location of implantations and the growth capacity of each DA neuron. When grafted to the rat striatum, the human DA neurons have exhibited a higher growth capacity than rat DA neurons, but the maximum extension of their axonal processes is not known. Based on the density of reinnervation at various distances from grafts of rat mesencephalon in rat striatum (32), and the assumption that each human DA neuron innervates a striatal volume tenfold larger than that of a rat neuron, the following estimations can be made: If human embryonic DA neurons are implanted along three tracts in the putamen (as in the patients of Lindvall et al. (90) and Widner et al. (162) still only about 25% of the total volume of this structure would be reached by a graft-derived reinnervation with a density 25% or more of normal (Fig. 6). In a nearly completely denervated human parkinsonian brain, a DA terminal density of 25% could represent a critical level for obtaining functional effects. Two strategies to obtain more complete reinnervation of the striatal complex might be envisaged: First, the graft material could be more efficiently distributed over larger areas and bilaterally, which may carry an additional surgical risk. Figure 6 illustrates schematically in a horizontal section the estimated effects of increasing the number of implantation sites from three to six in the putamen and from one to three in the caudate. This change in procedure will increase the area reached by an innervation density 25% or more of normal from 35% to 75% in the putamen and from 19% to 70% in the caudate nucleus. Second, the graft tissue

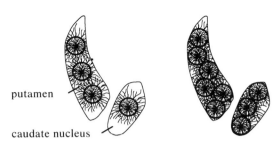

putamen

caudate nucleus

PRESENT
PROCEDURE

OPTIMAL
PROCEDURE

FIG. 6. Semischematic illustration of the estimated extent of graft-derived reinnervation with 25% or more of normal density from each human embryonic mesencephalic implant, as represented in a horizontal section through the caudate nucleus and putamen. With three implant sites in the putamen (90) as well as one implant site in the caudate (162) ("present procedure"), about 35% and 19%, respectively, of the cross-sectional area at this level of the two structures are reached by this density of innervation. To cover 70% to 75% of the area with the same density would require six implant sites in the putamen and three implant sites in the head of the caudate nucleus ("optimal procedure"). This is based on (1) the number of DA neurons projecting to the rat and human striatum and the calculated volume of innervation of each neuron; (2) a detailed analysis of the density of reinnervation at various distances from grafts of embryonic rat mesencephalon in rat striatum (32) (25% density 1.05 mm from the graft); and (3) the radius (3.32 mm) of a reinnervation with 25% or more of normal density from grafted human DA neurons, assuming a tenfold larger innervation volume than rat neurons.

might be supplied with some trophic factor, such as basic fibroblast growth factor (bFGF), platelet-derived growth factor (PDGF), or brain-derived neurotrophic factor (BDNF), before or after implantation, to enhance both survival and axonal outgrowth of mesencephalic DA neurons. These trophic factors have been shown to enhance DA uptake and the number of neurite-bearing cells in cultures of mesencephalic DA neurons (41,68,77,78,108). However, the effects of BDNF, bFGF, and PDGF after administration to DA grafts *in*

vivo still are unclear. Infusion of BDNF into the lateral ventricle or directly into the implant did not influence the survival of the grafted DA neurons or their axonal outgrowth in the striatum (130). Only minor effects of bFGF were found on sprouting of fetal DA neurons from intrastriatal grafts (142).

Graft Placement and Transmitter Production

Functional recovery has been obtained in animal experiments only when the mesencephalic DA-rich grafts have been placed near the denervated target area, that is, within or directly outside the striatum. This is most probably because of the inability of the grafted DA neurons to extend their axons over a great distance. However, in their ectopic striatal location, only part of the anatomic and functional connections characteristic of normal mesostriatal DA neurons are reestablished by the grafts [see chapter by Björklund, Dunnett, and Nikkhah (*this volume*)]. This might then lead to a situation where nigral grafts would be effective for some but not all symptoms of PD. Experiments in rats support this idea by showing, for example, that the impairment in skilled movement in the contralateral limb after a unilateral lesion of the mesostriatal DA system is not improved by embryonic nigral grafts (39). Furthermore, although such grafts reverse deficits in simple sensorimotor orientation observed in experimental PD, they do not ameliorate impairments in a more complex sensorimotor integrative task, in which the rat has to perform the orienting response while in the act of eating (100). Inability of a graft to reverse a DA-mediated behavior might reflect an insufficient integration of the graft into the host brain.

From the results of clinical trials it cannot be determined whether the incomplete recovery in patients is due to insufficient reinnervation or poor integration into the host striatum. Therefore, it is highly warranted to clarify in more detail to what extent nigral grafts are effective and ineffective, respectively, on particular parkinsonian deficits in nonhuman primates, and if a failure to compensate can be referred to a lack of integration or proper activation of the graft. More complete integration would probably require implantation of the grafts in the ventral mesencephalon (where the neurons could receive their normal afferent inputs), which, in turn, would necessitate elongated growth of DA axons to reach the striatum. Wictorin et al. (157) have shown that human embryonic DA neurons implanted into the substantia nigra of immunosuppressed rats are able to grow along the mesostriatal pathway and give rise to a terminal plexus in the denervated caudate–putamen. Although the implications for human-to-human grafting trials are as yet unclear, the results indicate that the activity of presumed growth-inhibiting factors present along the pathway might be overcome under certain conditions.

Most likely, the placement of the graft should be carefully selected to reverse a particular symptom in a patient with PD, and insufficient relief could be explained by inappropriate choice of implantation site. Studies in the rat brain have clearly shown that DA neurons implanted into specific subregions of the denervated striatum compensate for specific features of the hemiparkinsonian syndrome (37,38). Postural (rotational) asymmetry can be reversed by grafts reinnervating the dorsal caudate–putamen, whereas grafts innervating the ventrolateral part of the striatum ameliorate deficits in sensorimotor attention but have no effects on rotational asymmetry. Given numerous other similarities between the primate and rodent basal ganglia, such a topography probably exists in the primate brain, but it remains to be shown how it is organized. Dunnett and Annett (36) have reported that monkeys with caudate grafts (but not those with putamen grafts) showed good recovery of rotational asymmetry. In contrast, the data indicated that the monkeys with putamen grafts improved their skills in reaching into tubes, and showed reduced contralateral neglect.

In all human trials performed so far, embryonic nigral grafts have been placed either in the caudate nucleus, in the putamen, or in both structures. Although DA deficiency in the putamen and caudate nucleus is recognized as the major cause of motor abnormalities, it certainly is not responsible for all the symptoms in PD. Biochemical evidence from autopsy studies have indicated degeneration of mesencephalic DA neurons projecting to other forebrain regions (e.g., to frontal and limbic cortical areas, globus pallidus, nucleus accumbens, and subthalamic nuclei) (Fig. 7A) (2). Furthermore, an immunohistochemical study has shown a depletion of dopaminergic innervation in the superficial layer of the primary motor cortex in PD (52). It is conceivable that some of the symptoms in PD, including certain sensorimotor deficits, are caused by pathologic changes outside the caudate and putamen and, thus, are not likely to be influenced by DA grafts implanted in these structures. For example, implantation of DA-producing cells into the ventral striatum might be necessary in some patients because it has been reported (22) that grafts in the rat nucleus accumbens are important for the amplitude of locomotion. In patients with marked disturbances in the locomotor component of movement, maximal recovery therefore probably can be obtained only with multiple graft placements that also involve the nucleus accumbens.

The degree of degeneration of various parts of the patient's own DA system, as well as the rate of disease progression, also will influence both the short-term and long-term functional effects after neural transplantation. Assuming that 25% of the normal DA terminal density in the striatum represents the threshold between virtually normal striatal function and a major impairment, the clinical effects of a graft-derived

Dopamine content in Parkinson's disease

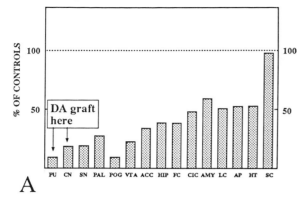

A

Other transmitters in Parkinson's disease

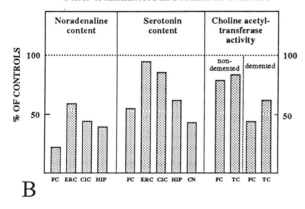

B

FIG. 7. Schematic illustration showing that the biochemical abnormalities in idiopathic PD are not confined to DA neurons innervating the caudate nucleus and putamen, which have been the target sites in all grafting attempts performed so far. Dopaminergic neurons outside the striatum (**A**) as well as noradrenergic, serotonergic, and cholinergic projections to the cortex and hippocampus from the brain stem and basal forebrain (**B**) also degenerate in PD. The symptomatology caused by these pathologic changes is unlikely to be influenced by intrastriatal DA-rich implants. ACC, nucleus accumbens; AMY, amygdala; AP, area postrema; CIC, cingulate cortex; CN, caudate nucleus; ERC, entorhinal cortex; FC, frontal cortex; HIP, hippocampus; HT, hypothalamus; LC, locus coeruleus; PAL, pallidum; POG, parolfactory gyrus; PU, putamen; SC, spinal cord; SN, substantia nigra; TC, temporal cortex; VTA, ventral tegmental area. Data from Agid et al. (2), Scatton et al. (133), Dubois et al. (35), and Ruberg et al. (126)

reinnervation of 10% of normal will be different if 10% or 20% of the patient's own DA system remains at the time of transplantation. Similarly, if disease-related degeneration of the intrinsic DA innervation in a grafted patient leads to a total striatal DA innervation below a critical threshold density, improvements observed after transplantation might decrease or disappear despite a well functioning graft. A similar deterioration is possible after degeneration of DA projections to nongrafted striatal regions if they are involved in or function as an amplifier of behaviors elicited from the grafted area (22). Optimal, long-term symptomatic relief in PD thus probably necessitates grafts both in severely DA-depleted structures, as well as in those striatal regions that have a more well preserved DA

innervation (as evidenced by PET scan) at the time of transplantation.

Idiopathic PD also affects other transmitter systems, including long ascending noradrenergic, serotonergic, and cholinergic systems from brain stem nuclei innervating the forebrain (Fig. 7B). Some of the symptoms in PD that therefore may not be alleviated by DA grafts in the striatum are depression, dementia, postural instability, and autonomic dysfunction. *Depression* is observed in about 40% of patients with PD during their illness (101), and may be related to dysfunction in cortical projections of noradrenergic locus coeruleus neurons and serotonergic raphe neurons (Fig. 7B). The incidence of *dementia* in PD is still unclear, and in recent reports ranges from 20% to 80% (136). Studies on autopsy ma-

of regrafting has been described in monkeys in which a prompt loss of graft function was observed on the previously implanted site (49). In contrast, rats subjected to sequential intrastriatal grafting of allogeneic mesencephalic tissue showed no rejection or impairment of function in either the first or the second graft (33,159). In a clinical setting, regrafting may be important by allowing for multiple implant sites in both hemispheres, as well as for adding more tissue if a previous graft gives insufficient symptomatic relief. The rat data indicate that regrafting with allogeneic tissue, as in clinical trials with embryonic human DA neurons, can be performed without major risks of graft rejection, provided that an atraumatic technique is used (33).

At present, it is not possible to give any general recommendations regarding the use of immunosuppression when grafting embryonic tissue to patients with PD. The arguments in favor of using immunsuppression can be summarized as follows (161): (1) Immunologic rejection can occur in the CNS, and immunization of the host against donor tissue has been observed after intracerebral neural grafting. (2) By minimizing the risk for possible immune reactions, immunosuppression allows for optimal conditions for the evaluation of the functional effects of neural grafting. No detrimental effects on the development of transplanted neural tissue caused by administration of the immunosuppressive drugs, cyclosporine and azathioprine, have been reported in rats. (3) Patients subjected to allografting of human CNS tissue should have the possibility of receiving a second graft at a later stage. Although the risk for immune reactions may be low (see above), the outcome of a second transplantation is much worse if the host is preimmunized (103), and immunosuppression reduces the degree of host immunization. (4) The risk of unexpected, adverse autoimmune reactions can be reduced by immunosuppression (106).

In ongoing clinical trials with neural grafting in PD, cyclosporin, either alone or in combination with steroids or azathioprine, is given as immunosuppressive treatment (see Table 1). One advantage of the triple-drug regimen is that the three components act on different mechanisms of the immune response. T-cell–mediated responses, which probably are the most critical ones for graft rejection in the brain as well as other tissues, are preferentially controlled by cyclosporin. The inflammatory events are minimized by steroids. The critical proliferation of activated lymphocytes can be partly controlled by azathioprine. Furthermore, the toxicity observed after higher doses of the different drugs is considerably reduced by the combination, in which lower doses are used without loss of efficacy.

The duration of immunosuppressive treatment to ensure long-term graft survival can only be speculated on because appropriate experimental and clinical data are lacking. With the uncertainty over the need for immunosuppression in intracerebral transplantation in humans, it is clear that if serious complications occur, the immunosuppressive treatment should be withdrawn. If patients have graft effects of significant therapeutical value, it seems at present that life-long immunosuppressive treatment should be expected. However, in one patient with idiopathic PD, cyclosporine was withdrawn at 31 months (89), and two patients with MPTP-induced parkinsonism were taken off cyclosporine at 12 months and azathioprine at 18 months (162) without evidence of graft dysfunction over at least the subsequent year.

If immunosuppression is necessary, the current inability to monitor rejection of grafted embryonic tissue reliably and noninvasively becomes a problem. A leaking BBB could indicate an early phase of rejection, and this might be detectable by MRI. If rejection were to precede any functional effects, it probably would pass unnoticed. If positive functional effects develop, rejection would lead to a partial or complete disappearance of such graft-induced improvements. In either situation, it would be desirable to detect the first signs of a rejection process in the brain to be able to prevent the complete destruction of the graft.

With the current survival rate of grafted DA neurons, tissue from more than one embryo is necessary to ensure a significant therapeutic effect. This raises the question of whether grafting of CNS tissue from several donors increases the risk for immunologic rejection. There are no conclusive experimental data supporting this being the case, which agrees well with clinical observations in patients who received tissue from four or more human embryos (90,132,162). With several donors at each transplantation, it seems more likely, considering major histocompatibility complex (MHC) I and II antigen disparity (see ref. 161 for discussion), that the risk for rejection is the same when the tissue from each of the embryos is implanted in the same host as it would be if it had been grafted to different recipients. This idea is supported by the finding that mixed grafts of embryonic mesencephalic tissue from two mouse donor strains showed no reduction in the number of DA cells after implantation into mice of a third strain (160). Although the data are sparse in nonhuman primates, they also suggest that pooling of tissue from several donors does not compromise graft viability (36). Immunologic rejection has been reported, however, after implantation of embryonic mesencephalic tissue from two donors into an MPTP-treated monkey (8). It seems most likely that the severe trauma caused by the cavitation technique in the caudate of this animal enhanced the immune reaction.

Storage of Fetal Tissue

Given the current survival rate of grafted DA neurons, it is most likely that mesencephalic tissue from several human embryos is needed to achieve major symptomatic relief in a patient with PD especially with multiple implantation sites. With a technique for storage of embryonic CNS tissue that does not significantly compromise graft viability, it may be possible to pool donor tissue obtained from routine abortions over several days and also perform bacteriologic examination of the tissue before implantation. Pretransplantation storage also could allow for preoperative manipulation of the graft tissue, such as addition of trophic factors (to increase graft survival and growth) or cell sorting. The latter technique would be intended to make a more or less "pure" population of DA neurons for implantation, but could also allow for removal of cells that have a negative influence on graft survival, such as glial and endothelial cells expressing MHC antigens and thereby initiating immune responses in the host.

Three major technical approaches are being explored for the storage of embryonic mesencephalic DA neurons, namely, freezing (27,28,122,125,131), refrigeration above freezing temperature (129), and cell culture (19,143). Although surviving DA grafts can be obtained by all these methods, the tissue preservation usually results in decreased DA neuron survival. Depending on the technique used, this could be due to different factors [for references, see (129)], such as rate of freezing and thawing, storage temperature and medium, increased vulnerability of the preserved cells to mechanical stress, donor age, and maturation of the embryonic tissue in culture. Cryopreservation of human embryonic mesencephalic tissue at the temperature of liquid nitrogen is used currently in clinical trials (140). In animal experiments, this technique has reduced the number of surviving DA neurons (28), but viable intrastriatal grafts have been observed after implantation of cryopreserved, dissociated mesencephalic tissue from rat, monkey, and human embryos into the monkey brain (28,122). In rat-to-rat transplantation experiments, the number of DA neurons in the graft at 6 weeks after surgery was about 60% lower with cryopreserved as compared to fresh donor tissue (131). To what extent cryopreserved human DA neurons survive in the brain of patients with PD is unknown (123).

An alternative approach that also is being tested in clinical trials is to store the embryonic mesencephalic tissue at 4°C in a "hibernation medium" (129). Rat tissue can be stored under such conditions and then grafted, within a few days, without significant morphologic and functional impairment compared to fresh tissue. Similarly, volume assessment of fresh and hibernated grafts prepared from human embryonic tissue and implanted into rats revealed no adverse effects of hibernation (129). This technique might be a convenient and simple tool for storage of mesencephalic tissue in clinical trials. Compared to cryopreservation, however, hibernation has the disadvantage of not allowing for prolonged storage of the tissue (more than 5 days).

Embryonic rat DA neurons also can be successfully grafted into the rat brain after short periods in culture, but after longer times (7 days), very poor graft survival has been observed (19). It has been proposed that the maturation of the DA neurons in the cell culture, particularly the formation of axonal processes, and the dissociation before implantation compromise their ability to survive cell suspension grafting. Interestingly, Strecker et al. (143) have obtained good survival and function of grafts of rat embryonic DA neurons cultured for 9 days in rotating flasks. These aggregate cultures could be implanted without dissociation, which might explain the good survival of the grafts despite the maturation that had taken place *in vitro*. No attempts to use cell culture techniques in clinical trials have been reported.

Alternative Sources of Donor Tissue

The most solid animal experimental basis supporting clinical trials with transplantation in PD exists for embryonic, DA-rich mesencephalic tissue. Long-lasting effects on behavioral deficits probably or definitely relevant for the human disorder have been well documented in several studies performed on rodents and nonhuman primates with experimental parkinsonism. Such deficits include asymmetries in spontaneous rotational behavior and sensorimotor neglect, as well as the cardinal symptoms of PD, tremor, rigidity, and hypokinesia [see chapters by Brundin and Annett (*this volume*)]. Furthermore, the functional capacity of the tissue actually implanted in patients has, in the case of human embryonic DA neurons, been characterized in the 6-OHDA-induced rat model of PD. Ventral mesencephalic tissue, prepared as a cell suspension from human aborted embryos aged 8 weeks postconception or younger, survives transplantation into immunosuppressed rats (21,23). When implanted as solid pieces, surviving DA neurons also were observed in tissue obtained from 12-week-old fetuses (144,146). The grafted DA neurons gave rise to an extensive terminal network in the whole of the rat striatum and formed synapses with host striatal neurons (23,26,144,145). The human mesencephalic grafts reversed both spontaneous and drug-induced motor asymmetry in recipient hemiparkinsonian rats (21,23,65,146), and also resulted in spontaneous DA release (23). Electrophysiologic recordings revealed spontaneously active dopaminergic neurons within the graft as well as host striatal firing rates consistent with those of DA-innervated cells (65,148).

From the theoretical point of view, it seems most likely that the most efficient functional restoration after nerve cell degeneration is achieved by neuronal grafts. These can act through a synaptic release of transmitter that, at least to some extent, is physiologically regulated because of autoreceptors and the integration of the grafted cells in host neuronal circuitries. However, it is highly warranted to find alternative sources of donor tissue, with the ultimate goal of becoming independent of a continuous supply of human embryonic tissue. This will become particularly important if, in the future, cell transplantation into the CNS will be performed in a large number of patients with PD and have a wider application to other neurologic disorders. The use of tissue from aborted human embryos will always be a controversial ethical issue, and in some countries this therapeutic approach will not be possible. Although several other types of implants may be interesting for future grafting studies in patients, their current potential clinical usefulness rests almost exclusively in the capacity to effect a short-term, partial reversal of apomorphine-induced rotational asymmetry in animals with a unilateral lesion of the mesostriatal DA system. This behavioral test can give a good measure of the tonic DA-secreting capacity of the graft, but its relevance for PD in humans is unclear—it does not provide any information on the ability of the graft to effect a symptomatic relief in clinical trials. A clinically useful alternative to embryonic mesencephalic tissue must have a long-lasting effect and a well documented capacity to reverse deficits in the animal models that resemble the symptoms in patients. In the following, some of the current research related to alternative sources of donor tissue is discussed from the clinical perspective.

Adrenal Medulla

Although there seems to be a moderate improvement that can be reproduced in some patients subjected to adrenal medulla autotransplantation, the widespread clinical use of this procedure is definitely premature. Continued clinical trials would require a substantial reduction in the mortality and morbidity rates, as well as a marked increase in both the degree and duration of the functional effects. Further development of the adrenal medulla transplantation procedure is, however, severely hampered by the fact that the mechanisms underlying

the reported improvements are largely unknown. The reduction of PD symptoms is most likely not the result of catecholamine release from the implanted cells, as originally thought (cf. above). It has been hypothesized that the adrenal medullary tissue contains some unknown trophic factor(s), or that the implantation surgery induces the formation of such a factor, stimulating axonal sprouting from the remaining DA neurons in the host (9,16,121). Morphologic support for this phenomenon has been reported in autopsy studies on two patients with PD subjected to adrenal medulla grafting (62,79). However, the functional importance of the presumed sprouting-derived new striatal DA innervation is unknown, and must be analyzed in animal experiments. If the trophic factor(s) can be isolated and found to be responsible for the improvement after adrenal medulla autotransplantation in patients, then this will create possibilities for new treatment strategies in PD; however, it seems unlikely that implantation of adrenal medullary tissue will be the most efficient way of delivering these factors. The possible involvement of bFGF has been suggested because this factor is present in the adrenal gland and brain, increases in areas of injury, and promotes survival and neurite extension of DA neurons in culture. In support of this idea, Otto and Unsicker (112) have shown that bFGF can stimulate recovery of nigral DA neurons in MPTP-treated mice.

The development of adrenal medulla autotransplantation into a therapy for PD necessitates a substantial improvement in the long-term survival of grafted adrenal medullary cells and their capacity to secrete DA and other catecholamines. Both in rats and monkeys, the survival of chromaffin tissue has been poor after grafting to the striatum, which agrees well with the modest clinical response and the findings in autopsy material from patients with PD subjected to adrenal medulla autotransplantation (see above). Implantation of chromaffin tissue as long, narrow "ribbons" into the monkey striatum has been reported to increase survival of grafted adrenal medullary cells (34). Another approach to improve the long-term survival of these cells is to supply the graft tissue with nerve growth factor (NGF). Animal studies have shown that NGF, supplied either by infusion (147) or by co-grafts of NGF-secreting peripheral nerve (80) or genetically engineered cells (29), induces a significant increase in the number of surviving chromaffin cells.

From the clinical perspective, a major problem with the adrenal medulla strategy is that functional effects after transplantation in rats and monkeys seem limited to amelioration of apomorphine-induced rotational asymmetry, and do not extend to spontaneous behaviors. The effects on rotational behavior are less pronounced with grafts of adrenal medulla compared to embryonic, DA-rich mesencephalic tissue (18). Furthermore, the functional effects of adrenal medulla grafts are transient over some weeks if NGF is not supplied, but infusion of NGF will increase the duration of the functional response (147). After cessation of the NGF infusion, the grafts tend to die and the functional effects disappear. It also has been proposed that adrenal grafts can ameliorate apomorpine-induced rotation by a nonspecific mechanism (18). Reductions in apomorphine-induced rotation similar to those obtained with adrenal medulla grafts were achieved with noncatecholaminergic grafts (adipose tissue or sciatic nerve) supplemented with NGF infusions (118). A limited number of studies on the functional capacity of adrenal medulla grafts in MPTP-treated monkeys have been reported. Plunkett et al. (121) found reduction of apomorphine-induced rotational asymmetry after adrenal medulla autotransplantation into a preformed cavity in the caudate nucleus, but the same effect was observed with cavitation alone. The improvement was not as complete as that seen after embryonic dopaminergic grafts. It seems highly war-ranted to document further the functional capacity of adrenal medulla grafts, with optimal survival after addition of NGF, in animal studies, especially with regard to behavioral deficits relevant to the human disorder.

Clinical programs with adrenal autotransplantation and addition of NGF recently have been initiated. One patient has received NGF via intrastriatal infusion for 4 weeks after stereotaxic implantation of adrenal medullary cells, and has been described as exhibiting improved motor function, although the therapeutic value was only modest (111). Other series of patients are receiving adrenal medulla–peripheral nerve double grafts (see, e.g., ref. 91), but no conclusive data are available yet.

Other Catecholamine-Producing Tissues

In addition to adrenal medullary cells, some other sources of catecholamine-producing tissue have been suggested to have a potential for clinical application. Superior cervical ganglion cells survive implantation into the monkey striatum and show axonal outgrowth (69). Furthermore, amelioration of parkinsonian symptoms was reported to occur in three MPTP-treated monkeys with bilateral implants of superior cervical ganglion cells in the caudate nucleus, but not in one nongrafted control animal (105). However, detailed analysis of the long-term functional capacity with complete animal groups needs to be performed to substantiate the clinical potential of this grafting approach. Immortalized cell lines like PC12 represent another potential source of graft tissue (13) that can provide a continuous supply of DA, but are unsuitable for clinical application because they either form tumors or are rejected after implantation. If the PC12 cells are enclosed in polymer capsules, both uncontrolled growth and rejection by the host may, however, be prevented, and long-term survival (at least up to 3 months) is then possible (1). However, their capacity to alleviate parkinsonian symptoms is not known.

Dopamine-Releasing Polymer

Controlled release of DA from a polymer matrix placed within the striatum in rats with a unilateral lesion of the mesostriatal DA system can reduce apomorphine-induced rotational asymmetry (11,63). This effect was maintained for the 2-month duration of the experiment (11). No data are available on the effect of these grafts on spontaneous behavioral deficits, relevant to PD in humans. Furthermore, the clinical usefulness of polymeric implants is unclear because the DA release occurs only during a limited time period.

Genetically Engineered Cells

Another exciting strategy is to implant cells that have been genetically engineered to synthesize and release dopa or DA. Such cells are made through insertion of the gene encoding TH, they can be produced in large numbers, and, if derived from the patient's own tissues, are not at risk for immunologic rejection. A possible advantage compared to embryonic neurons might be that genetically engineered cells are less likely to be affected by the disease process. In the first attempts at testing the functional capacity of such TH-expressing cells, immortalized fibroblastic, endocrine, or neuroblastoma cell lines (producing either L-dopa or DA) (63,64,164), primary fibroblasts (secreting L-dopa) (44), and myoblasts (secreting DA) (75) were shown to ameliorate apomorphine-induced rotational asymmetry after implantation into the DA-denervated rat striatum. Although these data support the potential usefulness of gene transfer in combination with the intracerebral transplantation approach, from the perspective of a clinical application three major issues

must be considered: *First,* there is the tumorigenic nature of the immortalized cells and the risk for production of wild-type virus when using a viral vector to introduce the TH gene. Cell division of the cell lines might possibly be controlled by pretreatment with mitosis inhibitors or by introduction of a temperature-sensitive oncogene. However, for human trials the use of primary cells clearly is more attractive. No tumors were found up to 6 months after implantation of TH-expressing primary myoblasts (75). Furthermore, plasmid DNA, which was used to transfect muscle cells in the study of Jiao et al. (75), is potentially safer than a viral vector. *Second,* the duration of the symptomatic relief produced by the implants is cause for concern. The limiting factor for the immortalized cells has been tumor formation and, therefore, functional effects have been recorded only up to 2 weeks after transplantation (63,64,164). With grafts of primary fibroblasts (44), another problem has become apparent, namely a decline in the expression of the inserted TH gene as well as in functional improvement over a 2-month period. It seems that this problem might have been overcome by the use of muscle cells, in which a stable and high level of TH gene expression was obtained for the 6-month duration of the experiment (75). *Third,* there is the question of the ability of genetically engineered cells to reverse functional deficits relevant to the human disorder. So far, only reduction of apomorphine-induced rotational asymmetry has been demonstrated. Critical issues for the ability of genetically engineered cells to reverse a particular functional deficit in patients with PD will include how important it is that the graft restores a well regulated or partly regulated synaptic release, and that it is anatomically and functionally integrated into the host brain. The use of progenitor cells isolated from the CNS (124) and proliferated *in vitro* may be particularly advantageous in this regard because they can differentiate into cells with neuronal properties and migrate from the implantation site, favoring structural integration with the host tissue.

In summary, it should be underscored that this research is still at a very early stage, and that transplantation of genetically engineered cells is far from application in patients. Before any clinical trials can be carried out in PD, it must be shown in rodents and nonhuman primates that long-term survival and function of genetically engineered cells after transplantation are possible without major risks, and that these grafts also can reverse motor deficits resembling the symptoms in the patient with PD.

CONCLUSIONS

The demonstration that embryonic, DA-rich neural grafts can survive and have functional effects in the human parkinsonian brain, similar to what has been described previously in rodents and nonhuman primates, represents an important step toward a transplantation therapy in PD. In the next phase, the grafting procedures need to be optimized to effect a major, long-term reversal of the most disabling parkinsonian symptoms in a majority of operated patients. Human embryonic mesencephalic tissue currently represents the best alternative for implantation in PD, but other sources of donor tissue must be explored, mainly in animal experiments. It is likely that the degree of recovery of individual symptoms after transplantation will depend on how the graft works. Possibly, grafts releasing DA or dopa in a diffuse manner ("biologic minipumps") can affect some more "simple" behavioral deficits, whereas reversal of "complex" symptoms will require synaptic release of DA, which, at least partly, is regulated by the host brain. If so, the choice of tissue for implantation in the future might be based to some extent on the symptomatology of the individual patient. The pattern of symptoms as well as the magnitude of the DA denervation in various forebrain structures (visualized by PET) will determine the optimal graft placement. However, the functional topography of the DA system in the human striatum is only partly understood. A major objective for studies in nonhuman primates therefore will be to elucidate how grafts placed in different subregions differentially affect various parkinsonian symptoms. Even with many implantation sites, however, the graft-derived DA reinnervation probably will not reach all denervated regions and, in addition, other symptoms might be unrelated to the DA deficit. Maximal improvement in these cases might be achieved only if grafting is combined with other forms of treatment such as L-dopa or thalamic stimulation (to alleviate tremor). Finally, in PD there is probably a continuous degeneration of the patient's own nigral DA neurons, and the disease process possibly could also damage the grafted cells. Although no evidence for such a mechanism has been found so far, if it occurs, new strategies to protect graft neurons will have to be developed. Obviously, for the further development of a transplantation therapy suitable for most patients with PD, more animal research is needed. However, particularly since idiopathic PD is not found in animals, progress in this field also will require clinical trials in a few patients who are closely monitored before and after transplantation, both functionally and with respect to graft survival.

ACKNOWLEDGMENTS

Our own research reviewed in this article was supported by the Swedish MRC (14X-8666), the Bank of Sweden Tercentenary Foundation, Magnus Bergvalls Stiftelse, Kocks Stiftelse, Åke Wibergs Stiftelse, and the Medical Faculty, University of Lund. I am most grateful to Gerd Andersson for valuable secretarial help and to Bengt Mattsson for the illustrations.

REFERENCES

1. Aebischer P, Tresco PA, Winn SR, Greene LA, Jaeger CB. Long-term cross-species brain transplantation of a polymer-encapsulated dopamine-secreting cell line. *Exp Neurol* 1991;111: 269–275.
2. Agid Y, Javoy-Agid F, Ruberg M. Biochemistry of neurotransmitter in PD. In: Marsden CD, Fahn S, eds. *Movement disorders 2.* London: Butterworth; 1987:166–230.
3. Alexander GE, Delong MR, Strick PL. Parallel organization of functionally segregated circuites linking basal ganglia and cortex. *Annu Rev Neurosci* 1986;9:357–381.
4. Allen GS, Burns RS, Tulipan NB, Parker RA. Adrenal medullary transplantation to the caudate nucleus in Parkinson's disease: initial clinical results in 18 patients. *Arch Neurol* 1989; 46:487–491.
5. Appel SH. A unifying hypothesis for the cause of amyotrophic lateral sclerosis, Parkinsonism, and Alzheimer disease. *Ann Neurol* 1981;10: 499–505.
6. Apuzzo MLJ, Neal JH, Waters CH, et al. Utilization of unilateral and bilateral stereotactically placed adrenomedullary–striatal autografts in parkinsonian humans: rationale, techniques and observations. *Neurosurgery* 1990; 26:746–757.
7. Backlund E-O, Granberg P-O, Hamberger B, et al. Transplantation of adrenal medullary tissue to striatum in parkinsonism: first clinical trials. *J Neurosurg* 1985;62:169–173.
8. Bankiewicz KS, Plunkett RJ, Jacobowitz DM, et al. The effect of fetal mesencephalon implants on primate MPTP-induced parkinsonism: histochemical and behavioral studies. *J Neurosurg* 1990;72:231–244.
9. Bankiewicz KS, Plunkett RJ, Kopin IJ, Jacobowitz DM, London WT, Oldfield EH. Transient behavioral recovery in hemiparkinsonian primates after adrenal medullary allografts. *Prog Brain Res* 1988;78:543–549.
10. Barbeau A, Roy M, Cloutier T, Plasse L, Paris S. Environment and genetic factors in the etiology of Parkinson's disease. *Adv Neurol* 1986;45:299–306.
11. Becker JB, Robinson TE, Barton P, Sintov A, Siden R, Levy RJ. Sustained behavioral recovery from unilateral nigrostriatal damage produced by the controlled release of dopamine from a silicone polymer pellet placed into the denervated striatum. *Brain Res* 1990;508:60–64.
12. Besson MJ, Gauchy C, Kemel ML, Glowinski J. In vivo release of ^{3}H-GABA synthesized from ^{3}H-glutamine in the substantia nigra and the pallido-entopeduncular nuclei in the cat. In: DiChiara G, Gessa GL, eds. *GABA and the basal ganglia.* New York: Raven Press; 1981: 95–103.
13. Bing G, Notter MFD, Hansen JT, Gash DM. Comparison of adrenal medullary, carotid body and PC12 cell grafts in 6-OHDA lesioned rats. *Brain Res Bull* 1988;20:399–406.
14. Björklund A, Stenevi U. Reconstruction of the nigrostriatal pathway by intracerebral nigral transplants. *Brain Res* 1979;177:555–560.
15. Blunt SB, Jenner P, Marsden CD. The effect of chronic L-DOPA treatment on the recovery of motor function in 6-hydroxydopamine-lesioned rats receiving ventral mesencephalic grafts. *Neuroscience* 1991;40:453–464.
16. Bohn MC, Cupit L, Marciano F, Gash DM. Adrenal medulla grafts enhance recovery of striatal dopaminergic fibers. *Science* 1987;237:913–916.
17. Broadwell RD, Charlton HM, Ebert PS, et al. Allografts of CNS tissue possess a blood–brain barrier: II. Angiogenesis in solid tissue and cell suspension grafts. *Exp Neurol* 1991;112:1–28.
18. Brown VJ, Dunnett SB. Comparison of adrenal and foetal nigral grafts on drug-induced rotation in rats with 6-OHDA lesions. *Exp Brain Res* 1989;78:214–218.
19. Brundin P, Barbin G, Strecker RE, Isacson O, Prochiantz A, Björklund A. Survival and function of dissociated rat dopamine neurons grafted at different developmental stages or after being cultured in vitro. *Dev Brain Res* 1988;39:233–243.
20. Brundin P, Björklund A, Lindvall O. Practical aspects of the use of human fetal brain tissue for intracerebral grafting. *Prog Brain Res* 1990;82:707–714.
21. Brundin P, Nilsson OG, Strecker RE, Lindvall O, Åstedt B, Björklund A. Behavioural effects of human fetal dopamine neurons grafted in a rat model of Parkinson's disease. *Exp Brain Res* 1986;65:235–240.
22. Brundin P, Strecker RE, Londos E, Björklund A. Dopamine neurons grafted unilaterally to the nucleus accumbens affect drug-induced circling and locomotion. *Exp Brain Res* 1987; 69:183–194.
23. Brundin P, Strecker RE, Widner H, et al. Human fetal dopamine neurons grafted in a rat model of Parkinson's disease: immunological aspects, spontaneous and drug-induced behaviour, and dopamine release. *Exp Brain Res* 1988;70:192–208.
24. Brundin P, Widner H, Nilsson OG, Strecker RE, Björklund A. Intracerebral xenografts of dopamine neurons: the role of immunosuppression and the blood–brain barrier. *Exp Brain Res* 1989;75:195–207.
25. Chalmers RME, Fine A. The influence of L-dopa on survival and outgrowth of fetal ventral mesencephalic dopaminergic neurons in vitro and after intracerebral transplantation. In: Lindvall O, Björklund A, Widner H, eds. *Intracerebral transplantation in movement disorders: experimental basis and clinical experiences.* Amsterdam: Elsevier; 1991:333–342.
26. Clarke DJ, Brundin P, Strecker RE, Nilsson OG, Björklund A, Lindvall O. Human fetal dopamine neurons grafted in a rat model of Parkinson's disease: ultrastructural evidence for

synapse formation using tyrosine hydroxylase immunocytochemistry. *Exp Brain Res* 1988; 73:115–126.

27. Collier TJ, Redmond DE Jr, Sladek CD, Gallagher MJ, Roth RH, Sladek JR Jr. Intracerebral grafting and culture of cryopreserved primate dopamine neurons. *Brain Res* 1987;436: 363–366.

28. Collier TJ, Sladek CD, Gallagher MJ, et al. Cryopreservation of fetal rat and non-human primate mesencephalic neurons: viability in culture and neural transplantation. *Prog Brain Res* 1988;78:631–636.

29. Cunningham LA, Hansen JT, Short MP, Bohn MC. The use of genetically altered astrocytes to provide nerve growth factor to adrenal chromaffin cells grafted into the striatum. *Brain Res* 1991;561:192–202.

30. Decombe R, Rivot JP, Aunis D, Abrous N, Peschanski M, Herman JP. Importance of catecholamine release for the functional action of intrastriatal implants of adrenal medullary cells: pharmacological analysis and *in vivo* electrochemistry. *Exp Neurol* 1990;107:143–153.

31. Dohan FC, Robertson JT, Feler C, Schweitzer J, Hall C, Robertson JH. Autopsy findings in a Parkinson's disease patient treated with adrenal medullary to caudate nucleus transplant. *Soc Neurosci Abstr* 1988;7:4.

32. Doucet G, Brundin P, Descarries L, Björklund A. Effect of prior dopamine denervation on survival and fiber outgrowth from intrastriatal fetal mesencephalic grafts. *Eur J Neurosci* 1990;2:279–290.

33. Duan W-M, Widner H, Björklund A, Brundin P. Sequential intrastriatal grafting of allogeneic embryonic dopamine-rich neuronal tissue in adult rats: will the second graft be rejected? 1993;57:261–274.

34. Dubach M, German DC. Extensive survival of chromaffin cells in adrenal medulla "ribbon" grafts in the monkey neostriatum. *Exp Neurol* 1990;110:167–180.

35. Dubois B, Ruberg M, Javoy-Agid F, Ploska A, Agid Y. A subcortico-cortical cholinergic system is affected in Parkinson's disease. *Brain Res* 1983;288:213–218.

36. Dunnett SB, Annett LE. Nigral transplants in primate models of parkinsonism. In: Lindvall O, Björklund A, Widner H, eds. *Intracerebral transplantation in movement disorders: experimental basis and clinical experiences*. Amsterdam: Elsevier; 1991:27–51.

37. Dunnett SB, Björklund A, Schmidt RH, Stenevi U, Iversen SD. Intracerebral grafting of neuronal cell suspensions: IV. Behavioural recovery in rats with unilateral 6-OHDA lesions following implantation of nigral cell suspensions in different forebrain sites. *Acta Physiol Scand (Suppl)* 1983;522:29–37.

38. Dunnett SB, Björklund A, Stenevi U, Iversen SD. Grafts of embryonic substantia nigra reinnervating the ventrolateral striatum ameliorate sensorimotor impairments and akinesia in rats

with 6-OHDA lesions of the nigrostriatal pathway. *Brain Res* 1981;229:209–217.

39. Dunnett SB, Whishaw IQ, Rogers DC, Jones GH. Dopamine rich grafts ameliorate whole body motor asymmetry and sensory neglect but not independent limb use in rats with 6-hydroxydopamine lesions. *Brain Res* 1987;415: 63–78.

40. Fazzini E, Dwork AJ, Blum C, et al. Stereotaxic implantation of autologous adrenal medulla into caudate nucleus in four patients with Parkinsonism: one-year follow-up. *Arch Neurol* 1991;48:813–820.

41. Ferrari G, Minozzi M-C, Toffano G, Leon A, Skaper SD. Basic fibroblast growth factor promotes the survival and development of mesencephalic neurons in culture. *Dev Biol* 1989; 133:140–147.

42. Fine A, Hunt SP, Oertel WH, et al. Transplantation of embryonic marmoset dopaminergic neurons to the corpus striatum of marmosets rendered parkinsonian by 1-methyl-4-phenyl-1,2,3,6-tetrahydropyridine. *Prog Brain Res* 1988; 78:479–489.

43. Finsen BR, Sørensen T, Gonzalez B, Castellano B, Zimmer J. Immunological reactions to neural grafts in the central nervous system. *Rest Neurol Neurosci* 1991;2:271–282.

44. Fisher LJ, Jinnah HA, Kale LC, Higgins GA, Gage FH. Survival and function of intrastriatally grafted primary fibroblasts genetically modified to produce L-dopa. *Neuron* 1991; 6:371–380.

45. Forno LS, Langston JW. Unfavorable outcome of adrenal medullary transplant for Parkinson's disease. *Acta Neuropathol* 1991;81: 691–694.

46. Franco-Bourland RE, Madrazo I, Drucker-Colin R, et al. Biochemical analyses of lumbar and ventricular CSF from parkinsonians before and after adrenomedullary autotransplantation to the caudate nucleus. *Soc Neurosci Abstr* 1988;5:10.

47. Freed CR, Breeze RE, Rosenberg NL, et al. Survival of implanted fetal dopamine cells and neurologic improvement 12 to 46 months after transplantation for Parkinson's disease. *N Engl J Med* 1992;327:1549–1555.

48. Freed CR, Breeze RE, Rosenberg NL, et al. Transplantation of human fetal dopamine cells for Parkinson's disease: results at 1 year. *Arch Neurol* 1990;47:505–512.

49. Freed CR, Richards JB, Hutt CJ, Kriek EH, Reite ML. Rejection of fetal substantia nigra allografts in monkeys with MPTP-induced Parkinson's syndrome. *Soc Neurosci Abstr* 1988; 7:7.

50. Frodl EM, Duan W-M, Sauer H, Kupsch A, Brundin P. Human embryonic dopamine neurons xenografted to the rat: effects of cryopreservation and varying regional source of donor cells on transplant survival, morphology and function. *Brain Res* 1994 (*in press*).

51. Garnett ES, Nahmias C, Firnau G. Central dopaminergic pathways in hemiparkinsonism ex-

amined by positron emission tomography. *Can J Neurol Sci* 1984;11:174–179.

52. Gaspar P, Duyckaerts C, Alvarez C, Javoy-Agid F, Berger B. Alterations of dopaminergic and noradrenergic innervations in motor cortex in Parkinson's disease. *Ann Neurol* 1991;30:365–374.

53. Goetz CG, Olanow CW, Koller WC, et al. Multicenter study of autologous adrenal medullary transplantation to the corpus striatum in patients with advanced Parkinson's disease. *N Engl J Med* 1989;320:337–341.

54. Goetz CG, Stebbins GT III, Klawans HL, et al. United Parkinson Foundation neurotransplantation registry multicenter US and Canadian data base: presurgical and 12 month follow-up. *Prog Brain Res* 1990;82:611–617.

55. Goetz CG, Stebbins GT III, Klawans HL, et al. United Parkinson Foundation Neurotransplantation Registry on adrenal medullary transplants: presurgical, and 1- and 2-year follow-up. *Neurology* 1991;41:1719–1722.

56. Goetz CG, Tanner CM, Penn RD, et al. Adrenal medullary transplant to the striatum of patients with advanced Parkinson's disease: 1-year motor and psychomotor data. *Neurology* 1990; 40:273–276.

57. Goldberg G. Supplementary motor area, structure and function: review and hypotheses. *Behav Brain Sci* 1985;8:567–615.

58. Graham DG, Tiffany SM, Bell WR Jr, Guthknecht WF. Autoxidation versus covalent binding of quinones as the mechanism of toxicity of dopamine, 6-hydroxydopamine and related compounds toward C1300 neuroblastoma cells in vitro. *Mol Pharmacol* 1978;14:644–653.

59. Guttman M, Burns RS, Martin WRW, et al. PET studies of Parkinsonian patients treated with autologous adrenal implants. *Can J Neurol Sci* 1989;16:305–309.

60. Hardebo J-E, Falck B, Owman Ch. A comparative study on the uptake and subsequent decarboxylation of monoamine precursors in cerebral microvessels. *Acta Physiol Scand* 1979; 107:161–167.

61. Henderson BTH, Clough CG, Hughes RC, Hitchcock ER, Kenny BG. Implantation of human fetal ventral mesencephalon to the right caudate nucleus in advanced Parkinson's disease. *Arch Neurol* 1991;48:822–827.

62. Hirsch EC, Duyckaerts C, Javoy-Agid F, Hauw J-J, Agid Y. Does adrenal graft enhance recovery of dopaminergic neurons in Parkinson's disease? *Ann Neurol* 1990;27:676–682.

63. Horellou P, Brundin P, Kalén P, Mallet J, Björklund A. In vivo release of DOPA and dopamine from genetically engineered cells grafted to the denervated rat striatum. *Neuron* 1990;5:393–402.

64. Horellou P, Marlier L, Privat A, Mallet J. Behavioural effect of engineered cells that synthesize L-dopa or dopamine after grafting into the rat neostriatum. *Eur J Neurosci* 1990; 2:116–119.

65. van Horne CG, Mahalik T, Hoffer B, et al. Behavioral and electrophysiological correlates of human mesencephalic dopaminergic xenograft function in the rat striatum. *Brain Res Bull* 1990;25:325–334.

66. Hornykiewicz O. Brain neurotransmitter changes in Parkinson's disease. In: Marsden CD, Fahn S, eds. *Movement disorders*. London: Butterworths; 1982:41–58.

67. Hurtig H, Joyce J, Sladek JR Jr, Trojanowski JQ. Postmortem analysis of adrenal-medulla-to-caudate autograft in a patient with Parkinson's disease. *Ann Neurol* 1989;25:607–614.

68. Hyman C, Hofer M, Barde Y-A, et al. BDNF is a neurotrophic factor for dopaminergic neurons of the substantia nigra. *Nature* 1991;350:230–232.

69. Itakura T, Kamei I, Nakai K, et al. Autotransplantation of the superior cervical ganglion into the brain: a possible therapy for Parkinson's disease. *J Neurosurg* 1988;68:955–959.

70. Jancovic J, Grossman R, Goodman C, et al. Clinical, biochemical, and neuropathologic findings following transplantation of adrenal medulla to the caudate nucleus for treatment of Parkinson's disease. *Neurology* 1989;39:1227–1234.

71. Javoy-Agid F, Ruberg M, Pique L, et al. Biochemistry of the hypothalamus in Parkinson's disease. *Neurology* 1984;34:672–675.

72. Jenkins IH, Fernandez W, Playford ED, et al. Impaired activation of the supplementary motor area in Parkinson's disease is reversed when akinesia is treated with apomorphine. *Ann Neurol* 1992;32:749–757.

73. Jenner P, Dexter DT, Sian J, Schapira AHV, Marsden CD. Oxidative stress as a cause of nigral cell death in Parkinson's disease and incidental Lewy body disease. *Ann Neurol* 1992; 32:S82–S87.

74. Jiao S-S, Ding Y-J, Zhang W-C, et al. Adrenal medullary autografts in patients with Parkinson's disease. *N Engl J Med* 1989;321:324–325.

75. Jiao S, Gurevich V, Wolff JA. Long-term correction of rat model of Parkinson's disease by gene therapy. *Nature* 1993;362:450–453.

76. Kelly PJ, Ahlskog JE, van Heerden JA, Carmichael SW, Stoddard SL, Bell GN. Adrenal medullary autograft transplantation into the striatum of patients with Parkinson's disease. *Mayo Clin Proc* 1989;64:282–290.

77. Knüsel B, Michel PP, Schwaber JS, Hefti F. Selective and nonselective stimulation of central cholinergic and dopaminergic development in vitro by nerve growth factor, basic fibroblast growth factor, epidermal growth factor, insulin and insulin-like growth factors I and II. *J Neurosci* 1990;10:558–570.

78. Knüsel B, Winslow JW, Rosenthal A, et al. Promotion of central cholinergic and dopaminergic neuron differentiation by brain-derived neurotrophic factor but not neurotrophin 3. *Proc Natl Acad Sci USA* 1991;88:961–965.

79. Kordower JG, Cochran E, Penn RD, Goetz CG. Putative chromaffin cell survival and enhanced host-derived TH-fiber innervation fol-

lowing a functional adrenal medulla autograft for Parkinson's disease. *Ann Neurol* 1991;29: 405–412.

80. Kordower JH, Fiandaca MS, Notter FD, Hansen JT, Gash DM. NGF-like trophic support from peripheral nerve for grafted rhesus adrenal chromaffin cells. *J Neurosurg* 1990;73:418–428.

81. Langston JW, Forno LS. The hypothalamus in Parkinson disease. *Ann Neurol* 1978;3:129–133.

82. Langston JW, Widner H, Brooks D, et al. Core assessment program for intracerebral transplantations (CAPIT). *Mov Disord* 1992;7:1–13.

83. Leenders KL, Palmer AJ, Quinn N, et al. Brain dopamine metabolism in patients with Parkinson's disease measured with positron emission tomography. *J Neurol Neurosurg Psychiatry* 1986;49:853–860.

84. Leenders KL, Salmon EP, Tyrrell P, et al. The nigrostriatal dopaminergic system assessed in vivo by positron emission tomography in healthy volunteer subjects and patients with Parkinson's disease. *Arch Neurol* 1990;47: 1290–1298.

85. Lindvall O, Backlund E-O, Farde L, et al. Transplantation in Parkinson's disease: two cases of adrenal medullary grafts to putamen. *Ann Neurol* 1987;22:457–468.

86. Lindvall O, Brundin P, Widner H, et al. Grafts of fetal dopamine neurons survive and improve motor function in Parkinson's disease. *Science* 1990;247:574–577.

87. Lindvall O, Rehncrona S, Brundin P, et al. Human fetal dopamine neurons grafted into the striatum in two patients with severe Parkinson's disease: a detailed account of methodology and a 6 month follow-up. *Arch Neurol* 1989;46:615–631.

88. Lindvall O, Rehncrona S, Brundin P, et al. Neural transplantation in Parkinson's disease: the Swedish experience. *Prog Brain Res* 1990; 82:729–734.

89. Lindvall O, Sawle G, Widner H, et al. Evidence for long-term survival and function of dopaminergic grafts in progressive Parkinson's disease. *Ann Neurol* 1994;35:172–180.

90. Lindvall O, Widner H, Rehncrona S, et al. Transplantation of fetal dopamine neurons in Parkinson's disease: 1-year clinical and neurophysiological observations in two patients with putaminal implants. *Ann Neurol* 1992;31:155–165.

91. López-Lozano JJ, Bravo G, Abascal J, et al. Co-transplantation of peripheral nerve and adrenal medulla in Parkinson's disease. *Lancet* 1992;339:430.

92. López-Lozano JJ, Bravo G, Abascal J, et al. Grafting of perfused adrenal medullary tissue into the caudate nucleus of patients with Parkinson's disease. *J Neurosurg* 1991;75:234–243.

93. López-Lozano JJ, Bravo G, Brera B, et al. Can an analogy be drawn between the clinical evolution of Parkinson's patients who undergo au-

toimplantation of adrenal medulla and those of fetal ventral mesencephalon transplant recipients? In: Lindvall O, Björklund A, Widner H, eds. *Intracerebral transplantation in movement disorders: experimental basis and clinical experiences.* Amsterdam: Elsevier; 1991:87–98.

94. Madrazo I, Drucker-Colin R, Diaz V, Martinez-Marta J, Torres C, Becerril JJ. Open microsurgical autograft of adrenal medulla to the right caudate nucleus in two patients with intractable Parkinson's disease. *N Engl J Med* 1987;316:831–834.

95. Madrazo I, Drucker-Colin R, Torres C, et al. Long term changes in Parkinson's disease patients with adrenal medullary autografts to the caudate nucleus. In: Bunney WE Jr, Hippius H, Lackman FG, Schmauss M, eds. *Proceedings of the XVIth C.I.N.P. Congress.* Berlin: Springer; 1990;118–132.

96. Madrazo I, Franco-Bourland R, Aguilera M, Ostrosky-Solis F. Hispanic registry of graft procedures for Parkinson's disease. *Lancet* 1989;2:751–752.

97. Madrazo I, Franco-Bourland R, Aguilera M, et al. Fetal ventral mesencephalon brain homotransplantation in Parkinson's disease: the Mexican Experience. In: Lindvall O, Björklund A, Widner H, eds. *Intracerebral transplantation in movement disorders: experimental basis and clinical experiences.* Amsterdam: Elsevier; 1991:123–129.

98. Madrazo I, Franco-Bourland R, Ostrosky-Solis F, et al. A Neural transplantation (auto-adrenal, fetal nigral and fetal adrenal) in Parkinson's disease: the Mexican experience. *Prog Brain Res* 1990;82:593–602.

99. Madrazo I, Franco-Bourland R, Ostrosky-Solis F, et al. Fetal homotransplants (ventral mesencephalon and adrenal tissue) to the striatum of Parkinsonian subjects. *Arch Neurol* 1990; 47:1281–1285.

100. Mandel RJ, Brundin P, Björklund A. The importance of graft placement and task complexity for transplant-induced recovery of simple and complex sensorimotor deficits in dopamine denervated rats. *Eur J Neurosci* 1990;2:888–894.

101. Mayeux R. Mental state. In: Koller WC, ed. *Handbook of Parkinson's disease.* New York: Marcel Dekker; 1987:127–144.

102. McDowell FH, Cedarbaum JM. Natural history of dopa treated Parkinson's disease: 18 years follow-up. In: Clifford Rose F, ed. *Parkinson's disease: clinical and experimental advances.* London: John Libbey & Company; 1987:119–125.

103. Medawar PB. Immunity to homologous grafted skin: III. The fate of skin homografts transplanted to the brain, to subcutaneous tissue, and to the anterior chamber of the eye. *Br J Exp Pathol* 1948;29:58–69.

104. Molina H, Quiñones R, Alvarez L, et al. Transplantation of human fetal mesencephalic tissue

in caudate nucleus as treatment for Parkinson's disease: the Cuban experience. In: Lindvall O, Björklund A, Widner H, eds. *Intracerebral transplantation in movement disorders: experimental basis and clinical experiences.* Amsterdam: Elsevier; 1991:99–110.

105. Nakai M, Itakura T, Kamei I, et al. Autologous transplantation of the superior cervical ganglion into the brain of parkinsonian monkeys. *J Neurosurg* 1990;72:91–95.

106. Nicholas MK, Arnason BGW. Immunological considerations in transplantation to the central nervous system. In: Seil FJ, ed. *Frontiers in clinical neuroscience. Vol 6: Neural regeneration and transplantation.* New York: Alan Liss; 1989;239–284.

107. Nieoullon A, Cheramy A, Glowinski J. Interdependence of the nigrostriatal dopaminergic systems on the two sides of the brain in the cat. *Science* 1977;198:416–418.

108. Nikkhah G, Odin P, Smits A, et al. Platelet-derived growth factor promotes survival of rat and human mesencephalic dopaminergic neurons in culture. *Exp Brain Res* 1993;92:516–523.

109. Olanow CW, Koller W, Goetz CG, et al. Autologous transplantation of adrenal medulla in Parkinson's disease, 18-month results. *Arch Neurol* 1990;47:1286–1289.

110. Olney JW. Excitatory amino acids and neuropsychiatric disorders. *Biol Psychiatry* 1989;26: 505–525.

111. Olson L, Backlund E-O, Ebendal T, et al. Intraputaminal infusion of nerve growth factor to support adrenal medullary autografts in Parkinson's disease: one-year follow-up of first clinical trial. *Arch Neurol* 1991;48:373–381.

112. Otto D, Unsicker K. Basic FGF reverses chemical and morphological deficits in the nigrostriatal system of MPTP treated mice. *J Neurosci* 1990;10:1912–1921.

113. Pakkenberg B, Møller A, Gundersen HJG, Mouritzen Dam A, Pakkenberg H. The absolute number of nerve cells in substantia nigra in normal subjects and in patients with Parkinson's disease estimated with an unbiased stereological method. *J Neurol Neurosurg Psychiatry* 1991;54:30–33.

114. Penn RD, Goetz CG, Tanner CM, et al. The adrenal medullary transplant operation for Parkinson's disease: clinical observations in five patients. *Neurosurgery* 1988;22:999–1004.

115. Perlow MJ, Freed WJ, Hoffer BJ, Seiger Å, Olson L, Wyatt RJ. Brain grafts reduce motor abnormalities produced by destruction of nigrostriatal dopamine system. *Science* 1979;204: 643–647.

116. Perry RH, Tomlinson BE, Candy JM, et al. Cortical cholinergic deficit in mentally impaired parkinsonian patients. *Lancet* 1983; 309:789–790.

117. Peterson DI, Price ML, Small CS. Autopsy findings in a patient who had an adrenal-to-brain transplant for Parkinson's disease. *Neurology* 1989;39:235–238.

118. Pezzoli G, Fahn S, Dwork A, et al. Non-chromaffin tissue plus nerve growth factor reduces experimental parkinsonism in aged rats. *Brain Res* 1988;459:398–403.

119. Pezzoli G, Motti E, Zecchinelli A, et al. Adrenal medulla autograft in 3 parkinsonian patients: results using two different approaches. *Prog Brain Res* 1990;82:677–682.

120. Pezzoli G, Silani V, Motti E, Ferrante C. Clinical and biochemical follow-up after adrenal medulla autograft in Parkinson's disease (abstract). In: *9th International Symposium on Parkinson's Disease* 1988:33.

121. Plunkett RJ, Bankiewicz KS, Cummins AC, Miletich RS, Schwartz JP, Oldfield EH. Long-term evaluation of hemiparkinsonian monkeys after adrenal autografting or cavitation alone. *J Neurosurg* 1990;73:918–926.

122. Redmond Jr DE, Naftolin F, Collier TJ, et al. Cryopreservation, culture, and transplantation of human fetal mesencephalic tissue into monkeys. *Science* 1988;242:768–771.

123. Redmond DE Jr, Spencer D, Naftolin F, et al. Cryopreserved human fetal neural tissue remains viable 4 months after transplantation into human caudate nucleus. *Soc Neurosci Abstr* 1989;54:2.

124. Reynolds BA, Weiss S. Generation of neurons and astrocytes from isolated cells of the adult mammalian central nervous system. *Science* 1992;255:1707–1710.

125. Robbins RJ, Torres-Aleman I, Leranth C, et al. Cryopreservation of human brain tissue. *Exp Neurol* 1990;107:208–213.

126. Ruberg M, Mayo W, Brice A, et al. Choline acetyltransferase activity and [³H]vesamicol binding in the temporal cortex of patients with Alzheimer's disease, Parkinson's disease, and rats with basal forebrain lesions. *Neuroscience* 1990;35:327–333.

127. Ruberg M, Ploska A, Javoy-Agid F, Agid Y. Muscarinic binding and choline acetyltransferase activity in Parkinsonian subjects with reference to dementia. *Brain Res* 1982;232:129–139.

128. Saper CB, Sorrentino DM, German DC, de Lacalle S. Medullary catecholaminergic neurons in the normal human brain and in Parkinson's disease. *Ann Neurol* 1991;29:577–584.

129. Sauer H, Brundin P. Effects of cool storage on survival and function of intrastriatal ventral mesencephalic grafts. *Rest Neurol Neurosci* 1991;2:123–135.

130. Sauer H, Fischer W, Nikkhah G, et al. Brain-derived neurotrophic factor enhances function rather than survival of intrastriatal dopamine cell-rich grafts. *Brain Res* 1993;686:37–44.

131. Sauer H, Frodl EM, Kupsch A, ten Bruggencate G, Oertel WH. Cryopreservation, survival and function of intrastriatal fetal mesencephalic grafts in a rat model of Parkinson's disease. *Exp Brain Res* 1992;90:54–62.

132. Sawle GV, Bloomfield PM, Björklund A, et al. Transplantation of fetal dopamine neurons in

Parkinson's disease: positron emission tomography [^{18}F]-6-L-fluorodopa studies in two patients with putaminal implants. *Ann Neurol* 1991;31:166–173.

133. Scatton B, Javoy-Agid F, Rouquier L, Dubois B, Agid Y. Reduction of cortical dopamine, noradrenaline, serotonin and their metabolites in Parkinson's disease. *Brain Res* 1983;275: 321–328.

134. Schulzer M, Mak E, Calne DB. The antiparkinson efficacy of deprenyl derives from transient improvement that is likely to be symptomatic. *Ann Neurol* 1992;32:795–798.

135. Segovia J, Tossman U, Herrera-Marschitz M, et al. γ-Aminobutyric acid release in the globus pallidus in vivo after a 6-hydroxydopamine lesion in the substantia nigra of the rat. *Neurosci Lett* 1986;70:364–368.

136. Selby G. Clinical features. In: Stern G, ed. *Parkinson's disease*. London: Chapman and Hall; 1990:333–388.

137. Shoulson I, and The Parkinson Study Group. Effect of deprenyl on the progression of disability in early Parkinson's disease. *N Engl J Med* 1989;321:1364–1371.

138. Sladek JR Jr, Redmond DE Jr, Collier TJ, et al. Fetal dopamine neural grafts: extended reversal of methylphenyltetrahydropyridine-induced parkinsonism in monkeys. *Prog Brain Res* 1988;78:497–506.

139. Sloan DJ, Wood MJ, Charlton HM. The immune response to intracerebral neural grafts. *TINS* 1991;14:341–346.

140. Spencer DD, Robbins RJ, Naftolin F, et al. Unilateral transplantation of human fetal mesencephalic tissue into the caudate nucleus of patients with Parkinson's disease. *N Engl J Med* 1992;327:1541–1548.

141. Steece-Collier K, Yurek DM, Collier TJ, Sladek JR Jr. Neuropharmacological interactions of levodopa and dopamine grafts: possible impaired development and function of grafted embryonic neurons. In: Lindvall O, Björklund A, Widner H, eds. *Intracerebral transplantation in movement disorders: experimental basis and clinical experiences*. Amsterdam: Elsevier; 1991: 325–331.

142. Steinbusch HW, Vermeulen RJ, Tonnaer JA. Basic fibroblast growth factor enhances survival and sprouting of fetal dopaminergic cells implanted in the denervated rat caudate–putamen: preliminary observations. *Prog Brain Res* 1990;82:81–86.

143. Strecker RE, Miao R, Loring JF. Survival and function of aggregate cultures of rat fetal dopamine neurons grafted in a rat model of Parkinson's disease. *Exp Brain Res* 1989;76:315–322.

144. Strömberg I, Almqvist P, Bygdeman M, et al. Human fetal mesencephalic tissue grafted to dopamine-denervated striatum of athymic rats: light- and electron-microscopical histochemistry and in vivo chronoamperometric studies. *J Neurosci* 1989;9:614–624.

145. Strömberg I, Bygdeman M, Almqvist P. Target-specific outgrowth from human mesencephalic tissue grafted to cortex or ventricle of immunosuppressed rats. *J Comp Neurol* 1992;315: 445–456.

146. Strömberg I, Bygdeman M, Goldstein M, Seiger Å, Olson L. Human fetal substantia nigra grafted to the dopamine-denervated striatum of immunosuppressed rats: evidence for functional reinnervation. *Neurosci Lett* 1986; 71:271–276.

147. Strömberg I, Herrera-Marschitz M, Ungerstedt U, Ebendal T, Olson L. Chronic implants of chromaffin tissue into the dopamine-denervated striatum: effects of NGF on graft survival, fiber growth and rotational behavior. *Exp Brain Res* 1985;60:335–349.

148. Strömberg I, van Horne C, Bygdeman M, Weiner N, Gerhardt GA. Function of intraventricular human mesencephalic xenografts in immunosuppressed rats: an electrophysiological and neurochemical analysis. *Exp Neurol* 1991; 112:140–152.

149. Svendgaard N-A, Björklund A, Hardebo J-E, Stenevi U. Axonal degeneration associated with a defective blood–brain barrier in cerebral implants. *Nature* 1975;255:334–337.

150. Takeuchi J, Tabeke Y, Sakakura T, Hara Y, Yasuda T, Imai T. Adrenal medulla transplantation into the putamen in Parkinson's disease. *Neurosurgery* 1990;26:499–503.

151. Tanner CM, Watts RL, Bakay RAE, Petruk KC. Adrenal medullary autografts in patients with Parkinson's disease. *N Engl J Med* 1989; 321:325.

152. Taylor JR, Elsworth JD, Roth RH, Sladek JR Jr, Collier TJ, Redmond DE Jr. Grafting of fetal substantia nigra to striatum reverses behavioral deficits induced by MPTP in primates: a comparison with other types of grafts as controls. *Exp Brain Res* 1991;85:335–348.

153. Tetrud JW, Langston JW. The effect of deprenyl (selegiline) on the natural history of Parkinson's disease. *Science* 1989;245:519–522.

154. Tyce GM, Ahlskog JE, Carmichael SW, et al. Catecholamines in CSF, plasma, and tissue after autologous transplantation of adrenal medulla to the brain in patients with Parkinson's disease. *J Lab Clin Med* 1989;114:185–192.

155. Weiner WJ, Lang AE. *Movement disorders: a comprehensive study*. New York: Futura; 1989.

156. Whitehouse P, Hedreen JC, White C, DeLong M, Price DL. Basal forebrain neurons in dementia of Parkinson's disease. *Ann Neurol* 1983;13:243–248.

157. Wictorin K, Brundin P, Sauer H, Lindvall O, Björklund A. Long distance directed axonal growth from human dopaminergic mesencephalic neuroblasts implanted along the nigrostriatal pathway in 6-hydroxydopamine lesioned adult rats. *J Comp Neurol* 1992;323: 475–494.

158. Widner H, Brundin P. Immunological aspects of grafting in the mammalian central nervous system: a review and speculative synthesis. *Brain Res Rev* 1988;13:287–324.

159. Widner H, Brundin P. Sequential intracerebral transplantation of allogeneic and syngeneic fetal dopamine-rich neuronal tissue in adult rats: will the first graft be rejected? *Cell Transplantation* 1993;2:307–317.

160. Widner H, Brundin P, Björklund A, Möller E. Survival and immunogenecity of fetal allogeneic neural grafts implanted into the adult brains of mice and rats. *Rest Neurol Neurosci* 1989;(Suppl 1):13.

161. Widner H, Brundin P, Lindvall O. Clinical trials with allogeneic fetal neural grafts in Parkinson's disease: theoretical and practical immunological aspects. In: Johansson BB, Owman C, Widner H, eds. *Pathophysiology of the blood–brain barrier.* Amsterdam: Elsevier; 1990: 593–608.

162. Widner H, Tetrud J, Rehncrona S, et al. Bilateral fetal mesencephalic grafting in two patients with parkinsonism induced by 1-methyl-4-phenyl-1,2,3,6-tetrahydropyridine (MPTP). *N Engl J Med* 1992;327:1556–1563.

163. Winn SR, Wahlberg L, Tresco P, Aebischer P. An encapsulated dopamine-releasing polymer alleviates experimental parkinsonism in rats. *Exp Neurol* 1989;105:244–250.

164. Wolff JA, Fisher LJ, Xu L, et al. Grafting fibroblasts genetically modified to produce L-dopa in a rat model of Parkinson disease. *Proc Natl Acad Sci USA* 1989;86:9011–9014.

165. Yurek DM, Steece-Collier K, Collier TJ, Sladek JR Jr. Chronic levodopa impairs the recovery of dopamine agonist-induced rotational behavior following neural grafting. *Exp Brain Res* 1991;86:97–107.

166. Zetterström T, Herrera-Marschitz M, Ungerstedt U. Simultaneous measurement of dopamine release and rotational behaviour in 6-hydroxydopamine denervated rats using intracerebral dialysis. *Brain Res* 1986;376:1–7.

Functional Neural Transplantation,
edited by S. B. Dunnett and A. Björklund.
Raven Press, Ltd., New York © 1994.

6

Trophic Mechanisms Mediating Functional Recovery Following Intrastriatal Implantation

*Don M. Gash, †Mara Bresjanac, †Fred Junn, and *Zhiming Zhang

*Department of Anatomy and Neurobiology, University of Kentucky College
of Medicine, Lexington, KY 40536; †Department of Neurobiology and Anatomy,
University of Rochester School of Medicine and Dentistry,
Rochester, NY 14642*

In many animal models of human neural diseases and in some parkinsonian patients, neural implants have been shown to mediate functional recovery. But, although recovery following neural transplantation has been unequivocally demonstrated, the mechanisms underlying improved behavioral performance are still being resolved. The present chapter critically examines the trophic factor hypothesis of functional recovery which we (13,80) and some others (15,62,67) have postulated accounts for much of the observed recovery. This hypothesis proposes that behavioral recovery occurs through graft-induced, trophic factor-mediated, regeneration–modulation of injured host neural systems. Other mechanisms, some of which no doubt are also contributing to functional recovery, are reviewed elsewhere in this volume.

There are compelling reasons to posit that trophic factors play a key role in recovery of motor functions following implantation into the parkinsonian brain. Trophic substances are intimately involved in the development and maintenance of the nervous system. This presumably includes the nigrostriatal system, which degenerates in Parkinson's disease. Neurotrophic factors have been identified that promote the survival of mesencephalic dopamine neurons. In addition, several of these trophic substances ameliorate neurotoxic effects on mesencephalic dopamine neurons in culture. Although the cause of Parkinson's disease remains unknown, the pattern of atrophy and degeneration of central catecholamine neurons, seen most prominently in the dopamine neurons that compose the substantia nigra in the mesencephalon, suggests that some impairment in trophic mechanisms contributes to the pathophysiology underlying parkinsonism. Finally, and most importantly, regeneration–modulation of host dopaminergic pathways has been demonstrated in animals and some patients following transplantation. The remainder of this chapter will be devoted to examining each of these lines of evidence in detail.

TROPHIC FACTORS REGULATING CENTRAL DOPAMINE NEURONS

Recent studies have revealed a number of chemically identified trophic factors that influence dopamine neuron viability (Table 1). Most of the published studies have used dispersed cell cultures of fetal rat mesencephalon, containing developing substantia nigra, and ventral tegmental area dopamine neurons to assay trophic activities. In a serum-free medium, dopamine neuron survival is quite limited. Hyman and coworkers (55) found that 8-day cultures contained

TABLE 1. *Trophic factors affecting dopamine neurons*

Factor[a]	Effect[b]	Refs.
BDNF	Increases dopamine uptake and survival of TH[+] cells in fetal rat mesencephalic cell cultures.	55 63
	Protects fetal rat dopamine neurons *in vitro* against MPP[+] and 6-OHDA neurotoxicity.	55 103
CNTF	Ameliorates the effects of a mechanical nigrostriatal lesion in adult rats, preserving nigral (presumably dopamine) perikarya but not TH immunoreactivity.	49
EGF	Increases survival of TH[+] cells and dopamine uptake in fetal rat mesencephalon cell cultures. Effect apparently mediated by glia cells.	63 18
	Ameliorates MPP[+] neurotoxicity in fetal rat mesencephalon cell cultures, increasing dopamine uptake.	47
	Ameliorates the effects of MPTP toxicity in the striatum of young adult mice, promoting recovery of TH activity and dopamine levels.	47
	Ameliorates the effects of a mechanical nigrostriatal lesion in young adult rats, increasing number of TH[+] nigral neurons and TH[+] striatal fibers on lesioned side.	93
aFGF	Increases the number of TH[+] cells in fetal rat mesencephalon cell cultures, an effect apparently mediated by glia cells.	32
	Ameliorates the effects of MPTP toxicity in the striatum of young adult rats, promoting recovery of TH[+] fibers and dopamine levels.	26
bFGF	Increases dopamine uptake and survival of TH[+] cells in fetal rat mesencephalon cell cultures. However, effect appears to be mediated through glial cells.	37 63 32
	Ameliorates the effects of MPTP neurotoxicity in the striatum of young adult mice, promoting recovery of TH[+] fibers, TH activity, and dopamine levels.	89
GDNF	Enhances survival of TH[+] cells in fetal rat mesencephalic cell cultures. Effects independent of glial cells.	73
	Increases high-affinity dopamine uptake in culture.	
Insulin, IGF-1, IGF-2	Increase dopamine uptake in fetal rat mesencephalon cultures.	63
PDGF	Reduces loss of fetal rat and human mesencephalic TH[+] cells in culture.	86

[a]BDNF, brain-derived neurotrophic factor; CNTF, ciliary neurotrophic factor; EGF, epidermal growth factor; aFGF, acidic fibroblast growth factor; bFGF, basic fibroblast growth factor; GDNF, glial cell-derived growth factor; IGF-1 and IGF-2, insulin-like growth factors I and II; PDGF, platelet-derived growth factor.
[b]TH[+], tyrosine hydroxylase-positive; MPTP, 1-methyl-4-phenyl-1,2,3,6-tetrahydropyridine.

about one-quarter of the number of tyrosine hydroxylase-positive (TH[+]) cells seen in 2-day cultures. Tyrosine hydroxylase is the rate-limiting enzyme in dopamine synthesis and, in the mesencephalon (which is free of other TH[+] catecholaminergic cells), can serve as a marker for dopamine neurons.

Six trophic factors have been shown to increase the survival of TH[+] neurons in fetal mesencephalon cultures: brain-derived neurotrophic factor (BDNF), epidermal growth factor (EGF), acidic fibroblast growth factor (aFGF), basic fibroblast growth factor (bFGF), glial cell line-derived neurotrophic factor (GDNF), and platelet-derived growth factor (PDGF) (see Table 1). However, the effects of EGF, aFGF, and bFGF appear to be indirect and mediated by glial cells, since inhibition of glial proliferation prevents their neurotrophic effects (18,32). PDGF may fall into this category. Nikkhah et al. (86) found that higher levels of the PDGF isoform PDGF-BB promoted survival of both human and rat fetal mesencephalic dopamine neurons in culture. Their study did not rule out the possibility that the results were indirect and were due to PDGF-BB stimulation of other cell types. The effects of PDGF do not appear to be robust; Engele and Bohn (32) did not see a significant effect using lower levels of PDGF. While PDGF was not effective in their study, Engels and Bohn did find that conditioned medium from mesencephalic glial cultures increases cultured dopamine neuron viability. This glial factor may be the newly identified trophic factor GDNF (73), which appears to be highly specific for midbrain dopamine neurons.

Since TH$^+$ immunocytochemical methods may identify only those cells with relatively high levels of antigen and, thus, fail to reveal dopamine neurons containing less enzyme, other methods to determine the dopaminergic properties of cultures are also used. High-affinity uptake of dopamine is a characteristic of functional dopamine neurons. A number of factors including BDNF, EGF, aFGF, bFGF, GDNF, insulin, and insulin-like growth factors I and II (IGF-1 and IGF-2) increase dopamine uptake in fetal mesencephalon cell cultures (see Table 1). Presumably, this increase correlates directly with increased cell size and elaboration of neuritic processes.

In studies that may shed light on the etiology of Parkinson's disease, some trophic factors have attenuated the effects of excitotoxicity on dopamine neurons; BDNF significantly reduces the number of cultured dopamine neurons lost after exposure to the potent neurotoxins 1-methyl-4-phenylpyridinium (MPP$^+$) (55) and 6-hydroxydopamine (6-OHDA) (103). 1-Methyl-4-phenylpyridinium is an active metabolite of 1-methyl-4-phenyl-1,2,3,6-tetrahydropyridine (MPTP). Similarly, EGF added to fetal mesencephalon cultures treated with MPP$^+$ increases dopamine uptake (47).

Trophic effects for some of these factors

have also been demonstrated *in vivo*. EGF (47), aFGF (26), and bFGF (89) promote recovery from MPTP toxicity in the adult mouse striatum. Intrastriatal administration of either aFGF or bFGF significantly increases the number of TH$^+$ fibers and striatal dopamine levels in MPTP-treated mice. Similarly, EGF has been reported to increase striatal dopamine levels and TH activity. Finally, there are preliminary indications that direct infusion of ciliary neurotrophic factor (CNTF) can rescue axotomized nigral dopamine neurons in the rat (49). This factor has potent inductive effects on glia, promoting the differentiation of type 2 astrocytes (72,104). Therefore, if CNTF does increase dopamine neuron viability, it may be by glial stimulation.

Finally, no discussion of trophic effects on central dopamine neurons would be complete without some commentary on GM$_1$ ganglioside activity. Although GM$_1$ is not a trophic factor in the traditional sense, it displays modest-to-moderate neuronal protective influences in the CNS under a variety of injury or neurotoxic situations (48,99,107). GM$_1$ promotes recovery of rodent dopamine neurons subjected to MPP$^+$ toxicity *in vitro* (22) and MPTP toxicity *in vivo* (23,48). Recently, Schneider and his colleagues (100) have reported that squirrel and cynomolgous monkeys exhibit partial behavioral recovery and modest increases in striatal dopamine levels over a 6-week period following acute MPTP toxicity. With the protocols they were using for MPTP administration (intravenous and intramuscular injections), spontaneous behavioral recovery has been seen by other investigators (31,110). One possibility is that GM$_1$ accelerated the functional recovery that would have occurred naturally over a longer period.

The problem in assessing interactions between GM$_1$ and midbrain dopamine neurons is that the ganglioside's mechanisms of action in the CNS remain hazy. GM$_1$ seems to have general and rather nonspecific effects and may work by insertion into the cell membrane or by antineurotoxic or pro-neurotrophin activities (22). Until more is known about how GM_1 protects or rescues injured cells, it is difficult to assign it a role other than as a general cofactor for neuronal growth and regeneration.

TROPHIC FACTOR DISTRIBUTION IN THE BRAIN

The next issue is biologic relevance. That is, which of the trophic factors with dopamine activities are present in the basal ganglia and, therefore, have the opportunity to affect dopamine neuron development, growth, and aging.

Epidermal growth factor and bFGF are expressed in the striatum. In evaluating the actions of EGF, it is important to note that transforming growth factor-alpha (TGF-α), a member of the EGF-urogastrone family, binds equally well to the EGF receptor and serves as a functional homologue to EGF (81). Lazar and Blum (69) have recently quantitated EGF and TGF-α mRNA levels in the mouse brain using a hybridization ribonuclease protection assay. Although modest levels of EGF mRNA (about 20 fg/μg cytoplasmic RNA) were measured in the adult striatum, striatal levels of TGF-α mRNA were several orders of magnitude higher, in the range of 2800 fg/μg cytoplasmic RNA. *In situ* hybridization studies indicate that TGF-α mRNA in the rodent striatum is primarily expressed in neurons (66,114), although immunocytochemical evidence has been presented indicating localization of TGF-α protein in astrocytes (36). Collectively, these data suggest that TGF-α is present in the basal ganglia in sufficient titers to exert significant effects on mesencephalic dopamine neurons.

There is general agreement that bFGF is present in many regions of the brain (33), including the striatum (10), and can be expressed by several cell types, including neurons, astroglia, and microglia (6,117). However, conflicting data exist for aFGF. Immunocytochemical studies have sug-gested the widespread presence of aFGF in glia (108), whereas immunoblots have failed to detect aFGF protein, and Northern blots have not identified aFGF mRNA in the adult rat striatum (10). BDNF mRNA does not appear to be expressed in the newborn or adult striatum (34,79,94). IGF-1 and IGF-2 mRNAs are expressed by many cell types, including neurons in the striatum and midbrain (42,100). CNTF receptor is expressed in the rat striatum and midbrain, indicating a role for CNTF or CNTF-like molecules in the basal ganglia (27). GDNF has just been identified, and the sites (and time course) of its expression in the brain have not been reported.

The finding of trophic factors in the striatum with dopamine neuron-promoting activities fits in well with the prevailing concept that CNS organization and function is largely sculpted by target-derived trophic substances that regulate neuronal survival, growth, and connectivity. However, recent studies indicate that trophic regulation of the nigrostriatal pathway is far more complex. Mesencephalic dopamine neurons express mRNA for at least three of the trophic factors that promote their survival. Gall and her associates (42,100) have demonstrated, by combined *in situ* hybridization and immunocytochemical methods that many dopamine neurons in the substantia nigra and ventral tegmental area possess mRNA for BDNF and another member of the nerve growth factor family, neurotrophin-3 (NT-3). In a similar vein, Bean and coworkers (10), using a combination of techniques, including immunocytochemistry, RNA and protein analysis, and *in situ* hybridization, have shown colocalization of aFGF and bFGF with dopamine neurons in the rat, monkey, and human substantia nigra. In their study, nearly all dopamine neurons expressed bFGF RNA and protein, but only a subset of neurons appeared to contain aFGF message and protein.

As discussed earlier, BDNF and GDNF are the two identified trophic factors that have been demonstrated to *directly* promote fetal dopamine neuron survival *in vi-*

tro. The effects of BDNF on mature dopamine neurons are being investigated by several groups. Lapchak et al. (68) have recently reported that chronic intranigral administration of BDNF not only fails to rescue axotomized nigral dopamine neurons, but also significantly reduces high-affinity dopamine uptake, TH activity, and dopamine content in the striatum of normal rats. Normal rats in their study rotated toward the BDNF-treated side. On the other hand, Altar et al. (4) found only a trend toward dopamine content reduction from prolonged infusion of BDNF into the supranigral region. In the latter study, supranigral BDNF infusion increased striatal dopamine turnover and potentiated amphetamine-induced rotational behavior away from the infused side. It is not yet clear how to reconcile the differences between these two studies.

The trophic actions of many of the factors appear to require the presence of glial cells. For example, both aFGF and bFGF promote oligodendrocyte and astrocyte proliferation (16). CNTF, EGF, IGF-1, IGF-2, and PDBF have not been shown to directly affect dopamine neurons and, presumably, they work by stimulating trophic factor production by other CNS cells. It is tempting to speculate that these factors work through a common pathway by stimulating increased availability of a dopaminergic trophic factor: GDNF may turn out to be this factor; however, this remains to be demonstrated. What is evident is that the trophic regulation of midbrain dopamine neurons is more complex than originally envisioned and may entail autocrine–paracrine mechanisms as well as modulation by supporting glia.

NIGROSTRIATAL DEGENERATION

McGeer and associates (82) were the first to quantify mesencephalic dopamine neuron loss in the course of normal human aging. In the same landmark study, the authors also noted qualitative differences between nigral dopamine neurons from children and from older individuals; neurons from children were large, whereas those from adults tended to appear atrophied.

Parkinson's disease is characterized by a loss of nigral dopamine neurons greater than that seen in normal aging. The loss in cell numbers ranges from 50 to 85%, compared with age-matched controls (for review, see 58). In the few quantitative studies reported, surviving dopamine neurons in the parkinsonian substantia nigra are atrophied relative to controls. For example, Bogerts and coworkers (12), compared nigral cells from six long-term parkinsonian patients with those of nine normal persons. The brains were collected before 1937 and, thus, the patients had not been treated with L-dopa. Cell depletion was most severe in the lateral substantia nigra where 66% of the neurons were lost. In this region, the volume of surviving nerve cell bodies was reduced by 39% and cell nucleus size by 60%. Similar trends, but of lesser magnitude, were evident in the medial substantia nigra.

Another line of evidence that significant components of the nigrostriatal dopaminergic system remain in Parkinson's patients comes from positron emission tomography studies (70). With use of two tracers to measure high-affinity dopamine uptake sites, [18F]fluorodopa and [11C]nomifensine, uptake in the putamen of Parkinson's patients averaged about 40% that of normal healthy volunteers. These were patients with moderate to severe parkinsonism (Hoehn and Yahr stages 2–4). Since striatal dopamine levels are depressed to 20% or less of normal values, this suggests that residual dopamine neurons in the parkinsonian brain are producing less dopamine than normal neurons. In support of this suggestion are recent data indicating that both TH mRNA and TH protein levels per neurons are reduced in nigral dopamine neurons compared with age-matched controls (60).

The cause(s) of Parkinson's disease is unknown, but current theories emphasize the potential involvement of oxidative stress, excitotoxicity, and mitochondrial abnormalities in nigrostriatal degeneration (59, 106). Until the sequelae of events leading to parkinsonism have been elucidated, the role of altered trophic mechanisms in the degenerative process cannot be determined. However, it is obvious that diminished trophic factor levels or decreased sensitivity to trophic stimulation would make dopamine neurons more vulnerable to excitotoxic or oxidative challenges.

GRAFT-INDUCED CHANGES IN STRIATAL DOPAMINERGIC INNERVATION

Recent results from animal experiments and clinical investigations lend support to the trophic factor hypothesis of functional recovery. Bohn and coworkers, in 1987 (13), were among the first to suggest a role for trophic factors in promoting recovery in the parkinsonian brain, based on their analysis of adrenal grafts in mice with MPTP-induced striatal dopamine depletion. Although adrenal chromaffin cell survival was minimal 6 weeks postimplantation, an extensive network of TH+ fibers could be visualized around the implant site in tissue-grafted, but not sham-grafted, animals. The TH+ fibers always appeared to be of host origin, suggesting that the implants had stimulated existing host dopamine neurons. It was hypothesized that trophic factors from the grafted adrenal had either induced collateral sprouting from residual dopaminergic fibers in the striatum or had up-regulated TH levels in residual terminals.

Other studies have confirmed this observation in mice and, in addition, have reported similar increases in TH+ fibers around striatal implant sites in rats (Fig. 1), nonhuman primates, and Parkinson's disease patients (Table 2). In monkeys, at least, some increase in TH+ fibers is evident following sham transplantation, indicating that injury to the striatum is sufficient to induce a response (38,95). How-

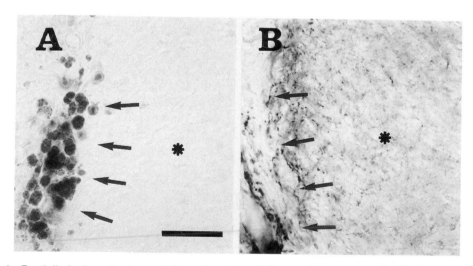

FIG. 1. Partially lesioned rats receiving adrenal medulla–sural nerve cografts display a marked increase in TH+ fibers. The response is illustrated in the following two animals 28 days posttransplantation. After sham transplantation (**A**) only macrophages are visible in the needle tract (*arrows*). TH fibers are not evident in the host striatum (*asterisk*). However, in the striatum of a cograft recipient (**B**), many fine varicose TH+ fibers can be visualized. The region shown in both animals is in the ventral striatum near the nucleus accumbens. TH immunocytochemistry; scale bar, 50 μm.

TABLE 2. *Implant induced increase in striatal TH⁺ fibers*

Species	Lesion[a]	Implant	Refs.
Mouse	MPTP	Adrenal medulla	13 24, 25
Mouse	MPTP	bFGF in Gelfoam	89
Mouse	MPTP	aFGF infusion	26
Mouse	MPTP	EGF infusion	47
Rat	6-OHDA	Activated leukocytes	35
Rat	6-OHDA	Peripheral nerve Adrenal medulla	119
Monkey	MPTP	Sham graft	38 95
Monkey	MPTP	Adrenal medulla	38 95 112
Monkey	MPTP	Fetal tissue	8, 9
Human	Idiopathic parkinsonism	Adrenal medulla	51 65

[a]MPTP, 1-methyl-4-phenyl-1,2,3,6-tetrahydropyridine; 6-OHDA 6-hydroxydopamine.

ever, experiments in mice (24,25) have demonstrated that increases in TH⁺ fiber density and striatal dopamine levels are directly related to the time course of survival and to the number of surviving grafted adrenal chromaffin cells (Table 3). Date and his associates (24,25) compared recovery in the nigrostriatal system between MPTP-treated mice receiving adrenal medulla xenografts, allografts, or isografts. They found that, even in animals receiving adrenal medulla xenografts and allografts that were rejected, TH⁺ fiber densities around the graft were several times greater than in sham-grafted recipients. Striatal dopamine levels were up 50% to 60% in the tissue recipients compared with sham-operated

mice. Isografts, which were not rejected, resulted in further enhanced fiber density and increased dopamine levels. Finally, cografting adrenal medulla with peripheral nerve minces (which provided trophic support and increased chromaffin cell survival by 150% over isografts alone) gave the best results, with over a sevenfold increase in TH⁺ fiber density, and a 150% increase in striatal dopamine levels.

A similar increase in TH⁺ fiber density surrounding intrastriatal graft sites has been identified in rats with partial nigrostriatal lesions (35,119). The use of partially lesioned rat hosts (17,91) may be necessary to visualize the TH⁺ fibers. The presence of intrastriatal dopaminergic processes of

TABLE 3. *Recovery following intrastriatal adrenal medulla grafts[a]*

Group	Increased TH⁺ fiber density (%)	Increased striatal dopamine levels (%)	Refs.
Xenograft	299	47	25
Allograft	267	60	25
Isograft	568	97	24
Cograft	766	157	24

[a]Recovery measured in mice with MPTP-induced striatal dopamine depletion. Average increases in TH⁺ fiber density next to the graft and striatal dopamine levels are shown for various adrenal medulla implant test groups, compared with sham-graft recipients. Striatal dopamine levels did not significantly differ between MPTP-treated only and MPTP-treated, sham-implanted animals. Cograft recipients received peripheral nerve implants with the adrenal medulla to increase chromaffin cell survival.

host origin has not been reported in rats with complete unilateral substantia nigra lesions, despite numerous studies by many different groups (e.g., see 41,56,78). The most likely explanation is the simplest. Dopaminergic projections to the striatum are overwhelmingly from the ipsilateral substantia nigra (90). Complete unilateral nigral lesions remove virtually all of the dopamine fibers in the striatum capable of regenerative sprouting or TH up-regulation. The other implication from this observation is that the TH$^+$ fiber increase seen in partially lesioned rats in response to implantation originates from surviving host mesencephalic dopamine neurons.

The time course of the regenerative response in rats is revealing. In partially lesioned rats receiving either sham or peripheral nerve–adrenal medulla cografts, a significant and nearly identical increase in intrastriatal TH$^+$ fibers was found 3 days postimplantation in both groups, compared with nonimplanted lesioned animals (119). However, TH$^+$ fiber density quickly declined in the sham-grafted animals. By 7 days postsurgery, it was less than half that of cograft recipients and, by 28 days, fiber density had nearly returned to presurgical baseline levels. In contrast, TH$^+$ fiber density remained elevated in cograft recipients, with no significant differences evident between 3-day, 7-day, 14-day, and 28-day test groups.

An increase in TH$^+$ fibers associated with intrastriatal implant sites in nonhuman primates and in humans has been documented by several groups. The primate response to implantation resembles that seen in the rodent brain, but there may be some differences. A number of stimuli (see Table 2) elicit the increase in detectable fibers: sham surgery, adrenal implants, nondopaminergic fetal implants, and fetal mesencephalic grafts. Some of the evidence, especially from studies by Bankiewicz and his colleagues (8,9,95), provide support for collateral sprouting contributing to the increased fiber number. They clearly demonstrate large numbers of TH$^+$ fibers streaming from the ventral striatum and nucleus accumbens region toward the implant site in the head of the caudate nucleus.

Behavioral recovery also has been associated with the increase in immunoreactive fibers. Plunkett and coworkers (95) and Bankiewicz and coworkers (8,9) have reported amelioration of bradykinesia, rigidity, and tremor in some fetal graft recipients and decreases in rotational behavior in other fetal-grafted and adrenal-implanted animals. Behavioral improvement was apparent within days to weeks following implantation.

Recently, efforts have been made to carefully chart the time course of behavioral recovery following intrastriatal grafting (D. M. Gash, et al., work in progress). From a computer-assisted system to continuously monitor home-cage activity and weekly ratings on a monkey parkinsonian rating scale, functional recovery was quantitated in a bilaterally parkinsonian monkey receiving an adrenal medulla autograft along with NGF infusion. By using a protocol similar to clinical procedures reported by Olson and colleagues (87) to promote long-term improvement in a parkinsonian patient, NGF was administered through a catheter implanted into the right putamen to enhance grafted chromaffin cell viability. One week after NGF infusion was initiated, adrenal medullary tissue was stereotactically autografted into three sites in the putamen surrounding the catheter. The animal began to improve within 24 hours following catheter placement (Fig. 2). Activity levels had increased by over 100% within 2 days following surgery. By the second week, bradykinesia, rigidity, and postural and gait abnormalities had been reduced almost by half. This level of recovery was maintained through the duration of the study, 20-weeks after adrenal implantation.

In general, the results from clinical adrenal medulla transplants conducted in the United States also support the trophic factor hypothesis of functional recovery. Re-

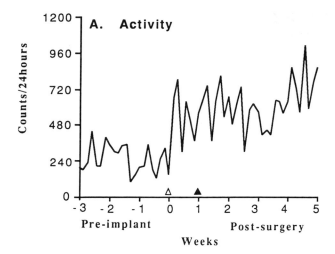

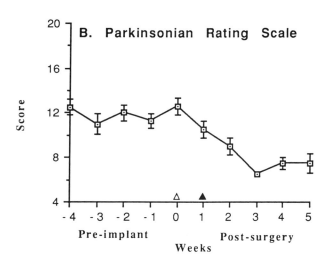

FIG. 2. Functional recovery in a bilaterally parkinsonian rhesus monkey following adrenal medulla implantation and NGF infusion. (**A**) Computer-assisted activity monitors were used to continuously record home-cage activity levels. Immediately following catheter implantation (*open triangles*) into the putamen and initiation of NGF infusion, activity levels doubled. Activity levels remained elevated and increased slightly following adrenal medulla autotransplantation (*solid triangles*) into the putamen a week later. (**B**) Parkinsonian features were rated from videotapes made weekly. The baseline for the 4-month period before transplantation was very stable, ranging from 11 to 14 points on the rating scale. Improvement was evident in the first week after catheter placement. The animal continued to improve through the third week and remained stable for the rest of the study.

ports evaluating functional recovery in over 100 patients receiving intrastriatal adrenal grafts for the treatment of Parkinson's disease have been published (1,2,5,45,46,57, 61,71). Many of the patients have been followed for up to 2 years after implantation. Transplant survival in this patient group appears to be poor. Surviving adrenal chromaffin cells could be identified in only two of six autograft recipients undergoing autopsy from 6 weeks to 30 months after grafting (51,54,57,65,92,111). Even in these two

cases, the number of surviving cells was small. Invariably, the graft sites largely consisted of macrophages, other blood-borne cells, and necrotic debris.

In spite of poor graft survival, over 40% of the patients experienced mild to moderate improvements in their symptoms, in some instances lasting for up to 2 years (1,2,5,45,46,57,61,71). The most commonly seen benefits were increased "on" time (the periods during the day in which antiparkinsonian drugs were effective), decreased severity of "off" time, and improved quality of life measures.

As graft survival was apparently minimal, it is tempting to suggest that the transplant procedures induced an up-regulation of host striatal dopamine fibers which was responsible for the functional recovery. Increased TH$^+$ fiber immunoreactivity surrounding the graft has been reported in two Parkinson's disease patients receiving adrenal medulla autografts into the head of the caudate nucleus. Kordower and co-workers (65), noted a robust enhancement of host-derived TH$^+$ fibers surrounding the implant in a patient who demonstrated functional improvement lasting for up to 18 months following grafting. Hirsh and colleagues (51), found a modest graft-associated fiber increase in a patient who experienced no improvement in symptoms following implantation. Thus, although alternative explanations are possible, the data support the thesis that functional recovery is mediated by trophic factors provided either by the graft during its transient survival or by the injury-stimulated host brain.

TROPHIC FACTOR AVAILABILITY FOLLOWING IMPLANTATION

There are three additional questions that need to be addressed to analyze the possible role of trophic factors in functional recovery: (a) The stimuli provided by grafted cells need to be determined. (b) The increased availability of trophic factors from host neural tissue in response to implantation or surgery needs to be delineated. (c) The nature of CNS dopaminergic plasticity needs to be defined. Although much remains to be learned in each of these areas, enough is known to form a broad outline of the effects of adrenal medulla and fetal tissue grafts on the host nigrostriatal system.

Doering and Tokiwa (29) have shown that the rat adrenal medulla appears to produce a factor that maintains nigral dopamine neuron viability. Although only between zero and 28 TH$^+$ neurons could be identified in individual fetal mesencephalic grafts into the sciatic nerve 1 year after transplantation, 20-fold more neurons, on the average, could be found in cografts of adrenal medulla and mesencephalon. Presumably, a critical trophic substance elaborated by adrenal chromaffin cells was responsible for this effect, although other cell types in the adrenal medulla (see 50) may have been involved. The list of biologically active substances produced by chromaffin cells is large and keeps growing. Adrenal chromaffin cells produce bFGF (11,113), leu- and met-enkephalin (88,96,115), neuropeptide Y (28), serotonin (52), a substance with molecular weight and biologic activity similar to CNTF (109), as well as dopamine, epinephrine, norepinephrine, and chromogranin A (115). Although bFGF promotes the survival of fetal mesencephalic dopamine neurons (at least indirectly through cytokine effects on glia), the individual and synergistic effects of the other molecules on central dopamine neurons are not clear.

Virtually all studies on fetal mesencephalon grafts have focused on the neuronal properties of the grafted dopamine neurons. However, it is important to keep in mind that the grafted mesencephalon consists primarily of glial cells. As discussed earlier, astrocytes produce several trophic substances, including factors that promote dopamine neuron survival. In addition, mesencephalic dopamine neurons synthesize at least four trophic factors: aFGF, bFGF, NT-3, and BDNF. Trophic influences of fetal mesencephalon grafts on aged mesencephalic dopamine neurons in the host are potentially significant and conceivably provide the principal impetus for functional recovery.

Several of the trophic factors that promote dopamine neuron survival have been shown to increase in the host brain following CNS injury (Table 4). Most of the published studies have focused on responses in the neocortex or hippocampus. In these brain regions, BDNF, bFGF, and IGF-1

TABLE 4. *Trophic factors increasing in response to injury*

Lesion	Site	Response	Refs.
Ischemia or hypoglycemia	Hippocampus	Increases BDNF mRNA within 2 hr	75
Kainic acid	Hippocampus, cortex	Increases BDNF mRNA within 30 min, increase also seen in contralateral hippocampus	30 7
Needle insertion, saline injection	Hippocampus	Increases BDNF mRNA within 1 hr	7
Tissue aspiration	Cortex	Increases bFGF mRNA within 4 hr, persists for 2 wk, bFGF protein paralleled mRNA	39 40
Knife cut	Cortex, corpus callosum	Increases bFGF mRNA within 1 d, highest expression at 7 d, bFGF protein paralleled mRNA	77
Electrolytic	Hippocampus	Increases IGF-1 at 7 and 14 d postlesion	118

levels increase following a variety of lesions: ischemia, hypoglycemia, kainic acid excitotoxicity, knife cuts, aspiration, and electrolytic lesions. Up-regulation occurs within hours, and the mRNA levels remain elevated from hours to days, depending on the insult, site, and trophic factor. Not all trophic factors increase in response to injury. For example, NT-3 levels are either not changed or actually decrease in the hippocampus in response to saline injections, kainic acid, or ischemia (7,76).

The foregoing studies extend the original findings of Nieto-Sampedro and Cotman (85) that trophic factor activities accumulate around the site of an aspiration lesion in the rat cortex. In their experiments, increased neurotrophic activity could be measured by 4 days after injury, reached a peak between 6 and 12 days, and was still evident by 15 days after lesion. Astrocytes appear to be responsible for much of this trophic activity (62,85).

NIGROSTRIATAL SYSTEM PLASTICITY

One of the more remarkable features of the nigrostriatal system is its extensive ability to compensate for lesions and cell loss.

An individual nigral dopamine neuron elaborates an extensive fiber field that may, in the rat, make 500,000 synaptic contacts (90). Parkinsonian symptoms are not manifest until striatal dopamine levels fall below 80% of normal and substantia nigra dopamine neuron loss exceeds 50% that of age-matched controls (53,58). The ability of the rat to compensate for nigral dopamine neuron loss appears to be even greater than for humans, at least for short periods. For example, Castaneda and colleagues (19), who used microdialysis to measure extracellular striatal levels of dopamine and its metabolites following bilateral nigral lesions, found that extracellular dopamine levels remained within normal values until greater than 80% of the substantia nigra neurons had been eliminated. Lesions that destroyed 80% to 95% of the nigra produced only a modest drop in extracellular dopamine concentrations. However, more complete lesions (greater than 95%) exceeded the capacity of surviving processes to compensate and resulted in a precipitous drop in extracellular levels of dopamine and its metabolites.

The increased number of TH$^+$ fibers and increased dopamine levels in the striatum following implantation are manifestations of nigrostriatal plasticity. In evaluating mechanisms to account for this plasticity, our group has considered two alternative hypotheses: (a) The increase is due to collateral sprouting from processes of surviving mesencephalic dopamine neurons; or (b) the increase is due to an upregulation of TH in residual axons and terminals in the striatum. One way to begin to distinguish between these two possibilities is by the time course of events.

Collateral sprouting in the rat brain has been carefully documented. In an elegant series of studies analyzing central catecholaminergic reinnervation of denervated irises grafted into either the caudal diencephalon or the internal capsule, Svendgaard and coworkers (105) found noradrenergic and dopaminergic fibers began to enter the graft as early as 5 days after implantation. The minimal growth rate of the reinnervating processes was calculated to be 0.5 to 0.8 mm/day. By 4 weeks after grafting, the irises were extensively innervated. Gilad and Reis (44) reported a similar sequence in evaluating collateral sprouting of dopamine fibers in the olfactory tubercle following unilateral olfactory bulbectomy. Olfactory bulbectomy eliminates a major source of nondopaminergic innervation to the olfactory tubercle, thereby providing denervated target sites for the intact dopaminergic system. Collateral sprouting from dopaminergic fibers began within 5 to 10 days after lesioning. By 7 days after the lesion, increased TH activity was measured. With a different paradigm involving excitotoxic lesions of the striatum, Roberts and DiFiglia (97) found synaptic reorganization and proliferation continued well beyond 7 weeks after lesioning. The pattern that emerges from this data is that collateral sprouting does not begin until 5 to 10 days after lesioning or implantation and then continues to progress for weeks to months.

Relatively normal extracellular dopamine levels are maintained in the striatum, even after an 80% loss of nigral dopamine neurons. Zigmond and coworkers (120,121)

have proposed two mechanisms to account for increased dopamine availability from residual dopamine fibers. Both involve changes in TH, the rate-limiting enzyme in dopamine synthesis. The first, which occurs within 60 hours after a partial lesion, entails increased activity of residual TH molecules by increased binding to the cofactor, tetrahydropterin. This effect disappears within days and is replaced beginning 5 to 7 days after the lesion by increased numbers of TH molecules in residual terminals (116). The increased TH levels persist for several months. As TH concentrations are normally between 1/100 and 1/1000 that of the other enzymes in the dopamine biosynthetic pathway (21), increases in TH activity or in the number of TH molecules can magnify dopamine production.

Whether by these or other mechanisms, compensatory changes occur bilaterally after unilateral lesions (3,74). Andersson and colleagues (3) reported that regulatory changes in dopamine turnover in the striatum contralateral to a kainic acid injection were not evident 2 days after the lesion, but were present by 10 days after the lesion. This observation is consistent with numerous other reports of regulatory interactions between the substantia nigra on both sides of the brain (20,83,84). Therefore, unilateral events, such as surgery or implantation affecting ipsilateral nigrostriatal dopamine regulation should be expected to produce regulatory changes in the contralateral nigrostriatal pathway. Importantly, bilateral increases in striatal dopamine levels have been demonstrated in MPTP-treated mice receiving unilateral intrastriatal grafts of adrenal medulla (14) and of Gelfoam containing bFGF (89). In addition, bilateral functional improvement is the rule, and not the exception, in parkinsonian patients receiving either adrenal or fetal grafts (e.g., see 2,45,46,71,76,102).

CONCLUSIONS

Nigral dopamine neurons retain extensive plasticity in the mature brain. Although there is a gradual loss of dopamine neurons in normal aging, the remaining neurons are able to compensate. Only when disease processes acerbates neuronal injury and striatal dopamine levels fall below 20% of normal, do the symptoms of parkinsonism appear. However, neuronal loss in the substantia nigra is often less severe than the dopamine depletion in the striatum suggests. Although the residual neurons are atrophied, the actual number of neurons may be within 50% of age-matched controls.

The trophic factor theory of functional recovery predicts that implantation stimulates the surviving host midbrain neurons to more effectively provide dopamine to the striatum. Several trophic factors have been reported to promote the survival of mesencephalic dopamine neurons, including BDNF, CNTF, EGF, aFGF, bFGF, GDNF, IGF-1, IGF-2, and PDNF. However, in many instances, the trophic effects may be indirect and depend on the presence of another cell type. Most of these factors exert stimulatory effects on glia cells which, in turn, may elaborate molecules with dopaminergic-promoting actions. Only BDNF and GDNF have been demonstrated to directly affect dopamine neurons.

Injury to the forebrain, including needle insertion and knife cuts, results in the increased expression of BDNF, bFGF, and IGF-1 within hours. Levels of these trophic factors may remain elevated for weeks. The long-term effects of intrastriatal implants on striatal trophic factor production are unclear.

Grafted cells are also capable of providing relevant trophic factors. Adrenal chromaffin cells synthesize bFGF and a factor similar in molecular weight and biologic activity to CNTF. Given the properties of mature neurons, dopamine neurons in fetal mesencephalon grafts should synthesize BDNF, NT-3, aFGF, and bFGF. The mesencephalic glial cells grafted along with the neurons may be even more important, as they seem to mediate many of the trophic effects on dopamine neurons.

Three mechanisms have been identified by which surviving dopamine processes in the striatum can increase dopamine levels: (a) stereotypic changes in TH molecules resulting in increased binding to the cofactor tetrahydropteridine and, therefore, increased activity; (b) increased numbers of TH molecules in residual dopamine terminals in the striatum; (c) collateral sprouting from surviving dopaminergic processes in the forebrain. The rapid time course of TH$^+$ fiber increase in the rat striatum following implantation can best be explained by the first mechanism. However, increased TH activity following injury appears to last for only a few days. It would not seem to account for the longer-term increases in TH$^+$ fibers observed in rodents, monkeys, and humans, as well as the functional recovery seen in monkeys and parkinsonian patients following grafting. Either or both of the other two mechanisms may be operating in graft recipients. On one hand, observations from implants and surgery in rhesus monkeys (8,9) support the interpretation of collateral sprouting. On the other hand, our studies on grafts in cebus monkeys (38) can best be explained as up-regulation of TH in residual axons and terminals. Obviously, carefully designed experiments will be needed to resolve this issue.

In summary, an extensive body of evidence from several sources supports trophic factor involvement in functional recovery. This is not to say that other mechanisms, such as the connectivity of grafted neurons, are not also involved in behavioral recovery. What remains to be resolved is the relative contribution of each of the proposed mechanisms to functional recovery in the parkinsonian brain.

ACKNOWLEDGMENTS

We thank Leja Allyn and Robin Lavy for assistance in manuscript preparation. Studies from our laboratory discussed in this review were supported by NIH grant P01 NS 25778.

REFERENCES

1. Ahlskog JE, Kelly PJ, van Heerden JA, et al. Adrenal medullary transplantation into the brain for treatment of Parkinson's disease: clinical outcome and neurochemical studies. *Mayo Clin Proc* 1990;65:305–328.
2. Allen GS, Burns RS, Tulipan NB, Parker RA. Adrenal medullary transplantation to the caudate nucleus in Parkinson's disease: initial clinical results in 18 patients. *Arch Neurol* 1989; 46:487–491.
3. Andersson K, Schwarcz R, Fuxe K. Compensatory bilateral changes in dopamine turnover after striatal kainate lesion. *Nature* 1980; 283:94–96.
4. Altar AC, Boylan B, Jackson C, Hershenson S, Miller J, Wiegand SJ, Lindsay RM, Hyman C. Brain-derived neurotrophic factor augments rotational behavior and nigrostriatal dopamine turnover in vivo. *Proc Natl Acad Sci USA* 1992;89:11347–11351.
5. Apuzzo MLJ, Neal JH, Waters CH, et al. Utilization of unilateral and bilateral stereotactically placed adrenomedullary–striatal autografts in parkinsonian humans: rationale, techniques, and observations. *Neurosurgery* 1990; 26:746–757.
6. Araujo DM, Cotman CW. Basic FGF in astroglial, microglial, and neuronal cultures: characterization of binding sites and modulation of release by lymphokines and trophic factors. *J Neurosci* 1992;12:1668–1678.
7. Ballarín M, Ernfors P, Lindefors N, Persson H. Hippocampal damage and kainic acid injection induce a rapid increase in mRNA for BDNF and NGF in the rat brain. *Exp Neurol* 1991; 114:35–43.
8. Bankiewicz KS, Plunkett RJ, Jacobowitz DM, Kopin IJ, Oldfield EH. Fetal nondopaminergic neural implants in parkinsonian primates. *J Neurosurg* 1991;74:97–104.
9. Bankiewicz KS, Plunkett RJ, Jacobowitz DM, et al. The effect of fetal mesencephalon implants on primate MPTP-induced parkinsonism. *J Neurosurg* 1990;72:231–244.
10. Bean AJ, Elde R, Cao Y, et al. Expression of acidic and basic fibroblast growth factors in the substantia nigra of rat, monkey, and human. *Proc Natl Acad Sci USA* 1991;88:10237–10241.
11. Blottner D, Westermann R, Grothe C, Böhlen, Unsicker K. Basic fibroblast growth factor in the adrenal gland: possible trophic role for preganglionic neurons *in vivo*. *Eur J Neurosci* 1989;1:471–478.
12. Bogerts B, Häntsch J, Herzer M. A morphometric study of the dopamine-containing cell groups in the mesencephalon of normals, Parkinson patients, and schizophrenics. *Biol Psychiatry* 1983;18:951–969.
13. Bohn MC, Cupit L, Marciano F, Gash DM. Adrenal medulla grafts enhance recovery of striatal dopaminergic fibers. *Science* 1987;237:913–916.
14. Bohn MC, Kanuicki M. Bilateral recovery of

striatal dopamine after unilateral adrenal grafting into the striatum of the 1-methyl-4-(2'-methylphenyl)-1,2,3,6-tetrahydropyridine (2'CH$_3$-MPTP)-treated mouse. *J Neurosci Res* 1990;25: 281–286.
15. Bregman BS, Reier PJ. Neural tissue transplants rescue axotomized rubrospinal cells from retrograde death. *J Comp Neurol* 1986; 244:86–95.
16. Burgess WH, Maciag T. The heparin-binding (fibroblast) growth factor family of proteins. *Annu Rev Biochem* 1989;58:575–606.
17. Carman LS, Gage FH, Shults CW. Partial lesion of the substantia nigra: relation between extent of lesion and rotational behavior. *Brain Res* 1991;553:275–283.
18. Casper D, Mytilineou C, Blum M. EGF enhances the survival of dopamine neurons in rat embryonic mesencephalon primary cell culture. *J Neurosci Res* 1991;30:372–381.
19. Castañeda E, Whishaw IQ, Robinson TE. Changes in striatal dopamine neurotransmission assessed with microdialysis following recovery from a bilateral 6-OHDA lesion: variation as a function of lesion size. *J Neurosci* 1990;10:1847–1854.
20. Castellano MA, Diaz MR. Nigrostriatal dopaminergic cell activity is under control by substantia nigra of the contralateral brain side: electrophysiological evidence. *Brain Res Bull* 1991;27:213–218.
21. Cooper JR, Bloom FE, Roth RH. *The biochemical basis of neuropharmacology*, 6th ed. New York: Oxford University Press; 1991.
22. Dalia A, Neff NH, Hadjiconstantinou M. GM$_1$ ganglioside improves dopaminergic markers of rat mesencephalic cultures treated with MPP$^+$. *J Neurosci* 1993;13:3104–3111.
23. Date I, Felten SY, Felten DL. Exogenous GM$_1$ gangliosides induce partial recovery of the nigrostriatal dopaminergic system in MPTP-treated young mice but not in aging mice. *Neurosci Lett* 1989;106:282–286.
24. Date I, Felten SY, Felten DL. Cografts of adrenal medulla with peripheral nerve enhance the survivability of transplanted adrenal chromaffin cells and recovery of the host nigrostriatal dopaminergic system in MPTP-treated young adult mice. *Brain Res* 1990;537:33–39.
25. Date I, Felten SY, Felten DL. The nigrostriatal dopaminergic system in MPTP-treated mice shows more prominent recovery by syngeneic adrenal medullary graft than by allogeneic or xenogeneic graft. *Brain Res* 1991;545:191–198.
26. Date I, Notter MFD, Felten SY, Felten DL. MPTP-treated young mice but not aging mice show partial recovery of the nigrostriatal dopaminergic system by stereotaxic injection of acidic fibroblast growth factor (aFGF). *Brain Res* 1990;526:156–160.
27. Davis S, Aldrich TH, Valenzuela DM, et al. The receptor for ciliary neurotrophic factor. *Science* 1991;253:59–63.
28. de Quidt ME, Emson PC. Neuropeptide Y in the adrenal gland: characterisation, distribu-

tion and drug effects. *Neuroscience* 1986; 19:1011–1022.

29. Doering LC, Tokiwa MA. Adrenal medulla and substantia nigra co-grafts in peripheral nerve: chromaffin cells survive for long periods and prevent degeneration of nigral neurons. *Brain Res* 1991;551:267–278.

30. Dugich–Djordjevic MM, Tocco G, Lapchak PA, et al. Regionally specific and rapid increases in brain-derived neurotrophic factor messenger RNA in the adult rat brain following seizures induced by systemic administration of kainic acid. *Neuroscience* 1992;47:303–315.

31. Eidelberg E, Brooks BA, Morgan WW, Walden JG, Kokemoor RH. Variability and functional recovery in the *n*-methyl-4-phenyl-1,2,3,6-tetrahydropyridine model of parkinsonism in monkeys. *Neuroscience* 1986;18:817–822.

32. Engele J, Bohn MC. The neurotrophic effects of fibroblast growth factors on dopaminergic neurons *in vitro* are mediated by mesencephalic glia. *J Neurosci* 1991;11:3070–3078.

33. Ernfors P, Lönnerberg P, Ayer-LeLievre C, Persson H. Developmental and regional expression of basic fibroblast growth factor mRNA in the rat central nervous system. *J Neurosci Res* 1990;27:10–15.

34. Ernfors P, Wetmore C, Olson L, Persson H. Identification of cells in rat brain and peripheral tissues expressing mRNA for members of the nerve growth factor family. *Neuron* 1990; 5:511–526.

35. Ewing SE, Weber RJ, Zauner A, Plunkett RJ. Recovery in hemiparkinsonian rats following intrastriatal implantation of activated leukocytes. *Brain Res* 1992;576:42–48.

36. Fallon JH, Annis CM, Gentry LE, Twardzik DR, Loughlin SE. Localization of cells containing transforming growth factor-α precursor immunoreactivity in the basal ganglia of the adult rat brain. *Growth Factors* 1990;2:241–250.

37. Ferrari G, Minozzi M–C, Toffano G, Leon A, Skaper SD. Basic fibroblast growth factor promotes the survival and development of mesencephalic neurons in culture. *Dev Biol* 1989; 133:140–147.

38. Fiandaca MS, Kordower JH, Hansen JT, Jiao S–S, Gash DM. Adrenal medullary autografts into the basal ganglia of cebus monkeys: injury-induced regeneration. *Exp Neurol* 1988;102:76–91.

39. Finklestein SP, Fanning PJ, Caday CG, et al. Increased levels of basic fibroblast growth factor (bFGF) following focal brain injury. *Restor Neurol Neurosci* 1990;1:387–394.

40. Frautschy SA, Walicke PA, Baird A. Localization of basic fibroblast growth factor and its mRNA after CNS injury. *Brain Res* 1991; 553:291–299.

41. Freund TF, Bolam JP, Björklund A, et al. Efferent synaptic connections of grafted dopaminergic neurons reinnervating the host neostriatum: a tyrosine hydroxylase immunocytochemical study. *J Neurosci* 1985;5:603–616.

42. Gall CM, Gold SJ, Isackson PJ, Seroogy KB. Brain-derived neurotrophic factor and neurotrophin-3 mRNAs are expressed in ventral midbrain regions containing dopaminergic neurons. *Mol Cell Neurosci* 1992;3:56–63.

43. Garcia-Segura LM, Perez J, Pons S, Rejas MT, Torres-Aleman I. Localization of insulin-like growth factor I (IGF-I)-like immunoreactivity in the developing and adult rat brain. *Brain Res* 1991;560:167–174.

44. Gilad GM, Reis DJ. Collateral sprouting in central mesolimbic dopamine neurons: biochemical and immunocytochemical evidence of changes in the activity and distribution of tyrosine hydroxylase in terminal fields and in cell bodies of A10 neurons. *Brain Res* 1979;160:17–36.

45. Goetz CG, Stebbins GT, Klawans HL, et al. United Parkinson Foundation Neurotransplantation Registry on adrenal medullary transplants: presurgical, and 1- and 2-year follow-up. *Neurology* 1991;41:1719–1722.

46. Goetz CG, Tanner CM, Penn RD, et al. Adrenal medullary transplant to the striatum of patients with advanced Parkinson's disease: 1-year motor and psychomotor data. *Neurology* 1990; 40:273–276.

47. Hadjiconstantinou M, Fitkin JG, Dalia A, Neff NH. Epidermal growth factor enhances striatal dopaminergic parameters in the 1-methyl-4-phenyl-1,2,3,6-tetrahydropyridine-treated mouse. *J Neurochem* 1991;57:479–482.

48. Hadjiconstantinou M, Rossetti ZL, Paxton RC, Neff NH. Administration of GM_1 ganglioside restores the dopamine content in striatum after chronic treatment with MPTP. *Neuropharmacology* 1986;25:1075–1077.

49. Hagg T, Varon S. Ciliary neurotrophic factor (CNTF) prevents axotomy-induced degeneration of adult rat substantia nigra dopaminergic neurons. *Soc Neurosci Abstr* 1992;18:390.

50. Hansen JT, Kordower JH, Fiandaca MS, Jiao S–S, Notter MFD, Gash DM. Adrenal medullary autografts into the basal ganglia of cebus monkeys: graft viability and fine structure. *Exp Neurol* 1988;102:65–75.

51. Hirsch EC, Duyckaerts C, Javoy-Agid F, Hauw J-J, Agid Y. Does adrenal graft enhance recovery of dopaminergic neurons in Parkinson's disease? *Ann Neurol* 1990;27:676–682.

52. Holzwarth MA, Brownfield MS. Serotonin coexists with epinephrine in rat adrenal medullary cells. *Neuroendocrinology* 1985;41:230–236.

53. Hornykiewicz O, Kish SJ. Biochemical pathophysiology of Parkinson's disease. In: Yahr MD, Bergmann KJ, eds. *Parkinson's disease. Adv Neurol* 1986;45:19–34.

54. Hurtig H, Joyce J, Sladek JR Jr, Trojanowski JQ. Postmortem analysis of adrenal-medulla-to-caudate autograft in a patient with Parkinson's disease. *Ann Neurol* 1989;25:607–614.

55. Hyman C, Hofer M, Barde Y-A, et al. BDNF is a neurotrophic factor for dopaminergic neurons of the substantia nigra. *Nature* 1991;350:230–232.

56. Jaeger CB. Cytoarchitectonics of substantia

nigra grafts: a light and electron microscopic study of immunocytochemically identified dopaminergic neurons and fibrous astrocytes. *J Comp Neurol* 1985;231:121–135.

57. Jankovic J, Grossman R, Goodman C, et al. Clinical, biochemical, and neuropathologic findings following transplantation of adrenal medulla to the caudate nucleus for treatment of Parkinson's disease. *Neurology* 1989;39:1227–1234.

58. Jellinger K. Overview of morphological changes in Parkinson's disease. In: Yahr MD, Bergmann KJ, eds. *Parkinson's disease. Adv Neurol* 1986;45:1–18.

59. Jenner P, Schapira AHV, Marsden CD. New insights into the cause of Parkinson's disease. *Neurology* 1992;42:2241–2250.

60. Kastner A, Hirsch EC, Agid Y, Javoy–Agid F. Tyrosine hydroxylase protein and messenger RNA in the dopaminergic nigral neurons of patients with Parkinson's disease. *Brain Res* 1993;606:341–345.

61. Kelly PJ, Ahlskog JE, van Heerden JA, Carmichael SW, Stoddard SL, Bell GN. Adrenal medullary autograft transplantation into the striatum of patients with Parkinson's disease. *Mayo Clin Proc* 1989;64:282–290.

62. Kesslak JP, Nieto-Sampedro M, Globus J, Cotman CW. Transplants of purified astrocytes promote behavioral recovery after frontal cortex ablation. *Exp Neurol* 1986;92:377–390.

63. Knüsel B, Michel PP, Schwaber JS, Hefti F. Selective and nonselective stimulation of central cholinergic and dopaminergic development *in vitro* by nerve growth factor, basic fibroblast growth factor, epidermal growth factor, insulin and the insulin-like growth factors I and II. *J Neurosci* 1990;10:558–570.

64. Knüsel B, Winslow JW, Rosenthal A, et al. Promotion of central cholinergic and dopaminergic neuron differentiation by brain-derived neurotrophic factor but not neurotrophin 3. *Proc Natl Acad Sci USA* 1991;88:961–965.

65. Kordower JH, Cochran E, Penn RD, Goetz CG. Putative chromaffin cell survival and enhanced host-derived TH-fiber innervation following a functional adrenal medulla autograft for Parkinson's disease. *Ann Neurol* 1991;29:405–412.

66. Kudlow JE, Leung AWC, Kobrin MS, Paterson AJ, Asa SL. Transforming growth factor-α in the mammalian brain: immunohistochemical detection in neurons and characterization of its mRNA. *J Biol Chem* 1989;264:3880–3883.

67. Labbe R, Firl A, Mufson EJ, Stein DG. Fetal brain transplant: reduction of cognitive deficits in rats with frontal cortex lesions. *Science* 1983;221:470–472.

68. Lapchak, PA, Beck KD, Araujo DM, Irwin I, Langston JW, Hefti F. Chronic intranigral administration of brain-derived neurotrophic factor produces striatal dopaminergic hypofunction in unlesioned adult rats and fails to attenuate the decline of striatal dopaminergic function following medial forebrain bundle transection. *Neuroscience* 1993;53:639–650.

69. Lazar LM, Blum M. Regional distribution and developmental expression of epidermal growth factor and transforming growth factor-α mRNA in mouse brain by a quantitative nuclease protection assay. *J Neurosci* 1992;12:1688–1697.

70. Leenders KL, Salmon EP, Tyrrell P, Perani D, Brooks DJ, Sager H, Jones T, Marsden CD, Frackowiak RSJ. The nigrostriatal dopaminergic system assessed in vivo by positron emission tomography in healthy volunteer subjects and patients with Parkinson's disease. *Arch Neurol* 1990;47:1290–1298.

71. Lieberman A, Ransohoff J, Berczeller P, et al. Adrenal medullary transplants as a treatment for advanced Parkinson's disease. *Acta Neurol Scand* 1989;126:189–196.

72. Lillien LE, Sendtner M, Rohrer H, Hughes SM, Raff MC. Type-2 astrocyte development in rat brain cultures is initiated by a CNTF-like protein produced by type-1 astrocytes. *Neuron* 1988;1:485–494.

73. Lin L-FH, Doherty DH, Lile JD, Bektesh S, Collins F. GDNF: a glial cell line-derived neurotrophic factor for midbrain dopaminergic neurons. *Science* 1993;260:1130–1132.

74. Lindefors N, Ungerstedt U. Bilateral regulation of glutamate tissue and extracellular levels in caudate–putamen by midbrain dopamine neurons. *Neurosci Lett* 1990;115:248–252.

75. Lindvall O, Ernfors P, Bengzon J, et al. Differential regulation of mRNAs for nerve growth factor, brain-derived neurotrophic factor, and neurotrophin 3 in the adult rat brain following cerebral ischemia and hypoglycemic coma. *Proc Natl Acad Sci USA* 1992;89:648–652.

76. Lindvall O, Widner H, Rehncrona S, et al. Transplantation of fetal dopamine neurons in Parkinson's disease: one-year clinical and neurophysiological observations in two patients with putaminal implants. *Ann Neurol* 1992, 31:155–165.

77. Logan A, Frautschy SA, Gonzalez A-M, Baird A. A time course for the focal elevation of synthesis of basic fibroblast growth factor and one of its high-affinity receptors (flg) following a localized cortical brain injury. *J Neurosci* 1992; 12:3828–3837.

78. Mahalik TJ, Finger TE, Stromberg I, Olson L. Substantia nigra transplants into denervated striatum of the rat: ultrastructure of graft and host interconnections. *J Comp Neurol* 1985; 240:60–70.

79. Maisonpierre PC, Belluscio L, Friedman B, et al. NT-3, BDNF, and NGF in the developing rat nervous system: parallel as well as reciprocal patterns of expression. *Neuron* 1990;5:501–509.

80. Marciano FF, Wiegand SJ, Sladek JR Jr, Gash DM. Fetal hypothalamic transplants promote survival and functional regeneration of axotomized adult supraoptic magnocellular neurons. *Brain Res* 1989;483:135–142.

81. Marquardt H, Hunkapiller MW, Hood LE, Todaro GJ. Rat transforming growth factor type 1: structure and relation to epidermal growth factor. *Science* 1984;223:1079–1082.

82. McGeer PL, McGeer EG, Suzuki JS. Aging and extrapyramidal function. *Arch Neurol* 1977; 34:33–35.

83. Nieoullon A, Chéramy A, Glowinski J. Interdependence of the nigrostriatal dopaminergic systems on the two sides of the brain in the cat. *Science* 1977;198:416–418.

84. Nieoullon A, Chéramy A, Leviel V, Glowinski J. Effects of the unilateral nigral application of dopaminergic drugs on the *in vivo* release of dopamine in the two caudate nuclei of the cat. *Eur J Pharmacol* 1979;53:289–296.

85. Nieto-Sampedro M, Cotman CW. Growth factor induction and temporal order in central nervous system repair. In: Cotman, ed. *Synaptic plasticity*. New York: Guilford Press; 1985:407–455.

86. Nikkhah G, Odin P, Smits A, Tingstrom A, Othberg A, Brundin P, Funa K, Lindvall O. Platelet-derived growth factor promotes survival of rat and human mesencephalic dopaminergic neurons in culture. *Exp Brain Res* 1993;92:516–523.

87. Olson L, Backlund E-O, Ebendal T, et al. Intraputaminal infusion of nerve growth factor to support adrenal medullary autografts in Parkinson's disease. *Arch Neurol* 1991;48:373–381.

88. Osamura RY, Tsutsumi Y, Yanaihara N, Imura H, Watanabe K. Immunohistochemical studies for multiple peptide-immunoreactivities and colocalization of met-enkephalin-Arg^6-Gly^7-Leu^8, neuropeptide Y and somatostatin in human adrenal medulla and pheochromocytomas. *Peptides* 1987;8:77–87.

89. Otto D, Unsicker K. Basic FGF reverses chemical and morphological deficits in the nigrostriatal system of MPTP-treated mice. *J Neurosci* 1990;10:1912–1921.

90. Paxinos G, ed. *The rat nervous system, vol 1; Forebrain and midbrain*. Sydney: Academic Press; 1985.

91. Perese DA, Ulman J, Viola J, Ewing SE, Bankiewicz KS. A 6-hydroxydopamine-induced selective parkinsonian rat model. *Brain Res* 1989;494:285–293.

92. Peterson DI, Price ML, Small CS. Autopsy findings in a patient who had an adrenal-to-brain transplant for Parkinson's disease. *Neurology* 1989;39:235–238.

93. Pezzoli G, Zecchinelli A, Ricciardi S, et al. Intraventricular infusion of epidermal growth factor restores dopaminergic pathway in hemiparkinsonian rats. *Mov Disord* 1991;6:281–287.

94. Phillips HS, Hains JM, Laramee GR, Rosenthal A, Winslow JW. Widespread expression of BDNF but not NT3 by target areas of basal forebrain cholinergic neurons. *Science* 1990; 250:290–294.

95. Plunkett RJ, Bankiewicz KS, Cummins AC, et al. Long-term evaluation of hemiparkinsonian monkeys after adrenal autografting or cavitation alone. *J Neurosurg* 1990;73:918–926.

96. Pruss RM, Mezey E, Forman DS, et al. Enkephalin and neuropeptide Y: two colocalized neuropeptides are independently regulated in primary cultures of bovine chromaffin cells. *Neuropeptides* 1986;7:315–327.

97. Roberts RC, DiFiglia M. Evidence for synaptic proliferation, reorganization, and growth in the excitotoxic lesioned adult rat caudate nucleus. *Exp Neurol* 1990;107:1–10.

98. Rotwein P, Burgess SK, Milbrandt JD, Krause JE. Differential expression of insulin-like growth factor genes in rat central nervous system. *Proc Natl Acad Sci USA* 1988;85:265–269.

99. Sable BA, Slavin MD, Stein DG. GM$_1$ ganglioside treatment facilitates behavioral recovery from bilateral brain damage. *Science* 1984; 225:340–341.

100. Schneider JS, Pope A, Simpson K, Taggart J, Smith MG, DiStefano L. Recovery from experimental parkinsonism in primates with GM$_1$ ganglioside treatment. *Science* 1992;256:843–846.

101. Seroogy KB, Lundgren KH, Guthrie KM, Tran TD, Isackson PJ, Gall CM. Dopaminergic neurons express NT-3 and BDNF mRNAs in rat mesencephalon. *Soc Neurosci Abstr* 1992;18:234.

102. Spencer DD, Robbins RJ, Naftolin F, et al. Unilateral transplantation of human fetal mesencephalic tissue into the caudate nucleus of patients with Parkinson's disease. *N Engl J Med* 1992;327:1541–1548.

103. Spina MB, Hyman C, Squinto S, Lindsay RM. Brain-derived neurotrophic factor protects dopaminergic cells from 6-hydroxydopamine toxicity. *Ann NY Acad Sci* 1992;648:348–350.

104. Stockli KA, Lillien LE, Naher-Noe M, et al. Regional distribution, developmental changes, and cellular localization of CNTF-mRNA and protein in the rat brain. *J Cell Biol* 1991; 115:447–459.

105. Svendgaard NA, Björklund A, Stenevi U. Regenerative properties of central monoamine neurons: studies in the adult rat using cerebral iris implants as targets. *Adv Anat Embryol Cell Biol* 1975;51/4:3–77.

106. Taylor R. A lot of "excitement" about neurodegeneration. *Science* 1991;252:1380–1381.

107. Toffano G, Savoini GE, Moroni F, Lombardi G, Calza L, Agnati LF. Chronic GM$_1$ ganglioside treatment reduces dopamine cell body degeneration in the substantia nigra after unilateral hemitransection in rat. *Brain Res* 1984;296:233–239.

108. Touyama I, Hara Y, Yasuhara O, et al. Production of antisera to acidic fibroblast growth factor and their application to immunohistochemical study in rat brain. *Neuroscience* 1991; 40:769–779.

109. Unsicker K, Stögbauer F. Screening of adrenal medullary neuropeptides for putative neurotrophic effects. *Int J Dev Neurosci* 1992; 10:171–179.

110. Waters CM, Hund SP, Jenner P, Marsden CD. An immunohistochemical study of the acute and long-term effects of 1-methyl-4-phenyl-1,2,3,6-tetrahydropyridine in the marmoset. *Neuroscience* 1987;23:1025–1039.

111. Waters C, Itabashi HH, Apuzzo MLJ, Weiner

LP. Adrenal to caudate transplantation—post-mortem study. *Mov Disord* 1990;5:248–250.

112. Watts RL, Bakay RAE, Herring CJ, et al. Preliminary report on adrenal medullary grafting and cografting with sural nerve in the treatment of hemiparkinsonian monkeys. In: Dunnett SB, Richards S-J, eds. *Neural transplantation: from molecular basis to clinical applications. Prog Brain Res* 1990;82:581–591.

113. Westermann R, Johannsen M, Unsicker K, Grothe C. Basic fibroblast growth factor (bFGF) immunorcactivity is present in chromaffin granules. *J Neurochem* 1990;55:285–292.

114. Wilcox JN, Derynck R. Localization of cells synthesizing transforming growth factor-alpha mRNA in the mouse brain. *J Neurosci* 1988; 8:1901–1904.

115. Winkler H, Apps DK, Fischer-Colbrie R. The molecular function of adrenal chromaffin granules: established facts and unresolved topics. *Neuroscience* 1986;18:261–290.

116. Wolf ME, Zigmond MJ, Kapatos G. Tyrosine hydroxylase content of residual striatal dopamine nerve terminals following 6-hydroxydopamine administration: a flow cytometric study. *J Neurochem* 1989;53:879–885.

117. Woodward WR, Nishi R, Meshul CK, Williams TE, Coulombe M, Eckenstein FP. Nuclear and cytoplasmic localization of basic fibroblast growth factor in astrocytes and CA_2 hippocampal neurons. *J Neurosci* 1992;12:142–152.

118. Yamaguchi F, Itano T, Miyamoto O, et al. Increase of extracellular insulin-like growth factor I (IGF-I) concentration following electrolytical lesion in rat hippocampus. *Neurosci Lett* 1991;128:273–276.

119. Zhang Z, Bresjanac M, Greenamyre JT, Olschowka J, Gash DM. Sprouting in partial nigrostriatal lesioned rats following adrenal medulla and sciatic nerve cografts. *Soc Neurosci Abstr* 1992;18:1321.

120. Zigmond MJ, Acheson AL, Stachowiak MK, Stricker EM. Neurochemical compensation after nigrostriatal bundle injury in an animal model of preclinical parkinsonism. *Arch Neurol* 1984;41:856–861.

121. Zigmond MJ, Stachowiak MK, Berger TW, Stricker EM. Neurochemical events underlying continued function despite injury to monoaminergic systems. *Exp Brain Res* 1986;13 (*suppl*):119–128.

Functional Neural Transplantation,
edited by S. B. Dunnett and A. Björklund.
Raven Press, Ltd., New York © 1994.

7

Functional Capacity of Striatal Transplants in the Rat Huntington Model

*Anders Björklund, *Kenneth Campbell, †D. J. Sirinathsinghji,
‡Rosemary A. Fricker, and ‡Stephen B. Dunnett

*Department of Medical Cell Research, University of Lund, S-223 62 Lund, Sweden,
†Merck Sharp & Dohme Research Laboratories, Neuroscience Research Centre, Harlow,
Essex CM20 2QR, United Kingdom, ‡Department of Experimental Psychology, University of
Cambridge, Cambridge CB2 3EB, United Kingdom

Intracerebral neural transplants may promote functional recovery in the lesioned CNS by several different mechanisms. On the simplest possible level, implanted cells can provide a local drug-delivery system, a "biologic minipump," which may have distinct advantages over systemic delivery in that it circumvents the blood–brain barrier and allows targeting of an active compound to a particular brain region. Cells releasing, for example, neurotransmitters, peptides, or growth factors may not require any sophisticated regulatory machinery to exert functional effects. In other instances, the grafts' physiologic actions may depend on regulated neuronal release mechanisms, synaptic connections, or more extensive anatomic integration with the host brain. As discussed in further detail in the last chapter of this book, the functional capacity of fetal CNS tissue grafts is likely to reflect a combination of these various mechanisms.

Neural grafting for the correction of basal ganglia dysfunction has been based on two principal strategies (i.e., neurotransmitter replacement and pathway reconstruction), which have been explored in two lesion models:

1. *The Parkinson-like condition* induced by 6-hydroxydopamine (6-OHDA)- or 1-methyl-4-phenyl-1,2,3,6-tetrahydropyridine (MPTP)-induced damage of the nigrostriatal dopamine pathway in rats and monkeys: Striatal dopamine depletion is likely to be the principal neurotransmitter deficit underlying the hypokinetic symptoms of parkinsonism. Destruction of the nigrostriatal dopamine system, or blockade of dopaminergic D_2 receptors, is thus sufficient to induce a hypokinetic state in rats and monkeys that closely resembles the condition seen in Parkinson's disease (PD). Dopaminergic drugs (L-dopa or dopamine receptor agonists) are effective in alleviating the symptoms of PD, at least in the early stages of the disease.

2. *The Huntington-like condition* seen in animals with excitotoxin-induced destruction of the neurons of the nucleus caudatus–putamen: In Huntington's disease (HD) the neuropathology is more complex, involving a disruption of some of the major input–output circuits of the basal ganglia. The principal symptoms include complex emotional and cognitive disturbances, coupled with incapacitating involuntary movements (chorea) that develop progressively over a 10- to 20-year period. The hyperkinetic symptoms of HD, and possibly also

some of the cognitive impairments, may be conceived as the result of a progressive destruction of the striatal projection neurons, of which the principal transmitter is γ-aminobutyric acid (GABA) (see 1 and 29, for recent reviews). Consistent with this view, Crossman et al. (19) have shown that injection of GABA antagonists into the lateral part of the globus pallidus (i.e., one of the primary target areas of the striatal GABAergic projection neurons) can induce hyperkinetic (choreic) movements in monkeys. Also, in rodents, local infusion of GABA–receptor-active drugs into striatal output structures, including the globus pallidus or substantia nigra pars reticulata, have been observed to induce substantial effects on motor behavior (40,81,89, 107).

These data suggest that defective GABA neurotransmission in critical striatal output structures might play an important role in the choreic symptoms of HD. Crossman et al. (19) and Albin et al. (1) have argued that degeneration of the GABAergic projection to the globus pallidus might be the most critical element, leading, first, to a hyperactivity of the GABAergic pallidosubthalamic pathway and, second, to a functional inactivation of the subthalamic nucleus. Nevertheless, it has proved difficult to alleviate the hyperkinetic symptoms of HD through systemic administration of GABA–receptor-active drugs. This is probably because GABA neurons are connected in series in the striatal output pathways (12). The effect of GABA receptor activation in one area (e.g., globus pallidus) may thus be counteracted by simultaneous receptor activation in another connected site (e.g., subthalamic nucleus). Local GABA delivery (e.g., into the globus pallidus) could provide a possible means to circumvent this problem.

The principal idea underlying neural transplantation in the rat HD model is to restitute a striatum-like structure at the site of the excitotoxic striatal damage and thereby replace some of the functions lost by the destruction of the striatal projection neurons. The striatal projection neurons, however, have quite different functional characteristics and play quite different roles in the functional processing of the basal ganglia than do the nigrostriatal dopamine neurons. The nigral dopamine neurons generally are considered to be a modulatory "level-setting" system, which may exert many of their functions in a tonic regulatory manner in the absence of specific patterned input–output signals. By contrast, the striatal projection neurons represent a site of convergence of topographically organized cortical and thalamic inputs that are conveyed downstream toward the subcortical motor systems. Thus, although the nigral dopamine neurons may be able to exert some of their functions in the absence of extrinsic afferent regulation, the striatal projection neurons are likely to require at least a minimum of regulatory afferent inputs. The goal of the neuronal replacement strategy in the rat HD model, therefore, is not only to restore striatal GABA neurotransmission, but to make use of the growth properties of the fetal striatal neurons and neuroblasts to restore some critical aspects of the lesioned host striatal circuitry.

THE EXPERIMENTAL MODEL

Injections of ibotenic acid (IA) or kainic acid (KA) into the head of the caudate–putamen in rats cause extensive (>90–95%) neuronal cell loss in the injected area, accompanied by reactive gliosis and a reduction of the transmitter-related enzymes, glutamic acid decarboxylase (GAD) and choline acetyltransferase (ChAT), by 70% to 85% (17,52,53,79,110). The magnitude of the atrophic changes that are seen after large doses of IA (16–20 µg) are similar to those reported for advanced cases of HD (6): Beginning at about 4 weeks after injection there is a progressive atrophy of the neuron-depleted area, resulting in up to 60% to 70% reduction in volume, and a 50% to 55% reduction in weight, of the head of the caudate–putamen by 3 to 4 months. Although the myelinated fiber bundles of the internal capsule are spared, the gray matter is replaced by a dense astrocytic glial scar (36). As a consequence of tissue shrinkage, the lateral ventricle is greatly enlarged. In addition, there are also signs of neuronal cell loss in those brain structures that are anatomically directly linked with the caudate–putamen (i.e., neocortex, globus pallidus, and the substantia nigra pars reticulata; 55,93,99). The dopamine neurons of the pars compacta, the target neurons of which are destroyed by the excitotoxic damage, exhibit shrinkage (by about 30%)— but no or minimal cell loss—that is fully developed within 2 to 3 months (71,91). Consistent with this, the density of the dopamine-containing terminal network in the lesioned striatum appears to be reduced over time (53).

In the cell suspension graft procedure, cells obtained from E14–15 rat fetuses are injected stereotaxically into the lesioned caudate–putamen. After implantation of $4–10 \times 10^5$ to 10×10^5 cells (corresponding to one to two striatal primordia) the grafts will grow to reach a final size of 5 to 12 mm^3 (52,53). As a consequence, the neuron-depleted, atrophic striatum increases in volume from about 30% to 50% to about 70% to 80% of its normal size. The intrastriatal striatal grafts develop and mature with a time course that is fairly close to that of the normal striatum: they increase five- to eightfold in volume over the first 3 weeks, and they appear to have reached their final size and anatomic maturation by 6 to 8 weeks (62). Interestingly, the growth and development of the grafts depend greatly on the conditions at the implantation site. Grafts implanted into the nonlesioned striatum were initially of the same size as those implanted into the neuron-depleted striatum (about 1 mm^3 at 4 days), but they did not grow in size at longer survival times (62), and grafts implanted into long-term lesioned (i.e., severely atrophic) striata grow to about 70% to 80% of the size obtained with control grafts implanted into recent le-

sions (61). Striatal grafts implanted into other brain regions, such as globus pallidus, substantia nigra, or neocortex, reach much smaller final sizes than those implanted into the recent or long-term excitotoxin-lesioned striatum (55). These observations indicate that trophic interactions between the implanted fetal tissue and the host brain environment play an important role in the growth and maturation of the fetal tissue implants.

MORPHOLOGIC FEATURES OF INTRASTRIATAL STRIATAL GRAFTS

The double protrusion area of the embryonic telencephalic ventricular wall, the so-called ganglionic eminences (Fig. 1), which is used as graft tissue in these studies, is a heterogeneous structure that gives rise not only to the striatal primordium, but also to other components of the basal forebrain. Thus, during normal embryogenesis, the ganglionic eminences are likely to contribute to the generation of neurons in, for example, the globus pallidus, amygdala and the piriform cortex. Consistent with this, the intrastriatal striatal grafts are morphologically heterogeneous. Mature grafts derived from dissections that include the combined lateral and medial ganglionic eminences from E14–E15 donors contain patches of striatum-like tissue, characterized by their DARPP-32 immunopositivity (Fig. 2A) (62,130) and dense acetylcholinesterase (AChE) staining (see Fig. 2B) (45,55). These areas, named "patch-zones" or *P-zones* by Graybiel et al. (45), also receive a characteristic dense tyrosine hydroxylase (TH)-positive innervation and express dopamine D$_1$ and D$_2$ receptors. The DARPP-32-negative, AChE-poor areas of the grafts (designated "nonpatch" or NP-zones by Graybiel et al.) are generally considered nonstriatal (see below). The striatum-like nature of the P-zones is further supported by the demonstration of the so-called striatum-enriched phosphatase (STEP) (68) exclusively within these areas

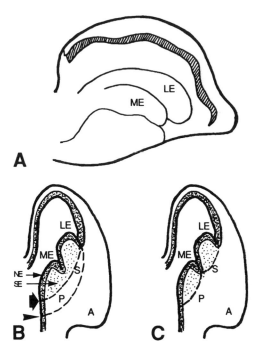

FIG. 1. Schematic representation of E14–15 fetal telencephalon showing areas that were dissected for transplantation. **A**: Medial view of the lateral ventricular wall showing both the medial and lateral elevations (*ME* and *LE*, respectively). **B**: Cross-section through the E14–15 telencephalon at the level of the medial and lateral elevations. The *dashed lines* indicate the minimal (*thick arrow*) and maximal extents of the dissection for striatal grafts derived from both the medial and lateral elevations. Note that the maximal dissection is likely to include both the striatal (*S*) and pallidal (*P*) primordia. **C**: *Dashed lines* denote the approximate extent of the regions dissected in grafts derived from either the medial or lateral elevation selectively. *A*, amygdalar primordium, *NE*, neuroepithelium; *SE*, subependymal layer. (Modified from Wictorin et al., 130)

of the striatal grafts (Fig. 3; R. A. Fricker and S. B. Dunnett, *unpublished observations*).

In a recent study, Pakhzeban et al. (90) have found that the proportion of the striatal grafts expressing striatal markers can be greatly enhanced (up to 80–90%) if the dissection is limited to the dorsal, superficial part of the lateral eminence (see Figs. 1C and 2C). Conversely, dissections limited to the superficial part of the medial eminence give rise to grafts that are essentially free of striatum-like tissue (see Fig. 2D) (90; K. Campbell et al., *unpublished observations*). However, grafts derived from the entire medial eminence, including its deep portion, do contain the usual mix of striatal and nonstriatal tissue (94). These results suggest that the nonstriatal graft compartment is contributed, in part, by the superficial part of the medial ganglionic eminence (which is the largest of the two in E14–15 rat embryos) and, in part, by the deeper portions of the lateral eminence that borders onto the cortical and amygdalar primordia.

The importance of donor age for the final size and morphologic composition of intrastriatal striatal grafts has only recently been addressed. In a direct comparison of grafts from four different donor ages, for which each graft comprised the amount of tissue obtained from one striatal primordium, Fricker and Dunnett (*unpublished observations*) have found that the P-zone (determined by AchE staining and STEP immunohistochemistry) is markedly reduced in

FIG. 2. P- and NP-zones in the grafts. Intrastriatal striatal grafts derived from both the medial and lateral elevations (see Fig. 1) display a heterogeneous (patchy) expression of the striatal markers DARPP-32 (**A**) and AChE (**B**). These two striatal markers are found within the same patch regions of the transplant (*T*) as shown on the adjacent sections in A and B. Both markers are distributed homogeneously within the host striatum (*H*). **C,D**: The pattern of DARPP-32 immunoreactivity within the transplant when selective dissections of the lateral (C) and medial (D) elevations are used. Note the considerable increase in the striatum-like regions (as measured by DARPP-32-immunohistochemistry) of the grafts in transplants derived solely from the lateral elevation. Transplants derived from the medial elevation are characteristically low in DARPP-32-immunoreactivity. *Arrowheads* in C and D delineate the borders of the transplant; *arrows* indicate small patches of DARPP-32-labeled neurons. *cc*, corpus callosum. *L*, lesioned striatum with densely packed myelin fiber bundles. Scale bars, 200 μm. (A,B: modified from ref. 130; C,D: *unpublished observations*.)

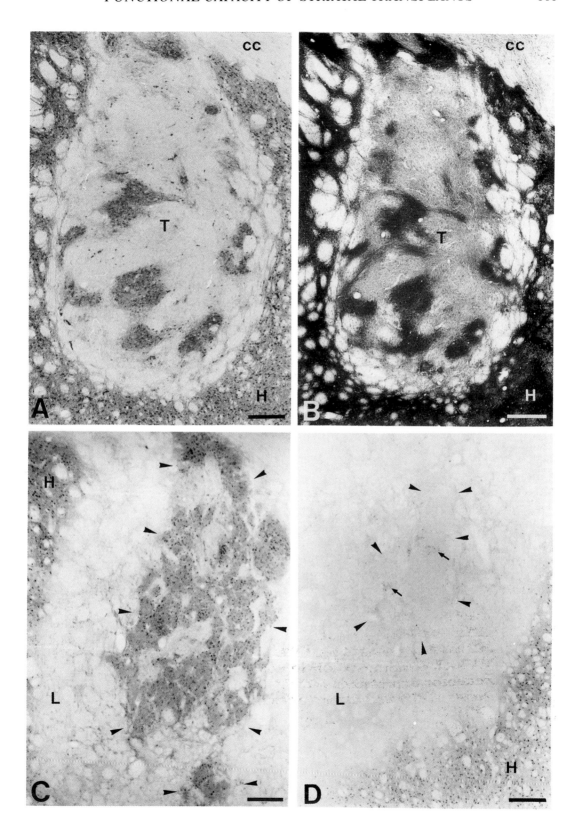

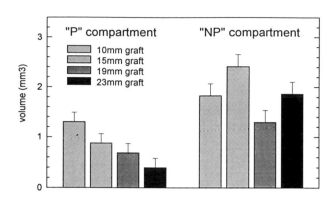

FIG. 3. Internal organization of striatal grafts depends on donor age. The volumes of the AChE-positive patches (the *P-zone compartment*) and the remaining AChE-negative areas (the *NP-zone compartment*) were measured in grafts derived from donors of four different embryonic ages, as indicated by the crown–rump lengths (CRL; 10–23 mm). For each donor age the amount of tissue grafted in each recipient corresponds to one striatal primordium. (Data from R. A. Fricker and S. B. Dunnett, *unpublished*.)

size in grafts taken from older donors, both in absolute volume and in percentage of the total graft volume. As illustrated in Fig. 3, the P-zone which constitutes about 40% of the cross-sectional area in E14 transplants [crown–rump length (CRL) 10 mm] is reduced to about 30% in grafts from E16–17 donors (CRL 15–19 mm) and 15% in grafts from E18 donors (CRL 23 mm). The total volume of the P-zone was reduced from about 1.3 mm³ to about 0.4 mm³ (i.e., by about 70%). Indeed, grafts from even older fetuses (E21) are very small and contain few surviving neurons (142; *authors' unpublished data*).

These age-of-donor differences, as well as differences in the principles used for dissection of the striatal eminence, are likely to explain the marked variation in morphologic features and histochemical characteristics of the striatal grafts reported by different investigators. For example, the grafts obtained by Deckel et al. (22,24,25) and Sanberg et al. (87,104,105), using tissue E17–18 donors, exhibited low levels of D₂-receptor expression and very sparse AChE staining, limited to a few small patches within the grafts, indicating that they contained little striatum-like tissue. Similarly, Helm et al. (51) observed no or very small patches of dopamine D₁ and D₂ receptor-binding in large-sized E15–16 striatal grafts. Although, in the first case, the small size of the striatum-like graft component may at

least be partly explained by the age of the donor tissue, the results obtained by Helm et al. are more likely to be due to the type of fetal dissection used.

The Striatum-like P-Zones

The morphologic features of neurons found in the striatum-like regions of the graft resemble those found in the normal striatum, including medium-sized, densely spiny neurons, as well as a number of interneuron subtypes (13–15,31,49,77,96,138). Electrophysiologic studies have shown that grafted striatal neurons possess some of the physiologic features characteristic for mature adult striatal neurons (19). In addition to the morphologic and physiologic similarities, grafted striatal neurons also express several neurotransmitter phenotypes observed in the normal adult striatum. The neuropeptides enkephalin, dynorphin, and substance P, and their respective mRNA transcripts are found within striatal grafts forming distinct patches that show close correlation with the DARPP-32 or AChE-positive striatum-like P-zones of the grafts (7,44,55,95,96,113,141) (Fig. 4A–C). *In situ* hybridization studies have demonstrated that the expression of these neuropeptide mRNAs in grafted striatal neurons is similar to or slightly higher than that in the normal striatum, and that their densities in the striatum-like P-zones are similar to those in the normal striatum (7,113). Although both enkephalin- and substance P-containing neurons are found within the same P-zones, the percentage cross-sectional area of expression for substance P mRNA in the graft (approximately 21–22%) is significantly lower than that for enkephalin mRNA (approximately 30–36%, which is similar to that for DARPP-32 mRNA; see 7 and 10). In addition, the relative level of enkephalin and substance P mRNA expression varies from patch to patch, with some patches expressing high levels of enkephalin mRNA and lower levels of substance P mRNA or vise versa (10). Markers for striatal interneurons such as NADPH-diaphorase, somatostatin, and neuropeptide Y, as well as ChAT, have also been observed in striatal grafts (45,50,65,95,96,113).

Neurons containing GABA and glutamatic acid decarboxylase (GAD; the synthetic enzyme for GABA) have also been demonstrated within striatal grafts both in the P-zones and the NP-zones, using either immunohistochemical methods or *in situ* hybridization (10,13,95,96,113,141). With GAD-immunohistochemistry, Clarke et al. (13) observed two types of medium-sized neurons within the P-zones: one with a smooth nuclear envelope, similar to the medium-sized spiny GABAergic projection neuron of the normal striatum; and one with deep nuclear indentations of the kind seen in striatal GABAergic interneurons. *In situ* hybridization has demonstrated that the percentage of the total cross-sectional area of the graft that exhibits GAD mRNA expression is almost twice that for DARPP-32 mRNA (10). Interestingly, (as illustrated in Fig. 4D,E) the areas of the grafts expressing low levels or GAD mRNA correlate with the striatal P-zones, as defined by DARPP-32 expression, whereas the high GAD mRNA levels are found in the nonstriatal areas (10). This is consistent with the pattern of GAD expression in the intact forebrain, which is markedly lower in striatal neurons than in those of surrounding areas, such as the neocortex and globus pallidus. In addition to lying outside of the striatal regions of the graft, neurons expressing high levels of GAD mRNA were of considerably larger diameter (i.e., similar to those in the cortex and pallidum) than the lower-expressing cells found in the striatum-like regions (10).

The intrastriatal striatal transplants express neurotransmitter receptors characteristic of the normal striatum. Both dopamine D_1 and D_2 receptors as well as their respective mRNA transcripts, which are highly expressed in the normal striatum, have been localized within the striatum-like regions of the grafts by ligand-binding autoradiography and *in situ* hybridization cytochemical methods (10,55,65,69,75). The expression of high levels of dopamine receptors is clearly confined to the striatum-like P-zones (see Fig. 4G–I). Although the level of expression of D_1 and D_2 receptors varies markedly from patch to patch, their expression is a constant feature of striatal grafts taken from E14–15 donors. As discussed above, striatal grafts with low levels of dopamine receptor expression (see, e.g., 22,24,25,51) are likely to contain little striatum-like tissue. In addition to dopamine receptors, opiate receptors and muscarinic acetylcholine receptors, which are found in high levels in the adult forebrain, have also been localized within the striatal grafts. Although the muscarinic receptors display a more homogeneous expression throughout the grafts, the opiate receptors are largely confined to the P-zones (51,55,65).

The Nonstriatal NP-Zones

Accumulating evidence indicates that the NP regions of the grafts are nonstriatal and may contain neurons of cortical, pallidal, and amygdalar origin, the primordia of which are likely to be included in the combined medial and lateral ganglionic eminence dissection used for transplantation (see above). Clarke et al. (15), by using

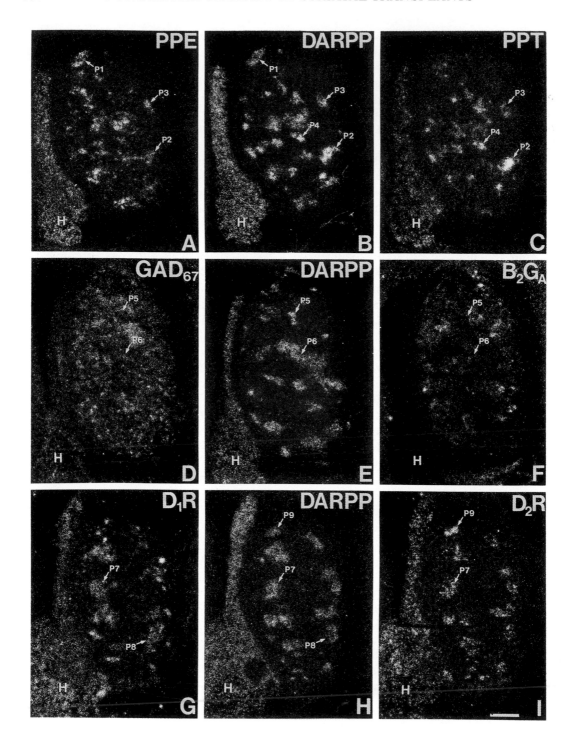

Golgi impregnation, have shown that neurons that express morphologic features similar to those of cortical pyramidal neurons and pallidal projection neurons are present within the NP-zones of the striatal grafts, and Walker et al. (123) and Zhou et al. (141) have reported the presence of low-expressing AChE neurons and large-sized GAD-positive neurons resembling those of the normal globus pallidus. At the ultrastructural level, DiFiglia et al. (31) and Clarke et al. (15) have reported synaptic features and arrangements of GAD-positive boutons, typical of the normal globus pallidus. Graybiel et al. (45) have described graft neurons expressing calbindin immunoreactivity in the NP regions, which have morphologic characteristics similar to those normally found in the pallidum, cortex, and amygdala, whereas the somatostatin-positive neurons in the NP zones resemble cortical somatostatin neurons. Finally, expression of cholecystokinin mRNA and mRNAs for the α_1 and β_2 GABA$_A$ receptor subunits, which constitute type I benzodiazepine binding (normally found in the cortex and pallidum, but not in the striatum), has been observed in the nonstriatal NP regions (see Fig. 4E,F) (15,115).

NEUROTRANSMITTER PROPERTIES

Excitotoxic striatal lesions result in severe losses of intrinsic striatal neurons, along with marked reductions in GAD and ChAT enzyme activity levels both in the striatum and its output structures, the globus pallidus and substantia nigra. Similarly, *in situ* hybridization studies show loss of GAD mRNA expression in the lesioned striatum (K. Campbell, unpublished data). Biochemical studies of intrastriatal striatal transplants have demonstrated a graft-induced normalization of both GAD and ChAT activity levels in KA- and IA-lesioned rats (53,108).

Consistent with the marked reductions in striatal, pallidal, and nigral GAD activity levels, the extracellular levels of GABA in the striatum, globus pallidus, and substantia nigra, as measured with push–pull perfusion or microdialysis, are also markedly reduced after striatal excitotoxic lesions (8,111). Basal extracellular GABA overflow is reduced by 60% to 80% and the K^+-evoked GABA release is almost completely abolished in the lesioned striatum, as measured by *in vivo* microdialysis (8,9). In addition, excitotoxic lesions result in 85% and

---

FIG. 4. Intrastriatal striatal grafts express neurotransmitter phenotypes characteristic of both the mature striatum as well as adjacent forebrain structures (e.g., cerebral cortex and globus pallidus). **A–C:** Negative prints from the autoradiographic film showing adjacent coronal sections through a striatal transplant processed using in situ hybridization histochemistry for the enkephalin precursor preproenkephalin (*PPE*) mRNA (A), *DARPP-32* mRNA (B) and the substance P precursor preprotachykinin (*PPT*) mRNA (C). Both PPE and PPT mRNA are found preponderantly in the striatum-like patches (*P*) of the graft as marked by the expression of DARPP-32 mRNA (*P1–4*). In certain patches both PPE and PPT mRNA are expressed (e.g., *P2* and *P3*), although rarely at the same level. All three genes are expressed rather homogeneously in the remaining host striatum (*H*). **D–F:** Adjacent graft section processed to visualize GAD_{67} mRNA (D), *DARPP-32* mRNA (E), and the mRNA encoding the β_2-subunit of the GABA$_A$ (B_2G_A) receptor (F). High levels of GAD$_{67}$ mRNA and β_2-subunit mRNA are found preponderantly outside the DARPP-32-positive striatal patch regions (*P5* and *P6*), GAD$_{67}$ mRNA levels are present also in the patch regions, but not in lower levels. Note lack of detectable B$_2$G$_A$ mRNA labeling in the remaining host striatum, which is characteristic for this gene; by contrast it is highly expressed in the globus pallidus and cerebral cortex. **G–I:** Adjacent sections through the graft processed to visualize the mRNA encoding the dopamine D$_1$ receptor (D$_1$R, G), DARPP-32, and the dopamine D$_2$ receptor (D$_2$R,I). The mRNA for D$_1$R (*P7* and *P8*) is expressed selectively in the striatal patch regions of the grafts, as is that for the D$_2$R (*P7* and *P9*). Both D$_1$R and D$_2$R mRNA are expressed in some patches (e.g., *P7*). (Scale bar in I, 750 μm.) (Data from ref. 10.)

95% reductions in pallidal and nigral GABA overflow, as measured by the push–pull perfusion technique (111).

These lesion-induced deficits in GABA overflow are partly reversed by intrastriatal striatal grafts. Both basal GABA overflow and K^+-evoked GABA release are restored to normal or supranormal levels within the grafted striatum (9). The GABA overflow in the globus pallidus and substantia nigra, as measured by push–pull perfusion, was restored to 34% and 60%, respectively, of control levels (111). The graft-derived GABA release appears to be vesicular, since the K^+-evoked GABA overflow was Ca^{2+}-dependent (9). Nishino et al. (84) have reported similar results in rats with ischemia-induced damage to the striatum and adjacent cortical areas. This lesion (induced by medial cerebral artery occlusion) caused a 50% to 60% reduction in GABA overflow in the globus pallidus, as measured by microdialysis. Striatal grafts, implanted into the lesioned striatum, restored pallidal GABA overflow to near-normal levels. Excitotoxic lesion-induced deficits in striatal acetylcholine release, as assessed with an *in vitro* slice perfusion technique, have also been at least partially restored by the intrastriatal striatal transplants (124).

FUNCTIONAL EFFECTS OF LESIONS AND TRANSPLANTS AS MONITORED BY REGIONAL GLUCOSE METABOLISM

Excitotoxic lesions of the striatum have profound long-lasting effects on regional glucose metabolism, not only within the striatum itself, but also in intact brain regions linked through one or several synapses with the lesioned striatum (58,59, 134). Reduced glucose consumption in the affected striatum has also been demonstrated in HD patients by positron emission tomography (PET) (60,63). In a study using the 2-deoxy[^{14}C]glucose autoradiographic technique, Isacson et al. (52) monitored the changes in regional glucose metabolism in rats subjected to a unilateral striatal ibo-

tenic acid lesion, and in lesioned rats receiving E13–15 striatal cell suspension grafts, implanted 1 week after the lesion. The rats were processed for analysis 10 weeks later. In the lesion-only rats, there was a 60% reduction in glucose utilization throughout the lesioned striatum, accompanied by significant unilateral or bilateral increases in the major primary and secondary striatal targets, as well as in the contralateral intact striatum. The strongest increases were seen in the pars reticulata of the substantia nigra (+49% ipsilaterally and +29% contralaterally), in the globus pallidus (+26% and +29%), in the subthalamic nucleus (+18% and +19%), and in the deep layers of the superior colliculus (+17% and +18%).

These lesion-induced hypermetabolic responses were normalized by the striatal grafts ipsilaterally in the globus pallidus and subthalamic nucleus and bilaterally in the deep superior colliculus. A significant transplant-induced effect was also seen in the contralateral intact striatum as well as in two functionally associated areas: the ventral tegmental area and the nucleus accumbens. Other striatum-related areas, such as substantia nigra, entopeduncular nucleus, and ventrolateral thalamus, were unaffected by the transplants.

These results clearly demonstrate that the intrastriatal grafts have a functional influence on the host brain, not only in the immediate vicinity of the transplant but also in areas remote from the graft site. The ability of the striatal grafts to normalize the lesion-induced hypermetabolic response in globus pallidus (a primary striatal target) and the subthalamic nucleus and superior colliculus (secondary striatal target areas), in particular, would seem compatible with the idea that the grafted neurons can establish functional connections with the host brain (*see below*).

STUDIES ON BEHAVIOR

The behavioral deficits seen in rats after axon-sparing excitotoxic lesions of the caudate–putamen can be broadly classified into four categories: (a) aspects of spontaneous locomotion and sensorimotor function; (b) the reactivity to drugs, such as effects of direct or indirect dopamine receptor agonists on locomotor behavior or catalepsy; (c) cognitive-type deficits in tests of conditioned behaviors; and (d) regulatory impairments (34,92,102; for review see 37 and 101). Most of these cognitive and regulatory deficits are well detectable only in animals with bilateral lesions, whereas some lateralized motor functions, such as drug-induced turning behavior and paw use, are also sensitive to unilateral lesions.

Table 1 summarizes the behavioral studies conducted so far in rats with intrastriatal excitotoxic lesions and striatal transplants. Most of these studies have used intrastriatal injections of KA or IA as excitotoxic agents. In two studies (47,69), the behavioral effects of transplants implanted into the nonlesioned striatum have been explored, and one recent study (38) has employed quinolinic acid (QA)-induced striatal lesions. Whether the choice of toxin is of any importance for the extent and characteristics of the lesion-induced behavioral syndrome is unclear. Different excitotoxins possess differences in potency for different types of neurons (18,30). Kainic acid is the most potent of the toxins used and causes the most extensive so-called remote damage (e.g., in thalamus, hippocampus, and amygdala), which is at least partly due to the high seizure-inducing potency of this drug (4,18). Ibotenic acid, which has to be given in an order of magnitude higher doses to induce lesions of comparable size, on the other hand, is less epileptogenic and causes less remote damage (18,110). Finally, QA has been reported to give relative sparing of the somatostatin-containing interneurons after injections into the striatum, which is somewhat analogous to the situation in HD (3). This feature of the drug, which has been best documented in primates is, however, less prominent in rats (5,20,30). Indeed, our own studies (S. B. Dunnett et al., *unpublished*) suggest that the selectivity may be due as much to the dose used for

each toxin, as to the specificity of the different toxins themselves. Nevertheless, striatal QA lesions seem to be different in that clearcut nocturnal locomotor hyperactivity is seen only in female rats, but not in male rats or in ovariectomized females (38). This is in contrast with KA- or IA-induced striatal lesions, for which the effect on locomotion is prominent in both males and females. Since only limited behavioral studies have been performed in QA-lesioned rats, it is not yet known whether these sex differences may also translate to other aspects of the lesion-induced behavioral syndrome.

Locomotor Activity

Deckel et al. (21,22,27) were the first to report effects of intrastriatal grafts on lesion-induced locomotor hyperactivity. They used single, bilateral injections of KA (0.8 μg/side) centered in the anterior part of the caudate–putamen. These moderate-sized lesions were reported to reduce the cross-sectional area of the anterior caudate–putamen by 17% (21) or 28% (23). Their grafts consisted of solid pieces of E17–18 striatal primordia (1.5–2 μl/side). These grafts remained relatively small, and judging from the low level of D_2-receptor-binding in the grafts (22,24,25) they may have contained little striatum-like tissue (see foregoing section on morphologic features). Nevertheless, the increase in daytime locomotor activity, which amounted to an approximately twofold increase in movement time or distance traveled over the 1- to 2-hr test period, was partly normalized in the grafted rats 3 to 5 months after transplantation. Consistent with the low level of D_2-receptor-binding, however, the exaggerated locomotor activity seen after amphetamine injection was unaffected (22,24).

Isacson et al. explored locomotor activity in rats with large, unilateral, IA lesions (4 × 5 μg in the head of caudate–putamen; 52), or moderate-sized bilateral lesions (2 × 5 μg into the anteromedial caudate–putamen; 54). These lesions resulted in an av-

TABLE 1. *Behavioral studies of fetal striatal transplants in the rat HD model*

Study (Ref.)	Lesion type	Graft type and donor age	Tests of motoric behaviors	Tests of cognitive functions
Deckel et al. (27)	Bil KA	Bil solid E18	Reduced hyperactivity	
Isacson et al. (52)	Uni IA	Uni susp E13–15	Reduced hyperactivity	
Isacson et al. (54)	Bil IA	Bil susp E14–15	Reduced hyperactivity; graft effect correlated with proximity to the host GP	Improvement in delayed alternation in T-maze; grafts in CP better than grafts in GP; effect correlated with graft size
Deckel et al. (21)	Bil KA	Bil solid E18	Reduced hyperactivity; no effect on deficits in sensorimotor orienting responses	Possible improvement in delayed alternation in T-maze (see text)
Deckel et al. (22,24)	Bil KA	Bil solid E17–18	Reduced hyperactivity; no effect on amph- or apo-induced activity. Grafts into intact CP induce lesion-like hyperactivity	
Deckel et al. (23)	Bil KA	Bil solid E17	No effect on deficits in sensorimotor-orienting responses; minor effects on locomotion	No effect on spontaneous alternation in T-maze
Giordano et al. (42)	Bil KA	Bil solid E17	Hyperactivity reduced to control levels on multiple parameters of locomotor behavior	
Sanberg et al. (100,104)	Bil KA	Bil solid E17	Hyperactivity reversed at 9, but not 3 wk; reversal of amph-induced hyperactivity; graft placed outside CP (lat ventr) without effect; no effect of control graft (sciatic nerve)	
Hagenmeyer-Houser (47)	None	Bil solid E17	Grafts into intact CP induce lesion-like hyperactivity	
Dunnett et al. (35)	Uni IA	Uni susp E14–15	Improved skilled paw use; reduced rotation in response to amph and apo	

Reference	Lesion	Graft	Effect	Effect
Norman et al. (85,87)	Uni KA	Bil solid E17–19	Reduced rotation in response to apo at 5 and 10 wk	
Sanberg et al. (103)	Bil KA	Bil solid E17	Reduced hyperactivity with grafts placed in CP, but not lat. ventr; effect partly abolished by lesion of the graft; no effect of control graft (sciatic nerve)	
Montoya et al. (82)	Uni IA	Uni susp E13–14	Improved skilled paw use; no effect of control graft (fetal nigral tissue)	
Valouskova et al. (121)	Bil KA	Uni solid E14	Effect on paw preference in a paw-reaching task	No detrimental effect on delayed alternation in T-maze (some effect by grafts of cortex tissue)
Lu et al. (70)	None	Bil solid E15–17	Transient lesion-like hyperactivity, at 3 and 6 wk, but not at 20 wk postgrafting; similar effects by control grafts (nigra, cortex)	
Giordano et al. (43)	Bil KA	Bil solid E15–16	Partial improvement in motor coordination and haloperidol-induced catalepsy; possible effects also of control grafts (cortex, tectum)	
Emerich et al. (38)	Bil QA	Bil solid E17	Lesion-induced hyperactivity in female rats reduced at 6 and 10 wk after grafting	
Mayer et al. (74)	Uni IA	Uni susp E15		Recovery in a visual reaction time task
Reading and Dunnett (94)	Bil IA in NAc	Bil susp E14–15	Reduced hyperactivity	Disinhibited responding in a differential reinforcement of low rates (DRL) test reversed by the grafts

Key: Bil, bilateral; Uni, unilateral; KA, kainic acid; apo, apomorphine; amph, amphetamine; susp, suspension; CP, caudate–putamen; GP, globus pallidus; lat ventr, lateral ventricle; IA, ibotenic acid; KA, kainic acid; QA, quinolinic acid.

erage of 65% and 45% reductions, respectively, in the volume of the head of caudate–putamen. As assessed in tests of nighttime locomotor activity (with or without food deprivation) both types of lesion caused an approximately twofold increase in overall activity, measured as total photobeam crossings. Cell suspension grafts obtained from E13–15-day fetuses were implanted as four 1-μl deposits (in the unilateral lesioned rats) or two 3-μl deposits (in the bilaterally lesioned rats). Each lesioned striatum received approximately the amount of tissue corresponding to one striatal primordium (lateral plus medial eminences combined). These grafts grew to an average final size of 4 to 7 mm³ and contained the characteristic AChE-dense patches, signifying a significant striatum-like component (see above).

The lesion-induced overnight hyperactivity was completely reversed by the striatal transplants in both the unilaterally and the bilaterally IA-lesioned rats. In their bilateral lesion and graft study, Isacson et al. (54) compared the effect of grafts implanted into the anteromedial caudate–putamen with grafts placed in the region of the globus pallidus. Although graft-induced damage to the globus pallidus and the adjacent internal capsule was a confounding factor in the pallidal graft group, grafts in both locations were effective. In fact, the graft-induced effect on overnight activity was highly correlated ($r = 0.74$) with the proximity of the

graft to the host globus pallidus. In all grafted animals with activity scores within or below the control range, the graft was located within 0.5 mm from the host globus pallidus. This was taken to indicate that the graft effect on the locomotor hyperactivity parameter may be mediated by an effect on the host globus pallidus.

Sanberg and collaborators (42,43,100, 103–105), in a series of papers, have analyzed lesion- and graft-induced locomotor hyperactivity changes in further detail. Similar to the Deckel et al. studies (see foregoing), they used bilateral KA lesions centered on the anteromedial caudate–putamen, and solid grafts of E17 fetal striatum. Sanberg et al., however, used multiple graft deposits (a total of 4–4.6 mm³ on each side, compared with 1–2 μl in the Deckel et al. studies), the interval between lesion and grafting was longer (3–4 weeks compared with 1 week), and they used male rats as recipients. Since the activity changes induced by excitotoxic striatal lesions are more consistent when analyzed during night-time (i.e., the rats' active period; 34, 102), Sanberg et al. tested their animals during the peak of the nocturnal activity period.

As illustrated in Figs. 5 and 6, Sanberg et al. (see Table 1) have, in several independent experiments, observed a complete reversal of nocturnal locomotor hyperactivity. This effect developed between 3 and 9 weeks after transplantation and was seen

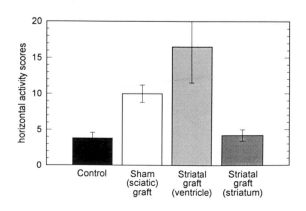

FIG. 5. Striatal grafts can ameliorate the hyperactivity induced by KA lesions of the striatum. Horizontal activity was monitored for unoperated control rats, and for rats with striatal lesions and either sham grafts (derived from sciatic nerve), striatal grafts implanted into the ventricle, or striatal grafts implanted into the lesioned striatal parenchyma. To be effective, the grafts must both comprise striatal tissue and be implanted into the striatum itself. (Redrawn from ref. 105, with permission.)

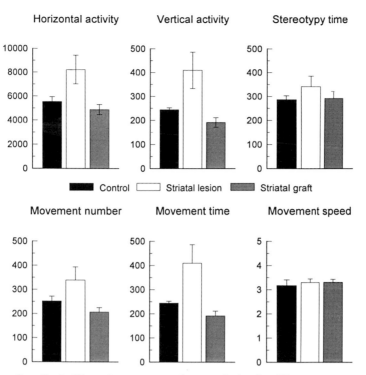

FIG. 6. Striatal grafts affect different measures of motor behavior. The rats were monitored in an automated test apparatus, as used by Sanberg and colleagues, to demonstrate the hyperactivity induced by KA lesions of the neostriatum and its alleviation by striatal grafts implanted into the denervated striatum. Only 6 of the 14 different measures used are shown. (Redrawn from data in ref. 43, with permission.)

only with grafts that were placed within the lesioned striatum, but not those in the adjacent lateral ventricle. Moreover, grafts of sciatic nerve were without effect (100,104) (see Fig. 5). As analyzed in further detail, virtually all aspects of locomotor behavior, as assessed by Digiscan activity monitors, were normalized by the intrastriatal striatal grafts (42,105). In contrast with the results of Deckel et al. (22,24) the exaggerated response to amphetamine was also completely reversed by the fetal striatal grafts, but not by the sciatic nerve control grafts (100,104). In one experiment, Sanberg et al. (103) observed that bilateral electrolytic lesions, placed to destroy part of the established striatal grafts (performed at 9 weeks after transplantation) partly reversed the graft-induced effect, such that the activity of the lesioned animals fell in between the

ones with intact grafts and the lesion-only controls. Although electrolytic lesions may not be ideal for this purpose, since they destroy only part of the graft at the same time as they may lesion host fibers passing through the area, these data are compatible with the idea that the graft-induced effect on hyperlocomotion, at least in part, is dependent on the continued presence of surviving graft tissue.

A more recent study reported the role of postlesion delay in rats with bilateral striatal QA lesions (38). The effect of the graft (E17 striatum) on locomotor hyperactivity was similar, regardless of the delay (1 week or 1 month) between lesion and grafting. The effect was fully established at 6 weeks after transplantation and, at that time, all movement variables were reduced to control level. At 10 weeks, three of seven or eight relevant parameters (vertical activity, movement time, and distance traveled) were again increased above control level. The rats were not tested at longer survival times.

Although locomotor activity testing has been highly useful for the evaluation of graft-induced behavioral effects in the rat HD model, it is clear that the effect of striatal excitotoxic lesions on both daytime and nighttime locomotor activity has a disturbing variability, particularly when tested long-term after lesion. Thus, both Deckel et al. (23; who used female rats) and Giordano et al. (43; who used male rats) observed only minor lesion-induced changes in either nocturnal spontaneous locomotion or amphetamine-induced hyperlocomotion in whole batches of rats that had received the same type of bilateral KA lesions that had produced sustained, marked hyperactivity in previous experiments. These rats seem to have had similar-sized lesions, and they showed significant deficits in other behavioral parameters. In fact, Deckel and Robinson (26) have reported significant daytime and nighttime locomotor *hypo*activity at 25 weeks after bilateral striatal KA lesions in male rats. In this experiment, locomotor *hyper*activity seems to have been expressed briefly after the lesion, suggesting that some of the locomotor changes induced by striatal KA lesions may be transient. More extensive studies, using repeated locomotor testing to monitor the time course of locomotor changes after lesion and transplant, are clearly warranted.

Sensorimotor Coordination

Two studies have applied a sensorimotor test battery in which the rats' orienting responses to sensory and olfactory stimuli and their muscle tone and limb strength were scored in a blind fashion (21,23). In the first experiment, the rats were tested every second week until 10 weeks after transplantation (i.e., 11 weeks after KA lesion). The bilateral KA lesion caused a re-

duction of the total sensorimotor score by an average of about 30%, and this reduction remained throughout testing. The rats receiving bilateral solid grafts of E18 striatum did not differ from the lesion-only controls at any time. In the locomotor activity test, however, as well as in the test for delayed-rewarded alternation in a T-maze (both performed at 3 months after operation), the same rats were reported to show significant recovery of the lesion-induced deficits (see Table 1). In the second experiment, the same sensorimotor test was applied at 8 months after surgery to KA-lesioned rats that had received larger volumes (2–3 μl) of E17 fetal striatum. A lesion-induced deficit was seen in the part of the test related to forelimb and middle body region responses, and again this deficit was not ameliorated by the transplants. However, the rats in this latter experiment also showed only minor transplant-induced effects in the overnight activity test performed at 6 months after transplantation.

Giordano et al. (43) compared the effects of different types of fetal CNS tissue (obtained from E15–16 rat fetuses) on two measures of motor function: motor coordination on a rotating rod, and catalepsy after dopamine receptor antagonist (haloperidol) treatment. The marginal statistical differences between the lesioned, grafted, and control groups preclude any safe conclusions from this experiment. However, the results did suggest a partial graft effect on both measures, but there was no clear-cut difference between the different types of grafts.

Skilled Paw Use

In the paw-use test, the rats are rated for their success in retrieving food pellets through a forelimb reaching-and-grasping movement. As shown by Whishaw et al. (125), this test is highly sensitive to excitotoxic lesions of the striatum (as well as to aspirative lesions of the sensorimotor cortex and 6-OHDA lesions of the nigrostriatal dopamine projection). This test appears to be highly useful for studies on functional recovery in the rat HD model, since the deficits are profound and stable over time, and since it can also be applied to rats with unilateral lesions.

In a first study, Dunnett et al. (35) compared the performance of rats with unilateral striatal IA lesions, with and without cell suspension grafts obtained from E15 striatal primordia, at 7 months after surgery. In the lesion-only rats, the success rate was significantly reduced for both paws, by about two-thirds on the side contralateral to the lesion and by about one-half on the ipsilateral side. When allowed to use either paw, the marked paw preference (for the ipsilateral paw) seen in the lesioned-only rats was unaffected by the grafts. However, when the rats were restricted to use only one paw at a time, the grafted rats showed significant improvement for both paws, up to a level that was no longer different from nonlesioned controls. That the striatal grafts can have an effect on paw preference is, however, indicated by a study of Valouskova et al. (121), who used unilateral E14 striatal transplants in rats with bilateral striatal KA lesions. As assessed at 3 months after surgery, the grafts induced a significant shift in paw preference toward the side contralateral to the transplant. In this study, any effect on the quality of paw use was difficult to evaluate, since almost all lesioned and grafted

rats reached control levels of performance, which may be due to the relatively small size of the lesions used.

In a second experiment, summarized in Fig. 7, Montoya et al. (82) compared the effect of two types of intrastriatal grafts (E14 striatum or E14 ventral mesencephalon) and two types of lesion (unilateral striatal IA lesion or 6-OHDA lesion of the nigrostriatal pathway). In this study, the rats were pretrained before the lesion was performed, and a modified paw-reaching test, with a so-called staircase box (83), was used. This test box makes it easier to make independent assessment of the performance of the two forelimbs. The IA lesion caused a marked paw-reaching deficit that was most pronounced for the limb contralateral to the lesion. The striatal grafts (but not the control ventral mesencephalic grafts) induced a marked, although incomplete recovery in both limbs. The effect was evident by 1 month after transplantation and was maintained throughout the 3-month observation period (see Fig. 7). Interestingly, neither type of graft had any effect on impaired paw use in the rats with 6-OHDA-induced lesions of the nigrostriatal dopamine pathway. Thus, in this experiment, the graft-induced functional effect appeared to be specific in two ways: for the type of fetal brain tissue implanted (striatum versus mesencephalon), and for the underlying anatomic defect (i.e., the striatal grafts were effective when the paw-reach-

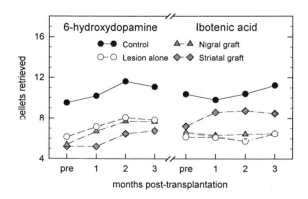

FIG. 7. Effects of nigral or striatal grafts on the performance of rats with 6-OHDA lesions of the dopaminergic nigrostriatal pathway (*left*) or ibotenic acid striatal IA lesions (*right*) in a skilled paw-reaching task. Note that the recovery induced by striatal grafts was specific: It was restricted to the striatal (but not the nigrostriatal) lesion deficit, and depended on implantation of embryonic striatal (but not nigral) tissues. (Redrawn from ref. 83.)

ing deficit was induced by a lesion of the striatal projection neurons, but not when it was induced by a lesion of the nigral dopamine afferents).

Drug-Induced Turning

Rats with unilateral excitotoxic lesions of the striatum exhibit unilateral turning in response to dopamine receptor agonists (e.g., apomorphine) or dopamine-releasing drugs (amphetamine). With large striatal lesions, the rats turn in the direction toward the lesioned side, signifying a preferential activation of the intact striatal neurons by the drugs (35,109). With more restricted lesions, however, the direction of apomorphine-induced rotation depends on which subfield of the striatum is involved: with more posterior lesions the rats turn ipsilaterally, but with the lesion restricted to the anteromedial caudate–putamen the rats turn in the opposite direction (16,86,88; S. B. Dunnett and L. E. Annett, *unpublished data*). However, the rats always turn ipsilaterally in response to amphetamine (S. B. Dunnett and L. E. Annett, *unpublished data*).

In two studies (35,85,87), intrastriatal striatal transplants reduced dopamine agonist turning by about 50% to 70%. In the study of Norman et al. (85,87), who used the type of anterior striatal KA lesions that induce contralateral turning, the effect was detected by 5 weeks after transplantation and was further developed by 10 weeks. A major effect of the graft in their test (which was performed in open-field boxes) was a change in the pattern of turning, from tight pivotal rotations to turning in wide circles.

In the study of Dunnett et al. (35), which used larger and more posterior IA lesions, the ipsilateral turning induced by either apomorphine or amphetamine was reduced by up to 70% when tested at 7 to 8 months after transplantation and lesion surgery. By contrast, turning in response to a nondopamine-active drug (atropine) was unaffected by the grafts. As discussed in further

detail in a later section on the function of graft–host connections, these data are compatible with the idea that the striatal grafts possess functional dopamine receptors (as demonstrated with receptor-binding and *in situ* hybridization techniques) as well as a functional dopaminergic afferent input. Indeed, the observations of Helm et al. (51) indicate that striatal grafts that express no or very sparse dopamine D_1 and D_2 receptors (probably because of the way the fetal tissue was dissected; see the earlier section on morphologic features) have no effect on apomorphine-induced turning in unilateral IA-lesioned rats. Further studies, however, are clearly warranted to substantiate this idea. Given that the importance of size and placement of the excitotoxic lesion for the magnitude and direction of turning has now been clarified, agonist-induced turning behavior should be a highly useful test for further studies of host–graft interactions in the rat HD model.

Conditioned Behaviors

As summarized in Table 1, there are six studies that have applied tests of conditioned behaviors in the functional analysis of transplants in the rat HD model. Isacson et al. (54) and Deckel et al. (21) have reported improved performance of grafted rats on delayed alternation in a T-maze. The Isacson et al. (54) study, which used bilateral IA lesions and E14–15 striatal cell suspension transplants, showed that grafts placed in the head of the caudate–putamen were more effective than grafts placed in the globus pallidus region (Fig. 8). Although the grafted rats acquired the task more slowly than the normal controls, three of the eight rats with grafts in the caudate–putamen reached criterion (>90% correct alternations), and the other five were close to criterion at the end of the 18-day test period. By contrast, all lesion-only rats remained at random level of performance (50%); the rats with grafts placed into the globus pallidus fell in between these two

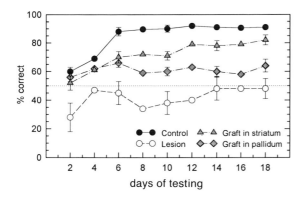

FIG. 8. Effects of striatal grafts on the cognitive deficit induced by bilateral IA lesions of the striatum. Rats were trained over 18 days in a paired-trial, delayed alternation task in a T-maze. Note that significantly greater recovery is obtained when the grafts were implanted back into the lesioned neostriatum itself, than when implanted into the deafferentated target areas of the globus pallidus. (Redrawn from ref. 54.)

groups. Spontaneous (i.e., nonrewarded) alternation was unaffected by either lesion or graft in this experiment.

In the Deckel et al. (21) study, using bilateral KA lesions and E18 solid transplants, the rats were pretrained on the test before lesion and transplant surgery. In the second test, applied 3 months after surgery, the performance of the lesion-only rats was significantly impaired, compared with the normal controls. The performance of the grafted rats fell in between the two groups, such that they did not differ from either the lesion-only or the normal controls. The difficulty in interpreting these data is partly because both the lesion-only and the grafted rats performed at a random level (i.e., 50% correct) by the end of the second test period. Moreover, the intact controls did not acquire the task very well, reaching about 75% correct alternations within the 10-day test period [i.e., well below the criterion (>85%) that had been applied in the pretest]. Thus, although it seems clear that grafts of younger (E14–15) striatal tissue can improve acquisition of delayed alternation in IA-lesioned rats, it remains unclear whether grafts from older donors (E18) can exert similar effects. In the Deckel et al. (21) study the same grafted rats showed significant graft-induced improvement on one of four measures in the locomotor hyperactivity test. In a later paper, Deckel et al. (23) reported an effect of the bilateral KA lesions on spontaneous T-

maze alternation, which was unaffected by E17 solid striatal transplants.

Mayer et al. (74) used a so-called visual-choice reaction time task in an automated nose-poke test apparatus (see Chapter 22). In this test, the rat has to learn to make a movement with the head away from a light stimulus applied in the left or right visual field. Rats trained to do this task will show substantial impairment in performing responses contralateral, but not ipsilateral, to a unilateral striatal IA lesion. Lesioned rats, receiving E15 striatal suspension grafts, were initially equally as impaired as the lesion-only rats when tested 6 months after surgery, but reacquired performance within 11 to 15 trials.

The test used in the Mayer et al. study (74), which involves both response initiation and response selection, is normally likely to be critically dependent on integrative functions within the striatal circuitry. The ability of the grafted rats to reacquire the performance on the lesioned side suggests not only that some critical aspects of lesioned striatal connectivity are reestablished by the graft, but also that the grafted rats need to learn to use the newly formed transplant circuitry for this particular purpose.

In a recent study, Reading and Dunnett (94) used bilateral IA lesions centered in the ventral striatum, including the nucleus accumbens, as opposed to the dorsal (caudate–putamen) placement used in the studies discussed so far. As discussed in further detail in Chapter 8, lesions of the ventral striatum have profound disinhibition effects on a range of both conditioned and unconditioned behaviors and, therefore, may be highly useful for studies on the functional capacity of striatal transplants. Reading and Dunnett (94) used the differential reinforcement of low rates responding (DRL) test to show that the IA-lesioned rats were unable to acquire performance that required them to inhibit a previously rewarded response. This deficit was substantially alleviated in rats with E15 cell suspension grafts implanted bilaterally into the lesioned area. Moreover, the sensitivity of the DRL performance to dopaminergic manipulation, which was abolished by the lesion, was reinstated by the transplants, again suggesting the presence of a functional dopaminergic afferent input. Also the lesion-induced locomotor hyperactivity induced by the lesion was reversed in the grafted rats.

Importance of Age of Donor Tissue for the Functional Efficacy of Striatal Transplants

From this survey of the behavioral studies, it seems clear that intrastriatal grafts of tissue taken from fetal striatal primordia are effective in reversing many aspects of the behavioral syndrome induced by unilateral or bilateral excitotoxic lesions of the caudate–putamen; that grafts placed outside the caudate–putamen or globus pallidus (i.e., in the lateral ventricle) are ineffective; and that grafts of other types of tissue (sciatic nerve or fetal mesencephalon) appear to have no significant effect. A close reading of the literature suggests, however, that the functional efficacy of striatal grafts is variable, and that this variability may depend, at least partly, on the age of the donor tissue as well as the internal composition of the striatal grafts.

In a first attempt to clarify this issue, Fricker and Dunnett (*unpublished obser-*

vations) have studied the effects of grafts of striatal primordia taken from four different donor ages on skilled paw use in rats with unilateral striatal IA lesions. To compensate for the progressive growth of the developing striatum, the grafts were matched such that each recipient received the amount of tissue corresponding to one striatal primordium. As illustrated in Fig. 9, only grafts taken from E14 donors (CRL 10 mm) had a substantial effect in the paw-reaching test. Grafts from E16 donors (CRL 15 mm) had a small effect (seen above all on the ipsilateral paw), whereas the oldest tissue (E18; CRL 23 mm) had, if anything, a negative effect. Interestingly, the decline in paw-reaching success across the groups matched well the decline in size of the striatum-like compartment (P-zone) in the grafts, as determined by TH- and STEP immunohistochemical methods (see discussion on morphologic features, above; Fig. 3). These data suggest that the ability of the striatal grafts to ameliorate lesion-induced deficits in skilled paw use is critically dependent on the size of the striatum-like compartment in the transplants. From the data in Fig. 3 it would appear that there is a critical minimum P-zone volume of about 1 mm for significant behavioral recovery to occur. In fact, a similar figure can be derived from the graft volume data of Isacson et al. (54). In this study a significant effect on delayed alternation in a T-maze (see previous section on conditioned behaviors) was seen in animals with graft sizes in the caudate–putamen of at least 2 to 3 mm^3, which corresponds to a P-zone volume of about 1 mm^3.

In view of these recent data, it is interesting that Deckel et al. (21–24) and Sanberg et al. (100,104,105) have obtained partial or complete reversal of lesion-induced locomotor hyperactivity in animals with grafts (from E17-18 donors) that contained little striatum-like tissue (as judged by D$_2$-receptor binding and AChE histochemistry). This suggests the possibility that effects on locomotor hyperactivity (in con-

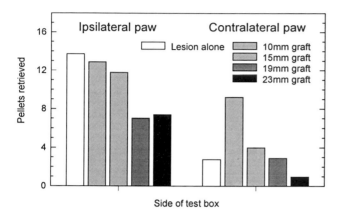

FIG. 9. Effects of graft donor age on recovery of paw-reaching deficits induced by unilateral striatal IA lesions. Performance on the side *ipsilateral* to the lesion is similar to the level attained by normal rats; this is unaffected by grants from the younger donors, but is disrupted by grafts from the older donors (19- and 23-mm CRL, equivalent to E17 and E18, respectively) donors. The lesions induce a marked deficit on the *contralateral* side of the body, which is not changed by the grafts from older donors, but is significantly reduced by the grafts from the younger donors (10-mm CRL is equivalent to E14 days of gestation). (Data from R. A. Fricker and S. B. Dunnett, *unpublished*.)

trast with paw-reaching and delayed alternation learning) can be obtained with much less striatum-like graft tissue, or indeed that effects on locomotor hyporeactivity can be achieved with grafts containing nonstriatal (NP-zone) tissue only. If so, the mechanisms by which striatal transplants influence characteristics of general locomotion activity, on one hand, and deficits in more specific motoric and cognitive functions, on the other, may be different.

ESTABLISHMENT OF NEURONAL CONNECTIVITY BETWEEN THE STRIATAL TRANSPLANTS AND THE LESIONED HOST BRAIN

Host Afferents to the Graft

The ability of the intrastriatal striatal grafts to restore not only simple metabolic and motoric activity, but also more complex conditioned behaviors and skilled motor tasks, suggests that the grafts may depend on some degree of functional integration with the host striatal circuitry. Normal striatal function is regulated by major afferent inputs from, above all, cortex, thal-

amus, and substantia nigra. The intrastriatal striatal grafts receive afferent inputs from all three systems. *Dopaminergic afferents,* originating in the host substantia nigra project densely and selectively to the striatal P-zones of the grafts and form synaptic contacts with the dendrites and spines of the medium-sized densely spiny neurons (13,14,62,65,66,93,127,130). *Cortical and thalamic afferents,* by contrast, innervate both the P-zones and the NP-zones, above all in the peripheral portions of the grafts (13,127–129,135,136); however, other studies have reported minimal graft–host connectivity (42,76,122). Differences in grafting protocols, composition of the graft tissue, or anatomic-tracing techniques used may account for these discrepancies. It seems clear from a large number of independent studies, reviewed below, that both afferent and efferent connectivity is a constant and reproducible feature of E14–15 striatal cell suspension grafts implanted into the IA-lesioned rat striatum.

The medium-sized spiny neurons represent the major subtype in the striatum. These neurons possess extensive efferent projections to the globus pallidus and substantia nigra, and they receive direct synaptic inputs from all major striatal afferent systems, including the dopamine neurons of the substantia nigra, and the glutaminergic afferents from the intralaminar thalamic nuclei and the cerebral cortex (for review, see 44 and 116). The ultrastructural organization of afferent connectivity with medium-sized spiny neurons in the striatum is such that dopaminergic and cortical terminals form synapses predominantly on the dendritic spines. These inputs make synapses on the more distal portions of the dendrites, whereas the local inputs from recurrent collaterals of the medium-sized cells and the cholinergic interneurons are found on, or close to, the cell bodies (116). The nigrostriatal dopaminergic fibers form mostly symmetric synapses on the dendritic shafts and spines (39), whereas the cortical afferents form asymmetric synaptic specializations on the dendritic spines, and the thalamic afferents on both shafts and spines, of the medium-sized striatal spiny neurons (33,118,135–136). As discussed later, some aspects of this complex connectivity appear to be reestablished in the striatal transplants.

Dopaminergic and Serotonergic Afferents

McGeer et al. (78) were the first to report that intrastriatal grafts receive a dopaminergic innervation. This observation has subsequently been substantiated in several studies using catecholamine histofluorescence (93) or tyrosine hydroxylase (TH) immunohistochemistry (14,28,62,65,67,69,106, 130,131,140). These dopaminergic fibers terminate in a patchy manner, specifically in the striatum-like P-regions of the graft (65,67,130,131) (Fig. 10A,B). In electron microscopic studies, Clarke and colleagues have shown that the TH terminals form symmetric synapses onto dendrites and spines of medium-sized spiny graft neurons (13,14). Some of these, at least, were GABAergic. Retrograde-tracing experiments, in which the injection sites were clearly confined inside the graft boundaries, have demonstrated that the dopaminergic innervation of the striatal implant indeed arises from the host substantia nigra (93,127,128). Consistent with this view, a 6-OHDA lesion of the host nigrostriatal dopamine pathway is efficient in removing the TH-positive innervation of the grafts (28,67,130). In certain cases, the number of cells retrogradely labeled in the host substantia nigra from the graft was greater than half of that seen after a similar injection into the intact striatum.

The serotonergic innervation from the mesencephalic raphe terminates in a rather diffuse manner not restricted to the striatum-like P-regions of the graft (127,140). The density of the serotonergic innervation approached the levels seen in the host striatum, above all in the peripheral graft regions. Retrograde tracing from the graft has identified labeled cells within the host raphe nuclei (127,128).

FIG. 10. Intrastriatal striatal grafts receive afferent inputs from the host brain. **A**: Tyrosine hydroxylase (TH) immunohistochemistry shows a patch-like distribution, with the transplant (*T*). **B**: TH-positive fibers (*black punctate labeling*) concentrate in the patch (*P*) regions of the grafts marked by DARPP-32 immunoreactive neurons (*gray diffuse label*) in graft sections reacted to simultaneously reveal TH and DARPP-32 immunoreactivities. Note the very sparse TH-positive innervation of the nonpatch (*NP*) regions. **C**: Darkfield photomicrograph showing PHA-L immunoreactive terminals within a striatal transplant following multiple iontophoretic injections of PHA-L into the ipsilateral frontal cortex. **D**: Higher magnification of the *dashed box* in C showing the punctate labeling indicative of cortical terminations preponderantly in the peripheral portions of the graft (*asterisks* denote blood vessels for orientation). *cc,* corpus callosum; *1,* area of lesion-induced gliosis and packed myelin bundles. (Scale bars in A, 180 μm; B, 100 μm.) (A,B: modified from ref. 130; C,D: from ref. 128.)

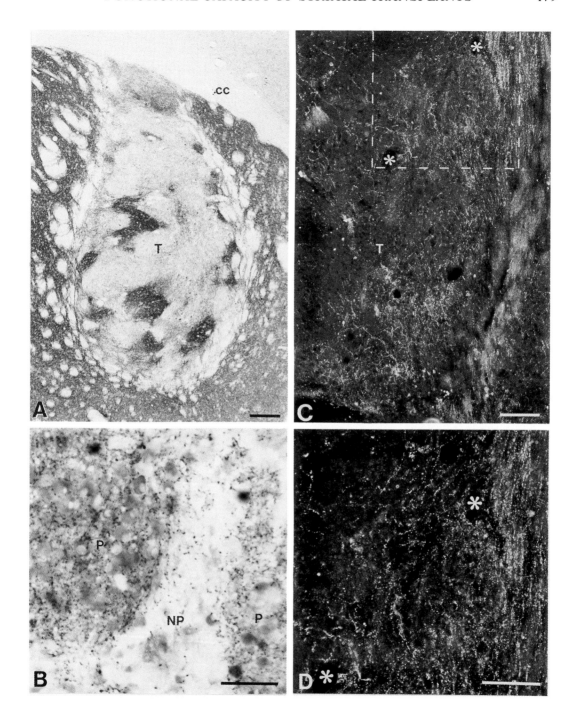

Cortical and Thalamic Afferents

Host cortical innervation of intrastriatal striatal grafts have been studied in retrograde and anterograde tracing experiments, tracer injections have been made into either the striatal implant or into the host frontal cortex. In a first study, using wheat germ agglutinin–horseradish peroxidase (WGA–HRP) injections into the transplant, some labeled cells in the host frontal cortex were observed (93), but they were few and were faintly labeled. In a subsequent experiment, employing small iontophoretic injections of the more sensitive tracer Fluoro–Gold (FG), a much more extensive labeling of host cortical neurons was obtained (128). In this study, the total number of retrogradely labeled cells amounted to about one-third of that seen after similar injections into the intact striatum. The cells labeled from the striatal grafts had regional and laminar distributions similar to those seen after similar FG injections into the striatum in intact animals.

With an anterograde tracing technique [multiple injections of phascolus vulgaris leucoagglutinin (PHA-L) into the frontal cortex], fibers arising from cells in the frontal cortex were observed to innervate the striatal graft most densely in the peripheral regions of the implants (128; see Fig. 10C,D). In electron microscopic studies, employing either PHA-L tracing or anterograde degeneration after focal cortical lesions, the cortical terminals form asymmetric synaptic specializations onto grafted striatal neurons (13,129,135). As in the normal striatum, these synapses were seen to contact both dendritic spines and shafts, but the proportion of shaft synapses appeared to be higher than normal. Approximately 50% of the identified contacts were onto spines in the graft, whereas in the host striatum, more than 90% were onto spines (135). In another study a considerably higher proportion, 87%, of cortical terminals were observed to contact dendritic spines within the graft, compared with 98% in the host striatum (129).

Retrograde tracing has confirmed the existence of a substantial thalamic innervation of the intrastriatal striatal grafts. Injections of either WGA-HRP or fluorescent tracers into the graft label cells in the intralaminar thalamic nuclei, including the centrolateral, parafascicular, and paracentral thalamic nuclei (93,127,128). With FG as a tracer, between 225 and 4960 host thalamic neurons were labeled from each tracer deposit (127), which corresponds to between 5% and 100% of the number of thalamic neurons labeled by similar injections in the intact striatum. The largest numbers of cells were seen from tracer deposits involving the peripheral portions of the grafts. Consistent with this, anterograde-tracing studies have shown that the thalamic innervation of the striatal grafts is dense in the peripheral portions of the graft, whereas the central regions appear to be considerably less innervated (127). Xu et al. (136) have examined the ultrastructure of the thalamic innervation of the grafted neurons. Similar to the thalamic innervation in the intact striatum, the thalamic axons innervating the grafts made synaptic contacts with both dendritic spines and shafts. In the intact animal, the thalamic input is specialized such that about 90% of the synapses coming from the parafascicular nucleus are onto shafts, whereas about 90% of axons labeled from the centromedian nucleus synapse with the dendritic spines. However, this anatomic specialization was not present in the grafts.

Graft Efferents to the Host Brain

The behavioral data, summarized in the foregoing, are consistent with the view that large striatal lesions (like the striatal degeneration seen in HD) remove a major inhibitory (probably largely GABAergic) control of downstream extrapyramidal motor centers and that the striatal transplants can reinstate at least a tonic inhibitory control over primary and secondary striatal target areas, including the globus pallidus, substantia nigra, and the subthalamic nucleus. Although this inhibitory action could be caused by a diffuse release of GABA from the grafted neurons (as detected in the microdialysis and push–pull perfusion experiments) there is direct anatomic evidence in support of the idea that the effect may be mediated by efferent graft–host connections formed by the medium-sized densely spiny (most probably GABAergic) neurons with the grafts.

The first anatomic evidence for grafted striatal neurons projecting to the host brain was obtained by Pritzel et al. (93). Anterogradely WGA–HRP-labeled fibers were found in the globus pallidus and, to a lesser extent, in the substantia nigra ipsilateral to the striatal graft in one of the five rats studied with this technique. Wictorin et al. (131), using the more sensitive PHA–L-tracing method, confirmed the presence of axonal projections from the graft to the nearby globus pallidus and, to a lesser extent, the entopeduncular nucleus using anterograde PHA–L tracing from the graft. However, in this study, no anterogradely labeled axons were found in the substantia nigra. Injection of retrograde tracers into the host globus pallidus resulted in labeling of large numbers of graft neurons, which were aggregated in patches that corresponded very closely to the striatal P-zones of the graft (130,131) (Fig. 11A). Indeed, when retrograde tracing was combined with immunocytochemistry or in situ hybridization for DARPP-32, over 90% of the retrogradely labeled cells were seen to be DARPP-32-expressing. In addition, graft neurons labeled with FG from the host globus pallidus have been observed to express both GAD, enkephalin, and substance P precursor mRNA (Campbell et al., *in preparation*; see Fig. 11B,C). Quantitative assessment indicates that about one-fourth of the neurons labeled with FG from the globus pallidus express enkephalin mRNA, and about one-half expresses substance P precursor mRNA. Over 90% of the retrogradely labeled neurons were GAD expressing. These data provide further support for the view that the efferent projecting graft neurons are striatum-like, that they most probably utilize the inhibitory neurotransmitter GABA, and that they constitute both the enkephalin-containing and the substance P-containing subtypes.

With use of cross-species neural markers and anterograde axonal tracers, the efferent axons projecting caudally from the striatal grafts have been traced along the myelinated fascicles of the internal capsule to establish direct synaptic connections with the neurons of the host globus pallidus (131–133) (see Fig. 11D). The GABA released from the outgrowing axons may thus be able to act directly on the denervated neuronal elements in the appropriate striatal target areas in the host brain.

The extent to which grafted striatal neurons send axonal projections to the damaged host brain appears to differ with the species of the donor. Studies using E13–14 mouse striatal primordia implanted into the excitotoxically lesions adult rat brain in combination with immunohistochemistry for the mouse neuron-specific marker M6 have demonstrated that grafted mouse striatal neurons can extend axons into the host brain for about 1 to 2 mm (133) (see Fig. 11E). Interestingly, these fibers travel along the myelinated bundles in the host internal capsule, reaching as far caudal as the globus pallidus. Striatal primordia derived from 6- to 8-week (postconception) human fetal tissue, grafted to the IA-lesioned adult rat striatum, possess a considerably greater growth capacity (126). The human fetal striatal grafts have been observed to extend axonal projections into the host brain as far as the rostral level of the spinal cord (i.e., approximately 2 cm). Here, both the globus pallidus and substantia nigra pars reticulata were in receipt of considerable innervation from the graft.

Although there is substantial light and electron microscopic evidence demonstrating the formation of extensive afferent and efferent graft–host connections, there are several other studies in which minimal connectivity has been reported between striatal grafts and the host brain. With the relatively insensitive WGA–HRP anterograde-

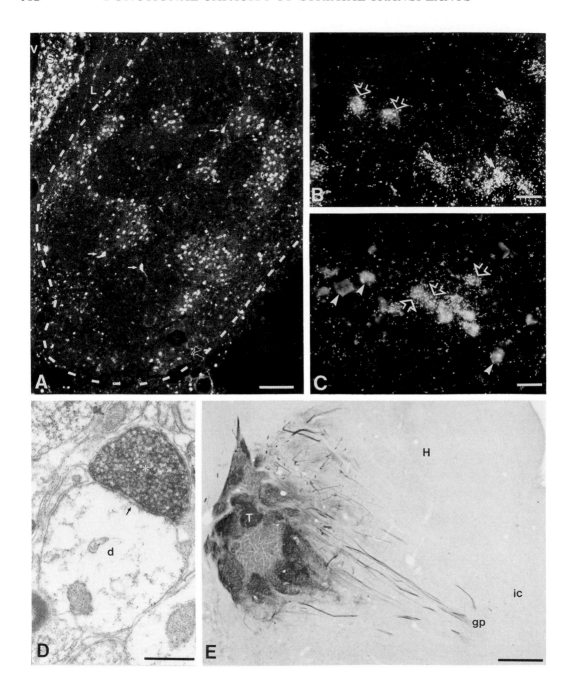

tracing technique, McAllister et al. (76) failed to observe any nigrostriatal afferents to grafts of E14 striatal primordia implanted into the KA-lesioned striatum. Similarly, Giordano et al. (42) have reported a lack of nigrostriatal projections to striatal grafts when using donor tissue from E17 rat embryos implanted into the KA-lesioned striatum. The latter grafts, however, appear to have contained very little striatum-like P-zone tissue, which is the primary target for the host nigral dopaminergic afferents (see section on morphologic features, above). In later studies, this group has, in fact, observed dopaminergic innervation of the grafts using the more sensitive technique of TH immunocytochemistry (69,106). Walker and McAllister (122) have also described a lack of efferent projections to the host globus pallidus. However, in this study, the transplants were relatively young (approximately 1–2 months old) and, again, WGA–HRP was employed as the anterograde tracer. Finally, several studies have reported scant efferent graft projections to the substantia nigra (76,122,140), which is consistent with our own observations showing that the major efferent projection of striatal grafts is to the globus pallidus, and that the entopeduncular nucleus and sub-stantia nigra receive considerably less input.

ARE GRAFT–HOST CONNECTIONS FUNCTIONAL?

The rich afferent innervation of the intrastriatal striatal transplants suggests that the grafted striatal neurons may be functionally regulated by the host brain. In particular, several lines of evidence indicate that the host-derived dopaminergic afferents, which specifically innervate the striatum-like graft P-regions and synapse directly onto medium-sized spiny neurons, are capable of modulating grafted striatal neuron activity.

One strategy to study the functional influence of the dopaminergic afferents on the striatal graft neurons has used dopamine receptor-mediated activation of the protooncogene product Fos as a cellular marker for dopamine-mediated postsynaptic responses within the transplants. In the normal striatum, dopamine-releasing drugs induce Fos expression in the striatal projection neurons, and this effect is abolished by removal in the nigrostriatal dopamine affer-

---

FIG. 11. Intrastriatal striatal transplants send efferents to the host brain. **A**: Retrogradely Fluoro-Gold (FG)-labeled graft neurons are distributed in patch-like compartments of the striatal transplants after FG injections into the ipsilateral globus pallidus. Over 90% of the FG-labeled neurons after pallidal injections were DARPP-32-positive and located within the P-zones of the graft. A few neurons of considerably larger size are indicated by *arrows*. **B,C**: Combining retrograde FG labeling from the pallidum with in situ hybridization for the enkephalin precursor PPE mRNA (B) and for the substance P precursor PPT (C) shows that a significant proportion of the efferent projecting graft neurons are enkephalin- and substance P-containing (*open arrows; small arrows* point to silver grain accumulations from PPE mRNA or PPT mRNA-expressing graft neurons not double-labeled with FG). **D**: Electron micrograph showing PHA-L-labeled bouton (*asterisk*) from an injection restricted to the striatal graft boundaries, forming a symmetric synapse on a dendrite (*d*) in the ipsilateral host globus pallidus. **E**: Efferent fiber outgrowth from an 8-day-old intrastriatal striatal transplant (*T*) derived from mouse E14–15 striatal primordia implanted into the lesioned rat host striatum (*H*) and visualized using an antibody against the mouse-specific protein, M6. Note the directed growth of axons specifically toward the host globus pallidus (*gp*) that extend along the internal capsule (*ic*). (Scale bars in A, 125 μm; B,C, 20 μm; D, 0.4 μm; E, 500 μm.) (Modified from refs. 9, 131–133.)

ents (11,46). A similar effect can be obtained with dopamine D$_1$ receptor agonists, but only in the absence of a functional dopaminergic innervation (11,97). In intrastriatal striatal grafts, dopamine-releasing drugs (amphetamine and cocaine) induced Fos expression selectively in the neurons located within the DARPP-32- and AChE-positive P-zones, and this effect is abolished by a 6-OHDA lesion of the host nigrostriatal input (66,73). As in the normal striatum, apomorphine had no effect in grafts with an intact host dopamine innervation, but induced strong Fos expression in the P-zone neurons in animals in which the dopamine innervation had been removed. Similar results have been obtained after haloperidol treatment (32).

Another approach has used dopamine receptor-mediated regulation of neuropeptide expression in striatal target neurons as a tool to explore host dopaminergic regulation of graft neuron function. In the intact striatum, dopamine exerts a differential regulation over striatal neuropeptide mRNA expression, such that the mRNA encoding for enkephalin is up-regulated in response to dopamine denervation or blockade of dopamine receptors, whereas that for substance P is dramatically down-regulated (41). Since enkephalin and substance P are thought to exist in separate populations of striatal projection neurons (i.e., striatopallidal and striatonigral neurons, respectively), dopamine is proposed to inhibit the enkephalinergic striatopallidal neurons, while exciting the substance P-ergic striatonigral neurons (41).

Striatal grafts subjected to dopamine-depleting conditions (i.e., dopaminergic lesion with 6-OHDA or prolonged treatment with haloperidol) also exhibit a differential regulation of neuropeptide mRNA expression. Following such treatment, the mRNA encoding for enkephalin is significantly increased, whereas that for substance P is markedly reduced, similar to what is seen in the normal striatum (Fig. 12) (7,14). As in the Fos experiment, these changes occurred selectively in the striatum-like P-re-

gions. In animals that are dopaminergically denervated before striatal grafting, enkephalin content (as detected by immunohistochemistry) is considerably increased in the striatal P-zone regions of the graft when compared with grafts placed into the dopamine-intact striatum (67). Thus, it appears that the host-derived dopaminergic innervation of the striatal grafts exerts a normal regulatory control of the expression of cellular activity markers, such as c-*fos* and neuropeptide mRNA expression in the grafted striatal neurons.

In the normal striatum, virtually all the efferent projection neurons, as well as some of the interneurons, employ the inhibitory neurotransmitter GABA. These neurons are known to receive a dopamine innervation from the substantia nigra, and there is evidence that GABA release within the striatum, as well as in its primary output structures globus pallidus and substantia nigra pars reticulata, is under a direct dopaminergic regulation. Striatal grafts restore GAD enzyme activity and GABA release in the lesioned striatum and also partially in the globus pallidus and substantia nigra. In addition, graft-derived GABA release is also modulated by host dopamine inputs to the graft. Dopamine-depleting 6-OHDA lesions of the normal striatum result in increased GABA levels after K$^+$-induced depolarization, as measured by intracerebral microdialysis (64,120). Similar dopamine-specific lesions result in a considerable potentiation of K$^+$-induced GABA release also from intrastriatal striatal grafts (9). Furthermore, amphetamine injections in animals bearing intrastriatal striatal transplants have been observed to induce significant increases in pallidal and nigral GABA levels by the push–pull perfusion method (111). Taken together, these data support the view that GABA release from the grafted striatal neurons is under a prominent dopaminergic control from the host nigrostriatal pathway. Interestingly, a recent study (112) has provided evidence for a reciprocal graft–host control-regulating dopamine release from the host dopaminergic

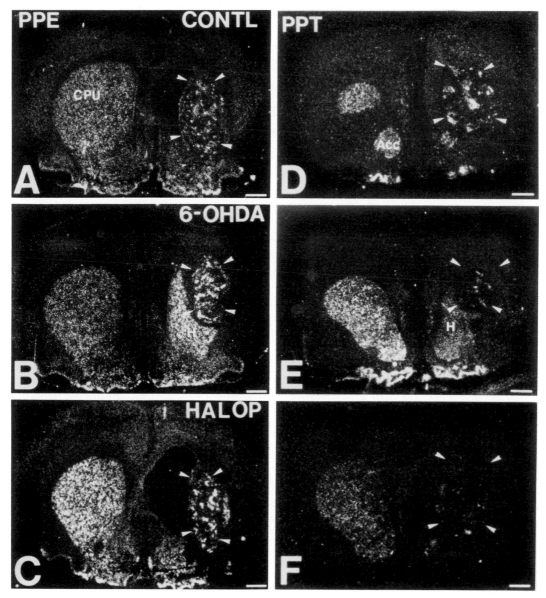

FIG. 12. Host dopaminergic fibers innervating the striatal grafts regulate neuropeptide mRNA expression. Negative prints of autoradiographic films showing *PPE* (**A–C**) and *PPT* (**D–F**) mRNA in the normal striatum (*left*) and in intrastriatal striatal grafts (*right:* indicated by *arrowheads*) after do-pamine-depleting 6-OHDA lesions of the host brain or chronic haloperidol (*HALOP*) treatment. (A and D) PPE and PPT mRNA expression in sections through the center of the control untreated grafts (*CONTL*). The increase in hybridization signal for PPE mRNA in (B) is seen in the striatal graft patches (P-zones) and in the ipsilateral host striatum (*H*) after unilateral 6-OHDA lesions, and in (C) it occurs in both the contralateral intact striatum and in the graft patches after prolonged haloperidol treatment. In contrast, the hybridization signal for PPT mRNA is reduced both in the graft patches (E) and in the spared portions of the host striatum ipsilateral to the 6-OHDA lesion. After prolonged haloperidol treatment, the reduction in PPT mRNA occurs in both the intact striatum and graft patches (F). *Acc,* nucleus accumbens. (Scale bars, 1 mm.) (Modified from ref. 7.)

fibers. In this experiment, the inhibitory effect of cholecystokinin on striatal dopamine release, which is abolished in the IA-lesioned striatum, was restored in the grafted striatum.

The functional properties of the cortical and thalamic graft afferents have been explored electrophysiologically (98,137). The results demonstrated functional connections between host cortical and grafted striatal neurons, as well as an input to grafted striatal neurons from the thalamic intralaminar nuclei. Grafted striatal neurons responded to cortical or thalamic stimulation in a manner similar to normal striatal neurons, but their responses were often smaller in magnitude and were frequently missing (137). These results may reflect that the grafts are heterogeneous for their striatal and nonstriatal compartments (the P- and NP-zones) and that the peripheral areas of the grafts are more densely innervated by the host cortical and thalamic inputs than the deep central portions.

Further evidence for host cortical regulation of the striatal grafts has been obtained in a microdialysis study of graft-derived GABA release, in which the graft was perfused with the glutamate analogue, kainic acid (139). Previous microdialysis studies have shown that KA added to the perfusion fluid induces an increase in extracellular glutamate levels, and that this effect is dependent on the integrity of the corticostriatal afferents (139). Perfusion of striatal grafts with KA induced a significant increase in extracellular GABA levels. As with the intact striatum, this effect was presumably due to stimulation of glutamate release from host-derived corticostriatal fibers, since prior decortication abolished the response (9).

CONCLUDING REMARKS AND CLINICAL PERSPECTIVE

In Fig. 13 we have summarized some of the principal results obtained in neuroanatomic studies of neuronal connectivity in intrastriatal striatal grafts. Figure 13A highlights the connectivity of the "patch cell" (i.e., the medium-sized neurons in the striatum-like, DARPP-32-positive and AChE-rich graft patches; P-zones), which appear to be the only neuronal elements in the striatal grafts giving rise to efferent connections with the host brain. Most of these efferent projecting cells, or possibly all of them, have the morphologic and chemical characteristics of medium-sized densely spiny neurons, which is the preponderant class of effector cell in the normal striatum. Most or all of them are DARPP-32-positive; the vast majority of them are GAD-positive and, hence, GABAergic; and they comprise two principal subtypes, one containing enkephalin and another containing substance P. Although most of the striatal substance P neurons normally project to the substantia nigra and the internal segment of the globus pallidus (i.e., the entopeduncular nucleus), few if any, of the substance P-containing graft neurons send axons all the way down to the substantia nigra. Instead, our recent studies, with in situ hybridization in combination with fluorescent retrograde tracing (10), indicate that both the enkephalin- and the substance P-containing graft neurons project to the globus pallidus. However, some of them may innervate the entopeduncular nucleus, which is a normal target for the substance P neurons. In addition, it is clear that the graft neurons have local axonal projections within the transplants that terminate, at least in part, in the nonstriatal NP-regions.

As illustrated in Fig. 13, we propose that the patch cell, being the only type of neuron projecting out of the graft, is the principal effector cell of the striatal transplants, and that these neurons are reached by some of the major striatal afferents that are of importance for regulation of striatal functions in the intact animal: the dopaminergic input from the pars compacta of the substantia nigra, and the glutamatergic afferents from the cortex and thalamus. Of the two principal striatal output pathways—the so-called indirect pathway by the external segment of the globus pallidus and the sub-thalamus nuclei, and the direct pathway to the substantia nigra pars reticulata and the entopeduncular nucleus (1,2,44)—only the indirect pathway seems to be reestablished to a significant extent with grafts of rat or mouse striatal neurons. Thus, although both principal types of striatal projection neurons, the striatonigral substance P-containing ones and the striatopallidal enkephalin-containing ones, are likely to be represented among the patch cells, both types seem to project to the globus pallidus in the grafted animals.

The situation may be slightly different in animals with grafts of fetal human striatal neurons, since these cells possess sufficient growth capacity to connect with both globus pallidus and substantia nigra (126). Whether the enkephalin- and substance P-projections in these animals are properly segregated in the two targets, however, is unknown.

The ability of the intrastriatal striatal grafts to provide a partial reconstruction of striatal circuitry, which is disrupted by the excitotoxic lesion, may be of critical importance for graft-induced behavioral recovery in the rat HD model, particularly relative to more complex sensorimotor and cognitive tasks. The evidence for this, however, is largely indirect. The best examples may be the graft-induced recovery in forelimb use in the paw-reaching task and delayed alternation learning in the T-maze. These behaviors are normally sensitive to lesions not only of the striatal projection neurons, but also to lesions of the nigrostriatal dopamine pathway and the frontoparietal cortex. For skilled paw use, at least, graft-induced recovery seems to be critically dependent on a minimum amount of striatal tissue (and, hence, patch cells) in the grafts. For effects on lesion-induced hyperlocomotion, the situation is less clear. It is notable that significant amelioration of locomotor hyperactivity has also been obtained with grafts that contain only small amounts of striatum-like tissue. This suggests that the mechanism underlying this effect is essentially indepen-

dent of the formation of graft–host connectivity and, accordingly, is also independent of the presence of patch cells in the graft. Alternatively, it seems possible that the effect on hyperlocomotion is a very sensitive measure for graft-induced functional effects in the HD model. If so, such effects may be possible to obtain with much smaller amounts of striatal tissue and with fewer patch cells than is true, for example, with skilled paw use and delayed alternation learning. These issues, which are of importance for the understanding of the mechanism(s) of action of the striatal grafts, will have to be addressed in future studies.

The data discussed so far have all been obtained in rodents. In the perspective of clinical application of striatal transplants in HD, studies in nonhuman primates are clearly needed to assess the validity of neural transplantation in a model that is more similar to the human condition. The conclusions one can draw from studies in the rat model are limited because the striatum is anatomically and functionally more complex in humans than in rats. The disturbances in motor function that are induced by striatal lesions in rodents are much more limited than those seen in patients with HD. Moreover, the human striatum is considerably larger (approximately 200 times) than that in the rat, thus presenting a greater challenge for any replacement strategy.

Studies in nonhuman primates are clearly needed to clarify these issues. Initial experiments performed by Isacson et al. (56,57) and Hantraye et al. (48) indicate that striatal excitotoxic lesions in monkeys can induce motor deficits that resemble, at least to some extent, the symptoms seen in HD patients. In particular, the abnormal movements and dyskinasias, which are observed after administration of the dopamine receptor agonist apomorphine, bear resemblance to the choreic symptoms in HD. The apomorphine-induced dyskinesias were reported to be stable over time and to correlate in severity with the size of the excitotoxic striatal damage in the lesioned monkeys. Is-

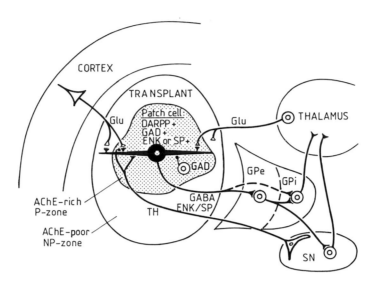

A

FIG. 13. Proposed connectivity model of striatal graft function. **A**: Summary of some of the principal neuroanatomic and histochemical data concerning the connectivity and phenotype of the efferent projecting neurons in the graft P-zones, the "patch cell." **B**: Schematic representation of basal ganglia circuitry (**I**) showing the proposed alterations in rats with excitotoxic lesions of the striatum (**II**) and in lesioned and striatal grafted animals (**III**). There exists two major pathways emanating from the *normal* intact *striatum* or *CPu* which are capable of influencing the output of the basal ganglia. First, the enkephalinergic "indirect" pathway projects to the *GPe* and employs GABA as a neurotransmitter. This projection provides an inhibitory influence (as illustrated by *solid black* neurons with *blunt ends*) over the activity of pallidosubthalamic (*STN*) and pallidonigral (*SNr*) projection neurons, the latter of which, in turn, are also GABAergic. The STN provides an excitatory (as shown by *open neurons with arrows ends*), presumably glutamatergic input to the SNr. The "direct" pathway, which contains substance P and also uses GABA, projects directly to the SNr and exerts an inhibitory influence over SNr output. The output neurons of the SNr also use GABA to inhibit thalamic neurons projecting to neurons of the cortex, which ultimately control output. After an excitotoxic lesion of the CPu (indicated by *hatching* and *dashed lines* in II), motor output is proposed to be increased owing to the loss of inhibitory control over GPe output. Loss of this inhibition is suggested to result in an increased inhibition of the STN and SNr by GABAergic GPe projection neurons (schematically depicted by the *increased thickness* of the axon). This increased inhibition of the STN would result in decreased excitatory drive (as illustrated by the *decrease in width* of the axon) to the SNr neurons as well. The cumulative effect of this would result in a severe reduction in the inhibition from SNr neurons to the thalamus, which may allow thalamic neurons to overexcite cortical neurons in control of motor output. In III, striatal grafts (*stippled box within the hatched CPu*) are proposed to reduce the increased motor output by providing reconnection of the "indirect" GABAergic pathway receiving appropriate regulatory inputs from the cortex and dopaminergic SNc. *CPu,* caudate–putamen; *Enk,* enkephalin; *GAD,* glutamic acid decarboxylase; *Glu,* glutamic acid; *GPe,* external segment of globus pallidus; *GPi,* internal segment of globus pallidus (entopeduncular nucleus); *IBO,* ibotenic acid; *SN,* substantia nigra (*c,* pars compacta, *r,* pars reticulata); *SP,* substance P; *STN,* subthalamic nucleus; *TH,* tyrosine hydroxylase; *Thal,* thalamus. (Modified from ref. 2.)

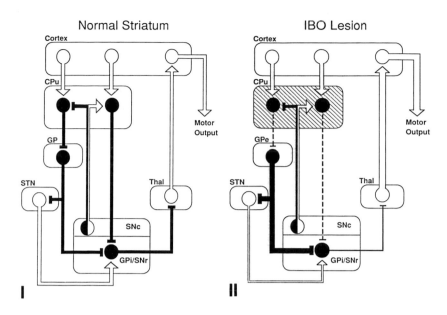

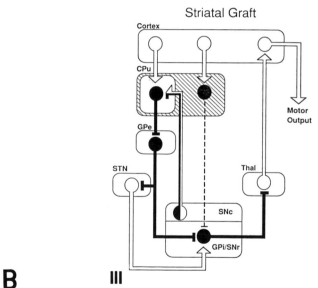

FIG. 13. (*Continued*)

acson et al. (56,57) have reported on five baboons in which cross-species grafts of fetal rat striatal tissue were implanted into the lesioned striatal area under immunosuppression. All five showed a gradual decline in apomorphine-induced dyskinesia, resulting in a 60% to 80% reduction in dys-kinesia scores by 7 to 10 weeks after transplantation. In two monkeys, in which immunosuppression was discontinued, the symptoms reappeared as the grafts were rejected. Studies using allografts of monkey striatal tissue are now in progress in several laboratories.

The remarkable capacity of striatal grafts for extensive functional recovery and circuitry reconstruction in rats subjected to striatal excitotoxic lesions provides a rational basis for the consideration of clinical trials in patients suffering from HD. Indeed, such trials have already been initiated (72). However, one should keep in mind that the validity of excitotoxic lesions of the striatum as a good experimental model of human HD is not yet fully established and, consequently, the results obtained in animal experiments may not be entirely relevant to the human condition. In the rat model, the degeneration of striatum occurs very rapidly, whereas in HD it occurs gradually over time. Since human HD is a progressive disease, there is also the risk that the, as yet unknown, disease process may also affect the implanted neurons. Noninvasive techniques, based on positron emission tomography or magnetic resonance imaging, that allow the assessment of graft survival should thus be an essential part of any clinical trial. Additionally, there are several important practical problems related to the procurement of embryonic human CNS tissue, such as those of obtaining enough tissue for transplantation, and of performing accurate and reproducible tissue dissections from the often severely disrupted forebrains of the fragmented embryonic material. This necessitates preclinical experimental trials to ensure that the criteria used for the identification of the striatal primordia are sufficiently reliable.

Although many problems remain to be solved, nevertheless, there are strong arguments that speak in favor of some limited and well-controlled clinical trials of neural transplantation in HD. First, there is at present no other effective treatment for this severe disorder. Second, the application of transplantation in parkinsonian patients (see Chapter 4) have not yet demonstrated any serious complications or adverse effects of intracerebral grafting of embryonic tissue into the human brain. In parallel with any clinical trials, however, it is essential that animal experiments continue to create a more solid experimental basis. In particular, more experiments in primates are needed to establish optimal technical parameters for neural grafting in the larger and more complex primate brain. Further studies in monkeys with excitotoxic striatal lesions should be highly useful for this purpose.

ACKNOWLEDGMENT

We thank Klas Wictorin for his kind help with illustrative material and Siv Carlson for excellent secretarial assistance.

REFERENCES

1. Albin RL, Young AB, Penney JB. The functional anatomy of basal ganglia disorders. *Trends Neurosci* 1989;12:366–375.
2. Alexander GE, Crutcher MD. Functional architecture of basal ganglia circuits: neural substrates of parallel processing. *Trends Neurosci* 1990;13:266–271.
3. Beal MF, Kowall NW, Ellison DW, Mazurek MF, Swartz KJ, Martin JB. Replication of the neurochemical characteristics of Huntington's disease by quinolinic acid. *Nature* 1986;321: 168–171.
4. Ben-Ari Y, Tremblay E, Ottersen P. Injections of kainic acid into the amygdaloid complex of the rat: an electrographic, clinical and histological study in relation to the pathology of epilepsy. *Neuroscience* 1980;5:515–528.
5. Boegman RJ, Smith Y, Parent A. Quinolinic acid does not spare striatal neuropeptide Y-immunoreactive neurons. *Brain Res* 1987;415: 178–182.
6. Bruyn GW. Huntington's chorea, historical, clinical and laboratory synopsis. In: Vinken PJ, Bruyn GW, eds. *Handbook of clinical neurology,* vol 6. Amsterdam: Elsevier North-Holland; 1968:298–378.
7. Campbell K, Wictorin K, Björklund A. Differential regulation of neuropeptide mRNA expression in intrastriatal striatal transplants by host dopaminergic afferents. *Proc Natl Acad Sci USA* 1992;89:10489–10493.
8. Campbell K, Kalén P, Lundberg C, Wictorin K, Rosengren E, Björklund A. Extracellular γ-aminobutyric acid levels in the rat caudate–putamen: monitoring the neuronal and glial contribution by intracerebral microdialysis. *Brain Res* 1993;614:241–250.
9. Campbell K, Kalén P, Wictorin K, Lundberg C, Mandel RJ, Björklund A. Characterization of

GABA release from intrastriatal striatal transplants: dependence on host-derived afferents. *Neuroscience* 1993;53:403–415.

10. Campbell K, Wictorin K, Björklund A. Neurotransmitter-related gene expression in intrastriatal striatal transplants. I. Phenotypical characterization of striatal and non-striatal graft regions. 1994 [*Submitted*].

11. Cenci MA, Kalén P, Mandel RJ, Wictorin K, Björklund A. Dopaminergic transplants normalize amphetamine- and apomorphine-induced Fos expression in the 6-hydroxydopamine lesioned striatum. *Neuroscience* 1992;46:943–957.

12. Chevalier G, Deniau JM. Disinhibition as a basic process in the expression of striatal functions. *Trends Neurosci* 1990;13:277–280.

13. Clarke DJ, Dunnett SB. Synaptic relationships between cortical and dopaminergic inputs and intrinsic GABAergic systems within intrastriatal striatal grafts. *J Chem Neuroanat* 1993;6:147–158.

14. Clarke DJ, Dunnett SB, Isacson O, Sirinathsinghji DJS, Björklund A. Striatal grafts in rats with unilateral neostriatal lesions. I. Ultrastructural evidence of afferent synaptic inputs from the host nigrostriatal pathway. *Neuroscience* 1988;24:791–801.

15. Clarke DJ, Wictorin K, Dunnett SB, Bolam P. Internal composition of striatal grafts: light and electron microscopy. In: Percheron G, McKenzie JS, Féger J, eds. *The basal ganglia IV. New ideas and data on structure and function.* New York: Plenum Press, 1994 [*in press*].

16. Concepcion EE, Low WC. Functional heterogeneity of the striatum in a rodent model of Huntington's disease: considerations for neurological transplantation. *J Neural Transplant Plast* 1992;3:185–186.

17. Coyle JT, Schwarcz R. Lesion of striatal neurones with kainic acid provides a model for Huntington's chorea. *Nature* 1976;263:244–246.

18. Coyle JT, Schwarcz R. The use of excitatory amino acids as selective neurotoxins. In: Björklund A, Hökfelt T, eds. *Handbook of chemical anatomy,* vol 1: Amsterdam: Elsevier; 1983:508–527.

19. Crossman IJ, Mitchell MA, Sambrook A, Jackson A. Chorea and myoclonus in the monkey induced by gamma-aminobutyric acid antagonism in the lentiform complex. *Brain* 1988;111:1211–1233.

20. Davies SW, Roberts PJ. Model of Huntington's disease. *Science* 1988;241:474–475.

21. Deckel AW, Moran TH, Coyle JT, Sanberg PR, Robinson RG. Anatomical predictors of behavioral recovery following striatal transplants. *Brain Res* 1986;365:249–258.

22. Deckel AW, Moran TH, Robinson G. Behavioral recovery following kainic acid lesions and fetal implants of the striatum occurs independent of dopaminergic mechanisms. *Brain Res* 1986;363:383–385.

23. Deckel AW, Moran TH, Robinson G. Receptor characteristics and recovery of function following kainic acid lesions and fetal transplants of the striatum. I. Cholinergic systems. *Brain Res* 1988;474:27–38.

24. Deckel AW, Moran TH, Robinson G. Receptor characteristics and recovery of function following kainic acid lesions and fetal transplants of the striatum. II. Dopaminergic systems. *Brain Res* 1988;474:39–47.

25. Deckel AW, Robinson G. Receptor characteristics and behavioral consequences of kainic acid lesion and fetal transplants of the striatum. *Ann NY Acad Sci* 1987;495:556–578.

26. Deckel AW, Robinson G. Transplantation of different volumes of fetal striatum: Effects of locomotion and monoamine biochemistry. *Soc Neurosci Abstr* 1986;16:1479.

27. Deckel AW, Robinson RG, Coyle JT, Sanberg PR. Reversal of longterm locomotor abnormalities in the kainic acid model of Huntington's disease by day 18 fetal striatal implants. *Eur J Pharmacol* 1983;93:287–288.

28. Defontaines B, Peschanski M, Onteniente B. Host dopaminergic afferents affect the development of DARPP-32 immunoreactivity in transplanted embryonic striatal neurons. *Neuroscience* 1992;48:857–869.

29. DeLong MR. Primate models of movement disorders of basal ganglia origin. *Trends Neurosci* 1990;13:281–285.

30. DiFiglia M. Excitotoxic injury of the neostriatum: a model for Huntington's disease. *Trends Neurosci* 1990;13:286–289.

31. DiFiglia M, Schiff L, Decker AW. Neuronal organization of fetal striatal grafts in kainate- and sham-lesioned rat caudate nucleus: light- and electronmicroscopic observations. *J Neurosci* 1988;8:1112–1130.

32. Dragunow M, Williams M, Faull RLM. Haloperidol induces Fos and related molecules in intrastriatal grafts derived from fetal striatal primordia. *Brain Res* 1990;530:309–311.

33. Dubé L, Smith AD, Bolam JP. Identification of synaptic terminals of the thalamic or cortical origin in contact with distinct medium-size spiny neurons in the rat neostriatum. *J Comp Neurol* 1988;267:455–471.

34. Dunnett SB, Iversen SD. Learning impairments following selective kainic acid-induced lesions within the neostriatum of rats. *Behav Brain Res* 1981;2:189–209.

35. Dunnett SB, Isacson O, Sirinathsinghji DJS, Clark DJ, Björklund A. Striatal grafts in rats with unilateral neostriatal lesions. III. Recovery from dopamine-dependent motor asymmetry and deficits in skilled paw reaching. *Neuroscience* 1988;24:813–820.

36. Dusart I, Marty S, Peschanski M. Glial changes following an excitotoxic lesion in the CNS—II: astrocytes. *Neuroscience* 1991;45:541–549.

37. Emerich DF, Sanberg PR. Animal models of Huntington's disease. In: Boulton A, Baker G, Butterworth R, eds. *Neuromethods,* vol 21; *Animal models of neurological disease.* Clifton, NJ: Humana Press; 1992:65–134.

38. Emerich DF, Zubricki EM, Shipley MT, Norman AB, Sanberg PR. Female rats are more sensitive to the locomotor alterations following quinolinic acid-induced striatal lesions: effects of striatal transplants. *Exp Neurol* 1991;111:369–378.

39. Freund TF, Powell JF, Smith AD. Tyrosine hydroxylase immunoreactive boutons in synaptic contact with identified striatonigral neurons, with particular reference to dendritic spines. *Neuroscience* 1984;13:1189–1215.

40. Gale K, Casu M. Dynamic utilization of GABA in substantia nigra: regulation by dopamine and GABA in the striatum and its clinical and behavioral implications. *Mol Cell Biochem* 1981;39:369–405.

41. Gerfen CR. The neostriatal mosaic: multiple levels of compartmental organization. *Trends Neurosci* 1992;15:133–139.

42. Giordano M, Hagenmeyer-Houser SH, Sanberg PR. Intraparenchyman fetal striatal transplants and recovery in kainic acid lesioned rats. *Brain Res* 1988;446:183–188.

43. Giordano M, Ford LM, Shipley MT, Sanberg PR. Neural grafts and pharmacological intervention in a model of Huntington's disease. *Brain Res Bull* 1990;25:453–465.

44. Graybiel AM. Neurotransmitters and neuromodulators in the basal ganglia. *Trends Neurosci* 1990;13:244–253.

45. Graybiel AM, Liu FC, Dunnett SB. Intrastriatal grafts derived from fetal striatal primordia. I. Phenotopy and modular organization. *J Neurosci* 1989;9:3250–3271.

46. Graybiel AM, Moratalla R, Robertson HA. Amphetamine and cocaine induce drug-specific activation of the c-*fos* gene in striosome–matrix compartments and limbic subdivisions of the striatum. *Proc Natl Acad Sci USA* 1990;87:6912–6916.

47. Hagenmeyer-Houser SH, Sanberg PR. Locomotor behavior changes induced by E-17 striatal transplants in normal rats. *Pharmacol Biochem Behav* 1987;27:583–586.

48. Hantraye P, Riche D, Maziere M, Isacson O. An experimental primate model for Huntington's disease: anatomical and behavioural studies of unilateral excitotoxic lesions of the caudate–putamen in the baboon. *Exp Neurol* 1990;108:91–104.

49. Helm GA, Palmer PE, Bennett JJ. Fetal neostriatal transplants in the rat: a light and electron microscopic Golgi study. *Neuroscience* 1990;37:735–756.

50. Helm GA, Palmer PE, Bennett JJ. Choline acetyltransferase- and substance P-like immunoreactive elements in fetal striatal grafts in the rat: a correlated light and electron microscopic study. *Neuroscience* 1992;47:621–639.

51. Helm GA, Robertson MW, Jallo GF, Simmons N, Bennett JP. Development of D_1 and D_2 dopamine receptors and associated second messenger systems in fetal striatal transplants. *Exp Neurol* 1991;111:181–189.

52. Isacson O, Brundin P, Kelly PAT, Gage FH, Björklund A. Functional neuronal replacement by grafted neurons in the ibotenic acid-lesioned striatum. *Nature* 1984;11:458–460.

53. Isacson O, Brundin P, Gage FH, Björklund A. Neural grafting in a rat model of Huntington's disease. Progressive neurochemical changes after neostriatal ibotenate lesions and striatal tissue grafting. *Neuroscience* 1985;16:799–817.

54. Isacson O, Dunnett SB, Björklund A. Graft-induced behavioural recovery in an animal model of Huntington's disease. *Proc Natl Acad Sci USA* 1986;83:2728–2732.

55. Isacson O, Dawbarn D, Brundin P, Gage FH, Emson PC, Björklund A. Neural grafting in a rat model of Huntington's disease: striosomal-like organization of striatal grafts as revealed by immunocytochemistry and receptor autoradiography. *Neuroscience* 1987;22:481–497.

56. Isacson O, Hantraye P, Riche D, Schumacher JM, Mazière M. The relationship between symptoms and functional anatomy in the chronic neurodegenerative diseases: from pharmacological to biological replacement therapy in Huntington's disease. In: Lindvall O, Björklund O, Widner H, eds. *Intracerebral transplantation in movement disorders*. New York: Elsevier Science Publishers; 1991:245–258.

57. Isacson O, Riche D, Hantraye P, Sofroniew MV, Mazière M. A primate model of Huntington's disease: cross-species implantation of striatal precursor cells to the excitotoxically lesioned baboon caudate–putamen. *Exp Brain Res* 1989;75:213–220.

58. Kelly PAT, Graham DI, McCulloch J. Specific alterations in local cerebral glucose utilization following striatal lesions. *Brain Res* 1982;201:695–696.

59. Kimura H, McGeer EG, McGeer PL. Metabolic alterations in an animal model of Huntington's disease using the ^{14}C-deoxyglucose methods. *J Neural Transm [Suppl]* 1981;16:103–109.

60. Kuhl DE, Phelps ME, Markham C. Winter J, Metter J, Riege W. Cerebral metabolism and atrophy in Huntington's disease determined by ^{18}FDG and computed tomographic scan. *Ann Neurol* 1982;12:425–434.

61. Labandeira-Garcia JL, Wictorin K. Development and integration of intrastriatal striatal grafts implanted into long-term ibotenate lesions. *J Neural Transplant Plast* 1992;3:181–182.

62. Labandeira-Garcia JL, Wictorin K, Cunningham ET Jr, Björklund A. Development of intrastriatal striatal grafts and their afferent innervation from the host. *Neuroscience* 1991;42:407–426.

63. Leenders KL, Frackowiak RJS, Quinn N, Marsden CD. Brain energy metabolism and dopaminergic function in Huntington's disease measured in vivo using positron emission tomography. *Mov Disord* 1986;1:69–77.

64. Lindefors N, Brodin E, Tossman J, Segovia J, Ungerstedt U. Tissue levels and in vitro release of tachykinin and GABA in striatum and substantia nigra of rat brain after unilateral striatal dopamine denervation. *Exp Brain Res* 1989;74:527–534.

65. Liu FC, Graybiel AM, Dunnett SB, Baughman RW. Intrastriatal grafts derived from fetal striatal primordia: II. Compartmental alignment of cholinergic and dopaminergic systems. *J Comp Neurol* 1990;295:1–15.

66. Liu FC, Dunnett SB, Robertson HA, Graybiel AM. Intrastriatal grafts derived from fetal striatal primordia: III. Induction of modular patterns of Fos-like immunoreactivity by cocaine. *Exp Brain Res* 1991;85:501–506.

67. Liu FC, Dunnett SB, Graybiel AM. Influence of mesostriatal afferents on the development and transmitter regulation of intrastriatal grafts derived from embryonic striatal primordia. *J Neurosci* 1992;12:4281–4297.

68. Lombroso PJ, Naegele JR, Sharma E, Lerner M. A protein tyrosine phosphatase expressed within dopaminoceptive neurons of the basal ganglia and related structures. *J Neurosci* 1993;13:3064–3074.

69. Lu SY, Shipley MT, Norman AB, Sanberg PR. Striatal, ventral mesencephalic and cortical transplants into the intact rat striatum: a neuroanatomical study. *Exp Neurol* 1991;113:109–130.

70. Lu SY, Giordano M, Norman AB, Shipley MT, Sanberg PR. Behavioral effects of neural transplants into the intact striatum. *Pharmacol Biochem Behav* 1990;37:135–148.

71. Lundberg C, Wictorin K, Björklund A. Retrograde degenerative changes in the substantia nigra pars compacta following an excitotoxic lesion of the striatum. *Brain Res [in press]*.

72. Madrazo I, Franco-Bourland RE, Castrejon H, Cuevas C, Ostrosky-Solis F, Aquilera M, Magallon E, Grijalva E, Guizar-Sahagun G. Fetal striatal brain homografting in two patients with Huntington's disease. *Soc Neurosci Abstr* 1993; 19:357.7.

73. Mandel RJ, Wictorin K, Cenci MA, Björklund A. Fos expression in intrastriatal grafts: regulation by host dopaminergic afferents. *Brain Res* 1992;583:207–215.

74. Mayer E, Brown VJ, Dunnett SB, Robbins TW. Striatal graft-associated recovery of a lesion-induced performance deficit in the rat requires learning to use the transplant. *Eur J Neurosci* 1991;4:119–126.

75. Mayer E, Heavens RP, Dunnett SB, Sirinathsinghji DJS. Autoradiographic localization of D_1 and D_2 dopamine receptors in primordial striatal tissue grafts. *Neurosci Lett* 1990;09:271–276.

76. McAllister JP, Cober SR, Schaible ER, Walker PD. Minimal connectivity between six month neostriatal transplants and the host substantia nigra. *Brain Res* 1989;476:345–350.

77. McAllister JI, Walker PD, Zemanick MC, Weber AB, Kaplan LI, Reynolds MA. Morphology of embryonic neostriatal cell suspensions transplanted into adult neostriata. *Dev Brain Res* 1985;23:282–286.

78. McGeer PL, Kimura H, McGeer EG. Transplantation of newborn brain tissue into adult kainic-acid-lesioned neostriatum. In: Sladek JR, Gash JR, eds. *Neural transplants: development and function.* New York: Plenum Press; 1984:361–371.

79. McGeer EG, McGeer PL. Duplication of biochemical changes of Huntington's chorea by intrastriatal injection of glutamic and kainic acids. *Nature* 1976;263:517–519.

80. McGeorge AJ, Faull RLM. The organization of the projection from the cerebral cortex to the striatum in the rat. *Neuroscience* 1989;29:503–537.

81. Mogenson GJ, Nielsen MA. Evidence that an accumbens to subpallidal GABAergic projection contributes to locomotor activity. *Brain Res Bull* 1983;11:309–314.

82. Montoya CP, Astell S, Dunnett SB. Effects of nigral and striatal grafts on skilled forelimb use in the rat. *Prog Brain Res* 1990;82:459–466.

83. Montoya CP, Campbell HL, Pemberton KD, Dunnett SB. The staircase test: a measure of independent forelimb reaching and grasping abilities in rats. *J Neurosci Methods* 1991;36:2–3.

84. Nishino H, Koide K, Aihara N, Kumazaki M, Sakurai T, Nagai H. Striatal grafts in the ischemic striatum improve pallidal GABA release and passive avoidance. *Brain Res Bull* 1993; 32:517–520.

85. Norman AB, Calderon SF, Giordano M, Sanberg PR. Striatal tissue transplants attenuate apomorphine-induced rotational behavior in rats with unilateral kainic acid lesions. *Neuropharmacology* 1988;27:333–336.

86. Norman AB, Calderon SF, Giordano M, Sanberg PR. A novel rotational behavior model for assessing the restructuring of striatal dopamine effector systems; are transplants sensitive to peripherally acting drugs? *Prog Brain Res* 1988;78:61–67.

87. Norman AB, Giordano M, Sanberg PR. Fetal striatal tissue grafts into excitotoxin-lesioned striatum: pharmacological and behavioral aspects. *Pharmacol Biochem Behav* 1989;34:139–147.

88. Norman AB, Norgren RB, Wyatt LM, Hildebrand JP, Sanberg PR. The direction of apomorphine-induced rotation behavior is dependent on the location of excitotoxin lesions in the rat basal ganglia. *Brain Res* 1992;569:169–172.

89. Ossowska K, Wedzony K, Wolfarth S. The role of the GABA mechanisms of the globus pallidus in mediating catalepsy, stereotopy and locomotor activity. *Pharmacol Biochem Behav* 1984;21:825–831.

90. Pakzaban P, Deacon TW, Burns LH, Isacson O. Increased proportion of AChE-rich zones and improved morphologic integration in host striatum of fetal grafts derived from the lateral but not the medial ganglionic eminence. *Exp Brain Res* 1993;97:13–22.

91. Pasinetti GM, Morgan DG, Finch CE. Disappearance of GAD-mRNA and tyrosine hydroxylase in substantia nigra following striatal ibotenic acid lesions: evidence for transneuronal regression. *Exp Neurol* 1991;112:131–139.

92. Pisa M, Sanberg PR, Fibiger HC. Striatal injec-

tions of kainic acid selectively impair serial memory performance in the rat. *Exp Neurol* 1981;74:633–653.

93. Pritzel M, Isacson O, Brundin P, Wiklund L, Björklund A. Afferent and efferent connections of striatal grafts implanted into the ibotenic acid lesioned neostriatum in adult rats. *Exp Brain Res* 1986;65:112–126.

94. Reading PJ, Dunnett SB. Embryonic striatal grafts reverse the disinhibitory effects of ibotenic acid lesions of the ventral striatum. *Exp Brain Res* 1994 [*in press*].

95. Roberts RC, DiFiglia M. Localization of immunoreactive GABA and enkephalin and NADPH diaphorase-positive neurons in fetal striatal grafts in the quinolinic-acid-lesioned rat neostriatum. *J Comp Neurol* 1988;274:406–421.

96. Roberts RC, DiFiglia M. Long-term survival of GABA–enkephalin, NADPH–diaphorase- and cabindin-d28k-containing neurons in fetal striatal grafts. *Brain Res* 1990;532:151–159.

97. Robertson HA, Peterson MR, Murphy K, Robertson GS. d-1-Dopamine receptor agonists selectively activate striatal c-*fos* independent of rotational behavior. *Brain Res* 1989;503:346–349.

98. Rutherford A, Garcia-Munoz M, Dunnett SB, Arbuthnott GW. Electrophysiological demonstration of host cortical inputs to striatal grafts. *Neurosci Lett* 1987;83:275–281.

99. Saji M, Reis DJ. Delayed transneuronal death of substantia nigra neurons prevented by gamma-aminobutyric acid agonist. *Science* 1987;235:66–69.

100. Sanberg PR, Calderon SF, Garver DL, Norman AB. Brain tissue transplants in an animal model of Huntington's disease. *Psychopharmacol Bull* 1987;23:476–482.

101. Sanberg PR, Coyle JT. Scientific approaches to Huntington's disease. *CRC Crit Rev Clin Neurobiol* 1984;1:1–44.

102. Sanberg PR, Fibiger HC. Body weight, feeding and drinking behaviors in rats with kainic acid lesions of the striatal neurons: with a note on body weight symptomatology in Huntington's disease. *Exp Neurol* 1979;66:444–466.

103. Sanberg PR, Giordano M, Henault MA, Nash DR, Ragozzino ME, Hagenmeyer-Houser SH. Intraparenchymal striatal transplants required for maintenance of behavioural recovery in an animal model of Huntington's disease. *J Neural Transplantation* 1989;1:23–31.

104. Sanberg PR, Henault MA, Deckel AW. Locomotor hyperactivity: effects of multiple striatal transplants in an animal model of Huntington's disease. *Pharmacol Biochem Behav* 1986;25:297–300.

105. Sanberg PR, Henault MA, Hagenmeyer-Houser SH, Giordano M, Russell KH. Multiple transplants of fetal striatal tissue in the kainic acid model of Huntington's disease. Behavioral recovery may not be related to acetylcholine esterase. *Ann NY Acad Sci* 1987;495:781–785.

106. Sanberg PR, Zubrycki E, Ragozzini ME, Giordano M, Shipley MT. Tyrosine hydroxylase-positive fibers and neurons in transplanted striatal tissue in rats with quinolinic acid lesions of the striatum. *Brain Res Bull* 1990;25:889–894.

107. Scheel-Krüger J. Dopamine–GABA interactions: evidence that GABA transmits, modulates and mediates dopaminergic functions in the basal ganglia and the limbic system. *Acta Neurol Scand [Suppl]* 1986;107:9–54.

108. Schmidt RH, Björklund A, Stenevi U. Intracerebral grafting of dissociated CNS tissue suspensions: a new approach for neuronal transplantation to deep brain sites. *Brain Res* 1981;218:347–356.

109. Schwartz R, Fuxe K, Agnati LF, Hökfelt T, Coyle JT. Rotational behaviour in rats with unilateral striatal kainic acid lesions: a behavioural model for studies on intact dopamine receptors. *Brain Res* 1979;170:485–495.

110. Schwartz R, Hökfelt T, Fuxe K, Jonsson G, Goldstein M, Terenius L. Ibotenic acid-induced neuronal degeneration: a morphological and neurochemical study. *Exp Brain Res* 1979;37:199–216.

111. Sirinathsinghji DJS, Dunnett SB, Isacson O, Clarke DJ, Kendrick K, Björklund A. Striatal grafts in rats with unilateral neostriatal lesions. II. In vivo monitoring of GABA release in globus pallidus and substantia nigra. *Neuroscience* 1988;24:803–811.

112. Sirinathsinghji DJS, Heavens RP, Torres EM, Dunnett SB. Cholycytokinin-dependent regulation of host dopamine inputs to striatal grafts. *Neuroscience* 1993;53;651–663.

113. Sirinathsinghji DJS, Morris BJ, Wisden W, Northrop A. Hunt SP, Dunnett SB. Gene expression in striatal grafts—I. Cellular localization of neurotransmitter mRNAs. *Neuroscience* 1990;34:675–686.

114. Sirinathsinghji DJS, Zivin M, Dunnett SB. Dopamine receptor and neuropeptide gene expression in dopamine denervated primordial striatal tissue grafts. *Restor Neurol Neurosci* 1992; 4:130.

115. Sirinathsinghji DJS, Mayer E, Fernandez JM, Dunnett SB. The localization of cholecystokinin mRNA in embryonic striatal tissue grafts: further evidence for the presence of non-striatal cells. Neuroreport 1993;4:659–662.

116. Smith AD, Bolam JP. The neural network of the basal ganglia as revealed by the study of synaptic connections of identified neurones. *Trends Neurosci* 1990;13:259–265.

117. Sofroniew MV, Isacson O, Björklund A. Cortical grafts prevent atrophy of cholinergic basal nucleus neurons induced by excitotoxic cortical damage. *Brain Res* 1986;378:409–415.

118. Somogyi P, Bolam JP, Smith AD. Monosynaptic cortical input and local axon collaterals of identified striatonigral neurons. A light and electron microscopic study using the Golgi-peroxidase transport-degenerative procedure. *J Comp Neurol* 1981;195:567–584.

119. Surmeier DJ, Xu ZC, Wilson CJ, Stefani A, Kitai ST. Grafted neostriatal neurons express a late-developing transient potassium current. *Neuroscience* 1992;48:849–856.

120. Tossman U, Segovia J, Ungerstedt U. Extracellular levels of amino acids in striatum and globus pallidus of 6-hydroxydopamine lesioned rats measured with microdialysis. *Acta Physiol Scand* 1986;127:547–551.

121. Valousková V, Brácha V, Bures J. Unilateral striatal grafts induce behavioral and electrophysiological asymmetry in rats with bilateral kainate lesions of the caudate nucleus. *Behav Neurosci* 1990;104:671–680.

122. Walker PD, McAllister JI. Minimal connectivity between neostriatal transplants and the host brain. *Brain Res* 1987;425:34–44.

123. Walker PD, Chovanes GI, McAllister JL. Identification of acetylcholinesterase-reactive neurons and neuropil in neostriatal transplants. *J Comp Neurol* 1987;259:1–12.

124. Wichmann T, Wictorin K, Björklund A, Starke K. Release of acetylcholine and its dopaminergic control in slices from striatal grafts in the ibotenic acid-lesioned rat striatum. *Naunyn Schmiedbergs Arch Pharmacol* 1988;338:623–631.

125. Whishaw IQ, O'Connor WT, Dunnett SB. The contributions of motor cortex, nigrostriatal dopamine and caudate–putamen to skilled forelimb use in the rat. *Brain* 1986;109:805–843.

126. Wictorin K, Brundin P, Gustavii B, Lindvall O, Björklund A. Reformation of long axonal pathways in adult rat CNS by human forebrain neuroblasts. *Nature* 1990;347:556–558.

127. Wictorin K, Isacson O, Fischer W, Nothias FH, Peschanski M, Björklund A. Connectivity of striatal grafts implanted into the ibotenic acid lesioned striatum. I. Subcortical afferents. *Neuroscience* 1988;27:547–562.

128. Wictorin K, Björklund A. Connectivity of striatal grafts implanted into the ibotenic acid lesioned striatum. II. Cortical afferents. *Neuroscience* 1989;30:297–311.

129. Wictorin K, Clarke DJ, Bolam JP, Björklund A. Host corticostriatal fibres establish synaptic connections with grafted striatal neurons in the ibotenic acid lesioned striatum. *Eur J Neurosci* 1989;1:189–195.

130. Wictorin K, Ouimet CC, Björklund A. Intrinsic organization and connectivity of intrastriatal striatal transplants in rats as revealed by DARPP-32 immunohistochemistry: specificity of connections with the lesioned host brain. *Eur J Neurosci* 1989;1:690–701.

131. Wictorin K, Simerly RB, Isacson O, Swanson LW, Björklund A. Connectivity of striatal grafts implanted into the ibotenic acid lesioned striatum. III. Efferent projecting graft neurons and their relation to host afferents with the grafts. *Neuroscience* 1989;30:313–330.

132. Wictorin K, Clarke DJ, Bolam JP, Björklund A. Fetal striatal neurons grafted into the ibotenate lesioned striatum: efferent projections and synaptic contacts in the host globus pallidus. *Neuroscience* 1990;37:301–315.

133. Wictorin K, Lagenaur CF, Lund RD, Björklund A. Efferent projections to the host brain from intrastriatal striatal mouse-to-rat grafts: time-course and tissue-type specificity as revealed by a mouse specific neuronal marker. *Eur J Neurosci* 1991;3:86–101.

134. Wooten GF, Collins RC. Regional brain glucose utilization following intrastriatal injections of kainic acid. *Brain Res* 1980;201:173–184.

135. Xu ZC, Wilson CJ, Emson PC. Restoration of the corticostriatal projection in rat neostriatal grafts: electron microscopic analysis. *Neuroscience* 1989;29:539–550.

136. Xu ZC, Wilson CJ, Emson PC. Restoration of thalamostriatal projections in rat neostriatal grafts: an electron microscopic analysis. *J Comp Neurol* 1990;303:2–14.

137. Xu ZC, Wilson CJ, Emson PC. Synaptic potentials evoked in spiny neurons in rat neurostriatal grafts by cortical and thalamic stimulation. *J Neurophysiol* 1991;65:477–493.

138. Xu ZC, Wilson CJ, Emson PC. Morphology of intracellularly stained spiny neurons in rat striatal grafts. *Neuroscience* 1992;82:441–458.

139. Young AMJ, Crowder JM, Bradford HF. Potentiation by kainate of excitatory amino acid release in striatum complementary in vivo and in vivo experiments. *J Neurochem* 1988;50:337–345.

140. Zhou FC, Buchwald N. Connectivities of the striatal grafts in adult rat brain; a rich afference and scant striatonigral efference. *Brain Res* 1989;504:15–30.

141. Zhou FC, Buchwald N, Hull C, Towle A. Neuronal and glial elements of fetal striatal grafts in the adult neostriatum. *Neuroscience* 1989;30:19–31.

142. Zhou FC, Pu CF, Finger S. Nimodipine-enhanced survival of suboptical neural grafts. *Restor Neurol Neurosci* 1991;3:211–215.

Functional Neural Transplantation,
edited by S. B. Dunnett and A. Björklund.
Raven Press, Ltd., New York © 1994.

8

Neural Transplantation in the Ventral Striatum

Paul J. Reading

*Department of Experimental Psychology, University of Cambridge,
Cambridge CB2 3EB, United Kingdom*

The once heretical notion of replacing adult central nervous tissue with functional transplants has gained increasing credibility since 1979. At this time, it was first demonstrated that transplanted embryonic neurons would not only survive and grow, but could also compensate for the behavioral asymmetries induced by unilateral nigrostriatal lesions in the rat (8,81). The majority of experimental studies involving embryonic neural grafts still continue to use the lesioned striatum as a substrate for functional analysis. Of these, most have concentrated on the dorsal striatum or caudate–putamen, with attempts to reverse the behavioral syndromes induced by either dopaminergic or intrinsic cell body lesions. This body of work has been fueled by the exciting possibility of direct application of the transplant technique to the crippling human conditions of Parkinson's disease and Huntington's disease. In both of these neurodegenerative disorders, it is the dorsal striatum that bears the brunt of early dysfunction in terms of dopaminergic deafferentation and striatal cell loss, respectively. This chapter focuses, however, on functional studies centered on the *ventral* striatum, an area comprising the nucleus accumbens, olfactory tubercle, and ventromedial caudate–putamen. Wherever possible, the results and conclusions reached from these studies are compared with those from work on the dorsal striatum, to which

the ventral striatum is intimately related, both anatomically and functionally.

Since the suggestion that the ventral striatum represented a functional subunit of the striatal complex (41), there has been an explosion of interest in the neurobiology of this enigmatic region of the basal forebrain. Several reasons can be expounded for this. First, from reconsiderations of its morphology and embryology, the proposed role of the nucleus accumbens in olfactory processes has been abandoned. Instead, renewed emphasis has been placed on the notion that it represents a specialized area of the caudate nucleus (107). Second, contemporary anatomical evidence that the ventral striatum receives descending afferentation from areas of the amygdala and allocortex, notably prefrontal cortex and hippocampus, has suggested anatomic routes whereby motivationally flavored limbic information could directly influence a subcortical motor structure (107). Since its inception, this intuitive "psychoanatomic" concept of the ventral striatum as a "limbic–motor" interface has been well rehearsed (e.g., 77). Third, a variety of techniques used to investigate the phenomena of intracranial self-stimulation (82,83) and the self-administration of abused psychostimulant drugs, such as amphetamine (46), have implicated reward processes with the action of the mesolimbic dopaminergic neurons that innervate the ventral striatum (10). Finally, a major incentive for research into the functions of the ventral striatum arose from its putative involvement in human disease. More specifically, the desire to delineate an anatomic locus for schizophrenia as apparently specific as the pharmacologic spectrum of the neuroleptic drugs used to treat it, implicated the nucleus accumbens and its attendant mesolimbic dopamine input (106). This concept has been developed and expanded by more recent formulations (39,108). From additional psychiatric perspectives, dysfunction of the ventral striatum has been suggested to play an important etiologic role in mania (84), depression (118), drug abuse (20), obsessive–compulsive behavior (86), as well as many cognitive and emotional aspects of Parkinson's disease (1,73,101,102).

Despite all this speculation, there have been no convincing demonstrations of abnormal morphologic structure nor biochemical function in the ventral striatum that could be construed as representing pathognomonic changes for a particular disease state. A possible exception to this is the report by Torack and Morris (113) that highlighted the unique neuropathology of an apparently new syndrome. It comprised a formidable combination of depression, parkinsonism, and dementia, and seemed to be characterized largely by pigmented cell loss from the ventral tegmental area (VTA), the origin of the dopaminergic innervation to the ventral striatum. In addition, a more recent immunohistochemical study on the brains of Alzheimer's disease sufferers provided strong evidence that, along with the more characterized neuropathologic changes of the disease, ventral striatal cholinergic neurons were particularly degenerate (63). This decrease in the number of cholinergic neurons, about 60%, was specific both to the striatal region, since dorsal areas were unaffected, and to the type of neuron, as neuropeptide Y-containing neurons in the ventral striatum were also spared.

THE FUNCTIONS OF THE VENTRAL STRIATUM

Evidence from Dopamine Lesions

With the foregoing background to the potential relevance of the ventral striatum to human disease, the question of its functional role in the intact brain arises. This will be addressed in some detail before the effects of neural grafts are considered, since an understanding of the functional role of the ventral striatum is an essential prelude to choosing and assessing tasks that probe the behavioral effects of transplants. Most theories of ventral striatal function have been based on the behavioral analysis of lesion syndromes in subhuman experimental subjects. Here, the administration of the catecholamine-depleting neurotoxin, 6-hydroxydopamine (6-OHDA), either to the terminal dopamine fields in the ventral striatum or to the dopamine cell bodies (A10) in the VTA has been most influential. By comparison with equivalent life-threatening bilateral lesions in the dorsal striatum or substantia nigra, animals with profound dopamine depletions of the ventral striatum appear relatively normal. The most consistent deficit has been the exaggeration and complete attenuation, respectively, of the activating effects of direct and indirect dopamine agonists, such as apomorphine and amphetamine, the former finding reflecting dopamine receptor supersensitivity (e.g., 58). From this, the vague concept arose that the ventral striatum might be a "locomotor" center, activated by mesolimbic dopamine release. However, after ventral tegmental lesions, rats may show *hyperactivity*, especially if observed overnight and if the lesion is made electrolytically (64). This paradoxical finding, in the light of the ventral striatum's proposed role in the expression of general locomotor activity, may be partly rationalized by consideration of factors such as the lesion technique and the involvement of prefrontal dopamine. For example, an electrolytic lesion, unlike 6-OHDA, largely spares the noradrenergic innervation of the limbic forebrain, which may influence the activity of the remaining dopamine neurons and the development of receptor supersensitivity (112). Additionally, Tassin points out that, of the postoperative biochemical correlations, it is the low prefrontal dopamine levels that are most predictive of hyperactivity (111). Since subsequent dopaminergic lesions of the nucleus accumbens attenuate the hyperactive aspects of the "ventral tegmental syndrome" (58), the high levels of activity may represent a form of functional overcompensation, especially since it occurs after damage with relatively low doses of neurotoxin (35). The foregoing discussion serves to indicate how measures of gross behaviors, such as locomotion, can produce confusing information that has little heuristic value, given the many potential underlying mechanisms to explain it.

Terminal depletions of dopamine from the ventral striatum produce even more subtle deficits. Gross locomotor hypoactivity (52,57); altered patterns of spontaneous lever-pressing, as revealed by operant schedules (95); and presumed attentional impairments (96) are apparent only transiently and disappear within about 2 weeks. The inherent plasticity of the mesolimbic dopamine system implied by such relatively rapid recovery may reflect the self-regulating properties of the mesocorticolimbic dopaminergic network (67). However, enduring changes in spontaneous behavior are observable, providing insightful comparisons with the effects of similar depletions in the dorsal striatum. Perhaps the most striking double dissociation relates to food consumption when a limited time is allowed for feeding (57). In such a situation, rats with ventral striatal depletions consumed more food than controls and were concurrently hypoactive. More dorsal depletions, in a subsequent complementary study, pro-

duced rats that were relatively hyperactive, but hypophagic (54).

This finding can be interpreted in terms of a ventral striatal lesion-induced deficit in time-sharing or switching between different classes of response category (94). This is supported by the observation that such rats also are apparently deficient at switching to classes of consummatory behaviors not controlled by obvious physiologic needs. More specifically, these rats fail to acquire control levels of schedule-induced polydipsia (93), an adjunctive behavior probably induced by the motivationally activating aspects of fixed-interval or fixed-time schedules (56). Interestingly, rats with caudate dopamine depletions show the same levels of excessive water consumption as control rats when placed on this type of schedule, but, in common with decorticate rats, have impaired lick efficiency, interpretable as a relatively pure motoric deficit (76).

A further example of a putative switching deficit shown by rats with ventral striatal lesions relates to their maladaptive perseverative responding in a variety of operant situations under conditions of extinction (97) or reversal (109,110). This reinforces the notion that the lesioned rats fail to switch between classes of behavior according to the presence of motivational influences signaling the appropriateness of such a switch. However, switching between separable responses that have similar topographies or eliciting stimuli does not seem to be so affected by ventral striatal dopaminergic lesions. For example, the lesion-induced hyperphagia induced by a limited feeding-time schedule is not accompanied by any deficit of behavioral switching between two individual food baskets (32). Similarly, complex two-lever schedules investigating the effects of lesions on tasks involving sequences of responses have revealed "higher-order" switching deficits (31). Thus, the lesioned rats exhibited lesion-induced strategical deficits when the correct solution of the task was altered, even when the nature of the change in response contingency necessitated perseveration on one of the levers. This type of *strategic*-switching deficit may correspond to the more cognitively flavored deficits seen in early parkinsonian and in frontal patients when performing, for example, the Wisconsin Card Sort Test (13,75). It contrasts with the more tangible problems of motor sequencing exhibited by subjects with preponderantly dorsal striatal dopamine depletions, including parkinsonian humans early in the course of their illness (6,72). Here, the fundamental deficit may reflect the inability to switch between individual relatively complex responses processed within the motor loop as part of an overall motor program, leading to a "motor" inflexibility. The relative inability of parkinsonians to stop walking or to change direction once started, unless the stimulus configuration of their environment changes dramatically, would reflect this type of switching difficulty. This implies that the general concept of *response switching* may constitute a basic correlate of dopamine activity throughout the striatum, as originally implied by the Lyon and Robbins (69) theory of amphetamine action and the behavioral data of Cools and colleagues (18). However, the nature of the switch may reflect the subregion of the striatal complex being considered, ranging from a strategic or volitional shift of motor plan to one more obviously involving relatively automatic motor sequences as part of a motor plan already selected.

Intrinsic Lesions

The behavioral consequences of lesions to the intrinsic neurons of the ventral striatum caused by electrolytic, radiofrequency, or excitotoxic amino acid techniques have been less extensively investigated than those following dopamine depletions. One of the earliest studies emphasized the similarity between the behavioral changes ob-

tained by bilateral electrode-induced damage to the accumbens and that to nearby septal lesions (66). In particular, hyperactivity, increased sensitivity to electric shock, and more rapid acquisition of a conditioned avoidance response were obtained. The prescient conclusion reached was that the accumbens could be functionally related to the limbic system. Although the lesion technique can be criticized on the grounds of nonspecificity, it is less nonspecific than comparable lesions to the dorsal striatum, for example, which, unlike the accumbens, is traversed by internal capsule fibers (40). The hyperactivity resulting from electrolytic lesions has been documented in a variety of situations, including spontaneous wheel-running in the home cage (59). In this study, the intrinsic lesions increased activity by a factor of 230% compared with sham-operated on controls.

Other early studies investigating the effects of similar bilateral intrinsic lesions to the accumbens have used a variety of behavioral indexes to characterize aspects of the lesion syndrome. In an early study, Wirtshafter and colleagues (120) described the attenuation of amphetamine-induced hyperthermia, but not, interestingly, hyperactivity following electrolytic lesions to the accumbens. In a series of reports, Albert's group have emphasized the hyperreactivity of rats with bilateral electrolytic lesions of the accumbens that appears additive to the similar effects of neighboring septal lesions (2–4). Lee and colleagues have also described the aggressive tendencies of lesioned rats (62). Smith and Holland (100), on the other hand, have documented the impaired lactational performance and consequent disrupted maternal behavior exhibited by similarly lesioned rats. Most recently, Rivas and Mir (91) have examined the sexual interactions of lesioned female rats. Following the lesion, they report various changes in the sexual preferences of the female rats and higher rates of mount rejections. However, since soliciting activity and lordosis were unimpaired, the results were interpreted not as reflecting alterations in sexual motivation, but again, as a hyperreactive syndrome, in this instance to the copulatory stimuli. A common theme relating most of the behavioral deficits mentioned in the foregoing seems to reflect the disruption or disorganization of innate response patterns. In particular, prepotent behaviors or habits, perhaps under dorsal striatal control, appear to have been "released" to an abnormal extent by the ventral striatal lesion.

In an operant setting, a recent study by Rawlins' group investigated extinction effects after small electrolytic lesions to the medial accumbens (14). Rats trained on a continuous reinforcement schedule were slower to extinguish than controls, whereas those lesioned rats trained on a partial reinforcement schedule were correspondingly *faster*. This attenuation of the so-called partial reinforcement extinction effect (PREE) was interpreted in terms of a disconnection of ventral subicular connections to the accumbens. It was noted that previous studies implicating the lateral septum in the PREE may have been misguided. In addition, the similarity of the performance of amphetamine-treated rats and lesioned rats was emphasized.

With more specific excitotoxic lesions to the nucleus accumbens, further studies have produced deficits interpretable as a loss of behavioral flexibility. On the basis of water and T-maze testing, Annett and colleagues (5) described the lesioned rats as showing inflexibility to external change. A further study has also confirmed this aspect of the excitotoxic lesion syndrome (89). Similarly, with use of bilateral ibotenic acid lesions, centered on the nucleus accumbens, they investigated the animals' ability to perform a delayed matching-to-position task. This operant task is classically a test of short-term memory and requires the animals to remember the location of a sample lever in a Skinner box over a random time period of up to 40 seconds in each trial. Three striking observations were noted.

First, the animals were markedly impaired at performing the basic task in a delay-dependent manner, suggestive of a short-term memory deficit. However, careful analysis of the error pattern implied that the deficit was not necessarily mnemonic, but that the animals had an intrusive bias to respond to a particular lever in the chamber. This inflexible tendency was apparent only when the attentional control exerted by the short-term memory trace was weak (i.e., at longer delays). The second finding was that the lesioned rats had great difficulty in switching their response strategy to a nonmatching schedule, in contrast with control animals that learned the switch in about four sessions. Finally, the lesioned rats were remarkably resistant to an extinction procedure, performing the unrewarded task literally thousands of times before attenuating their response rate, again in stark contrast to control rats. This resistance to extinction is also seen either after dopaminergic (97,109,110) or excitotoxic (5) lesions to the ventral striatum, at least on a continuous reinforcement schedule. It appears, then, that rats with bilateral damage to the ventral striatum are inflexible, performing complex operant tasks with a high degree of automaticity.

Excitotoxic lesions to the ventral striatum in primates have received very little attention. Stern and Passingham (103,104) have produced a series of abstracts concerned with the effects of bilateral ibotenic lesions to the ventral striatum in macaque monkeys. Briefly, their lesioned animals were impaired at hoarding peanuts and at employing a strategy for retrieving peanuts from four adjacent food wells (103). This latter deficit contrasted with the performance of control animals that quickly developed a stereotyped or habitual sequence (e.g., right to left) when retrieving the peanuts. A further report showed lesion-induced impairments specifically in the reversal stage of a spatial discrimination task (104). Finally, they have commented on the markedly increased frustration exhibited by the lesioned monkeys and hypothesize that this aspect of the syndrome may lie behind extinction effects observed in the operated on group (105). This latter result mirrors that obtained by Chih-Ta and colleagues in rats (14), since the lesioned monkeys were, in fact, *faster* to extinguish compared with controls on a *partial* reinforcement schedule (FR-15). The characteristics of the behavioral syndrome seen in the lesioned monkeys were best described as "bizarre." The animals exhibited hyperreactivity and ill-defined stereotypic behavior patterns, possibly reflecting disconnection of hippocampal or anterior cingulate cortical afferents.

Role of the Ventral Striatum

From this body of experimental data, some broad conclusions can be proposed concerning the role of the ventral striatum in normal brain function. Simplistically, it is proposed that the ventral striatum provides an indirect pathway for altering behavior in terms of strategy, rather than precise response topography. Dopamine activity in the ventral striatum is associated with increased activation or incentive motivation. This can be expressed either as general hyperactivity or as increased vigor of a goal-directed response that might be expected to expedite acquisition of the goal. However, whenever conditions dictate that routine or habitual behavior patterns must be inhibited, neural activity in the ventral striatum can also lead to a switch. This might occur during signals of novelty, nonreward, punishment, or intense arousal, when habitual or automatic behavior guided by previous stimulus–response learning must be overcome. Dorsal striatal processing probably plays a key role in the performance of such automatic behavior, allowing the smooth running of subconsciously selected motor plans. In this scheme, the ventral striatum acts as a relay between either frontal or limbic cortex and subcortical motor systems in the caudate–putamen, perhaps allowing ef-

fortful analysis and flexibility in performance when environmental contingencies change or are unexpected. This general role may go some way to explaining the paradoxical involvement of dopamine release in the ventral striatum under conditions of either reward or punishment. In both situations, motor activation is elicited, and ongoing behavior is either inhibited or enhanced, depending, perhaps, on previous stimulus–response and stimulus–reward learning.

TRANSPLANTATION INTO THE LESIONED VENTRAL STRIATUM

Dopamine Grafts

Whatever the precise functional significance of the behavioral syndromes induced by lesions of the ventral striatum, the advent of techniques to replace neurons with transplanted embryologic tissue raises the possibility of functional repair. Aside from the potential applications and intrinsic interest of being able to restore disrupted neural circuitry, it may also be hoped that the consequences of such embryonic neural grafts could provide additional clues about the normal functioning of the area concerned. In the dopamine-lesioned dorsal striatum, the specificity and time course of graft-induced functional recovery has been increasingly defined, both in terms of anatomy and biochemistry. In particular, dorsomedial striatal grafts have been the most effective in ameliorating the amphetamine-induced ipsilateral rotational response, whereas grafts in ventrolateral regions restore the lesion-induced sensorimotor deficits to a greater degree (25). This has been replicated and extended to include the investigation of more complex spontaneous behaviors (70). Of importance is that specifically dopamine-rich tissue is essential for the development and sustainment of recovery (29). In addition, the time course and extent of recovery is coincident and is correlated with the appearance and ramification of a dopaminergic fiber system that has appropriate ultrastructural connectivity with the striatal target tissue (9,34).

The theoretical and practical limitations of functional recovery following dopaminergic grafts have also been further defined. It has become apparent that a restored dopaminergic innervation of the dorsal striatum sufficient to reverse drug-induced behavioral phenomena completely is less effective when considering spontaneous behaviors. Notable examples of graft "failures" concern paw-reaching deficits and regulatory aspects of feeding and drinking seen after unilateral and bilateral lesions, respectively (23a,26,28). Many reasons can be expounded for the insufficiency of grafts in these situations. One of the most important probably relates to the ectopic position of the grafted dopamine cell bodies away from the midbrain where they would normally receive afferentation from a variety of brain sites in the intact animal. Additionally, only part of the dopamine system is replaced following relatively extensive lesions. This could represent the limiting factor concerning full recovery of more complex behaviors that require coordinated dopamine release onto various terminal areas. For example, the lack of dopaminergic innervation to ventral striatal and hypothalamic areas may lie behind the failure of dorsal striatal grafts to affect, respectively, the akinetic and regulatory deficits of the aphagic–adipsic syndrome seen after bilateral lesions to the medial forebrain bundle. Recently, the failure of dorsal grafts to restore paw-reaching deficits has been speculated to reflect the lack of motivational influences that may be subserved by ventral striatal dopamine function (71). This was based on a lesion and graft study implying that specific (dorsal) striatal dopamine depletions were not deficient on a paw-reaching task.

There has been a limited number of studies that have specifically assessed the ability of neural grafts to restore deficits induced by depletions of *ventral* striatal dopamine. However, these have revealed a very similar story to the earlier investigations involving more dorsal striatal areas. Early studies showed that the reliable attenuation of amphetamine-induced hyperactivity seen after bilateral dopaminergic lesions is reversed by appropriate implants into the nucleus accumbens (27,78). Intriguingly, as is routinely seen with dorsal striatal grafts and amphetamine-induced rotation, a degree of apparent overcompensation is reliably seen in the grafted animals. The study by Dunnett and colleagues (27) also addressed the effects of concomitant implantation of dopaminergic grafts into prefrontal cortex. Contrary to the theory that dopamine release in prefrontal and ventral striatal regions has opposing and competing effects on overall behavior (53, 68,85), the grafts in the two sites had additive effects on restoring drug-induced activity. This study also provided evidence for the reversal of lesion-induced dopamine receptor hypersensitivity, since the hyperactivity of the lesioned animals after low-dose apomorphine was attenuated by the presence of the grafts. Further studies have confirmed the ability of grafts to reverse the effects of lesions on drug-induced levels of activity, either at the level of the ventral tegmental area (15,45) or terminally in the ventral striatum (16,43–45).

The restitution of spontaneous behaviors, conditioned or unconditioned, has also been addressed in a handful of studies. Spontaneous activity during the day was lower in VTA-lesioned rats, yet restored by ventral striatal dopaminergic grafts in one study (45). However, the disappearance of stable behavioral effects in lesioned rats has been a serious confound in assessing graft-induced recovery. Dopaminergic grafts have not been observed to influence recovery on measures of hoarding or exploration that appear to be affected for longer periods after bilateral VTA lesions (45). Nevertheless, when grafts were used to replace the dopamine innervation following local terminal lesions, recovery of hoarding behavior was observed if the animals were administered systemic low-dose amphetamine

(44). From the same model, however, it has been suggested that the grafts may even inhibit the inherent capacity for spontaneous functional recovery (16). In this study, behavioral recovery in the rats with lesions alone occurred over 10 to 12 months and was suggested to reflect collateral sprouting of dopamine terminals spared by the initial lesion. It was noteworthy that the grafts appeared to inhibit this recovery, despite restoring absolute dopamine levels in the accumbens to values higher than those seen in animals with lesions alone. This would suggest that the smaller, but more appropriate, dopamine reinnervation in the rats with lesions alone may have been more functionally effective than the ectopic grafts. Further studies that used the more stable VTA lesion model have failed to demonstrate any significant graft-induced recovery on more complex behaviors. The indexes used in these experiments included spatial orientation (15), schedule-induced polydipsia (15), and the Morris water-maze task (11). The latter pilot study is important because it is the first to address the ameliorative effects of ventral striatal grafts on a conditioned or learned behavior.

At least one study has examined the ability of dopaminergic grafts in the accumbens to restore biochemical indexes of recovery following bilateral VTA lesions. By using microdialysis techniques in freely moving rats, Ishida and colleagues (51) demonstrated that amphetamine-induced release of dopamine 3,4-dihydroxyphenylacetic acid (DOPAC) and homovanillic acid (HVA) were increased significantly above the levels seen in the lesion-alone group, as little as 4 weeks postgrafting. The behavioral correlates of the biochemical recovery, namely, daily locomotor activity, were also ameliorated by the presence of the graft, although overcompensation was not seen in this study.

We have used the bilateral VTA lesion model in two experimental situations to assess the functional capacity of embryonic dopaminergic grafts in the dopamine-depleted ventral striatum. The first study used rats performing a simple operant schedule in the Skinner box. Termed a fixed-interval (FI) schedule, food is delivered on each trial to hungry rats following a lever press only if a certain interval of time has passed since food was last delivered (30 seconds in the experiment here). A highly reliable behavior pattern emerges after prolonged training, characterized by a so-called scalloped response profile. This term dates back to the earliest descriptions of the phenomenon, when cumulative lever responses were recorded as a function of the time elapsed during the fixed interval, averaged over a session. Trained experimental animals, in some sense, learn to anticipate the ending of the interval. This engenders a form of motor excitement, evidenced by consistent time-dependent increased levels of operant behavior. Put another way, as the interval nears its end, the rate of lever-pressing increases to maximal levels at the actual point of reward delivery, reflecting a process of increasing incentive motivation. Depletions of dopamine from the nucleus accumbens attenuates this accelerated rate of lever pressing, albeit relatively transiently, without altering the overall shape of the response profile curve (95). This can be interpreted as reflecting a diminution of the incentive motivational effects engendered by the schedule, leaving the timing aspects and general motoric abilities of the rats intact. Additionally, the lesion blocked the characteristic effects of low-dose amphetamine on performance of the schedule (95).

By using bilateral VTA dopaminergic lesions, we aimed to produce a longer-lasting behavioral deficit against which to compare the effects of bilateral grafts of dopaminergic-rich embryonic tissue into the terminal regions of the ventral striatum. The results are shown in Fig. 1. The group of lesioned rats had a stable response profile consisting of reduced terminal rates of responding on the schedule. In contrast, the group with additional grafts behaved almost identically to control sham-operated rats. Addition-

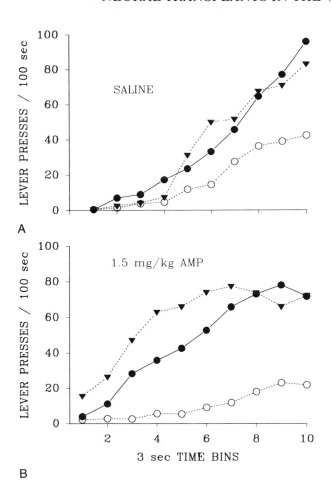

A

B

FIG. 1. A: The response rates of the three groups of rats averaged over ten 40-min sessions according to the time bin of the 30-sec fixed interval (*solid circle,* sham; *solid triangle,* graft; *open circle,* lesion). The *lesion* group had bilateral 6-OHDA lesions to the VTA and the *graft* group had subsequent bilateral dopaminergic grafts transplanted to the ventral striatum. **B**: The effects of low-dose amphetamine on the response profile of the three groups. Data were averaged from two sessions.

ally, the grafted rats were hypersensitive to the effects of amphetamine, whereas lesioned rats failed to show any activation following administration of the drug. The two important conclusions reached were, first, that dopamine grafts in this lesion model could restore aspects of a learned simple behavior without the need for pharmacologic intervention. Second, the apparent hypersensitivity of dopamine-grafted rats to amphetamine on tests of locomotor activity and rotation appears to extend to conditioned behavior controlled by an operant schedule.

The second study addressed the phenomenon of conditioned hyperactivity. This occurs when rats are repeatedly given an activating drug, such as amphetamine, specifically in a distinctive environment and are then given a placebo injection in that same environment. Compared with control groups that have experienced the same quantity of drug in a separate environment, the experimental group exhibit hyperactivity when given the placebo. Such activation can be loosely interpreted as reflecting the animals' "expectation" of receiving the drug and, like the activating effects of the drug itself, there is evidence that this "conditioned activity" is consequent to presynaptic dopamine release in the ventral striatum (38). We chose to investigate whether bilateral grafts in the ventral striatum would sustain such conditioned activity, given that they reliably restore the unconditioned activating effects of the drug to lesioned animals.

The results are summarized in Fig. 2. Briefly, the lesioned group failed to show locomotor hyperactivity, conditioned or unconditioned, after amphetamine administration. The control group that had repeatedly experienced amphetamine in the distinctive environment of the activity cages exhibited relatively high levels of activation when given a subsequent injection of saline. The grafted group, however, showed a unique profile of responding. When compared with control rats, a degree of overcompensated hyperactivity was evident when the grafted rats were under the influence of amphetamine. In contrast, when conditioned activity was assessed, they failed to show any significant level of heightened activity. From this, one can tentatively conclude that dopamine grafts in the region of the ventral striatum will reliably restore the activating effects of amphetamine, yet fail to restore behavior dependent on spontaneous dopamine release, a conclusion reached from many studies that used the dorsal striatal model. Similarly, the inevitable disruption of circuitry following grafting may explain the inadequacy of ventral striatal dopaminergic grafts in this situation.

The results of the study just outlined also have implications for the analysis of ventral striatal dopamine function. One possible conclusion from the negative effects of the dopamine grafts on spontaneous-conditioned activity is that the neuronal signals corresponding to the environmental cues associated with drug administration exert an effect through excitatory connections to dopamine neurons at the level of the VTA, rather than in the terminal regions of the dopaminergic field.

An experiment by Brundin and coworkers, which used ventral and dorsal striatal dopamine grafts in a rotation paradigm, also claimed to have implications for the theories concerning the functional role of ventral striatal dopamine release (12). The study used a group of rats with nigrostriatal bundle lesions together with bilateral terminal dopamine depletions from the nucleus accumbens. After amphetamine administration, these rats rotated ipsilaterally to the bundle lesion to a lesser degree than a group with a bundle lesion alone and no specific accumbens dopamine depletions. This was in accordance with earlier data of Kelly and Moore (55), from which the influential theory arose that ventral striatal dopamine release has a facilitatory effect on rotational behavior, rather than a directional one. The interesting finding of Brun-

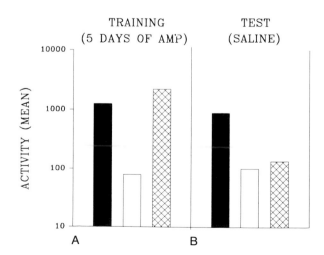

FIG. 2. **A**: The effects of administering amphetamine (1.5 mg/kg) to the three groups of rats in a distinctive two-beam photocell activity cage. Activity refers to the number of beam-to-beam crossings made in 1 hour. **B**: "Conditioned" activity after a subsequent placebo saline injection. *Solid bars,* sham; *open bars,* lesion; *hatched bars,* lesion plus graft.

din was that dopamine grafts implanted into the nucleus accumbens of the side with near complete forebrain dopamine depletion induced the rats to rotate more *ipsilaterally* to the graft. It was pointed out, although not actually demonstrated, that a dorsal striatal graft would have had the opposite effect (i.e., to reduce the ipsilateral bias). Brundin interpreted the result as reflecting the amplification of a dorsal striatal directional bias by the subsequent addition of a dopamine input to the accumbens unilaterally, albeit contralaterally.

Intrinsic Striatal Grafts

The mixed picture of success with striatal dopamine grafts and spontaneous behaviors contrasts with the remarkable emerging body of data concerning the functional capacities of embryonic grafts that replace intrinsic dorsal striatal circuitry disrupted by excitotoxic neuronal damage. Such grafts dissected from striatal primordial tissue restore many anatomic (42) and biochemical (49) aspects when transplanted homotopically to lesioned striata in rats. Quantitative analyses have implied that a marker for γ-aminobutyric acid (GABA) in the lesioned neostriatum, namely, the level of glutamic acid decarboxylase (GAD), was increased from 20% to 50% to 70% of control values by the presence of the grafts. Additionally, there was normalization of GAD in the previously denervated globus pallidus. Moreover, the restored levels of GABA in the globus pallidus, as measured by microdialysis, were influenced by amphetamine, implying that the grafts were responsive to an active dopaminergic innervation (99). Indeed, morphologically, there is strong evidence that dopaminergic fibers innervate the grafts in patchy formations and that these neurons originate in the substantia nigra pars compacta (17,65,115). Further findings implying the presence of thalamic and cortical afferents, together with anatomic demonstrations of efferent projections to the globus pallidus and, to a degree, the substantia nigra, suggest an elaborate integration of the striatal grafts within the host brain (116,117). One further index of graft-induced recovery comes from a study that examined c-*fos* induction within the transplant. More specifically, systemic administration of haloperidol was seen to induce c-*fos* molecules and Fos-related antigens in transplanted striatal tissue, with a time course and magnitude indistinguishable from controls (21).

Functional studies investigating the ability of embryonic striatal tissue to reverse the behavioral deficits caused by cell body damage have, so far, produced promising results in the dorsal striatum (see 79 for review). Hyperactivity, whether nocturnal (36,47,98) or diurnal (19), and deficits in maze alternations (19,48) have been reversed by the presence of bilateral grafts. Furthermore, drug-induced asymmetries, deficits in paw-reaching, and lesion-induced paw preferences have been influenced to significant extents by unilateral grafts (30,114). Finally, in a primate lesion model, the striatal grafts reduced the dyskinetic or choreiform symptomology of lesioned animals following dopamine receptor agonist administration (50). Detailed behavioral analysis of striatal lesions and grafts, however, is difficult for several reasons. First, large bilateral lesions to the dorsal striatum tend to produce severely incapacitated animals, with profound regulatory deficits (e.g., 236,24). This is problematic, since the animals must survive for about 20 weeks for the grafts to become fully established. Moreover, the deficits may be seen as relatively nonspecific, affecting all aspects of observable behavior. Furthermore, easily quantifiable behavioral tests, sensitive to lesion effects, are deceptively difficult to devise, especially if unilateral lesions are used when the animal must be forced to use the paw contralateral to the lesion and subsequent graft. In addition, unilateral lesions can produce bilateral effects, making assessment of the graft more difficult. For the bilateral dorsal striatal model, quantifiable deficits are equally difficult to obtain. For example, part of a recent study examined the ability of striatal grafts to reverse the functional effects of bilateral kainic acid (KA) striatal lesions. The rats were trained to remain on a rotating rod as a test of motor coordination. Lesion effects were seen when the rod was rotating at low, but not at high, speeds and, even then, only transiently (37).

The bilateral ventral striatal lesion and graft model has advantages in some of these aspects. The animals are not grossly impaired, surviving for long periods without the need for special feeding regimens. Furthermore, relatively subtle, but stable, behavioral deficits are produced on well-established computerized operant schedules, specifically those using the Skinner box (22,88,89). In addition, the question of whether the grafted tissue can be functionally activated by pharmacologic means can be addressed, given that low-dose amphetamine exerts most of its behavioral effects by a release of dopamine in the ventral striatum (33). There have as yet been no published functional studies that have used striatal grafts specifically in the region of the ventral striatum, although Olson has demonstrated that such grafts do receive dopaminergic innervation from embryonic ventral mesencephalon in the *in oculo* preparation (80).

We have completed one study (90) that investigated ventral striatal graft effects following bilateral excitotoxic lesions. As outlined previously, the lesion syndrome can be described as disinhibitory in which the animals are hyperactive and inflexible, perhaps reflecting disconnection of limbic and prefrontal cortical influences on subcortical motor output. We used a lever-pressing schedule with differential reinforcement of low rates of responding (DRL). This schedule necessitates that rats will be rewarded by food delivery after a lever press *if and only if* 20 seconds have elapsed since the previous response. Rats find it particularly difficult to acquire efficient levels of responding on this schedule, since they must inhibit the previously rewarded tendency to lever-press. However, extensive training does lead to very stable patterns of responding in which about 30% to 50% of an animal's responses are rewarded (i.e., are separated by at least 20 seconds). Amphetamine administered to such rats disrupts performance by disinhibiting lever responding, rather than a more specific inability to "time" the requisite 20 second interval (92). In a pilot study, the effects of ventral striatal excitotoxic lesions using ibotenic acid (IA) injected bilaterally into the region of the nucleus accumbens produced a remarkably similar syndrome to that induced by low-dose amphetamine given to normal rats. Analysis of the pattern of responding using signal detection indexes revealed that those rats with bilateral ventral striatal lesions, like amphetamine-treated animals, had a general disinhibited tendency to lever-press (87). One way of interpreting the lesion-induced deficit is that it reflects a problem in switching between response categories. Such an explanation arises from consideration of the strategies normal rats have been observed to adopt when performing on the differential reinforcement of low rates (DRL) task. It has been proposed that stereotyped mediating or collateral behaviors, such as gnawing or tail-licking, are exhibited by normal rats in a time-locked fashion after receiving reinforcement (74, 119). These mediating behaviors are somewhat idiosyncratic and perhaps represent an empirical means of "filling in time." If rats are prevented or dissuaded from exhibiting them, performance on the DRL schedule becomes less efficient, giving credence to their integral importance (60,61). It is conceivable that both the ventral striatal lesion and the effects of amphetamine on normal rats disrupt this aspect of behavior to produce the profound impairment on task performance.

We investigated the ability of three groups of rats to learn the DRL schedule and then assessed the effects of amphetamine. The groups consisted of sham-op-

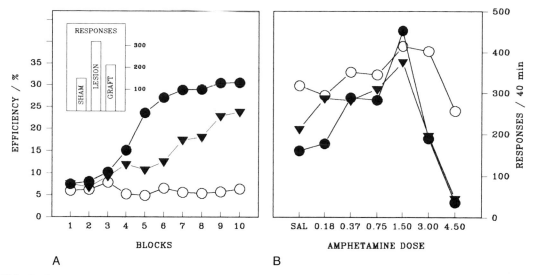

FIG. 3. *Lesion* (*open circles*) refers to the group of rats with bilateral ibotenic acid lesions centered on the nucleus accumbens. The *graft* group (*solid triangles*) received subsequent bilateral striatal transplants (*solid circles,* sham group). **A**: The acquisition of the DRL task over 50 training sessions. The performance of the three groups is expressed as efficiency (i.e., the percentage of rewarded lever presses exhibited in a 40-min session). Data are averaged over blocks of five sessions. **Insert**: The mean number of responses per session over the last training block. **B**: The effects of a range of doses of amphetamine on the number of responses per session.

erated controls, bilaterally lesioned rats following microinjections of ibotenic acid into the ventral striatum, and rats with lesions and subsequent homotopic implantations of embryonic striatal tissue. By using the more medial of the two eminences constituting the developing striatal primordia, the dissection for the embryonic tissue attempted to select that area destined to become mature ventral striatum.

The results are shown in Fig. 3. The grafted animals behaved significantly different from those with lesions alone on the acquisition of the task and when they were given amphetamine. In both cases the grafted group's behavior was more similar

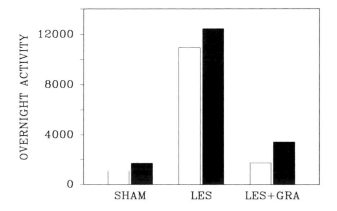

FIG. 4. The overnight activity of the three groups in terms of the total number of beam crossings in a photocell activity cage. Data were collected when the rats were either 85% of their free-feeding weight (*deprived, solid bars*) or after 1 week of free access to food (*satiated, open bars*).

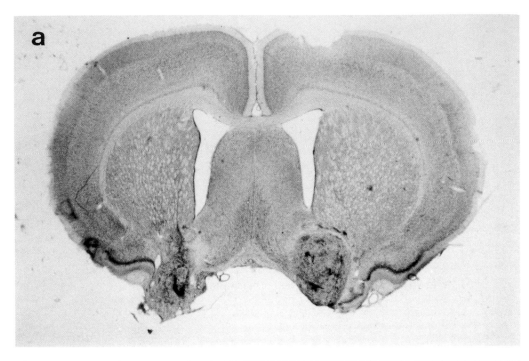

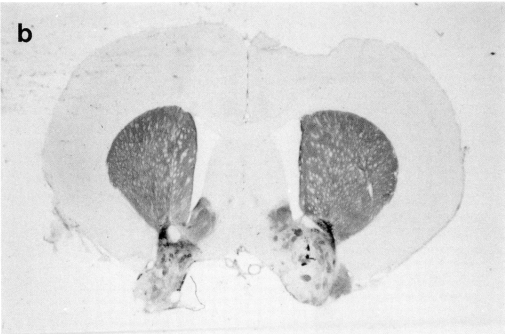

FIG. 5. a: A typical ventral striatal transplant centered on the nucleus accumbens stained with cresyl violet. **b**: The same graft stained for tyrosine hydroxylase immunoreactivity.

to the control group's. Precisely what aspect of the lesioned rats' behavior the grafts were partly able to reverse remains a matter of conjecture. However, it is possible that the grafted rats were more efficient at switching away from lever-pressing to other "mediating" behaviors. A final test of overnight activity also demonstrated reversal of lesion-induced hyperactivity by the presence of the grafts (Fig. 4).

The successful graft-induced amelioration of these aspects of the lesion syndrome might well reflect restored connectivity. Although detailed histologic analyses were not undertaken, standard cresyl violet and immunohistochemical stains against tyrosine hydroxylase revealed large surviving grafts that had typical dopaminergic-rich islands of tissue (Fig. 5). The restoration of amphetamine-induced effects also encourages the belief that functional dopamine fibers had reinnervated the transplant.

CONCLUSIONS

The relatively small number of studies that have assessed the functional capacity of embryonic neural implants to reverse the effects of lesions to the ventral striatum allow some conclusions to be made. As with the behavioral data from graft experiments, of dopaminergic tissues in the dorsal striatum, all but the simplest of spontaneous behaviors are not restored. One exception to this is the study, outlined above, that observed recovery of the abnormal patterns of behavior on a lever-pressing schedule following dopaminergic lesions to the ventral tegmental area. This possibly reflects that ventral striatal dopamine release is necessary and sufficient for the activational aspects of the fixed-interval behavior. In the other cases of graft "failure," it is conceivable that dopamine depletion in other terminal areas of the mesocorticolimbic pathway contributes to the lesion syndrome. Whether a more complete recovery would result from multiple-grafted sites, for

example, including the prefrontal cortex, septum, and amygdala, remains speculative. The contrasting complete restoration of some drug-induced behaviors is also concordant with the picture that has emerged from dorsal striatal transplant studies. In addition, the equally promising results obtained from the one study using striatal transplants to the excitotoxic-lesioned ventral striatum adds to the growing evidence of functional recovery of spontaneous behaviors induced by dorsal striatal grafts.

The use of computerized testing of animals with ventral striatal lesions and grafts has provided a particularly useful approach for several reasons. First, the lesion, whether dopaminergic or to intrinsic circuitry, leaves the animals with relatively subtle yet long-lasting deficits that do not significantly compromise survival or regulatory aspects of behavior. Second, there is a rich and developing database from physiologic psychology on the nature of behavioral deficits after such lesions. Third, the computerized nature of the tests allows the collection of large amounts of objective data. Finally, perhaps counterintuitively, animals, once trained on the type of behavioral paradigms described, behave with remarkable stability from day to day, providing an appropriate baseline from which to compare lesion and graft effects.

Credible functional studies of embryonic transplantation have necessarily lagged behind those investigating anatomic and biochemical aspects of recovery. However, the ultimate question of whether grafts are able to "work" in brain-damaged hosts, as well as the use of grafts as functional "tools" (7), should encourage the increasing development of their behavioral assessment in the respective arenas of applied and basic neurobiology.

ACKNOWLEDGMENT

The author was supported by a MRC Training Fellowship.

REFERENCES

1. Agid Y, Ruberg M, Dubois B, Javoy-Agid F. Biochemical substrates of mental disturbances in Parkinson's disease. *Adv Neurol* 1984;40: 211–218.
2. Albert DJ, Richmond SE. Septal hyperreactivity: a comparison of lesions within and adjacent to the septum *Physiol Behav* 1975;15:339–347.
3. Albert DJ, Walsh ML, Longley W. Medial hypothalamic and medial accumbens lesions which induce mouse killing enhance biting and attacks on inanimate objects. *Physiol Behav* 1985;35: 523–527.
4. Albert DJ, Walsh ML, Zalys C, Dyson E. Defensive agression towards an experimenter: no difference between males and females following septal, medial accumbens or medial hypothalamic lesions in rats. *Physiol Behav* 1986; 38:11–14.
5. Annett LE, McGregor A, Robbins TW. The effects of ibotenic acid lesions of the nucleus accumbens on spatial learning and extinction in the rat. *Behav Brain Res* 1989;31:231–242.
6. Benecke R, Rothwell JC, Dick JPR, Day BL, Marsden CD. Disturbance of sequential movements in patients with Parkinson's disease. *Brain* 1987;110:361–379.
7. Björklund A. Neural transplantation—an experimental tool with clinical possibilities. *Trends Neurosci* 1991;14:319–322.
8. Björklund A, Stenevi U. Reconstruction of the nigrostriatal dopamine pathway by intracerebral nigral transplants. *Brain Res* 1979;177: 555–560.
9. Björklund A, Dunnett SB, Stenevi U, Lewis ME, Iversen SD. Reinnervation of the denervated striatum by substantia nigra transplants: functional consequences as revealed by pharmacological and sensorimotor testing. *Brain Res* 1980;199:307–333.
10. Björklund A, Lindvall O. Catecholamine-containing brain stem regulatory systems. In: Bloom FE, ed. *Handbook of physiology: the nervous system,* vol 4. Baltimore: Williams & Wilkins; 1986.
11. Brundin P, Gage FH, Dunnett SB, Björklund A. Long-term locomotor and cognitive deficits in rats with 6-OHDA lesions of the VTA: a model for transplantion studies. In: Woodruff GN, Poat JA, Roberts PJ, eds. *Dopaminergic systems and their regulation.* London: Macmillan; 1986.
12. Brundin P, Strecker RE, Londos E, Björklund A. Dopamine neurons grafted unilaterally to the nucleus accumbens affect drug-induced circling and locomotion. *Exp Brain Res* 1987; 69:183–194.
13. Canavan AGM, Passingham RE, Marsden CD, Quinn N, Wyke M, Polkey CE. The performance of learning tasks of patients in the early stages of Parkinson's disease. *Neuropsychologica* 1989;27:141–156.
14. Chih-Ta Tai, Clark AJM, Feldon J, Rawlins JNP. Electrolytic lesions of the nucleus accumbens in rats which abolish the PREE enhance the locomotor response to amphetamine. *Exp Brain Res* 1991;86:333–340.
15. Choulli K, Herman J-P, Abrous N, Le Moal M. Behavioral effects of intraaccumbens transplants in rats with lesions of the mesocorticolimbic dopamine system. *Ann NY Acad Sci* 1987;495:497–509.
16. Choulli K, Herman J-P, Rivet M, Simon H, LeMoal M. Spontaneous and graft-induced behavioral recovery after 6-hydroxydopamine lesions of the nucleus accumbens in the rat. *Brain Res* 1987;407:376–380.
17. Clarke DJ, Dunnett SB, Isacson O, Sirinathsinghji DJS, Björklund A. Striatal grafts in rats with unilateral neostriatal lesions: immunocytochemical and ultrastructural evidence of dopaminergic ingrowth. *Neuroscience* 1987;24: 791–801.
18. Cools AR, Jaspers R, Schwartz M, Sontag K-H, Vrijmoed-de-Vries M, van den Bercken J. Basal ganglia and switching motor programs. In: McKenzie JS, Kemm RE, Wilcock LN, eds. *The basal ganglia.* New York: Plenum Press; 1984.
19. Deckel AW, Moran TH, Coyle JT, Sanberg PR, Robinson RG. Anatomical predictors of behavioral recovery following fetal striatal transplants. *Brain Res* 1986;365:249–258.
20. Di Chiara G, Acquas E, Carboni E. Role of mesolimbic dopamine in the motivational effects of drugs: brain dialysis and place preference studies. In: Willner P, Scheel-Krüger J, eds. *The mesolimbic dopamine system: from motivation to action.* Chichester: John Wiley & Sons; 1991.
21. Dragunow M, Williams M, Faull RL. Haloperidol induces *fos* and related molecules in intrastriatal grafts derived from fetal striatal primordia. *Brain Res* 1990;530:309–311.
22. Dunnett SB. Role of prefrontal cortex and striatal output systems in short-term memory deficits associated with ageing, basal forebrain lesions, and cholinergic-rich grafts. *Can J Psychol* 1990;44:210–232.
23a. Dunnett SB, Björklund A, Stenevi U, Iversen SD. Behavioural recovery following transplantation of substantia nigra in rats subjected to 6-OHDA lesions of the nigrostriatal pathway. II. Bilateral lesion. *Brain Res* 1981;229:457–470.
23b. Dunnett SB, Iversen SD. Learning impairments following selective kainic acid-induced lesions within the neostriatum of rats. *Behav Brain Res* 1981;2:189–209.
24. Dunnett SB, Iversen SD. Sensorimotor impairments following localized kainic acid and 6-hydroxydopamine lesions of the neostriatum. *Brain Res* 1982;248:121–127.
25. Dunnett SB, Björklund A, Schmidt RH, Stenevi U, Iversen SD. Behavioural recovery in rats with unilateral 6-OHDA lesions following implantation of nigral cell suspensions in different brain sites. *Acta Physiol Scand [Suppl]* 1983;522:29–37.
26. Dunnett SB, Björklund A, Schmidt RH, Stenevi U, Iversen SD. Intracerebral grafting of

neuronal cell suspensions. V. Behavioural recovery in rats with bilateral 6-OHDA lesions following implantation of nigral cell suspensions. *Acta Physiol Scand [Suppl]* 1983;522:39–47.

27. Dunnett SB, Bunch ST, Gage FH. Björklund A. Dopamine-rich transplants in rats with 6-OHDA lesions of the ventral tegmental area. I. Effects on spontaneous and drug induced locomotor activity. *Behav Brain Res* 1984;13:71–82.
28. Dunnett SB, Whishaw IQ, Rogers DC, Jones GH. Dopamine-rich grafts ameliorate whole body motor asymmetry and sensory neglect but not independent limb use in rats with 6-hydroxydopamine lesions. *Brain Res* 1987;415: 63–78.
29. Dunnett SB, Hernandez TD, Summerfield A, Jones GH, Arbuthnott G. Graft-derived recovery from 6-OHDA lesions: specificity of ventral mesencephalic graft tissues. *Exp Brain Res* 1988;71:411–424.
30. Dunnett SB, Isacson O, Sirinathsinghji DJS, Clarke DJ, Björklund A. Striatal grafts in rats with unilateral neostriatal lesions III. Recovery from dopamine-dependent motor asymmetry and deficits in skilled paw-reaching. *Neuroscience* 1988;24:813–820.
31. Evenden JL. *A behavioural and pharmacological analysis of response selection. [Dissertation]* University of Cambridge, 1983.
32. Evenden JL, Carli M. The effects of 6-hydroxydopamine lesions of the nucleus accumbens and caudate nucleus of rats on feeding in a novel environment. *Behav Brain Res* 1985; 15:63–70.
33. Evenden JL, Ryan CN. Behavioral responses to psychomotor stimulant drugs: localization in the central nervous system. *Pharmacol Ther* 1988;36:151–172.
34. Freund TF, Bolam JP, Björklund A, Stenevi U, Dunnett SB, Powell JF, Smith AD. Efferent synaptic connections of grafted dopaminergic neurons reinnervating the host neostriatum: a tyrosine hydroxylase immunocytochemical study. *J Neurosci* 1985;5:603–616.
35. Galey D, Simon H, LeMoal M. Behavioral effects of lesions of the A10 DA area of the rat. *Brain Res* 1977;124:83–97.
36. Giordano M, Houser SH, Sanberg PR. Intraparenchymal fetal striatal transplants and recovery in kainic acid lesioned rats. *Brain Res* 1988;446:183–188.
37. Giordano M, Ford LM, Shipley MT, Sanberg PR. Neural grafts and pharmacological intervention in a model of Huntington's disease. *Brain Res Bull* 1990;25:453–465.
38. Gold LH, Swerdlow NR, Koob GF. The role of mesolimbic dopamine in conditioned locomotion produced by amphetamine. *Behav Neurosci* 1988;102:544–552.
39. Gray JA, Feldon R, Rawlins JNP, Helmsley DR, Smith AD. The neuropsychology of schizophrenia. *Behav Brain Sci* 1991;14;1–84.
40. Gurdjian ES. The corpus striatum of the rat. *J Comp Neurol* 1928;45:249–281.
41. Heimer L, Wilson RD. The subcortical projec-

tions of the allocortex: similarities in the neural associations of the hippocampus, the piriform cortex and the neocortex. In: Santani MM, ed. *The Golgi centennial symposium: perspectives in neurobiology.* New York: Raven Press, 1975.

42. Helm GA, Palmer PE, Bennett JP Jr. Fetal neostriatal transplants in the rat: a light and electron microscopic Golgi study. *Neuroscience* 1990;36:735–756.
43. Herman J-P, Choulli K, LeMoal M. Hyperreactivity to amphetamine in rats with dopaminergic grafts. *Exp Brain Res* 1985;60:521–526.
44. Herman J-P, Choulli K, Geffard M, Nadaud D, Taghzouti K, LeMoal M. Reinnervation of the nucleus accumbens and frontal cortex of the rat by dopaminergic grafts and effects on hoarding behavior. *Brain Res* 1986;372:210–216.
45. Herman J-P, Choulli K, Abrous N, Dulluc J, LeMoal M. Effects of intraaccumbens grafts on behavioral deficits induced by 6-OHDA lesions of the nucleus accumbens or A10 dopaminergic neurons: a comparison *Behav Brain Res* 1988; 29:73–83.
46. Hoebel BG, Monaco AP, Hernandez L, Aulisi EF, Stanley BG, Lenard L. Self-injection of amphetamine directly into the brain. *Psychopharmacology* 1983;81:158–163.
47. Isacson O, Brundin P, Kelly P, Gage FH, Björklund A. Functional neural replacement by grafted striatal neurons in the ibotenic acid-lesioned rat striatum. *Nature* 1984;311:458–460.
48. Isacson O, Dunnett SB, Björklund A. Graft induced behavioral recovery in an animal model of Huntington's disease. *Proc Natl Acad Sci USA* 1986;83:2728–2732.
49. Isacson O, Dawbarn D, Brundin P, Gage FH, Emson PC, Björklund A. Neural grafting in a rat model of Huntington's disease: striostromal-like organization of striatal grafts as revealed by immunocytochemistry and receptor autoradiography. *Neuroscience* 1987;22:481–497.
50. Isacson O, Hantraye P, Riche D, Schumacher JM, Maziere M. The relationship between symptoms and functional anatomy in the chronic neurodegenerative diseases: from pharmacological to· biological replacement therapy in Huntington's disease. In: Lindvall O, Björklund A, Widner H, eds. *Intracerebral transplantation in movement disorders: restorative neurology,* vol. 4. Amsterdam: Elsevier; 1991.
51. Ishida Y, Hashitani T, Kumazaki M, Ikeda T, Nishino H. Behavioral and biochemical effects of intra-accumbens dopaminergic grafts. *Brain Res Bull* 1990;24:487–492.
52. Iversen SD, Koob GF. Behavioural implications of dopaminergic neurons in the mesolimbic system. *Adv Biochem Psychopharmacol* 1977;19:209–214.
53. Jaskiw GE, Weinberger DR, Crawley JN. Micro-injection of apomorphine into the prefrontal cortex of the rat reduces dopamine metabolite concentrations in micro-dialysate from the caudate nucleus. *Biol Psychiat* 1991;29:703–706.

54. Joyce EM, Iversen SD. Dissociable effects of 6-OHDA-induced lesions of neostriatum on anorexia, locomotor activity and stereotopy: the role of behavioural competition. *Psychopharmacology* 1984;83:363–366.

55. Kelly PH, Moore KE. Mesolimbic dopaminergic neurones in the rotational model of nigrostriatal function. *Nature* 1976;263:695–696.

56. Killeen P. On the temporal control of behavior. *Psychol Rev* 1975;82:89–115.

57. Koob GF, Riley SJ, Smith C, Robbins TW. Effects of 6-hydroxydopamine lesions of the nucleus accumbens septi and olfactory tubercle on feeding, locomotor activity and amphetamine anorexia in the rat. *J Comp Physiol Psychol* 1978;92:917–927.

58. Koob GF, Stinus L, LeMoal M. Hyperactivity and hypoactivity produced by lesions to the mesolimbic dopamine system. *Behav Brain Res* 1981;3:341–359.

59. Kubos KL, Moran TH, Robinson RG. Differential and asymmetrical behavioral effects of electrolytic or 6-hydroxydopamine lesions in the nucleus accumbens. *Brain Res* 1987;401:147–151.

60. Laties VC, Weiss B, Clark RL, Reynolds MD. Overt "mediating" behavior during temporally spaced responding. *J Exp Anal Behav* 1965;8:107–116.

61. Laties VC, Weiss B, Weiss AB. Further observations on overt "mediating" behavior and the discrimination of time. *J Exp Anal Behav* 1969;12:43–57.

62. Lee SC, Yamamoto T, Ueki S. Characteristics of aggressive behavior induced by nucleus accumbens septi lesions in rats. *Behav Neural Biol* 1983;37:237–245.

63. Lehericy S, Hirsch EC, Cervera P, Hersh LB, Hauw J-J, Ruberg M, Agid Y. Selective loss of cholinergic neurons in the ventral striatum of patients with Alzheimer's disease. *Proc Natl Acad Sci USA* 1989;86:8580–8584.

64. LeMoal M, Cardo B, Stinus L. Influence of ventral mesencephalic lesions on various spontaneous and conditioned behaviours in the rat. *Physiol Behav* 1969;4:567–574.

65. Liu FC, Graybiel AM, Dunnett SB, Baughman RW. Intrastriatal grafts derived from fetal striatal primordia II. Reconstitution of dopaminergic and cholinergic systems. *J Comp Neurol* 1990;205:1–14.

66. Lorens SA, Sorenson JP, Harvey JA. Lesions in the nuclei accumbens septi of the rat: behavioral and neurochemical effects. *J Comp Physiol Psychol* 1970;73:284–290.

67. Louilot A, Taghzouti K, Deminiere JM, Simon H, LeMoal M. Dopamine and behavior: functional and theoretical considerations. In: Sandler M, et al. eds. *Neurotransmitter interactions in the basal ganglia.* New York: Raven Press; 1987.

68. Louilot A, LeMoal M, Simon H. Opposite influences of dopaminergic pathways to the prefrontal cortex or the septum on the dopaminergic transmission in the nucleus accumbens.

An in vivo voltammetric study. *Neuroscience* 1989;29:45–56.

69. Lyon M, Robbins TW. The action of central nervous system stimulant drugs: a general theory concerning amphetamine effects. In: Essman WB, Valzelli L, eds. *Current developments in psychopharmacology,* vol 2. New York: Spectrum, 1975:81–163.

70. Mandel RJ, Brundin P, Björklund A. The importance of graft placement and task complexity for transplant-induced recovery of simple and complex sensorimotor deficits in dopamine denervated rats. *Eur J Neurosci* 1990;2:888–894.

71. Mandel RJ, Brundin P, Wictorin K, Björklund A. Evaluation of the functional mechanism of fetal mesencephalic grafts placed in the dopamine denervated striatum. Presented at Third IBRO Congress, Montreal, 1991.

72. Marsden CD. Which motor disorder in Parkinson's disease indicates the true motor function of the basal ganglia? In: Evered D, O'Connor M, eds. *Functions of the basal ganglia. Ciba Found. Symp.* 1984;107:225–237.

73. Mayeux R, Stern Y, Rosen J, Levanthal J. Depression, intellectual impairment and Parkinson's disease. *Neurology* 1981;31:645–650.

74. Mechner F, Latranyi M. Behavioral effects of caffeine, metamphetamine, and methylphenidate in the rat. *J Exp Anal Behav* 1963;6:331–342.

75. Milner B. Some effects of frontal lobe lesions in man. In: Warren JM, Akert K, eds. *The frontal granular cortex and behavior.* New York: McGraw-Hill; 1964.

76. Mittleman G, Whishaw IQ, Jones GH, Koch M, Robbins TW. Cortical, hippocampal, and striatal mediation of schedule-induced behaviours. *Behav Neurosci* 1990;104:399–409.

77. Mogenson GJ, Jones DL, Yim CY. From motivation to action: functional interface between the limbic system and the motor system. *Prog Neurobiol* 1980;14:69–97.

78. Nadaud D, Herman J-P, Simon H, Le Moal M. Functional recovery following transplantion of ventral mesencephalic cells in rats subjected to 6-OHDA lesions of the mesolimbic dopaminergic neurons. *Brain Res* 1984;304:137–141.

79. Norman AB, Lehman MN, Sanberg PR. Functional effects of fetal striatal transplants. *Brain Res Bull* 1989;22:163–171.

80. Olson L, Vanderhaeghen J-J, Freedman R, Henschen A, Hoffer A, Seiger A. Combined grafts of the ventral tegmental area and nucleus accumbens in oculo. Histochemical and electrophysiological characterization. *Exp Brain Res* 1985;59:325–337.

81. Perlow MI, Freed WJ, Hoffer BJ, Seiger A, Olson L, Wyatt RJ. Brain grafts reduce motor abnormalities produced by destruction of nigrostriatal system. *Science* 1979;204:643–647.

82. Phillips AG, Fibiger HC. Long-term deficits in stimulation-bound behavior and self-stimulation after 6-hydroxydopamine administration in the rat. *Behav Biol* 1978;16:127–143.

83. Phillips AG, Fibiger HC. The role of dopamine in maintaining intracranial self-stimulation in the ventral tegmentum, nucleus accumbens and medial prefrontal cortex. *Can J Psychol* 1978; 32:58–66.

84. Post RM, Weiss SRB, Pert A. Animal models of mania. In: Willner P, Scheel-Krüger J, eds. *The mesolimbic dopamine system: from motivation to action.* Chichester: John Wiley & Sons; 1991.

85. Pycock CJ, Kerwin RW, Carter CJ. Effects of lesions of cortical dopamine terminals on subcortical dopamine receptors in rats. *Nature* 1980;286:74–77.

86. Rapoport JL. Obsessive compulsive disorder and basal ganglia dysfunction. *Psychol Med* 1990;20:465–470.

87. Reading PJ, Dunnett SB. The effects of excitotoxic lesions of the nucleus accumbens on response inhibition. Presented at the 14th Annual Meeting of the European Neuroscience Association, Cambridge, 1991.

88. Reading PJ, Dunnett SB, Robbins TW. Dissociable roles of the ventral, medial and dorsal striatum in the acquisition and performance of complex visual stimulus-response habit. *Behav Brain Res* 1992;45:147–161.

89. Reading PJ, Dunnett SB. The effects of excitotoxic lesions of the nucleus accumbens on a matching to position task. *Behav Brain Res* 1992;46:17–29.

90. Reading PJ, Dunnett SB. Embryonic striatal grafts ameliorate the disinhibitory effects on operant and unconditioned behaviour following excitotoxic lesions to the ventral striatum [*submitted*].

91. Rivas RJ, Mir D. Effects of nucleus accumbens lesion on female rat sexual receptivity and proceptivity in a partner preference paradigm. *Behav Brain Res* 1990;41:239–250.

92. Robbins TW, Iversen SD. Amphetamine-induced disruption of temporal discrimination by response disinhibition. *Nature* 1973;245:191–192.

93. Robbins TW, Koob GF. Selective disruption of displacement behaviour by lesions of the mesolimbic dopamine system. *Nature* 1980;285:409–412.

94. Robbins TW, Everitt BJ. Functional studies of the central catecholamines. *Int Rev Neurobiol* 1982;23:303–365.

95. Robbins TW, Roberts DCS, Koob GF. Effects of *d*-amphetamine and apomorphine upon operant behavior and schedule-induced licking in rats with 6-hydroxydopamine-induced lesions of the nucleus accumbens. *J Pharm Exp Ther* 1983;224:662–673.

96. Robbins TW, Evenden JL, Ksir C, Reading P, Wood S, Carli M. The effects of D-amphetamine, alpha-flupenthixol, and mesolimbic dopamine depletion on a test of attentional switching in the rat. *Psychopharmacology* 1986;90:72–78.

97. Robbins TW, Giardini V, Jones GH, Reading PJ, Sahakian BJ. Effects of dopamine depletion from the caudate–putamen and nucleus accumbens septi on the acquisition and performance of a conditional discrimination task. *Behav Brain Res* 1990;38:243–261.

98. Sanberg PR, Henault MA, Deckel AW. Locomotor hyperactivity: effects of multiple striatal transplants in an animal model of Huntington's disease. *Pharmacol Biochem Behav* 1986;25:297–300.

99. Sirinathsinghji DJS, Dunnett SB, Isacson O, Clarke DJ, Björklund A. Striatal grafts in rats with unilateral neostriatal lesions. II. In vivo monitoring of GABA release in globus, pallidus and substantia nigra. *Neuroscience* 1988;24:803–810.

100. Smith MO, Holland RC. Effects of lesions of the nucleus accumbens on lactation and postpartum behavior. *Physiol Psychol* 1975;3:331–336.

101. Starkstein SE, Preziosi TJ, Berthier ML, Bolduc PL, Mayberg HS, Robinson RG. Depression and cognitive impairment in Parkinson's disease. *Brain* 1989;112:1141–1153.

102. Starkstein SE, Bolduc PL, Mayberg HS, Preziosi TJ, Robinson RG. Cognitive impairments and depression in Parkinson's disease: a follow up study. *J Neurol Neurosurg Psychiatry* 1990;53:597–602.

103. Stern CE, Passingham RE. The nucleus accumbens and the organization of behavioral sequences in monkeys. *Macaca fascicularis. Soc Neurosci Abstr* 1989;15:1244.

104. Stern CE, Passingham RE. Nucleus accumbens lesions selectively impair spatial but not visual or motor reversal learning in monkeys *Macaca fascicularis. Soc Neurosci Abstr* 1990;15:617.

105. Stern CE, Passingham RE. The nucleus accumbens in monkeys *Macaca fascicularis:* incentive and emotion. *Soc Neurosci Abstr* 1991; 17:664.

106. Stevens JR. An anatomy of schizophrenia? *Arch Gen Psychiatry* 1973;29:177–189.

107. Swanson LW, Cowan WM. A note on the connections and development of the nucleus accumbens. *Brain Res* 1975;92:324–330.

108. Swerdlow NR, Koob GF. Dopamine, schizophrenia, mania, and depression: toward a unified hypothesis of cortico-striato-pallidothalamic function. *Behav Brain Sci* 1987;10:197–245.

109. Taghzouti K, Louilot A, Herman JP, LeMoal M, Simon H. Alternation behaviour, spatial discrimination, and reversal disturbances following 6-hydroxydopamine lesions in the nucleus accumbens of the rat. *Behav Neural Biol* 1985;44:354–363.

110. Taghzouti K, Simon H, Louilot A, Herman JP, LeMoal M. Behavioural study after local injection of 6-hydroxydopamine into the nucleus accumbens in the rat. *Brain Res* 1985;344:9–20.

111. Tassin J-P, Stinus L, Simon H, Blanc G, Thierry, LeMoal M, Cardo B, Glowinski, J. Relationship between the locomotor hyperactivity induced by A_{10} lesions and the destruction of fronto-cortical DA innervation in the rat. *Brain Res* 1978;141:267–281.

112. Tassin J-P, Herve D, Vezina P, Trovero F, Blanc G, Glowinski J. Relationships between mesocortical and mesolimbic neurons: functional correlates of D_1 receptor heteroregulation. In: Willner P, Scheel-Krüger J, eds. *The mesolimbic dopamine system: from motivation to action.* Chichester: John Wiley & Sons; 1991.

113. Torack RM, Morris JC. The association of ventral tegmental area histopathology with adult dementia. *Arch Neurol* 1988;45:497–501.

114. Valouskova V, Bracha V, Bures J, Hernandez-Mesa N, Macias-Gonzales R, Mazurova Y, Nemecek S. Unilateral striatal grafts induce behavioral and electrophysiological asymmetry in rats with bilateral kainate lesions of the caudate nucleus. *Behav Neurosci* 1990;104:671–680.

115. Wictorin K, Isacson O, Fischer W, Nothias F, Peschanski M, Björklund A. Connectivity of striatal grafts implanted into the ibotenic acid-lesioned striatum. I. Subcortical afferents. *Neuroscience* 1988;27:547–562.

116. Wictorin K, Björklund A. Connectivity of striatal grafts implanted into the ibotenic acid-lesioned striatum. II. Cortical afferents. *Neuroscience* 1989;30:297–311.

117. Wictorin K, Simerly RB, Isacson O, Swanson LW, Björklund A. Connectivity of striatal grafts implanted into the ibotenic acid-lesioned striatum. III. Efferent projecting graft neurons and their relation to host afferents within the graft. *Neuroscience* 1989;30:313–330.

118. Willner P, Muscat R, Papp M, Sampson D. Dopamine depression and anti-depressant drugs. In: Willner P, Scheel-Krüger J, eds. *The mesolimbic dopamine system: from motivation to action.* Chichester: John Wiley & Sons; 1991.

119. Wilson MP, Keller FS. On the selective reinforcement of spaced responding. *J Comp Physiol Psychol* 1953;46:190–193.

120. Wirtshafter D, Asin KE, Kent EW. Nucleus accumbens lesions reduce amphetamine hyperthermia but not hyperactivity. *Eur J Pharmacol* 1978;51:449–452.

Functional Neural Transplantation,
edited by S. B. Dunnett and A. Björklund.
Raven Press, Ltd., New York © 1994.

9

Strategies for Testing Learning and Memory Abilities in Transplanted Rats

Stephen B. Dunnett

Department of Experimental Psychology, University of Cambridge,
Cambridge CB2 3EB, United Kingdom

CAN NEURAL TRANSPLANTS INFLUENCE COGNITIVE FUNCTION?

The first experiments into the functional viability of neural transplants investigated performance of grafted rats tested on a variety of simple and easily quantified behaviors reflecting the status of animals' motor and neuroendocrine function (17,68,72,73, 119). However, once it had been established that neural grafts could influence simple unconditioned behaviors, it was natural to ask whether they may have a similar capacity to influence more complex functions, in particular those associated with higher cortical centers involved in various aspects of cognition.

This pragmatic interest in expanding the range of tests for analysis of the breadth and extent of neural transplant function occurred at the time of a resurgence of interest in the neuropathologic processes involved in aging and dementia. In particular, Perry and colleagues (120) observed that the decline in mental test function in Alzheimer's disease patients correlated with a decline in cholinergic activity in the neocortex postmortem. In parallel, psychopharmacologic studies highlighted the similarity between cognitive deficits induced by anticholinergic drugs in young subjects and the memory impairments seen in aging (32). These two lines of research converged with the formulation of "the cholinergic hypothesis of geriatric memory dysfunction," which, in its simplest form, states that the cognitive (and especially the mnemonic) deficits observed in aging and dementia are attributable to a functional decline in forebrain cholinergic neurons and, in particular, in the magnocellular cells of the basal forebrain that give rise to the cholinergic innervation of the neocortical mantle (26,123).

The cholinergic hypothesis has stimulated widespread attention as the basis for optimism that cholinergic replacement could provide a rational strategy for developing an effective therapy for dementia. Although it is now clear that the cholinergic hypothesis overemphasizes the role of cholinergic systems in the neuropathology of dementia, it has nevertheless been important in reviving interest in the role of cholinergic neurons and other systems of the isodendritic core in regulating cortical function. Moreover, although cholinergic degeneration is almost certainly not primary in the pathogenesis of Alzheimer's disease, nevertheless, it may contribute to the more modest decline in intellectual functions (including memory) associated with natural aging and some other neurodegenerative conditions such as Parkinson's disease.

Thus, the last decade has seen a growing number of studies into the effects of neural transplants on learning and memory perfor-

TABLE 1. *Learning tasks used to assess the effects of neural transplants on cognitive function*

Learning test	Nature of test
Hebb-Williams mazes; Lashley mazes, etc.	Classic sets of complex enclosed mazes in which a rat must learn a sequence of turns to reach food at the goal compartment.
T-maze alternation	A maze shaped in the form of a T with a start arm, a single choice point, and two alternative side arms (see Fig. 1A). The correct choice is to alternate the response choices either on consecutive trials, or using a paired trial format with sample and choice trials.
Radial mazes	A "sunburst" design, with several arms (4,8,17 in different versions) radiating from a central platform (see Fig. 3A). At the start of each daily run, all arms are baited. The animal is free to enter the arms until all pellets are collected. In some versions, certain arms are never baited to enable distinction between reference and working memory.
Water mazes	An escape learning task: the rat swims in a large circular tank of water to find a hidden platform (submerged below surface) onto which it can climb to escape from the water (see Fig. 4A). Spatial navigation based on salient cues in the external environment.
Passive avoidance	A one-trial shock avoidance task: the rat receives electric footshock when it steps into an enclosed part of the test apparatus (see Fig. 6). Memory for the shock is tested by measuring avoidance (as latency to reenter) on retest 24 or 48 hr later.
Escape and active avoidance	Rats learn to escape from footshock by moving to a second compartment of the test box. Active avoidance involves learning to move in response to a warning signal (tone or light) that precedes the shock. In two-way active avoidance the rat learns to shuttle between two compartments in response to a series of warning signals.
Taste aversion	Rats are exposed to a distinctive taste, followed by injection of LiCl to induce emesis and sickness. They subsequently avoid foods or fluids with that taste.
Operant lever pressing	Operant tasks generally involve training rats to press levers for food or water reward in automated chambers ("Skinner boxes") (see Fig. 7). "Schedules of reinforcement" are programmed conditions for delivering reward (e.g., fixed ratio 5 rewards every fifth lever press, variable interval 1-min rewards on average one press per minute, etc.).
DRL	"Differential reinforcement of low rates" is an operant schedule of reinforcement which rewards spaced responding. A fixed time must have elapsed since the last press (e.g., 20 sec) for a lever press to be rewarded (see Fig. 8).
DMTP/DNMTP	"Delayed matching to position" and "delayed nonmatching to position" are operant versions of the paired-trial matching and alternation tasks in the T maze (see Fig. 9). First, one of the two retractable levers in a Skinner box is presented as the sample. Then after a variable delay interval, both levers are presented. The rat is rewarded for pressing the sample (matching) or the opposite (nonmatching) lever in the two tasks.
Win–stay/lose–shift	Rats tend to repeat a response that has previously been reinforced, and to switch a response that is not reinforced. In a two-lever chamber, reinforcement may be random (to investigate spontaneous switching), or the contingencies may be arranged so that a repeat or a switch response is reinforced contingent upon whether reinforcement was delivered on the preceding response.

Advantages of test	Disadvantages of test	Refs.
The traditional concept of a "maze": conceptually straightforward tests of complex learning capacities.	Performance susceptible to many complex variables. Difficult to disentangle the nature of any underlying deficit.	3,77,84
A maze pared to its minimum components. Analysis based on a single-choice response. Classic sensitivity to frontal cortex dysfunction.	As in all maze tasks, requires prolonged training. Difficult to distinguish spatial, working, and reference memory deficits.	44,76,81 82,88,121
Originally designed as a test of "working memory," the task design can be manipulated to distinguish working from reference memory and spatial-based from cue-based learning.	Complex (and largely unquantifiable) factors determine sequence and selection of arm choices. Relatively small differences between chance and perfect scores, requiring large groups to detect significant graft effects.	5,6,74–76 92,111 115
Originally designed as a test of allocentric spatial learning. Does not require shock or food deprivation to motivate the animals. Very sensitive to detect deficits.	Sensitivity of task leads to a difficulty in obtaining significant treatment effects, and to a lack of neural specificity, since disrupted following many different types of damage.	59,62,98 99,91,104 136–138 141–143
Quick and simple to test. Very widely used in psychopharmacologic and aging research.	Susceptible to confounds from motivational sensory and motor differences. Great variability of response needs large group sizes.	3,8,24,25 48,77,97 131
Simple to train. Generates multitrial learning curves over a single day. Shock motivation is effective even in seriously impaired animals.	Difficult to match groups and to eliminate sensory, motor, and motivational impairments underlying deficits in task performance.	3,4,90,97
Preparedness: rats readily associate health to taste and can be learned in a single exposure.	Proper control of exposure to taste and sickness can be difficult in lesion experiments.	12,50,53 66,67
Operant tasks yield large quantities of data under standardized, automated (and, hence, unbiased) conditions. The effects of different schedules have been well characterized.	It is easy to overlook unrecorded features of the animals' behavior that, nevertheless, contribute importantly to normal performance or to deficits following lesion.	30,54,93
The DRL schedule is sensitive to impairment in internal inhibition. It provides a classic test of hippocampal dysfunction.	Very sensitive to level of motivation. Distinction between deficits in inhibition vs timing require complex analysis.	20,45,49 54,64,80 132
Delay-dependent deficits in working memory can be distinguished from delay-independent changes in learning, attention, or motivation.	Ceiling effects at short delays can confound delay-dependent profile. Task requires prolonged training to asymptote. Specific deficit is restricted to selected lesions and ageing.	33,34,36– 38,41,46
The tests reflect an animal's strategies for sequencing responses in the context of reward and nonreward. Sensitive to basal forebrain and hippocampal damage.	Prolonged training is required for rats to learn the contingent task, and for responding to stabilize in the noncontingent task. Performance variable. Lesion deficits can be quite small.	51,131

mance based on cholinergic cell replace-ment. In many cases, this has been in the context of seeking to alleviate deficits as-sociated with aging or dementia, but in other cases, a more general analysis of the organization and repair of higher cognitive function associated with a variety of fore-brain sites—in particular the neocortex, al-locortex, amygdala, and hippocampus—has provided the focus.

A variety of test paradigms have been used to evaluate the influence of neural transplants on animals' cognitive capaci-ties. The first studies used simple maze-learning tasks, but these have been supple-mented with tests based on avoidance learning and, most recently, the introduc-tion of tests of learning and memory based on operant paradigms (Table 1).

MAZE STUDIES: T-MAZE TASKS

Rationale for Maze Alternation Tasks

The first demonstration that grafts can in-fluence a learned behavior involved testing rats with cholinergic-rich septal grafts for the maze-learning deficits associated with disruption of cholinergic innervation of the hippocampus. It was well known that le-sions of the hippocampal system disrupted the ability of rats to learn a variety of spa-tial maze tasks (83). One classic task that has been particularly widely employed is delayed spatial alternation in a T-maze (Fig. 1A). In this, the rat is required to alternate its responses to the two sides on consecu-tive trials to find food reward. The rat must remember which side it had entered on the immediately preceding trial, with responses on earlier trials being irrelevant. This task challenges a number of features of an ani-mal's cognitive performance—including the abilities of rule-learning, spatial navigation, and short-term memory—and is sensitive to damage in a variety of forebrain systems, including prefrontal cortex, hippocampus, and basal ganglia.

Rawlins and Olton introduced a paired-trial version of the T-maze alternation task (121). In this, the rat is given trials in pairs. On the first trial (the "sample"), one arm is baited and the other blocked off, so the rat can enter only the open arm to retrieve food. Then, on the second trial of the pair (the "choice") the previously closed arm is baited. The rat has a free choice between the two arms, both of which are now open, and it must select the arm opposite that previously entered to find the food. The paired-trial alternation task provides greater experimental control over exactly what the rat must remember than does the classic de-layed alternation task. Thus, the interval between the sample and choice trials (the within-pairs interval) can be manipulated to influence short-term remembering of the sample, independent of any interference from previous trials that would be depen-dent on the interval between the pairs of trials. The between-pairs interval may be quite long so that each pair of trials can be separated from previous pairs by a substan-tial delay (minutes, hours, or even days), which will reduce extraneous interference of the short-term memory trace to a mini-mum. The paired-trial alternation task was the first to be used to investigate the effi-cacy of transplantation on cognitive func-tion.

Fimbria–Fornix Lesions and Septal Grafts

In the first functional study, rats received lesions of the fimbria–fornix (FF) to deaf-ferent the hippocampus of its main cholin-ergic (as well as adrenergic and serotoner-gic) inputs, followed by grafts into the hippocampus of either embryonic ventral forebrain (rich in cholinergic neurons) or of embryonic locus coeruleus (rich in norad-renergic neurons) (49). The lesions pro-duced a profound deficit both in sponta-neous exploratory behavior (measured in terms of spontaneous alternation in a T-maze) and in the animals' abilities to learn a spatial alternation task in the T-maze (see Fig. 1B). Whereas the noradrenergic grafts had no effect whatsoever on the animals' maze-learning deficit, the cholinergic-rich

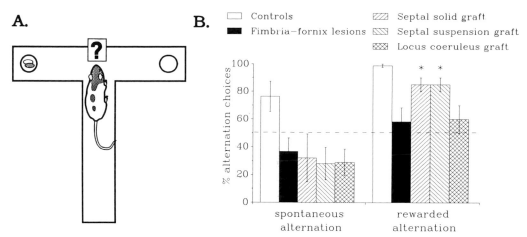

FIG. 1. A: Schematic illustration of the T-maze used to test rats in conventional delayed alternation and paired-trial alternation tasks. **B**: Performance in the paired-trial alternation test of control rats, rats with fimbria–fornix lesions and rats with lesions plus one of three alternative tissues implanted into the hippocampus. The grafts were cholinergic-rich septal grafts, implanted as solid pieces of tissue into the lesion cavity; noradrenergic-rich locus coeruleus grafts, also implanted as solid pieces of tissue; or cholinergic-rich septal grafts injected as dissociated cell suspensions directly into the host hippocampus. The *dotted line* indicates a chance (50%) level of performance. Cholinergic-rich grafts provide a partial alleviation of the rewarded alternation deficit induced by fimbria–fornix lesions. (Data from ref. 44.)

grafts provided a substantial and significant improvement in their ability to learn the alternation task (see Fig. 1B).

Several features of this experiment are of note:

1. The cholinergic-rich septal grafts were effective whether made by the solid or the cell suspension methods. This might suggest that a cholinergic reinnervation of the denervated hippocampus may be sufficient to restore a limited degree of function, even though the full septohippocampal circuitry is not reconstructed. However, several other features of the results complicate this interpretation.

2. Cholinergic reinnervation of the host hippocampus appeared to be a necessary, but not a sufficient, condition for functional repair. Thus, whereas the degree of recovery correlated with the extent of restitution of acetylcholinesterase staining in the host hippocampus over the whole group, there were individual cases for which a substantial return of acetylcholinesterase staining was

seen in the absence of functional recovery.

3. Although the effective grafts improved performance significantly, even the best-grafted animals still learned the task substantially slower than the rate achieved by control animals. Thus, even though the septal grafts can restore a normal density of cholinergic fiber inputs (13,16) and the ingrowing axons make fully normal synaptic contacts with the appropriate targets in the host hippocampus (23), function was not fully restored. This may reflect that, although the grafted rats did eventually relearn the task, they showed only very limited spontaneous alternation in the initial phase of habituation to the T-maze environment. Consequently, their acquisition of the alternation contingency commenced from a very different baseline from that of the control rats (44).

These observations suggest that establishment of the cholinergic inputs alone is insufficient to restore normal performance.

Rather, a more extensive reconstruction of the damaged neuronal circuitry may be necessary for full functional repair. This may require a better integration of the grafted neurons into the host neuronal network, or restitution of other neural systems disrupted by the lesions (e.g., noradrenergic or serotonergic afferents to the hippocampus, or efferent projections coursing through the fimbria–fornix to subcortical sites). Whatever the precise mechanism, several subsequent studies have replicated the basic efficacy of septal grafts to alleviate the deficits in T-maze alternation induced by hippocampal cholinergic deafferentation (29, 76).

Prefrontal Lesions and Cortical Grafts

Delayed alternation in a T-maze was again selected as the test of choice for evaluating the effects of neural grafts on cognitive function in another intriguing series of studies. In 1983, Labbe and coauthors reported that cortical grafts could alleviate alternation learning deficits in rats with large aspirative lesions of the prefrontal cortex (88). In this study, embryonic frontal cortex was implanted into an aspirative cavity of prefrontal cortex, closely followed by training the rats in a T-maze alternation task for water reward. The rats with cortical grafts were able to learn the task to criterion more rapidly than either rats with lesions alone or rats with control grafts of embryonic cerebellar tissue. The authors then went on to use horseradish peroxidase (HRP) as an anatomic tracer to demonstrate that these functional grafts established connections with the host brain. These results appeared remarkable because the data seemed to suggest that cortical tissue grafts could reconnect and reconstruct cortical damage and, thereby, restore cortical processing of complex cognitive information, although the authors were careful not to propose a specific mechanism.

However, only 7 days separated the lesion and transplantation surgeries in the Labbe et al. (88) study; behavioral training then commenced 4 days later. By contrast, the analysis of anatomic connectivity was not conducted until some months later. This difference in timing is important if we are to understand the nature of the functional recovery. In particular, the rapid testing of the animals immediately after transplantation has been critical in subsequent replications for the amelioration of T-maze alternation learning by cortical grafts (47, 81,135). For example, in my own laboratory, we have found that, whereas cortical grafts would improve the alternation learning of rats with prefrontal lesions when training commenced 7 days after lesion, when the same rats were retested 4 months later, they were now significantly impaired compared with the animals with lesions alone (Fig. 2; 47).

In fact, the recovery induced by cortical grafts in the prefrontal cavity model is almost certainly not due to reconstruction involving incorporation of the graft neurons into the host neural circuitry, but rather, is due to some as yet unidentified trophic stimulation of intrinsic recovery processes within the host brain (for review, see 35). As a clear demonstration of this, a similar pattern of recovery in delayed alternation learning can be achieved by simply implanting purified astrocytes, derived from embryos, or adult tissue that comprises preponderantly glia (81,82). Conversely, using a different behavioral test, once animals with cortical grafts manifested clear recovery, subsequently removing the grafts did not abolish the recovery (as would be expected if the grafts replaced some essential neuronal connections), but rather, the rats' improvement was left unaffected (134).

In summary, the importance of these observations is twofold. First, they suggest that recovery on these cognitive and learning tasks induced by grafting in the prefrontal cortex may be only a transient phenomenon. Second, they suggest that, in this

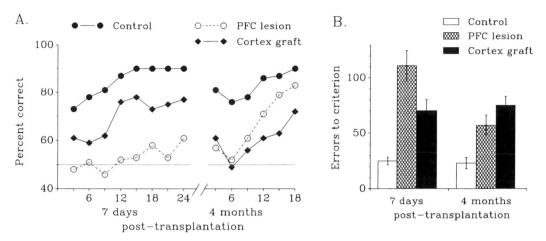

FIG. 2. Effect of cortical grafts in rats with aspirative lesions of the prefrontal cortex on performance in the paired-trial alternation test. The blocks of training commenced 7 days and again at 4 months following transplantation. **A**: Percentage correct performance in consecutive 3-day blocks of trials. **B**: Total errors to reach a criterion of 90% correct over 3 days, or the end of testing, whichever came first. The grafts alleviated the acute profound lesion deficit, but resulted in a long-term deficit over and above the improving lesion baseline. (Data from ref. 47.)

particular model system, the grafts exert their effects not by reestablishing essential graft–host circuits, but by providing some trophic influence on the development of the lesion and spontaneous recovery processes within the host brain itself (see Chapter 6). Consequently, the demonstration of reformation of connections is not a sufficient basis for concluding that the grafts necessarily work by a mechanism of circuit reconstruction. Indeed, a variety of different mechanisms of functional action have been identified (14). Each different model system needs separate analysis to identify its own necessary and sufficient conditions for recovery to be achieved (see Chapter 21).

THE RADIAL-ARM MAZE

Rationale for Radial Maze Tasks

Although the T-maze delayed alternation task has provided a sensitive test for assessing general cognitive impairments in rats, performance depends on many different abilities. The T-maze task provides little information on the specific nature of the underlying deficit. In the light of the long tradition in human neuropsychology that views the hippocampus as a critical site in the formation of memory (127,133), Olton and colleagues introduced a novel maze task—the radial maze—that enables particular aspects of a rats' memory capacities to be distinguished (111,115). The essence of the radial maze is that it provides a stable set of multiple choices, from which the available correct options change continually, depending on the animal's previous choices.

In the simplest version of the task the maze has eight equally spaced arms radiating from a central platform (Fig. 3A) (115). The maze is set in the center of a test room, the arms are open (a runway with only a small lip to stop the rat from falling off), and the animal can locate itself by reference to the many external stimuli in the room. At the start of a trial, all eight arms are baited with a single food pellet placed at the end of each arm. The task for the rat is to visit each of the arms, in turn, to collect and consume the food pellet, but not to return

A.

B.

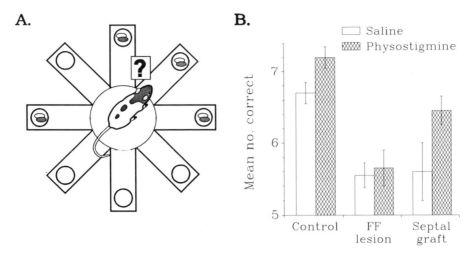

FIG. 3. **A**: Schematic illustration of the Olton eight-arm radial maze. **B**: Performance of control, fimbria–fornix lesioned and septal graft rats on the radial maze task following injections of saline and of 0.05 mg/kg physostigmine. Cholinergic grafts alleviated the lesion-induced deficit in radial maze performance only when supplemented with injections of the cholinesterase-inhibitor physostigmine. (Data from ref. 92.)

to any arm that has already been visited, since it has already eaten all the available food there. A well-trained rat will remember where it has already been and select each of the eight arms in turn, without returning to a previously visited arm. Performance is typically scored in terms of how many errors (repeat visits) are made in the first eight choices, or how many choices are required to collect all eight food pellets.

To perform accurately, therefore, the rat must remember exactly which arms have just been visited on the daily trial and which arms are still baited. The animal must maintain a constantly changing checklist of its recent actions. Olton argues that this requires a separate *working memory* system, which is quite distinct from the more general semantic knowledge that the animal has learned about the world in general, and the basic task demands in particular, which he terms *reference memory* (111).

The power of the radial maze task is enhanced by several different variations that identify different aspects of performance, in particular, the distinction between reference and working memory, and the differ-

ent cues that a rat may use to solve the task. For example, Olton and Pappas (114) used a 17-arm version of the radial maze in which only eight arms were baited on each daily trial (the same eight on each consecutive day), and the remaining arms were never baited. By avoiding the never-baited set of arms, well-trained rats showed that they were able to distinguish spatial location and to have learned the basic task demands (i.e., reference memory). Entry into one of the arms of the never-baited set constituted a reference memory error. Conversely, repeated entries into arms of the baited set at a higher rate than errors from the never-baited set indicated failures of working memory. Other variants of the radial maze task have used enclosed arms and distinctive internal cues. (113). This then permitted evaluation of the extent to which failures in performance (in both the reference and the working memory components) is due to a memory failure per se, independently from the heavy spatial contribution of the original versions of the task.

Olton and colleagues first demonstrated that hippocampal lesions disrupt performance of the basic eight-arm maze task, and then went on to show that the deficit is specifically in the working memory component, whereas rats with hippocampal lesions can make the spatial discriminations, show spared reference memory, and avoid the never-baited set (111,114,116).

Fimbria–Fornix Lesions and Septal Grafts

Low and colleagues (92) first used the eight-arm radial maze to investigate septal graft function in an extension of their studies, described earlier, in the T-maze task. In this experiment, no spontaneous recovery was seen in the rats with septal grafts unless the animals were treated additionally with the cholinesterase inhibitor physostigmine (which had no effect on the rats with lesions alone). By contrast, septal grafts have been effective in the absence of pharmacologic treatment in this task when electrolytic lesions of the septum or injections of AF64A have been used to make (possibly more selective) cholinergic denervations of the hippocampus (76,118).

More than two decades ago, O'Keefe and Dostrovsky (109) identified "place cells" in the hippocampus that changed their firing patterns when the animal moved through particular locations in the maze, an observation that was at the heart of the development of the cognitive map theory of hippocampal function (107,110). Shapiro and colleagues (130) recorded complex unit spike activity in the hippocampus of freely moving rats in the attempt to identify specific changes induced by cholinergic deafferentation and graft-derived reinnervation that may underlie the functional changes in grafted rats. As expected, lesions of the fimbria–fornix produced marked disturbance of the normal pattern of stable, reliable, spatially clustered place fields observed in the normal hippocampus. More remarkably, a considerable restitution of the place fields was observed in the hippocampus of grafted rats—the fields were more reliable, more tightly clustered in

space, and more stable when the maze was changed (130). These results suggested that septal grafts may ameliorate the effects of cholinergic deafferentation by influencing critical aspects of the ongoing electrophysiologic activity of the host hippocampus, an observation that is in line with reports of restitution of other electrophysiologic changes, such as in theta activity (130).

In a subsequent series of studies, Dalrymple-Alford and colleagues (28) compared the effects of septal grafts in rats with more selective lesions of the fimbria alone or the fornix alone as well as with the extensive combined lesion. To their surprise, they found that the grafts actually impaired performance in all three lesioned groups over and above the deficits induced by the lesions alone, when tested 7 months after transplantation. However, in these animals, the grafts were seen to grow extremely large, which may have contributed to a rather nonspecific disturbance of CNS function. In a subsequent analysis of the time course of behavioral effects in this model, septal grafts produced recovery only in rats with the combined lesion when tested 1 to 2 months after transplantation, whereas other groups tested at 5 to 6 and 10 to 11 months were without effect (22). Since the size of the grafts and the cholinergic fiber ingrowth were comparable in the different groups, the authors concluded that noncholinergic factors almost certainly provided a major contribution to graft effects in this model.

Basal Forebrain Lesions and Septal Grafts

The most elegant analysis of graft function using the radial maze has been provided by the series of studies from Sinden and colleagues (see also Chapter 10). They have taken advantage of the distinctive features of the Olton task to develop a multidimensional factorial analysis of the different influences on lesion and graft effects on task performance. First, they have used two versions of the eight-arm radial maze.

In one the maze is open and all arms are the same, so that the rat must learn the task based on external spatial cues, whereas in the other the arms are characterized by distinctive patterns, textures, and smells, and are shuffled between each trial, so that the rat must learn the task based on intramaze sensory cues. Second, in each maze, only four of the eight arms are baited on each trial, so that the task has both reference memory and working memory components. Third, in addition to making lesions by procedures that induce somewhat generalized disruptions of central cholinergic or hippocampal function (e.g., long-term alcohol ingestion or ischemia), they have compared the effects of lesions in different parts of the basal forebrain cholinergic system, in the septum, in the nucleus basalis, or in both areas combined. Fourth, in addition to the use of control grafts (of noncholinergic tissues or cholinergic tissues implanted in nontarget areas), they have compared the effects of implanting cholinergic-rich basal forebrain grafts either into the neocortex, or into the hippocampus, or into both areas combined. Fifth, the selective cholinergic nature of the graft effects has been challenged with pharmacologic probes using agonists and antagonists at both the muscarinic and nicotinic receptors.

In the light of such a powerful multifactorial design, the results have generally proved positive, but rather disappointing. In the first reports using this approach, alcohol intoxication produced deficits in maze performance, disrupting both reference and working memory components of both the spatial and cue-based task. All aspects of this generalized deficit were alleviated by septal grafts, whether implanted into the hippocampus or into the neocortex, with combined graft placements yielding even greater benefit across the board than either placement alone (5,6). The subsequent studies have found comparable deficits to be induced by both nucleus basalis magnocellularis (NBM) and by septal lesions, with greater deficits induced by combined lesions (5), and for the combined lesion deficit to be alleviated in all aspects by grafts into either the neocortex or the hippocampus (74). The lesioned rats were more sensitive than controls to the disrupting effects of both nicotinic and muscarinic antagonists and showed a greater improvement than control rats in response to both nicotinic and muscarinic agonists (75). Whereas nicotine significantly disrupted the performance of behaviorally recovered graft rats, all other drugs had an influence on the rats with grafts similar to that on the rats with lesions alone. A detailed account of these studies is given in Chapter 10.

Thus, the general pattern of disruption produced by the lesions and drugs was "indiscriminate" relative to the type of error (reference vs working memory; spatial vs associative cues) and to lesion placement, and the grafts were "equipotent" in whichever target region they were placed. Hodges et al. (74) concluded that it is unlikely that the observed effects are due to influences on specific cognitive or mnemonic processes. Rather, they propose the more plausible hypothesis that the results are due to general, relatively nonspecific functional changes (e.g., involving up- or down-regulation of attentional processes).

THE MORRIS WATER MAZE TASK

Rationale for the Water Maze

Richard Morris (98) introduced the water maze task that is now associated with his name in response to a theoretical debate about the essential function of the hippocampus. On the one hand, Olton was popularizing the working memory theory of hippocampal function and offered supporting data from the radial maze tasks described earlier (111,112). On the other hand, O'Keefe and Nadel (110) had developed a theory of hippocampal function based on spatial or "cognitive mapping," in which the hippocampus was considered to provide the neural circuitry necessary for animals to compute their location specifically in space and, more generally, in the cognitive world. O'Keefe and colleagues based much of their reasoning on the basis of electrophysiologic recording of units in the hippocampus as animals moved about open arenas or navigated through simple mazes, such as the "plus maze" (which was equivalent to a four-arm version of Olton's radial maze) (108–110).

The issue confronting Morris was how to evaluate the cues that an animal uses to navigate. Is there any basis for believing that rats have the capacity to generate an internal representation (or map) of the external world, or are they simply heading toward particular stimulus cues or adopting set sequences of responding to reach their goals? The solution was to design a maze in which a rat must reach its goal in the absence of any local cues to guide it. This he achieved by constructing the maze out of a large tank of water in which only distant stimuli external to the maze were available for navigation (98). The task confronting a rat swimming in the pool is to locate a hidden platform that provides an island onto which it can climb to escape from the water (Fig. 4A). The platform is positioned with its top just below the water surface, so that the rat cannot use visual or olfactory cues for localization. The rat might escape by swimming at random until it bumped into the platform by chance; however, if the platform is kept in a fixed location, Morris found that after a few trials normal rats are able to learn the platform location and swim directly to it (see Fig. 4B). A series of transfer and probe trials were used to confirm that indeed the rats were computing and navigating toward a place, rather than to the hidden platform per se. Morris reasoned that the rats must be generating an internal map of its environment from a variety of distal cues outside the maze as the basis for accurate navigation (98).

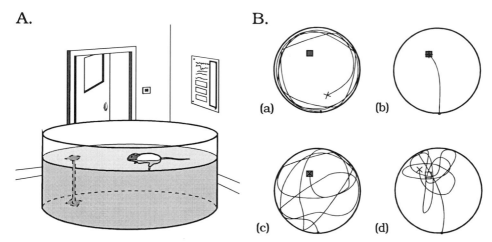

FIG. 4. A: Schematic illustration of the Morris water maze, comprising a hidden escape platform submerged below the surface in a tank of opaque milky water. The maze is surrounded by diverse objects by which the animal can navigate. **B**: Patterns of performance in the water maze. **a**: When first placed in the tank all rats initially swim around the edge of the pool seeking a route to escape. **b**: Within 10 to 20 trials, a control rat learns to swim directly to the submerged platform. **c**: Animals that have not learned the platform location tend to search at random. **d**: When the platform is removed in a probe trial, a well-trained rat continues to search in the location where the platform had previously been located.

Morris and colleagues (99) went on to show that spatial navigation in the water maze is severely disrupted by bilateral ablation of the hippocampus, an effect that has been replicated many times (104,137,138). Morris points out that, in contrast with Olton's various maze paradigms, the water maze task is dependent entirely on learning to navigate using spatial information (a *reference memory task,* in Olton's parlance), and has no working memory component. In fact, like the T-maze and radial mazes, it is now apparent that the water maze is sensitive to damage in a number of forebrain structures in addition to the hippocampus (including the neocortex and basal ganglia; 85,86,143), in specific neurotransmitter systems (including the dopaminergic and cholinergic projections; 71,136,141,142,144), and in aging itself (56,57,62,63,65).

Septal Grafts in Aged Rats

Azmitia et al. (7) first showed that serotonergic-rich grafts of embryonic raphe survived transplantation to the hippocampus of aged rats as well as in young adult rats. Many subsequent studies have showed that an aging brain environment is not incompatible with graft survival, although, in some circumstances, the reinnervation and reformation of connections are not as precise as in the young brain (60).

These structural observations were closely followed by a series of studies by Gage and colleagues (59,61) that neural grafts could alleviate some of the functional deficits associated with aging (see Chapter 11). However, there is a particular difficulty with testing the cognitive performance of aged animals: Quite apart from changes in sensory sensitivity and motor coordination and vigor, how can one match the motivational capacities of the animals? Thus, for example, if we are to test rats in a maze for food reward, how then does one establish levels of food deprivation that yield equivalent motivation in young and healthy rats com-pared with old, obese rats that may be two or three times the body weight? Similarly, if learning is to be motivated by aversive stimuli, such as footshock, again there are difficulties in matching the sensory effect of footshock when the footpads become hardened and calloused in old animals. It has turned out that the Morris water maze is particularly suitable for assessing cognitive functions of aged rats, once the few old animals with motor swimming difficulties are screened out: All rats, young and old alike, will then swim vigorously to escape from the pool. Moreover, probe trials with a visible escape platform can be used to confirm that the old animals swim as fast and as accurately as young rats when the cognitive challenge is removed. From this task, it has been found that a subpopulation of aged rats manifested quite distinctive impairments in learning the Morris water maze task that correlated well with a decline of metabolic activity in two particular areas of the brain: the various subfields of the hippocampus and the medial prefrontal neocortex (65).

Gage and colleagues went on to show that the water maze deficit can be alleviated by implantation of cholinergic-rich septal grafts into the hippocampus of impaired aged rats (61) (Fig. 5). Indeed, in this study 8 of 11 grafted, aged rats had good surviving grafts, and substantial improvement was observed in all 8 animals, whereas the remaining 3 grafted animals only had poorly surviving grafts, and these 3 cases were all uncompensated and indistinguishable from the control group of aged impaired rats without grafts. Recovery of aged rats with septal grafts implanted into the hippocampus on the Morris water maze task has subsequently been replicated in a number of studies (59). In particular, the recovered performance of aged animals with grafts is abolished following injections of relatively low doses of atropine, suggesting that the graft-derived recovery is itself based on a neural mechanism that involves restitution of functional cholinergic transmission (59).

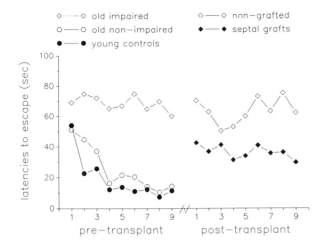

FIG. 5. Cholinergic grafts can alleviate deficits in the Morris water maze task. Performance of aged-impaired rats, with and without grafts. The aged rats were initially trained on the task and the subpopulation that were impaired were divided into two subgroups, one to receive septal grafts implanted into the hippocampus and the other to remain as nongrafted aged-impaired controls. Then all rats were retested 3 months later. For clarity, on the retest only the data from the aged-impaired subgroups are shown. The septal grafts provided a large and significant alleviation of the age-related impairment. (Data from ref. 61.)

Septal Grafts in Lesioned Rats

By contrast with the dramatic and reproducible effects in aged rats, the effects of septal grafts on the spatial navigation deficits of rats with basal forebrain lesions have proved more variable and difficult to demonstrate. In the first such study, we saw impairments as well as improvements following transplantation in rats with fimbria–fornix lesions that did not appear to relate in any coherent way to particular patterns of cholinergic reinnervation (43).

However, more detailed analysis of water maze performance by Nilsson et al. (104) revealed subtle benefits from septal grafts in the navigation skills of the transplanted animals. As in the previous T-maze alternation tasks, rats with septal grafts manifested a moderate recovery in their ability to learn the water maze task. However, by the end of training, the performance of grafted rats was still greatly impaired, even though they located the platform significantly more quickly than rats with lesions alone. By contrast clearer differences were observed on probe trials in which the escape platform was removed from the pool. The grafted rats showed a more precise initial heading angle toward the trained platform location and a greater concentration of their search in the training quadrant than

did the lesioned rats. In subsequent experiments, Nilsson and colleagues went on to demonstrate that the lesions also induced mild deficits, even when the platform was visible, that this also could be alleviated by septal grafts, and that the improvements shown by the grafted rats in both the spatial- and cue-based versions of the task were sensitive to disruption by atropine and, hence, were dependent on a presumed cholinergic mechanism (104).

Nevertheless, the recovery observed following implantation of septal grafts in rats with fimbria–fornix lesions still remains moderate in the Morris water maze as well as in other maze learning tasks, when contrasted with the occasionally, almost complete, reversal of deficits that has been achieved with similar grafts in aged animals. This highlights two principles. First, the fimbria–fornix lesion (or indeed any other experimental lesion) is not a true model of the neurodegeneration associated with aging, but reproduces just one aspect of the natural syndrome *in extremis*. Second, although the septal graft studies were initially formulated in the context of the cholinergic hypothesis of dementia, the fimbria–fornix lesion does not produce a specific cholinergic lesion. Rather, fimbria–fornix lesions disrupt noradrenergic, GABAergic, and serotonergic afferents and other subcortical efferents of the hippocampus, in addition to disruption of the cholinergic afferents from the septum.

One approach to this problem has been the attempt to make more circumscribed lesions within the medial septum or fimbria than is provided by gross transection of the fimbria–fornix. Thus, for example, Segal and colleagues (128) have compared the effects of septal grafts in rats that had sustained septohippocampal damage either by fimbria–fornix transection or by electrolytic lesion of the medial septal nucleus. Both lesions severely disrupted acquisition of the Morris water maze task. Whereas the grafts provided no significant change in learning deficits in rats with fimbria–fornix damage, they provided significant amelioration of the deficit in rats with more circumscribed medial septal damage. These authors speculated that sparing of the hippocampal efferents in the septal lesion, in combination with the graft-derived replacement of cholinergic afferents, is necessary for functional benefit.

Cholinergic–Serotonergic Interactions in Lesioned Rats

An alternative approach to the lack of specificity provided by the classic fimbria–fornix lesion has been to consider combinations of treatments to replace serotonergic as well as cholinergic afferents into the hippocampus. Vanderwolf (140) first demonstrated that combined cholinergic and serotonergic blockade (with scopolamine and p-chlorophenylalanine, respectively) produced a substantially greater disruption of rats' acquisition of swimming escape tests than did either treatment alone. Richter-Levin and Segal (125) replicated these observations of performance deficits following a similar combined pharmacologic blockade using the standard Morris water maze task, whereas neither drug had any substantial effect when administered on its own. This observation suggested a degree of redundancy such that either serotonergic

or cholinergic grafts might be able to reverse deficits associated with combined cholinergic and serotonergic dysfunction.

In a first test of this hypothesis Richter-Levin and Segal (124) depleted the forebrain serotonergic system with intraventricular injection of the serotonergic toxin 5,7-dihydroxytryptamine (5,7-DHT). Half of the lesioned rats received additional raphe grafts in the hippocampus, and then all rats were trained in the water maze. The single lesions alone produced no deficits, and the three groups (control, 5,7-DHT lesion, 5,7-DHT lesion plus raphe graft) did not differ in acquisition. However, the animals were then given injections of atropine before the daily trials to provide an additional blockade of cholinergic transmission. As previously, atropine treatment had no effect on the intact control rats, but severely disrupted performance in the lesion group. This deficit was alleviated in the rats with additional raphe grafts. The serotonergic reinnervation provided by a raphe graft can be seen to replace the intrinsic innervation in protecting the rats from the disruption provided by combined serotonergic and cholinergic depletion.

Along similar lines Nilsson et al. (105) have provided a more systematic analysis of components of the classic fimbria–fornix transection by using more selective lesions of distinct subsets of afferents. Septohippocampal cholinergic neurones were lesioned by electrolytic lesions of the septum, and the forebrain serotonergic system was depleted with intraventricular 5,7-DHT. Again, the rats with the combined lesions had far more profound deficits in the Morris water maze task than did rats with either lesion alone. Although, in the absence of any pharmacologic treatment, the 5,7-DHT lesions depleted norepinephrine as well as serotonin, this did not appear to contribute to the animals' deficits, since an identical pattern of performance was seen in rats that had been pretreated with the uptake blocker desmethylimipramine to protect the noradrenergic system from 5,7-DHT toxicity (105).

In an attempt to confirm the relevance of combined cholinergic and serotonergic denervation to the water maze deficits, Nilsson et al. (101) have gone on to compare the efficacy of cholinergic (septal), serotonergic (raphe) or combined grafts in rats with combined septal–5,7-DHT lesions. Although few effects were seen 4 months after transplantation, by 10 months, the rats with combined grafts showed substantial improvement in the water maze task and were not distinguishable from unlesioned controls on several measures. By contrast, no improvement over lesion baseline was seen in the rats with either septal or raphe grafts alone.

These studies agree in the observation that combined serotonergic and cholinergic lesions or receptor blockade are necessary to produce profound deficits on spatial navigation tasks. However, they are not entirely consistent: the Nilsson et al. study (101) suggest that combined septal and raphe grafts are necessary to reverse the deficits of the combined lesion, whereas the data of Richter-Levin and Segal (124) suggest that the serotonergic reinnervation alone may be sufficient. However, these studies differ in several important procedural respects. In particular, the Richter-Levin and Segal study employed pharmacologic means to block cholinergic receptors briefly. Consequently, the animals were tested for performance of a task that had previously been learned in the presence of an intact cholinergic system. By contrast, in the Nilsson et al. study, the animals had a permanent cholinergic as well as serotonergic denervation, and the grafted animals were tested in the more-demanding context of task acquisition (101).

Other Lesion and Graft Models

The Morris water maze task has proved to be useful in a number of other lesion and graft paradigms, in particular ones associated with neocortical and hippocampal function. Thus, it first provided an impor-

tant complement to the T-maze alternation task in the studies of the functional effects of cortical grafts implanted into prefrontal lesion cavities (47,52,134). Second, the Morris water maze has been used to demonstrate the functional capacity of cortical grafts in congenital microcephalic rats (89). Third, it has proved useful for evaluating hippocampal grafts in rats with ischemic damage of the hippocampus (117) (see Chapter 14).

By contrast, other studies indicate that, whereas many different lesions can disrupt spatial navigation function, structural repair by grafts does not always provide clear functional benefit. Thus, whereas cholinergic-rich septal grafts in the neocortex are effective in alleviating passive avoidance deficits following basal forebrain lesions that disrupt the cholinergic innervation of the neocortex (see next section under Graft Effects in Aged Rats), the same animals show only rather modest changes in the water maze task (48). In particular, as in the studies of Nilsson et al. (104), the greatest benefits were seen in the accuracy of performance during the probe trials, rather than in the marked deficits seen in basic task acquisition (48). Moreover, dopaminergic grafts in the striatum yield little benefit in the navigation deficits induced by neonatal forebrain dopamine depletion (1), and hippocampal grafts can actually further impair the performance of rats with total hippocampectomy (145).

These various applications reflect the ease and efficiency of testing in the Morris water maze task and its flexibility for application to a variety of different functional systems. We can, therefore, expect to see its application in the development of other graft models in the near future, for example, in the cognitive deficits associated with striatal lesions or more global forebrain ischemia. Nevertheless, the basis for the functional recovery in the different model systems is still not clear, and the Morris water maze task is likely to prove more useful as a test for pragmatic screening of lesion-induced deficits and graft-derived recovery, rather than for the precise behavioral analysis of the underlying functional impairments.

PASSIVE AND ACTIVE AVOIDANCE TASKS

Rationale Behind Passive Avoidance Tasks

Maze-learning studies have proved effective in illustrating general learning and cognitive impairments in old or lesioned animals. However, often the primary experimental interest is in whether a particular experimental treatment is associated with explicit memory impairments (11,87). Perhaps the most widely studied test of memory in both the aging and the psychopharmacologic literatures involves passive

avoidance acquisition and retention by rodents (4,39). In passive avoidance training, a rat or mouse is punished immediately if it engages in some spontaneous behavior. Typically, this involves placing the animal in a position where it would not usually stay (e.g., on a small raised platform or in the middle of a bright open arena). The animal is given a brief sharp footshock as soon as it steps off the platform onto a grid floor (a "step-down" task) or it enters from the brightly lit into the dark compartment of a two-compartment test box (a "step-through" passive avoidance task; Fig 6A). Then, at some later time, the animal is replaced in the same situation: on the platform or in the bright arena. Memory for the previous aversive event is manifested by inhibition of the spontaneous behavior (i.e., the animal stays where it is initially placed).

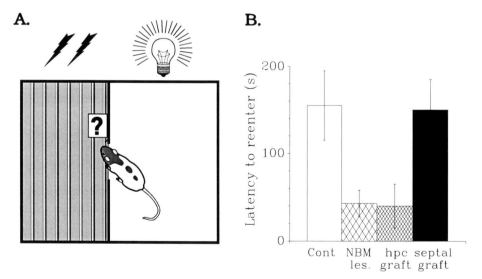

FIG. 6. **A**: Schematic illustration of the two compartment "step-through" apparatus used in passive avoidance tests. The *right compartment* has a solid floor, and is brightly illuminated, open, and exposed. The *left compartment* is dark, enclosed and has a grid-floor. The two compartments are separated by a sliding door that may be closed before administering footshock when the rat steps through into the dark compartment. **B**: Latency to reenter the dark compartment by control rats, rats with basal forebrain lesions, and rats with septal or hippocampal grafts implanted into the denervated neocortex. All rats had received mild footshock on first entering the dark compartment 2 days previously. On the test day, the lesioned rats rapidly reenter, indicating a poor retention (forgetting) of the original training. This deficit is alleviated by cholinergic-rich septal grafts, but not by cholinergic-poor hippocampal grafts. (Data from ref. 48.)

Graft Effects in Aged Rats

Aged rats manifest marked impairments in passive avoidance tests of memory (39,69,150). In particular, these impairments in avoidance learning have been seen to correlate with a decline in the numbers of noradrenergic neurons in the locus coeruleus and with a loss of noradrenergic activity in the hippocampus in aged rats and mice (91,149). Locus coeruleus grafts can provide an extensive fiber reinnervation of the hippocampus, the laminar pattern of which is normal, when the grafts are implanted into or adjacent to the deafferentated hippocampus of young rats (15,18). Therefore, in an attempt to compensate the age-related deficit, Collier and colleagues implanted embryonic locus coeruleus grafts into the ventricles of aged rats and found that the grafts could alleviate the aged animals' impairments in passive avoidance learning (24,25). Of particular note in these studies was the different approaches taken by the authors to address the issue of the noradrenergic specificity of the grafts' functional effects in the aged brain. First, they found that no similar benefit was provided by control grafts of cerebellar tissues. Second, the recovery was mimicked by chronic intraventricular infusion of norepinephrine. Third, the recovery in grafted rats was reversed by treatment with the β-blocker propranolol. However, although the grafts in this study provided a limited fiber ingrowth into the host hypothalamus, the ventricular placement of the grafts and the parallel recovery following intraventricular infusion of norepinephrine suggest that the recovery in the aged rats was attributable to a more diffuse mechanism of systemic norepinephrine release, perhaps influencing mechanisms of arousal (25).

Graft Effects After Basal Forebrain Lesions

Passive avoidance tests have also been used as an adjunct to maze-learning tests for evaluating the deficits in animals with basal forebrain lesions. Most studies have used injections of excitotoxins, such as kainic acid or ibotenic acid, focused on the cortically projecting cholinergic neurons of the nucleus basalis to make the lesions.

Several studies have used the basal forebrain model system to investigate the extent to which basal forebrain grafts implanted into the neocortex could ameliorate deficits in passive avoidance-learning tests. Thus, for example, as shown in Fig. 6B, ibotenic acid lesions of the basal forebrain result in more rapid reentry into the dark chamber in a step-through test of passive avoidance (48). The deficit is substantially alleviated by cholinergic-rich septal grafts implanted in multiple cortical sites, whereas control grafts devoid of cholinergic neurons (here, hippocampal tissue) were without detectable functional effect. Similar patterns of recovery have been demonstrated in several different studies (3,48,55,77,131).

However, we should be cautious about the specificity of the deficits and recovery in these experiments (42). Ibotenic or kainic acid lesions induce a range of regulatory, neurologic, and sensorimotor deficits, in addition to the deficits in passive avoidance and water maze learning (144,147). Several of these noncognitive deficits, such as contralateral sensory neglect, were also reversed by cortical septal grafts, whereas the grafted animals remained as impaired as those rats with lesions alone on some other learning tasks (48,131). Thus, both the behavioral and the neurotransmitter specificity of the basal forebrain lesion model are currently the subjects of detailed reexamination (42), and it appears increasingly likely that the nature of the lesioned animals' deficits involve some general attentional or arousal function, rather than a primary cognitive dysfunction in the classic sense.

Advantages and Disadvantages of Passive Avoidance Tests

The passive avoidance test has several advantages. First, is that the test is quick and extremely simple to administer. Second, if the training stimulus (i.e., the footshock) is sufficiently aversive, most control animals learn the consequences in a single trial. Thus, the time of initial learning can be determined precisely and, as a consequence, it is possible to evaluate memory (and its complement, forgetting) over different controlled retention intervals between training and testing. Third, in contrast with many other maze-learning tasks, passive avoidance tests require no long-term food-deprivation, which can stress an animal's health and are difficult to standardize in some experimental situations, such as those using aged rats.

Corresponding to the advantage of one-trial training of the passive avoidance test, a key disadvantage is that whether or not the animal avoids the previously shocked location the outcome of the test trial will profoundly influence an animal's beliefs and knowledge of the task situation. Because of this, the rat can be tested only once, and comparisons of different treatments (e.g., different retention intervals, drug doses, and such) therefore must be tested in separate groups of animals. In addition, the traditional measure of remembering—the latency to step down or to reenter the dark chamber—can be quite variable among animals. Thus, passive avoidance testing requires large numbers of animals for valid statistical comparison and, consequently, is extremely inefficient. This may prove acceptable when conducting experiments on the effects of aging or of different drugs, in which there is little surgical or time investment in each individual animal, but it can prove unacceptably inefficient in many lesion and transplantation studies that involve a high cost in time and resources for the preparation of each subject.

A more fundamental disadvantage of the passive avoidance paradigm is that, whereas a decline in performance may indeed reflect a disruption of memory, performance may be disturbed by a variety of other noncognitive changes, such as the animal's level of arousal, sensitivity to the footshock, attention to the environmental stimuli at the time of training or retest, or its level of general motor activity. One resolution of this issue is to first train an intact animal and then to administer the experimental treatment so that it is clear that all rats will indeed have received equivalent learning. This works well when the experimental treatment acts briefly, such as protein inhibitor drugs or electroconvulsive shock, both of which will still disrupt the subsequent storage and retrieval of new memories. However, since the interval between training and test is typically between 1 and 7 days, such a strategy cannot be used to evaluate long-term treatments involved in neural transplantation. In fact, it turns out to be extremely difficult to demonstrate that graft-derived recovery from passive avoidance deficits are indeed attributable to a restitution of some specific mnemonic or other cognitive ability.

Lesion and Graft Effects on Active Avoidance Tests

Active avoidance, in which the rat learns to move away from a given location to avoid shock, is related to passive avoidance, in which a rat must refrain from moving to avoid shock. The most common version of active avoidance training is the so-called two-way active avoidance test. This, typically also involves a two-compartment box (as in step-through passive avoidance), but the two sides are identical and separated by a door or low barrier. In an active avoidance test, a warning light or tone signals the impending occurrence of a footshock, which is then turned on 5 or 10 seconds later. The rat can escape the footshock by moving over to the other side. Then after an interval, the warning signal is again presented, and the rat escapes the shock by returning back to the first side. Although the rat can escape each footshock when it occurs by moving over to the other side, it can completely avoid receiving the shock by moving across as soon as the warning signal is presented. Thus, in a series of trials, the rat moves back and forth between the two sides, as soon as the signal is turned on, to avoid the shock, which underlies the common name for the training apparatus as a "shuttle" box. A normal rat will learn to avoid virtually all shocks within 20 or 30 training trials in the apparatus, and it provides a quick and efficient test of simple learning.

Several of the studies of basal forebrain lesions and cholinergic transplants have complemented conventional passive avoidance tests with parallel tests of active avoidance learning (3,4,90,97). In particular, Arendash and Mouton (3,4) evaluated the effects of cholinergic-rich grafts implanted into the neocortex of rats with basal forebrain lesions on active as well as passive avoidance. The lesions produced marked deficits in both acquisition and extinction of the two-way active avoidance task, which were equally severe in a group of rats with control grafts of noncholinergic (thalamic) tissue. By contrast the group of rats with cholinergic-rich grafts showed a substantial and significant alleviation, in particular in the deficit in extinction (3,4). However, in addition to the issue of the possible nonspecificity of the lesions in these studies (see above), the authors also note that there has been difficulties in replicating the graft-derived alleviation of active avoidance deficits in subsequent studies using larger groups of animals (3).

The apparatus and use of aversive training stimuli are similar in active and passive avoidance tests, and the two tasks suffer from some similar difficulties; for example, in how to match the aversive nature of the footshocks in different experimental groups of rats. However, active avoidance does not have the advantage of acquisition in a single trial, and the two tasks are, in many ways, logically quite distinct. Thus, whereas the focus in passive avoidance is on retention (memory) of a single training event over a period of some hours or days, active

avoidance is one of a wide range of learning tests, based on the principles of conditioning. These manifest many common phenomena (e.g., in the demonstration of gradual acquisition and extinction), which can better be studied in the more-controlled environment of the operant chamber.

CLASSICAL AND OPERANT CONDITIONING

Principles of Conditioning Paradigms

The neurobiologic tradition of neural transplantation studies has led to a preponderance of use of mazes and avoidance learning for both simple and more complex tests of animals' learning capacities. By contrast, the classical (Pavlovian) and operant (Skinnerian) conditioning techniques that have been widely used by psychologists for the analysis of animals' learning capacities (30,93) have been relatively neglected as a tool for assessing neural transplants.

Classical conditioning is based on the principle that animals can learn associations between stimuli when they are predictive of consequences of importance to the animal. For example, in the original Pavlovian experiments, if a tone was predictive of the subsequent presentation of food, dogs would salivate to the tone in anticipation of the food. The passive avoidance experiments we have considered are a form of classical conditioning—the animal learns in a single trial that the dark compartment is associated with painful footshock, and responds accordingly by subsequently avoiding that place.

Operant conditioning is based on the principle that if certain behaviors result in important (good or bad) consequences for animals, then the frequency with which the animal expresses those behaviors changes accordingly. The consequences can be any significant change in the environment, but are typically the presentation or removal of relevant reinforcing stimuli. By definition, a *reinforcer* is any stimulus that can change an animal's behavior—they may be positive (e.g., food) or aversive (e.g., footshock), and in addition to the more obvious ones such as food, water, a receptive sexual partner, or pain, more diffuse stimuli, such as "novelty," and stimuli that allow the opportunities for exploration or play can serve as reinforcers.

B. F. Skinner first designed the operant chamber (colloquially known as a "Skinner box"), which is an automated test apparatus for analyzing the conditions of learning in rats (Fig. 7). The requirements for any operant chamber are something on which an animal can respond (the "manipulandum"), and some way of delivering reinforcing stimuli. Typical manipulanda are levers for the rat to press or a chain to pull. Similarly, the reinforcement dispenser can be a food well or a drinking tube into which pellets of food or drops of water are delivered, respectively, or a grid floor to which can be applied footshocks. The major contribution of the field of operant conditioning has been the analysis of

the effects of different contingencies of reinforcement on changes in an animal's behavior (54). The contingency can be simple (e.g., every lever press results in the immediate delivery of one food pellet—known as a *continuous reinforcement* schedule) or quite complex (e.g., if a warning light is off then one lever press every 2 minutes on average results in a food pellet and other presses have no consequence; when the light is switched on then lever-pressing still produces food pellets, but there is an added probability of receiving additional footshocks). This latter example is not far-fetched—indeed, it is known as the Geller-Seifter schedule. It is used to evaluate rats' responses to situations of conflict, and it has proved extremely powerful in testing drugs and other treatments that have anxiolytic properties (78).

Advantages and Disadvantages of Operant Tests

The techniques of operant and classical conditioning offer several distinct advan-

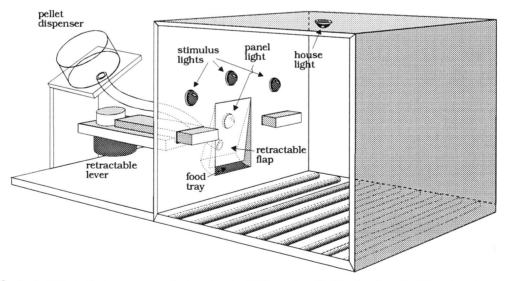

FIG. 7. A retractable lever operant chamber (a "Skinner box"). The front wall of the chamber contains a food well covered by a retractable Perspex flap. Two retractable response levers are positioned one on either side of the central food well. Three stimulus lights are located above each lever and the food well. The detection of the rat's responses (pressing of response levers or the food well panel), the delivery of food pellets, and the switching on and off of the stimulus and house lights, are all under the online control of a microcomputer.

tages over maze tasks as tests of an animal's learning capacity. First the tasks are defined in great detail, with a precise relationship established between relevant and otherwise neutral environmental stimuli, and the animal's responses. Second, they are generally automated and run under computer control, with the double advantage of efficiency and the precision of data collection. Third, there is an extensive psychological literature on the ways animals behave under different sets of controlled conditions, and there is now a well-established theoretical framework within which animal-learning processes can be analyzed.

There are three main disadvantages of the standard-conditioning approaches, which may account for their relatively limited use in the neural transplantation field. First, they require a range of computer and testing equipment that is well established in psychology departments, but is not common in other neurobiology laboratories. This is merely an inconvenience and is the easiest to overcome. Second, and perhaps more critically, is that operant and classical conditioning approaches can appear to carry a substantial theoretical framework, which can prove daunting to researchers without a formal psychological training. However, it is quite feasible to use the powerful techniques of operant and classical conditioning as pragmatic tests of neural function and dysfunction, without needing to become involved in the sometimes complex discussions about the logical basis of particular aspects of conditioning theory. Third, and perhaps most critically, it has often been difficult to identify circumscribed and specific lesions that disrupt either basic classical or operant-conditioning processes—indeed, even the decerebrate preparation can learn some basic classic associations (106). As a consequence, simple classical or operant conditioning paradigms can prove relatively insensitive to the experimental models of interest. However, a few notable exceptions have recently been developed, as will be illustrated in the remainder of this chapter.

TASTE AVERSION LEARNING

Rationale for Conditioned Taste Aversion Tests

Pavlov and Skinner considered that the principles of conditioning would apply equally for establishing associations with or between initially neutral stimuli, the selection of which is, therefore, arbitrary. This has turned out not to be true. Rather, it is easier to make certain associations than others. For example, it is easier to associate flashing lights with footshock and the taste of a food with subsequent illness, than to make the converse associations (67). In particular, taste aversion—the phenomenon whereby animals avoid eating foods that have made them sick on previous occasions—is of particular interest (66). It demonstrates a number of distinctive properties, including that the association can be established even when an hour or more separate the experience of the taste and subsequent nausea, whereas other classic associations, such as between lights or tones and shock or food, typically have to cooccur within seconds of each other for good conditioning to be established. Thus Seligman concludes that animals have a particular biologic propensity or "preparedness" to make certain associations in preference to others (129).

Of more interest in the present context is that the neural analysis of taste-related stimuli is critically dependent on the integrity of the amygdala and of the gustatory areas of neocortex, such that lesions in these areas can disrupt the learning of conditioned taste aversions (19).

Graft Effects on Conditioned Taste Aversion

Bermudez-Rattoni and colleagues first evaluated the effects of cortical grafts on the taste aversion learning of rats with electrolytic lesions in either the amygdala or the gustatory neocortex (12). Testing was conducted in two separate stages, the first of which assessed the effects of the lesions. The animals were water-deprived and allowed to drink for only 30 minutes a day. Baseline drinking was established over 10 days. Then on the 11th day, the rat was allowed to drink a sweet saccharin solution, followed 30 minutes later by an injection of lithium chloride to make the animals sick. On the next 2 days, the animals were given water and then on the third and sixth days tested with saccharin again. Whereas, the control rats avoided the sweet-tasting liquid, the lesions disrupted learning, and both lesion groups drank as much saccharin as the baseline levels of water intake. Half of each lesion group then received isotopic grafts (fetal cortex into the site of the cortical lesions, fetal amygdala into the site of the amygdala lesions), and were then retested for conditioned taste aversion 8 weeks later. Conditioning recovered spontaneously in the rats with amygdala lesions, whether or not they received grafts, so that the changing baseline made it impossible to evaluate the effects of the grafts. By contrast, the deficit following the cortical lesions was more stable and was equally apparent at this long test interval. However, the rats with additional cortical grafts showed a significant recovery of their ability to learn the taste aversion, and these grafted rats avoided the sweet-tasting solution when subsequently given the opportunity to drink it, as did the controls.

These observations of graft-derived recovery following cortical grafts may prove no more specific than the earlier studies in frontal cortex that turned out to be due to essentially trophic mechanisms (see section on prefrontal lesions under earlier T-maze discussion). However, Bermudez-Rattoni and colleagues have gone some way to ruling out a simple trophic explanation. First, the recovery was seen only following implantation of cortical tissues that established connections between the graft and host brain, but not in rats bearing unconnected tectal grafts (50). Furthermore, the time course of the recovery was gradual—nonexistent at 15 days postgrafting then pro-

gressively greater recovery up to 2 months—and over the same time period as the establishment of graft–host connectivity (53).

There is a more general issue about the extent to which these studies demonstrate restoration of a learning capacity *per se*. The authors certainly conclude that "fetal transplants can restore functional losses of behavior in lesioned adult animals, including cognitive functions" (12). It should be noted, however, that the effective lesions disrupt a primary sensory, rather than an association, area of neocortex, and the results do not indicate whether the deficit on this learning task is due to an intrinsic disruption of the animals' cognitive capacities, or whether otherwise intact cognitive processing is disturbed through the animals' inability to discriminate the relevant discriminative stimuli. It was clear when considering the passive avoidance tests that any interpretation based on a memory deficit must exclude the failure of lesioned animals simply being due to insensitivity to the aversive footshock. In exactly the same way, if we are to conclude a true cognitive deficit (and cognitive recovery) in conditioned taste aversion, it must first be shown that the lesioned animals can still discriminate the relevant tastes. This is unlikely to be so, at least following gustatory neocortex lesions, although the deficit following lesions of the amygdala may indeed be related to a disruption of conditioning processes (58).

DIFFERENTIAL REINFORCEMENT OF LOW RATES OF RESPONDING

Rationale for Use of the DRL Schedule

Whereas the general acquisition of basic operant-learning schedules has not proved particularly informative in neurobiologic analyses of the neural substrates of learning, operant schedules dependent on certain discrimination rules have been useful for the analysis of specific neural subsystems. For example, animals with hippo-campal damage have particular difficulty with tasks that require them to modify their responses to changing circumstances, with-holding responding at one moment and then switching or recommencing responding at another (70). The deficits manifested by hippocampal rats have been described as "perseverative" (31), have been considered to be due to a particular failure in inhibitory processes (83), and are particularly sensi-tive to tests that require switching or accu-rate timing of responding (70,94,122).

Perhaps the simplest operant schedule of reinforcement for revealing timing deficits is differential reinforcement of low rates of responding (DRL) (54). The task contin-gency is: "a response is reinforced if and only if a given minimum time (e.g., 20 sec-onds) has elapsed since the last response" (Fig. 8A). Any response made less than 20 seconds after the last resets the control timer, so that the rat has now to wait a fur-ther 20 seconds. Although the task rule it-self is simple to describe, it takes a consid-

erable length of training for rats to learn the DRL schedule with any degree of effi-ciency, because it must withhold repeating what has just proved successful. Moreover, there are no external cues to guide the ani-mal toward when it may now respond again; it must rely entirely on internal rep-resentations of the passage of time. Lesions within the hippocampal circuitry produce a major and lasting disruption in animals' abilities to perform efficiently on the DRL task (20,64,80,132). Rather, they continue high rates of responding and only infre-quently wait long enough to earn a food pel-let.

Grafts and Hippocampal Damage

Several studies have used the operant DRL task to evaluate the effects of neural grafts in rats with hippocampal damage. First, Woodruff and colleagues demon-strated a modest recovery of the profound

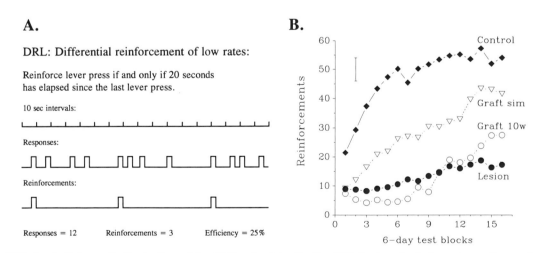

FIG. 8. A: Schematic illustration of the DRL schedule. On the DRL task a single lever is continuously available in the operant chamber. A lever press is rewarded by a food pellet if and only if >20 seconds has elapsed since the last lever press. **B**: Reinforcements earned during DRL training of controls, rats with fimbria–fornix lesions, and rats with additional septal grafts implanted into the hippocampus. Grafts implanted at the same time as making the lesions (*sim*) showed a significant alleviation of the deficit, whereas grafts implanted into the intact hippocampus, 10 weeks before the lesions (*10w*), were without benefit. (Data from ref. 49.)

DRL deficits manifested by animals, with extensive aspirations of the hippocampus, following implantation of hippocampal tissue into the cavities (146). This seemed to take place independently of the grafts becoming connected with the host brain, and subsequent graft removal studies suggested that the recovery in this particular model system was mediated by nonspecific or trophic influences (145).

Other studies have examined the effects of cholinergic grafts on the DRL deficits induced by fimbria–fornix lesions in rats. In the first of these, we found that an improved efficiency of DRL performance could be established by septal grafts taken from embryos of 13–14 days of gestational age, but not by grafts derived from older donors (45). This was not withstanding the fact that older embryos still provided a good acetylcholinesterase-positive reinnervation of the host hippocampus. Indeed, grafts derived from the oldest embryos actually disrupted performance beyond the level of deficit observed in rats with lesions alone. Thus, although cholinergic reinnervation of the host hippocampus by the graft was a necessary factor in recovery, this was not a sufficient explanation for the differences between graft groups, but rather, suggested that the presence or absence of other (unidentified) connections may be critical to the development of functional changes, whether beneficial or detrimental.

In a subsequent study using the same paradigm, the interval between conducting the lesion and transplantation surgeries also exerts an important influence on graft viability (see Fig. 8B) (49). The septal grafts alleviated the fimbria–fornix lesion deficit only when the grafts were implanted simultaneously with, or 11 days after, making the lesions and not when the transplants were implanted a couple of months before or after making the lesions. Again, good grafts and extensive cholinesterase-positive connections were established in all groups, indicating that reformation of new cholinergic inputs is not alone sufficient to sustain good functional recovery.

DELAYED MATCHING AND NONMATCHING TESTS

Rationale Behind Delayed Response Tasks

Another type of operant task that has proved powerful for evaluating cognitive functions of grafted rats, in particular relative to the animals' short-term memory capacities, is the delayed matching and nonmatching to position tests (DMTP/DNMTP) for rats. Unlike the DRL task, the DMTP/DNMTP tests were not originally derived from within the operant literature. Rather, they reflect an adaptation of delayed response procedures originally designed for evaluating short-term memory in monkeys to the rodent operant test apparatus. In particular, delayed matching and delayed nonmatching to sample tests have proved particularly powerful and flexible, and lend themselves to automated operant test procedures in addition to the conventional hand-testing approach in the Wisconsin general test apparatus (27,79,96) (also see Chapter 13).

The basic design of the delayed matching to sample task is as follows: At the start of each trial the animal is shown a sample object to remember. After a variable delay interval, the animal then indicates its memory for the sample information by choosing among several presented alternatives, and is rewarded for selecting the same stimulus or object as had been presented as sample earlier in the trial (in delayed matching to sample; Fig. 9A) or for selecting the stimulus or object that differs from the sample (in delayed nonmatching to sample; see Fig. 9B) (27,79).

The essential feature of the delayed matching and nonmatching tasks is that performance accuracy can be evaluated over different delay intervals, separating the sample and choice stages of each trial. The decline in performance at increasing delays then indicates the loss or decay of the relevant information from memory. When represented graphically (see Fig. 9C), the rate of forgetting is indicated by

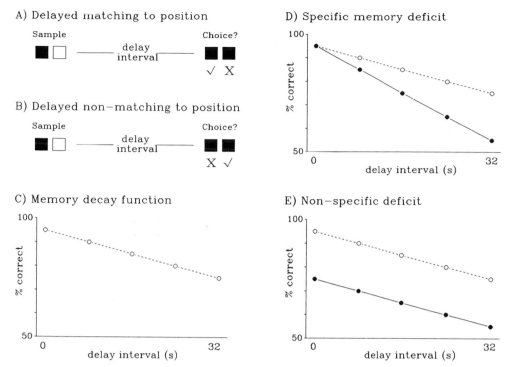

FIG. 9. Schematic representation of the design and alternative outcomes in delayed-matching and nonmatching to position tasks. **A**: In the DMTP task for rats, one of two levers is extended into the test chamber (*black square*) to denote the sample. When the rat responds, the lever is removed for a variable delay interval, and then both levers are presented. The correct response is to choose the sample lever (*tick*), whereas pressing the other lever is punished with time out (*cross*). **B**: In DNMTP, the converse contingencies apply. **C**: Theoretical outcome in a control experiment, in which the memory trace weakens so that the accuracy of performance declines as the delay interval is increased. The slope of the curve indicates the rate of forgetting. **D**: A specific impairment in short-term memory is manifested by an absence of impairment at the shortest delay, but performance declines more rapidly, and the slope of the function is greater, than in the control condition. **E**: A nonspecific impairment is manifested by a disruption of performance at all delays equally. The delayed matching and nonmatching to sample are conceptually similar, other than that the sample is one of two discrete objects rather than one of two positions. (Redrawn from ref. 37.)

the slope of the graph plotting the percentage correct performance against the delay interval.

The importance of this memory decay function is that it enables experimental treatments that enhance or disrupt memory specifically to be distinguished from the plethora of manipulations that disturb other nonspecific aspects of performance. Thus, an increase in the slope of the forgetting function (Fig. 9D), indicates a specific impairment in the animal's short-term memory as information is lost more rapidly. In

this situation, the experimental animal shows normal performance at the shortest delays when the memory load is minimal, which indicates that it has learned the discrimination rule, it can distinguish and is attending to the relevant stimuli, it is motivated to respond, and it has no marked motor impairment or bias that inhibits making the correct response. Conversely, a generalized delay-independent disturbance of performance at all delays (see Fig. 9E) indicates a nonspecific impairment (i.e., one that cannot be attributed to a dysfunction in memory *per se*), since the animal is impaired even at the shortest delays when the memory load is minimal. Alternative interpretations of the precise nature of this non-mnemonic deficit in terms of attention, discrimination learning, motivation, or sensory–motor function cannot be resolved from these results alone. Not surprisingly, most treatments that disturb performance of delayed matching and nonmatching tasks induce delay-independent deficits (37). By contrast both aging and lesions in the hippocampal system produce delay-dependent deficits in delayed matching or nonmatching to sample in monkeys (9,10,95,96,148), suggesting that these particular treatments can induce a relatively selective impairment in short-term memory functions.

By contrast with monkeys, it has been extremely difficult to train rats in operant versions of delayed matching and nonmatching to sample tasks using visual stimuli, perhaps because of the relative inattention of this species to the visual modality. One approach has been to use maze versions of delayed response and delayed matching tasks with highly distinctive three-dimensional junk objects or goal boxes as the samples (2,126). An alternative approach has used spatial locations as the sample information in delayed matching to position and delayed nonmatching to position tasks (DMTP/DNMTP) (33,139), and this has yielded a test paradigm that has been used more widely to evaluate lesion and graft function.

Rats are trained on the DMTP and DNMTP tasks in conventional operant chambers with two retractable levers and central food collection panel (see Fig. 7) (33,34). On each trial one lever is extended into the chamber as the sample and is then retracted as soon as the rat presses it. After a variable delay (typically between 0 and 64 seconds), both levers are extended again into the test chamber, and the rat must make a choice response. The rat is rewarded with a food pellet delivered to the central food well if it makes a correct choice by pressing the sample lever (in

DMTP) or the opposite lever (in DNMTP), whereas the converse response is punished by a "time out" period during which the chamber lights are switched off.

Rats are trained on either the DMTP or the DNMTP version of the task. They first learn the discrimination rule without delays, which is generally achieved within 1 to 2 weeks of daily training sessions. They are then switched to a range of random delay intervals, and trained until they reach an asymptotic level of performance, which generally requires a further 4 to 6 weeks of training. Although the rate of acquisition of the task is informative about the animals' general learning abilities (46), the most valuable data is provided by the memory decay functions obtained once the animals have reached asymptote. These provide the data both for evaluating changes in short-term memory and forgetting, and for testing the effects of drugs or other manipulations against a stable baseline (37).

Basal Forebrain Lesions and Cholinergic Grafts

Several studies have indicated that lesions both of the basal forebrain cholinergic innervation of the neocortex and of the septohippocampal projections to the hippocampus produce deficits in the DMTP task (33,36,37,46).

Several experiments have been conducted to evaluate the efficacy of cholinergic-rich grafts into the neocortex of rats with basal forebrain lesions on the DMTP and DNMTP tasks. The results have so far been disappointing. In one study, a significant delay-independent deficit induced by basal forebrain lesions was seen to be reversed by cholinergic grafts implanted in multiple cortical sites (34). However, in the NBM–cortical model system, the deficits made by quisqualic acid lesions are small, and they are not specifically mnemonic (42).

Of more interest in any model investigating the role of central cholinergic systems in memory deficits would be restitution of the fimbria–fornix lesion deficit, since this lesion produces a delay-dependent deficit indicative of a specific impairment in short-term memory. However, in three separate studies of the effects of cholinergic and noncholinergic grafts implanted in the hippocampus of such animals, the delay-dependent deficits that are observed in the DMTP/DNMTP task when tested immediately after making fimbria–fornix lesions have recovered over a period of 2 to 4 months (S.B. Dunnett, unpublished data). Since this length of time is necessary to allow the grafts to become established and form extensive connections with the host brain, there have been no residual deficits when the grafted animals come to testing, even though the lesioned animals remain impaired on the operant DRL tasks that are responsive to the same graft treatments (see previous section).

Cholinergic Grafts in Aged Rats

The efficacy of grafts in aged rats has been more encouraging. We first evaluated the effects of age on performance of the DMTP and the DNMTP tasks in rats of three different aged groups: 6, 15, and 24 months (41). Both tests revealed a highly significant deficit in the old rats (Fig. 10A). Of particular importance, the age-related deficit was delay-dependent. Thus, there was no impairment at short delays, indicating that the old rats had learned the decision rule, were able to discriminate the relevant stimuli, and were motivated to respond appropriately. By contrast, a progressively greater impairment was apparent only at longer delays, indicative of a specific short-term memory deficit in the old rats. The DMTP task appeared somewhat more sensitive and revealed deficits in the 15-month as well as the 24-month group, whereas only the eldest group was deficient on the DNMTP task. However, the variability of performance within each group was less for the DNMTP task, so this has been the version more widely used in subsequent experiments.

We then went on to evaluate the effect of cholinergic-rich septal grafts implanted into old rats at 20 months of age (38). Three groups of old rats received bilateral implants either into the neocortex, into the

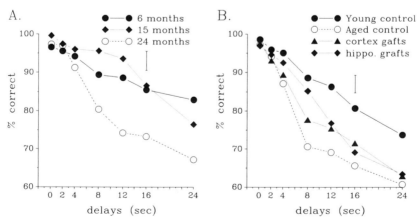

FIG. 10. A: Delay-performance function of young, middle-aged, and aged rats (6, 15, and 24 months old, respectively) in the delayed nonmatching to sample task. The aged rats manifest faster forgetting than the young rats, as shown by the increased slope of the delay-performance function. **B**: Effect of cholinergic-rich septal grafts implanted into the neocortex or hippocampus. Both graft placements yield a moderate, but significant, alleviation of the delay-dependent age-related deficit. (Data from refs. 38,41.)

hippocampus, or remained as sham-grafted old controls. Three months later all three old groups and an additional group of young animals were trained on the DNMTP task. The age- and delay-dependent deficit in DNMTP performance was replicated in the old control group. Moreover, this short-term memory deficit of aged rats was significantly alleviated in both cholinergic-rich graft groups (see Fig. 10B) (38). Although the benefit was somewhat greater following implantation to the hippocampus, the effect in the group receiving cortical implants was also significant.

However, the benefit was only partial in either graft group. Several alternative strategies may be possible to increase the level of benefit. First, a more extensive recovery may be achieved by combining the cortical and hippocampal placements in the same animal, as was seen to benefit recovery of radial maze learning in rats with cholinergic cell damage from alcohol intoxication (6) (see earlier section and Chapter 10). Second, it may be that the efficacy of cholinergic grafts is promoted by cotransplantation with serotonergic tissues, which was seen to enhance recovery in the Morris water maze task by rats with septal lesions (104) (see earlier section). Third, it is likely that other cortical–hippocampal systems are also implicated in the maintenance of normal learning and memory function, and might also be susceptible to graft-derived amelioration in aged animals. In fact, it is likely that each of these alternative strategies will be found to contribute to the profile of deficits manifested by different individual aged animals.

CONCLUSIONS

Comparison of Behavioral Test Strategies

Over the course of the last 10 years, a variety of different classes of tests have been introduced to evaluate the learning and memory performance of rats bearing neuronal grafts. The tests vary considerably in their efficiency, sensitivity and specificity.

Efficiency

Thus, at one extreme, passive avoidance tests are extremely easy to administer and take very little time for each animal, but at the cost of being highly variable, so that many animals must be included in each group, and of being susceptible to a wide range of noncognitive as well as cognitive influences. At the other extreme, several operant tests provide great precision and yield great stability of performance, with relatively low levels of variability. However, they require extensive training and testing, often on a daily basis over several months until the animals attain stable levels of performance. This can partly be alleviated if the test apparatus is entirely automated and large volumes of data are collected for little personal effort, but the prolonged nature of testing can result in insensitivity to deficits that recover with practice. In many ways the maze tasks provide a compromise of sensitivity and efficiency, at least when the requirement is for an empirical measure of a deficit, rather than a theoretical analysis of the underlying functional impairment. Although maze tasks generally require hand-testing that can be extremely tedious for the experimenter, generally each particular experiment can be completed within a time framework of only a few weeks.

Sensitivity

Passive avoidance tests are relatively insensitive both on a within- and a between-animals basis. Thus there is typically very wide variability of performance among different animals of each group, with some reentering the dark compartment rapidly and others staying out even up to the maximum cutoff point. Because each animal can be tested only once, it is not possible to obtain a more precise measure of an individual rat's performance by taking the mean of multiple trials. In addition the wide scatter and frequent skew of the collected data can restrict the analysis to use of less powerful nonparametric statistical tests. By contrast, maze tests by and large yield similar, gradual acquisition curves across the different animals of an experimental group, and blocks of trials can generally be averaged to provide relatively tighter variance of performance within each group for parametric analysis. The capacity of operant tests to provide large quantities of data on a fully automated basis means that such tests can provide the tightest variance and can be the most sensitive to small changes within animals (e.g., in dose–response studies of drug effects). However, this is dependent both on there being a clear operant deficit associated with the particular experimental treatment and on the deficit being stable (rather than recovering) over prolonged periods of testing.

Specificity

A wide range of lesions can disrupt performance on both passive avoidance and maze tasks, which therefore are useful for screening deficits and recovery in a wide range of paradigms. By contrast, although operant tests can provide high sensitivity and precision in the nature of the performance deficit, their specificity to lesions in particular neural systems and the fact that many experimental treatments produce no deficits on many conditioned behaviors, means that the breadth of their application can frequently be quite limited.

Do Neural Grafts Influence Cognitive Function?

All the tasks considered in this chapter are "cognitive," in the sense that they require learning, memory, or some other aspect of problem-solving for their successful performance. There is now substantial evidence that neuronal degeneration associated with a variety of explicit lesions as well as with the intrinsic aging process can produce profound deficits in the performance in a wide range of these cognitive tasks. Moreover, those deficits can be alleviated (and in some cases completely abolished) by neuronal transplants. However, underlying the present account and, in particular, in the occasional challenges to the neurochemical or functional specificity of the different model systems in particular behavioral tasks is the principle that a distinction must be drawn between a deficit in the performance of a cognitive task and a cognitive impairment *per se*. In many of the examples that have been considered, the particular tasks could not resolve the extent to which deficits in performance are due to an underlying impairment that is essentially noncognitive. Thus, if an animal has a primary sensory deficit, it will be impaired in its ability to detect the training stimuli and, hence, performance of the cognitive task will decline. In fact, a wide variety of sensory, motor, sensorimotor, attentional, and motivational impairments, all of which are essentially noncognitive, can each result in deficits in complex tasks that require additional cognitive processes for their successful completion.

Consequently, we need to address the somewhat more difficult question of whether there is any evidence that the underlying deficits and their alleviation by grafts involve essentially cognitive processes. Usually, this is not possible. Resolution of this issue requires the manipulation of particular features of a task to provide its own internal controls for nonspecific deficits, and in only a few cases has that been achieved. For example, a variety of probe trials and control procedures have been introduced both in the Morris water maze and in the radial maze to exclude the possibility of sensory and motor impairments. It is notable that, in both examples, the lesion deficits and graft-derived recovery have been seen not only on trials where the animal must use essentially spatial information, but also on trials based on explicit visual cues (74,104). Perhaps, the clearest evidence of an explicit cognitive deficit and its alleviation in any of the studies reviewed lies in the age-related impairment in operant delayed nonmatching to position tasks, which was seen to be partially alleviated by cholinergic-rich grafts implanted into the neocortex and hippocampus (38,41). The delay-dependent nature of the performance deficit in this task suggests a specific impairment in some aspect of short-term memory encoding, storage, or retrieval, and enables a wide variety of noncognitive interpretations to be excluded. As was noted earlier, this task has proved somewhat unstable in response to lesions of the central cholinergic systems, and its precise neuroanatomic basis is still far from clear (36). Nevertheless, we can conclude that whereas the cognitive nature of the majority of graft effects has not been demonstrated, nor in many instances is it excluded, at least in particular cases the evidence clearly favors a direct influence of a neuronal graft on an animal's cognitive abilities.

How Do Neural Grafts Influence Cognitive Function?

A second underlying theme of the present discussion has been the mechanism(s) by which grafts can exert their functional effects. This issue is frequently posed as if the alternatives are mutually exclusive and, in particular, that if graft-derived recovery is by a relatively nonspecific mechanism in one circumstance, then this supports nonspecific hypotheses about all graft function. In fact it has turned out that neuronal grafts can (and do) exert their effects by a wide variety of different mechanisms, from nonspecific effects of the surgery to the reformation of reciprocal axonal connections between the grafted neurons and the host

brain, and including trophic stimulation, pharmacologic release, and diffuse reinnervation as intermediate levels of action (14,40). It is apparent that some of the model systems considered in the present chapter, including many of the cortical grafts in animals with gross cortical lesions, exert their effects by relatively less specific trophic mechanisms. By contrast, in most other model systems, the mechanisms have not yet been analyzed in sufficient detail to resolve the issue. At present, the clearest evidence for the reformation of regulated connections with the host brain as the basis for graft function in cognitive tests comes from *in vivo* electrophysiologic and neurochemical studies of cholinergic-rich grafts in the hippocampus (21,100,102,103). However, analysis of the mechanisms of graft function has been considered in greater detail in the context of the role of nigral and striatal grafts in restoration of motor function (see Chapters 2, 3, and 7) and will be considered in greater detail in the final chapter of this volume.

ACKNOWLEDGMENTS

Studies from the author's own laboratory have been funded by the Mental Health Foundation and the Medical Research Council.

REFERENCES

1. Abrous DN, Choulli K, Simon H, Le Moal M, Herman JP. Behavioural effects of intracerebral dopaminergic grafts after neonatal destruction of the mesencephalic dopaminergic system. *Prog Brain Res* 1990;82:481–487.
2. Aggleton JP. One-trial object recognition by rats. *Q J Exp Psychol* 1985;37:279–294.
3. Arendash GW, Mouton PR. Transplantation of nucleus basalis magnocellularis cholinergic neurons into the cholinergic-depleted cerebral-cortex—morphological and behavioral-effects. *Ann NY Acad Sci* 1987;495:431–443.
4. Arendash GW, Strong PN, Mouton PR. Intracerebral transplantation of cholinergic neurons in a new animal model for Alzheimer's disease. In: Hutton TJ, Kenny AD, eds. *Senile demen-*

tia of the Alzheimer type. New York: Alan R Liss; 1985:351–376.

5. Arendt T, Allen Y, Marchbanks RM, Schugens MM, Sinden J, Lantos PL, Gray JA. Cholinergic system and memory in the rat—effects of chronic ethanol, embryonic basal forebrain brain transplants and excitotoxic lesions of cholinergic basal forebrain projection system. *Neuroscience* 1989;33:435–462.

6. Arendt T, Allen Y, Sinden J, Schugens MM, Marchbanks RM, Lantos PL, Gray JA. Cholinergic-rich brain transplants reverse alcohol-induced memory deficits. *Nature* 1988;332:448–450.

7. Azmitia EC, Perlow MJ, Brennan MJ, Lauder JM. Fetal raphe and hippocampal transplants in adult and aged C57BL/6N mice: an immunohistochemical study. *Brain Res Bull* 1981;7:703–710.

8. Bammer G. Pharmacological investigations of neurotransmitter involvement in passive avoidance responding: a review with some new results. *Neurosci Biobehav Rev* 1982;6:246–296.

9. Bartus RT, Dean RL, Beer B. Memory deficits in aged cebus monkeys and facilitation with central cholinomimetics. *Neurobiol Aging* 1980; 1:145–152.

10. Bartus RT, Fleming D, Johnson HR. Aging in the rhesus monkey: debilitating effects on short-term memory. *J Gerontol* 1978;33:858–871.

11. Bartus RT, Flicker C, Dean RL. Logical principles for the development of animal models of age-related memory impairments. In: Crook T, Ferris S, Bartus RT, eds. *Assessment in geriatric psychopharmacology.* New Canaan, CT: Mark Powley; 1983.

12. Bermudez-Rattoni F, Fernandez J, Sanchez MA, Aguilar-Roblero R, Drucker-Colin R. Fetal brain transplants induce recuperation of taste-aversion learning. *Brain Res* 1987;416: 147–152.

13. Björklund A, Gage FH, Stenevi U, Dunnett SB. Intracerebral grafting of neuronal cell suspensions. VI. Survival and growth of intrahippocampal implants of septal cell suspensions. *Acta Physiol Scand* (Suppl) 1983;522:49–58.

14. Björklund A, Lindvall O, Isacson O, Brundin P, Wictorin K, Strecker RE, Clarke DJ, Dunnett SB. Mechanisms of action of intracerebral neural implants—studies on nigral and striatal grafts to the lesioned striatum. *Trends Neurosci* 1987;10:509–516.

15. Björklund A, Nornes H, Gage FH. Cell suspension grafts of noradrenergic locus coeruleus neurons in rat hippocampus and spinal cord—reinnervation and transmitter turnover. *Neuroscience* 1986;18:685–698.

16. Björklund A, Stenevi U. Reformation of the severed septohippocampal cholinergic pathway in the adult rat by transplanted septal neurons. *Cell Tissue Res* 1977;185:289–302.

17. Björklund A, Stenevi U. Reconstruction of the nigrostriatal dopamine pathway by intracerebral transplants. *Brain Res* 1979;177:555–560.

18. Björklund A, Stenevi U, Svendgaard N-A. Growth of transplanted monoaminergic neurones into the adult hippocampus along the perforant path. *Nature* 1976;262:787–790.

19. Braun JJ, Lasiter PS, Kiefer SW. The gustatory neocortex of the rat. *Physiol Psychol* 1982;10: 13–45.

20. Brookes S, Rawlins JNP, Gray JA, Feldon J. DRL performance in rats with medial or lateral septal-lesions. *Physiol Psychol* 1983;11:178–184.

21. Buzsaki G, Gage FH, Czopf J, Björklund A. Restoration of rhythmic slow activity (theta) in the subcortically denervated hippocampus by fetal CNS transplants. *Brain Res* 1987;400:334–347.

22. Cassel JC, Kelche C, Will B. Time-dependent effects of intrahippocampal grafts in rats with fimbria–fornix lesions. *Exp Brain Res* 1990; 81:179–190.

23. Clarke DJ, Gage FH, Björklund A. Formation of cholinergic synapses by intrahippocampal septal grafts revealed by choline acetyltransferase immunocytochemistry. *Brain Res* 1986; 369:151–162.

24. Collier TJ, Gash DM, Bruemmer V, Sladek JR. Impaired regulation of arousal in old age and the consequences for learning and memory: replacement of brain noradrenaline via neuron transplants improves memory performance in aged F344 rats. In: Davis BB, Wood WG, eds. *Homeostatic function and aging.* New York: Raven Press; 1985:99–110.

25. Collier TJ, Gash DM, Sladek JR. Transplantation of norepinephrine neurons into aged rats improves performance in a learned task. *Brain Res* 1988;448:77–87.

26. Coyle JT, Price DL, DeLong MT. Alzheimer's disease: a disorder of cortical cholinergic innervation. *Science* 1983;219:1184–1190.

27. D'Amato MR. Delayed matching and short-term memory in monkeys. *Psychol Learn Motiv* 1973;7:227–269.

28. Dalrymple-Alford J, Kelche C, Eclancher F, Will B. Preoperative enrichment and behavioral recovery in rats with septal lesions. *Behav Neural Biol* 1988;49:361–373.

29. Daniloff JK, Bodony RP, Low WC, Wells J. Cross-species embryonic septal transplants—restoration of conditioned-learning behavior. *Brain Res* 1985;346:176–180.

30. Dickinson A. *Contemporary animal learning theory.* Cambridge: Cambridge University Press; 1980.

31. Douglas RJ. The hippocampus and behavior. *Psychol Bull* 1967;67:416–442.

32. Drachman DA, Sahakian BJ. Memory, aging and pharmacosystems. In: Stein D, ed. *The psychobiology of aging: problems and perspectives.* Amsterdam: Elsevier; 1980:347–368.

33. Dunnett SB. Comparative effects of cholinergic drugs and lesions of nucleus basalis or fimbria–fornix on delayed matching in rats. *Psychopharmacology* 1985;87:357–363.

34. Dunnett SB. Anatomical and behavioral con-

sequences of cholinergic-rich grafts to the neocortex of rats with lesions of the nucleus basalis magnocellularis. *Ann NY Acad Sci* 1987; 495:415–430.

35. Dunnett SB. Is it possible to repair the damaged prefrontal cortex by neural tissue transplantation? *Prog Brain Res* 1990;85:285–297.

36. Dunnett SB. Role of prefrontal cortex and striatal output systems in short-term memory deficits associated with ageing, basal forebrain lesions, and cholinergic-rich grafts. *Can J Psychol* 1990;44:210–232.

37. Dunnett SB. The role and repair of forebrain cholinergic systems in short-term memory. Studies using the delayed matching-to-position task in rats. *Adv Neurol* 1993;59:53–65.

38. Dunnett SB, Badman F, Rogers DC, Evenden JL, Iversen SD. Cholinergic grafts in the neocortex or hippocampus of aged rats—reduction of delay-dependent deficits in the delayed nonmatching to position task. *Exp Neurol* 1988; 102:57–64.

39. Dunnett SB, Barth TM. Animal models of Alzheimer's disease and dementia (with an emphasis on cortical cholinergic systems). In: Willner P, ed. *Behavioural models in psychopharmacology.* Cambridge: Cambridge University Press; 1991:359–418.

40. Dunnett SB, Björklund A. Mechanisms of function of neural grafts in the adult mammalian brain. *J Exp Biol* 1987;132:265–289.

41. Dunnett SB, Evenden JL, Iversen SD. Delay-dependent short-term-memory deficits in aged rats. *Psychopharmacology* 1988;96:174–180.

42. Dunnett SB, Everitt BJ, Robbins TW. The basal forebrain cortical cholinergic system—interpreting the functional consequences of excitotoxic lesions. *Trends Neurosci* 1991;14:494–501.

43. Dunnett SB, Gage FH, Björklund A, Stenevi U, Low WC, Iversen SD. Hippocampal deafferentation—transplant derived reinnervation and functional recovery. *Scand J Psychol* 1982;1:(Suppl)104–111.

44. Dunnett SB, Low WC, Iversen SD, Stenevi U, Björklund A. Septal transplants restore maze-learning in rats with fornix–fimbria lesions. *Brain Res* 1982;251:335–348.

45. Dunnett SB, Martel FL, Rogers DC, Finger S. Factors affecting septal graft amelioration of differential reinforcement of low rates (DRL) and activity deficits after fimbria–fornix lesions. *Restor Neurol Neurosci* 1989;1:83–92.

46. Dunnett SB, Rogers DC, Jones GH. Effects of nucleus basalis magnocellularis lesions in rats on delayed matching and non-matching to position tasks—disruption of conditional discrimination-learning but not of short-term-memory. *Eur J Neurosci* 1989;1:395–406.

47. Dunnett SB, Ryan CN, Levin PD, Reynolds M, Bunch ST. Functional consequences of embryonic neocortex transplanted to rats with prefrontal cortex lesions. *Behav Neurosci* 1987; 101:489.

48. Dunnett SB, Toniolo G, Fine A, Ryan CN, Björklund A, Iversen SD. Transplantation of embryonic ventral forebrain neurons to the neocortex of rats with lesions of nucleus basalis magnocellularis. 2. Sensorimotor and learning impairments. *Neuroscience* 1985;16:787–797.

49. Dunnett SB, Wareham AT, Torres EM. Septal graft amelioration of DRL after fimbria–fornix lesions in rats: role of the interval between lesion and transplantation surgeries. *Restor Neurol Neurosci* 1993;5:110–122.

50. Escobar M, Fernandez J, Guevara-Aguilar R, Bermudez-Rattoni F. Fetal brain grafts induce recovery of learning deficits and connectivity in rats with gustatory neocortex lesion. *Brain Res* 1989;478:368–374.

51. Evenden JL, Robbins TW. Win–stay behaviour in the rat. *Q J Exp Psychol* 1982;36B:1–26.

52. Fantie BD, Kolb B. An examination of prefrontal lesion size and the effects of cortical grafts on performance of the Morris water task by rats. *Psychobiology* 1990;18:74–80.

53. Fernandez-Ruiz J, Escobar ML, Pina AL, Diaz-Cintra S, Cintra-McGlone FL, Bermudez-Rattoni F. Time-dependent recovery of taste-aversion learning by fetal brain transplants in gustatory neocortex-lesioned rats. *Behav Neural Biol* 1991;55:179–193.

54. Ferster CB, Skinner BF. *Schedules of reinforcement.* New York: Appleton-Century-Crofts; 1957.

55. Fine A, Dunnett SB, Björklund A, Clarke DJ, Iversen SD. Transplantation of embryonic ventral forebrain neurons to the neocortex of rats with lesions of nucleus basalis magnocellularis. 1. Biochemical and anatomical observations. *Neuroscience* 1985;16:769.

56. Fischer W, Chen KS, Gage FH, Björklund A. Progressive decline in spatial learning and integrity of forebrain cholinergic neurons in rats during aging. *Neurobiol Aging* 1992;13:9–23.

57. Fischer W, Gage FH, Björklund A. Degenerative changes in forebrain cholinergic nuclei correlate with cognitive impairments in aged rats. *Eur J Neurosci* 1989;1:34–45.

58. Gaffan D, Harrison S. Amygdalectomy and disconnection in visual learning for auditory secondary reinforcement by monkeys. *J Neurosci* 1987;7:2285–2292.

59. Gage FH, Björklund A. Cholinergic septal grafts into the hippocampal formation improve spatial learning and memory in aged rats by an atropine-sensitive mechanism. *J Neurosci* 1986; 6:2837–2847.

60. Gage FH, Björklund A, Stenevi U, Dunnett SB. Intracerebral grafting of neuronal cell suspensions. VIII. Survival and growth of implants of nigral and septal cell-suspensions in intact brains of aged rats. *Acta Physiol Scand* (Suppl) 1983;522:67–75.

61. Gage FH, Björklund A, Stenevi U, Dunnett SB, Kelly PAT. Intrahippocampal septal grafts ameliorate learning impairments in aged rats. *Science* 1984;225:533–536.

62. Gage FH, Dunnett SB, Björklund A. Spatial learning and motor deficits in aged rats. *Neurobiol Aging* 1984;5:43–48.

63. Gage FH, Dunnett SB, Björklund A. Age-related impairments in spatial memory are independent of those in sensorimotor skills. *Neurobiol Aging* 1989;10:347–352.

64. Gage FH, Evans SH. Exploratory analysis of deficits in DRL performance induced by medial and lateral fornix damage. *Physiol Psychol* 1981;9:49–53.

65. Gage FH, Kelly PAT, Björklund A. Regional changes in brain glucose metabolism reflect cognitive impairments in aged rats. *J Neurosci* 1984;4:2856–2865.

66. Garcia J, Hankins WG, Rusinak KW. Behavioral regulation of the milieu interne in man and rat. *Science* 1974;185:824–831.

67. Garcia J, Koelling R. Relationship of cue to consequence in avoidance learning. *Psychon Sci* 1966;4:123–124.

68. Gash D, Sladek JR, Sladek CD. Functional development of grafted vasopressin neurons. *Science* 1980;210:1367–1369.

69. Gold PE, McGaugh JL, Hankin LL, Rose RP, Vasquez BJ. Age-dependent changes in retention in rats. *Exp Aging Res* 1981;8:53–58.

70. Gray JA. *The neuropsychology of anxiety.* New York: Oxford University Press; 1983.

71. Hagan JJ, Alpert JE, Morris RGM, Iversen SD. Effects of neostriatal and mesocorticolimbic dopamine depletions on learning in a water maze. *Behav Brain Res* 1982;5:103.

72. Halasz B, Pupp L, Uhlarik S, Tima L. Growth of hypophysectomised rats bearing pituitary transplants in the hypothalamus. *Acta Physiol Acad Sci Hung* 1963;23:287–292.

73. Halasz B, Pupp L, Uhlarik S, Tima L. Further studies on the hormone secretion of the anterior pituitary transplanted into the hypophysiotrophic areas of the rat hypothalamus. *Endocrinology* 1965;77:343–355.

74. Hodges H, Allen Y, Kershaw T, Lantos PL, Gray JA, Sinden J. Effects of cholinergic-rich neural grafts on radial maze performance of rats after excitotoxic lesions of the forebrain cholinergic projection system. 1. Amelioration of cognitive deficits by transplants into cortex and hippocampus but not into basal forebrain. *Neuroscience* 1991;45:587–607.

75. Hodges H, Allen Y, Sinden J, Lantos PL, Gray JA. Effects of cholinergic-rich neural grafts on radial maze performance of rats after excitotoxic lesions of the forebrain cholinergic projection system. 2. Cholinergic drugs as probes to investigate lesion-induced deficits and transplant-induced functional recovery. *Neuroscience* 1991;45:609–623.

76. Ikegami S, Nihonmatsu I, Hatanaka H, Takei N, Kawamura H. Transplantation of septal cholinergic neurons to the hippocampus improves memory impairments of spatial-learning in rats treated with AF64A. *Brain Res* 1989; 496:321–326.

77. Itakura T, Umemoto M, Kamei I, Imai H, Yokote H, Yukawa Sh, Komai N. Autotransplantation of peripheral cholinergic neurons into the brains of Alzheimer model rats. *Acta Neurochir* 1992;115:127–132.

78. Iversen SD, Iversen LL. *Behavioral pharmacology.* New York: Oxford University Press; 1981.

79. Jarrard LE, Moise SL. Short-term memory in the monkey. In: Jarrard LE, ed. *Cognitive processes of nonhuman primates.* New York: Academic Press; 1971:1–24.

80. Johnson CT, Olton DS, Gage FH, Jenko PG. Damage to hippocampus and hippocampal connections: effects on DRL and spontaneous alternation. *J Comp Physiol Psychol* 1977;91: 508–522.

81. Kesslak JP, Brown L, Steichen C, Cotman CW. Adult and embryonic frontal cortex transplants after frontal cortex ablation enhance recovery on a reinforced alternation task. *Exp Neurol* 1986;94:615–626.

82. Kesslak JP, Nieto-Sampedro M, Globus J, Cotman CW. Transplants of purified astrocytes promote behavioral recovery after frontal cortex ablation. *Exp Neurol* 1986;92:377–390.

83. Kimble DP. Hippocampus and internal inhibition. *Psychol Bull* 1968;70:285–295.

84. Kimble DP, Bremiller R, Stickrod G. Fetal brain implants improve maze performance in hippocampal-lesioned rats. *Brain Res* 1986; 363:356–363.

85. Kolb B, Pittman K, Sutherland RJ, Whishaw IQ. Dissociation of the contributions of the prefrontal cortex and dorsomedial thalamic nucleus to spatially guided behavior in the rat. *Behav Brain Res* 1982;6:365–378.

86. Kolb B, Sutherland RJ, Whishaw IQ. A comparison of the contributions of the frontal and parietal association cortex to spatial localization in rats. *Behav Neurosci* 1983;97:13–27.

87. Kubanis P, Zornetzer SF. Age-related behavioral and neurobiological changes: a review with an emphasis on memory. *Behav Neural Biol* 1981;31:115–172.

88. Labbe R, Firl A, Mufson EJ, Stein DG. Fetal brain transplants—reduction of cognitive deficits in rats with frontal-cortex lesions. *Science* 1983;221:470–472.

89. Lee MH, Rabe A. Functional consequences of neocortical transplants in rats with a congenital brain defect—electrophysiology and behavior. *Prog Brain Res* 1990;82:377–384.

90. Lerer B, Warner J, Friedman E, Vincent G, Gamzu E. Cortical cholinergic impairment and behavioral deficits produced by kainic acid lesions of rat magnocellular basal forebrain. *Behav Neurosci* 1985;99:661–677.

91. Leslie FM, Loughlin SE, Sternberg DB, McGaugh JL, Young LE, Zornetzer SF. Noradrenergic changes and memory loss in aged mice. *Brain Res* 1985;359:292–299.

92. Low WC, Lewis PR, Bunch ST, Dunnett SB, Thomas SR, Iversen SD, Björklund A, Stenevi U. Function recovery following neural transplantation of embryonic septal nuclei in adult rats with septohippocampal lesions. *Nature* 1982;300:260–262.

93. Mackintosh NJ. *The psychology of animal learning.* New York: Academic Press: 1974.

94. Meck WH, Church RM, Olton DS. Hippocam-

pus, time and memory. *Behav Neurosci* 1984; 98:3–22.

95. Mishkin M. Memory in monkeys severely impaired by combined but not by separate removal of amygdala and hippocampus. *Nature* 1978;273:297–298.

96. Mishkin M. A memory system in the monkey. *Philos Trans R Soc Lond Ser B Biol Sci* 1982;298:85–95.

97. Miyamoto M, Shintani M, Nagaoka A, Nagawa Y. Lesioning of the rat basal forebrain leads to memory impairments in passive and active avoidance. *Brain Res* 1985;328:97–104.

98. Morris RGM. Spatial localisation does not depend on the presence of local cues. *Learn Motiv* 1981;12:239–260.

99. Morris RGM, Garrud P, Rawlins JNP, O'Keefe J. Place navigation impaired in rats with hippocampal lesions. *Nature* 1982;297:681–683.

100. Nilsson OG, Björklund A. Behavior-dependent changes in acetylcholine release in normal and graft-reinnervated hippocampus—evidence for host regulation of grafted cholinergic neurons. *Neuroscience* 1992;49:33–44.

101. Nilsson OG, Brundin P, Björklund A. Amelioration of spatial memory impairment by intrahippocampal grafts of mixed septal and raphe tissue in rats with combined cholinergic and serotonergic denervation of the forebrain. *Brain Res* 1990;515:193–206.

102. Nilsson OG, Kalén P, Rosengren E, Björklund A. Acetylcholine-release in the rat hippocampus as studied by microdialysis is dependent on axonal impulse flow and increases during behavioral activation. *Neuroscience* 1990;36:325–338.

103. Nilsson OG, Leanza G, Björklund A. Acetylcholine-release in the hippocampus—regulation by monoaminergic afferents as assessed by in vivo microdialysis. *Brain Res* 1992;584:132–140.

104. Nilsson OG, Shapiro ML, Gage FH, Olton DS, Björklund A. Spatial-learning and memory following fimbria–fornix transection and grafting of fetal septal neurons to the hippocampus. *Exp Brain Res* 1987;67:195–215.

105. Nilsson OG, Strecker RE, Daszuta A, Björklund A. Combined cholinergic and serotonergic denervation of the forebrain produces severe deficits in a spatial learning task in the rat. *Brain Res* 1988;453:235–246.

106. Norman RJ, Buchwald JS, Villablanca JR. Classical conditioning with auditory discrimination of the eyeblink in decerebrate cats. *Science* 1977;196:551–555.

107. O'Keefe J. A review of hippocampal place cells. *Prog Neurobiol* 1979;13:419–439.

108. O'Keefe J. Spatial memory within and without the hippocampal system. In: Seifert W, ed. *Neurobiology of the hippocampus.* New York: Academic Press; 1983:375–403.

109. O'Keefe J, Dostrovsky J. The hippocampus as a spatial map. Preliminary evidence from unit activity in the freely moving rat. *Brain Res* 1971;34:171–175.

110. O'Keefe J, Nadel L. *The hippocampus as a cognitive map.* London: Oxford University Press; 1978.

111. Olton DS. Memory functions and the hippocampus. In: Seifert W, ed. *Neurobiology of the hippocampus.* New York: Academic Press; 1983:335–373.

112. Olton DS, Becker JT, Handelmann GE. Hippocampus, space and memory. *Behav Brain Sci* 1979;3:313–365.

113. Olton DS, Feustle WA. Hippocampal function required for nonspatial working memory. *Exp Brain Res* 1981;41:380–389.

114. Olton DS, Pappas BC. Spatial memory and hippocampal function. *Neuropsychologia* 1979; 17:669–682.

115. Olton DS, Samuelson RJ. Remembrance of places past: spatial memory in rats. *J Exp Psychol Anim Behav Proc* 1976;2:97–116.

116. Olton DS, Walker JA, Gage FH. Hippocampal connections and spatial discrimination. *Brain Res* 1978;139:295–308.

117. Onifer SM, Low WC. Spatial memory deficit resulting from ischemia-induced damage to the hippocampus is ameliorated by intrahippocampal transplants of fetal hippocampal neurons. *Prog Brain Res* 1990;82:359–366.

118. Pallage V, Toniolo G, Will B. Effects of septal grafts and neurotrophic factors on behavior in rats with medial septal-lesions. *Behav Brain Res* 1986;20:128–129.

119. Perlow MJ, Freed WJ, Hoffer BJ, Seiger Å, Olson L, Wyatt RJ. Brain grafts reduce motor abnormalities produced by destruction of nigrostriatal dopamine system. *Science* 1979;204: 643–647.

120. Perry EK, Tomlinson BE, Blessed G, Bergmann K, Gibson PH, Perry RH. Correlation of cholinergic abnormalities with senile plaques and mental test scores in senile dementia. *Bri Med J* 1993;2:1457–1459.

121. Rawlins JNP, Olton DS. The septo-hippocampal system and cognitive mapping. *Behav Brain Res* 1982;5:331–358.

122. Rawlins JNP, Tsaltas E. The hippocampus, time and working memory. *Behav Brain Res* 1983;10:233–262.

123. Ray J, Gage FH. Gene-transfer into established and primary fibroblast cell-lines—comparison of transfection methods and promoters. *Biotechniques* 1992;13:598.

124. Richter-Levin G, Segal M. Raphe cells grafted into the hippocampus can ameliorate spatial memory deficits in rats with combined serotonergic cholinergic deficiencies. *Brain Res* 1989; 478:184–186.

125. Richter-Levin G, Segal M. Spatial performance is severely impaired in rats with combined reduction of serotonergic and cholinergic transmission. *Brain Res* 1989;477:404–407.

126. Rothblat LA, Hayes LL. Short-term object recognition memory in the rat—nonmatching with trial-unique junk stimuli. *Behav Neurosci* 1987;101:587–590.

127. Scoville WB, Milner B. Loss of recent memory

after bilateral hippocampal lesions. *J Neurol Neurosurg Psychiatry* 1957;20:11–21.

128. Segal M, Greenberger V, Milgram NW. A functional analysis of connections between the grafted septal neurons and the hippocampus. *Prog Brain Res* 1987;71:349–357.

129. Seligman MEP. On the generality of the laws of learning. *Psychol Rev* 1979;77:406–418.

130. Shapiro ML, Simon DK, Olton DS, Gage FH, Nilsson O, Björklund A. Intrahippocampal grafts of fetal basal forebrain tissue alter place fields in the hippocampus of rats with fimbria–fornix lesions. *Neuroscience* 1989;32:1–18.

131. Sinden JD, Allen YS, Rawlins JNP, Gray JA. The effects of ibotenic acid lesions of the nucleus basalis and cholinergic-rich neural transplants on win–stay/lose–shift and win–shift/lose–stay performance in the rat. *Behav Brain Res* 1990;36:229–249.

132. Sinden JD, Rawlins JNP, Gray JA, Jarrard LE. Selective cytotoxic lesions of the hippocampal formation and DRL performance in rats. *Behav Neurosci* 1986;100:320.

133. Squire LR. *Memory and brain.* Oxford: Oxford University Press; 1987.

134. Stein DG. Transplant-induced functional recovery without specific neuronal connections. *Prog Res Am Paralysis Assoc* 1987;18:4–5.

135. Stein DG, Palatucci D, Kahn D, Labbe R. Temporal factors influence recovery of function after embryonic brain tissue transplants in adult rats with frontal cortex lesions. *Behav Neurosci* 1988;102:260.

136. Sutherland RJ. Cholinergic receptor blockade impairs spatial localization using distal cues. *J Comp Physiol Psychol* 1982;96:563–573.

137. Sutherland RJ, Kolb B, Whishaw IQ. Spatial mapping—definitive disruption by hippocampal or medial frontal cortical damage in the rat. *Neurosci Lett* 1982;31:271–276.

138. Sutherland RJ, Whishaw IQ, Kolb B. A behavioral analysis of spatial localization following electrolytic, kainate-induced or colchicine-induced damage to the hippocampal formation in the rat. *Behav Brain Res* 1983;7:133–153.

139. van Haren F, van Hest A. Spatial matching and nonmatching in male and female Wistar rats: effects of delay-interval duration. *Anim Learn Behav* 1989;17:355–360.

140. Vanderwolf CH. Near-total loss of learning and memory as a result of combined cholinergic and serotonergic blockade in the rat. *Behav Brain Res* 1987;23:43–57.

141. Whishaw IQ. Cholinergic receptor blockade impairs locale but not taxon strategies for place navigation in a swimming pool. *Behav Neurosci* 1985;99:979–1005.

142. Whishaw IQ, Dunnett SB. Dopamine depletion, stimulation or blockade in the rat disrupts spatial navigation and locomotion dependent upon beacon or distal cues. *Behav Brain Res* 1985;18:11–29.

143. Whishaw IQ, Mittleman G, Bunch ST, Dunnett SB. Impairments in the acquisition, retention and selection of spatial navigation strategies after medial caudate–putamen lesions in rats. *Behav Brain Res* 1987;24:125–138.

144. Whishaw IQ, O'Connor WT, Dunnett SB. Disruption of central cholinergic systems in the rat by basal forebrain lesions or atropine—effects on feeding, sensorimotor behavior, locomotor activity and spatial navigation. *Behav Brain Res* 1985;17:103–115.

145. Woodruff ML, Baisden RH, Nonneman AJ. Transplantation of fetal hippocampus may prevent or produce behavioral recovery from hippocampal ablation and recovery persists after removal of the transplant. *Prog Brain Res* 1990;82:367–376.

146. Woodruff ML, Baisden RH, Whittington DL, Benson AE. Embryonic hippocampal grafts ameliorate the deficit in DRL acquisition produced by hippocampectomy. *Brain Res* 1987;408:97–117.

147. Wozniak DF, Stewart GR, Finger S, Olney JW. Comparison of behavioral effects of nucleus basalis magnocellularis lesions and somatosensory cortex ablation in the rat. *Neuroscience* 1989;32:685–700.

148. Zola-Morgan S, Squire LR, Mishkin M. The neuroanatomy of amnesia—amygdala–hippocampus versus temporal stem. *Science* 1982;218:1337–1339.

149. Zornetzer SF. Catecholaminergic involvement in age-related memory dysfunction. *Ann NY Acad Sci* 1985;444:242–254.

150. Zornetzer SF, Thompson R, Rogers J. Rapid forgetting in aged rats. *Behav Neural Biol* 1982;36:49–60.

Functional Neural Transplantation,
edited by S. B. Dunnett and A. Björklund.
Raven Press, Ltd., New York © 1994.

10

Cholinergic Grafts and Cognitive Function

John D. Sinden, Jeffrey A. Gray, and Helen Hodges

Department of Psychology, Institute of Psychiatry, London SE5 8AF, United Kingdom

Acetylcholine (ACh) was the first compound in the mammalian central nervous system (CNS) to satisfy most of the pharmacologic criteria for neurotransmitter status (59). Although studies early this century demonstrated the actions of ACh in the peripheral nervous system as either muscarine- or nicotine-like, and psychopharmacologic experimentation beginning after World War II demonstrated powerful behavioral effects from the administration of anticholinergics (28,187), a detailed analysis of ACh's functional role in the brain has had to wait for more recent developments in the neurosciences. The development of immunohistochemical and *in situ* hybridization techniques has enabled the unequivocal identification of CNS cholinergic projection systems by, for example, use of antibodies to the synthesizing enzyme choline acetyltransferase (ChAT). Furthermore, studies of the action of ACh or its many receptor ligands at physiologic levels on single cells and pathways both *in vivo* and in brain slices have defined many of the actions of ACh at both the single-cell and the neural circuit level.

These developments have led to a rational approach for lesioning and drug studies, and fed directly into burgeoning neural transplantation research. As a direct consequence, over the last 15 years there has been a spectacular expansion of research directed toward an understanding of the functional role of brain cholinergic systems. This research has largely been driven by the search for an effective treatment for Alzheimer's disease. Like some of the early reports of the acute effects of administration of anticholinergic drugs, the symptoms of Alzheimer's disease are wide-ranging, with a progressive deterioration in language, perceptuospatial orientation and skills, as well as judgment (141,149). From a neurobiologic point of view, the nature of the impairments suggests damage to systems responsible for several aspects of cognitive function, including orientation to environmental stimuli, attention, learning, motor planning, and emotional responsiveness. Nevertheless, the prominent early sign seized on as a suitable case for treatment was impairment in memory, especially working or short-term memory (146). *Post mortem,* the damage to the Alzheimer brain is equally wide-ranging (209), characterized microscopically by the pathognomonic signs of neurofibrillary tangles in neurons of the cortex, hippocampus, and amygdala, and extracellular deposits of β-amyloid-containing plaques in cerebral parenchyma and around blood vessels (20). Neurochemically, a variety of reports have suggested both selective and nonselective depletions in a variety of classic and putative peptidergic neurotransmitter markers in the cortical mantle (18). However, the best *postmortem* neurochemical correlate of the degree of dementia measured in life was the extent of loss of cholinergic markers in the forebrain cholinergic projection system (FCPS), in both the areas containing the neuronal cell bodies: namely, the nucleus basalis of Meynert, the medial septal area, and the nucleus of the diagonal band (225); and in the cholinergic terminals of these neurons: namely, neocortex, the hippocampal formation, and amygdala (19, 170). This was, therefore, one strand in a network of evidence implicating forebrain cholinergic systems in cognitive function. Other evidence came from the deleterious effects of cholinergic antagonists, and beneficial effects of agonists, on cognitive function in both animals and humans (39). In its explicit form, the "cholinergic hypothesis of geriatric memory dysfunction" (13) has spawned a profusion of experiments on the effects of lesions of the basal nucleus in rodents on avoidance and maze learning and memory as "animal models of Alzheimer's disease" (see 46,172,202, for reviews).

Given the variety of neuropathologic changes and neurochemical deficits seen in Alzheimer's and other dementing neurodegenerative diseases, with hindsight, it now seems oversimplistic to attribute the global cognitive decline exclusively to cholinergic dysfunction. Nevertheless, where possible, specific lesions of the cholinergic neurochemical systems may permit the fractionation of those aspects of the symptomatology that relate to the activity of these systems. Similarly, experiments using transplantation of cholinergic cells (with noncholinergic grafts as controls) can permit a positive experimental approach to understanding the neurochemical and structural conditions that underlie different experimental models of neurodegenerative conditions, as well as providing the conditions for the development of potential therapies.

In this chapter, we will consider in detail the functional effects of transplants rich in cholinergic cells. Our focus will be on transplants in rodents with both relatively specific (chemical) and nonspecific (mechanical) experimental lesions of one or more branches of the ascending forebrain cholinergic projection system. As well, we

will include data from our own laboratory on rats following a lengthy period of repeated alcohol administration, which produces damage to the FCPS analogous to excitotoxic lesions of the medial septal area and basal nucleus (7,98); cholinergic grafts in the aging rodent (Gage), in nonhuman primates (Ridley), and in more specific tests of memory function (Dunnett) are discussed in greater detail elsewhere in this volume. When possible, we will attempt to relate behavioral data to that known about graft-induced restoration of damaged or depleted cholinergic fiber projections, ACh release, and its physiologic functions on target neurons or circuits. Thus, before directly considering the data on cholinergic graft effects, we will consider two essential preliminary questions. First, what is the nature of cholinergic neuronal systems in terms of morphology and physiology; in particular what are their special features in comparison with both other neurochemically specific ascending projection systems and the target neurons they innervate, and how might these account for the role of the cholinergic system (and eventually the cholinergic synapse) in cognitive function? Second, given the widespread distribution of cholinergic cell bodies within a range of subcortical structures, what are the special problems in interpreting cognitive deficits following lesions to the source areas of cholinergic projections? Answers to both these questions may have considerable bearing on our interpretation of current data on the behavioral effects of cholinergic-rich grafts and may suggest alternative experimental approaches for studying the effects of these grafts.

CHOLINERGIC ANATOMY

Overlapping Systems

The diversity and complexity of cholinergic projections throughout the brain and spinal cord were first suspected from the earliest chemical neuroanatomy studies using histochemical identification of the degradative enzyme for ACh, acetylcholinesterase (AChE) (196). The development of sensitive immunohistochemical markers for ChAT, sometimes in combination with cytotoxic or mechanical lesions, or tract-tracing techniques, led to definitive identification, in a range of species, of the cholinergic projection systems, particularly those forebrain pathways degenerating in, and thereby implicated in, the cognitive decline associated with, neurodegenerative disease (11,144,188,189).

As seen in their broadest view (Fig. 1A; 230), cholinergic neurons form continuous columns of cells extending rostrally from the striatum (including nucleus accumbens, olfactory tubercle, islands of Calleja, and the caudate–putamen complex) through the basal forebrain (including medial septal nucleus, vertical and horizontal limbs of the diagonal band nucleus, nucleus basalis, substantia innominata, and nucleus ansa reticularis). Caudally, these columns extend through basal diencephalic regions (including the posterior hypothalamus and motor neurons of cranial nerves III and IV) into the pedunculopontine and laterodorsal tegmental nuclei of the midbrain. In the brain stem, these columns continue through the various cranial nerve motor nuclei in a scattered fashion. Finally, ChAT-positive motor neurons show columnar organization throughout the length of the spinal cord. Seen from this global view, the entire cholinergic system appears to be linked into a "unified complex of contiguous subsystems" (230); however, in spite of morphologic continuity, cholinergic subsystems have regionally specific innervation patterns. In the rostral striatal complex, cholinergic cell bodies extend their axons only locally and, hence, display features of interneurons; however, nearby morphologically similar basal forebrain somata, like nearly all other cholinergic neurons, project their axons distally. The only other evidence for intrinsic cholinergic interneurons

lies in various reports of ChAT-like immunoreactivity in the rat cerebral cortex and hippocampus (100,124), in the absence of AChE reactivity (124). The ChAT-immunopositive cells are not seen in the cerebral cortex of cats or primates (114,191). Recent studies with *in situ* hybridization of ChAT mRNA in rats, although confirming the basic immunohistochemical findings, have failed to identify intrinsic ChAT mRNA-positive somata in the cortex and hippocampus (162,219).

The contiguous nature of cholinergic cell bodies throughout the mammalian CNS is exemplified by confluence and overlap of each subsystem's dendritic plexus (230). Dendritic arbors from ChAT-positive neurons intermingle not only within, but also between, traditional cytoarchitectonic boundaries. This is as true of subsystems with only projection neurons (e.g., the different nuclei of the basal forebrain) as of nearby interneuronal and projection cells (e.g., dendrites from nucleus accumbens cholinergic neurons readily interconnect with dendrites from diagonal band cells). The various cranial and spinal motor nuclei also make substantial dendritic contacts (230). Contiguity between regions is also aided by isolated, apparently ectopic ChAT-positive neurons appearing to form continuity bridges between clusters of cholinergic cells (230); this latter feature makes targeted lesions of entire cholinergic cell subsystems extremely difficult.

Most regions of the CNS receive a cholinergic innervation derived from one subsystem of ChAT-positive cells (see Fig. 1B). Although cholinergic projection neurons throughout the brain have very similar morphologic characteristics, the degree of topographic specificity of their projections varies. The major cholinergic projection from the pedunculopontine and laterodorsal tegmental nuclei is a diffuse and divergent one to a large variety of thalamic nuclei, as well as a variety of other midbrain, diencephalic, and basal forebrain structures, including the substantia nigra (83,90,168).

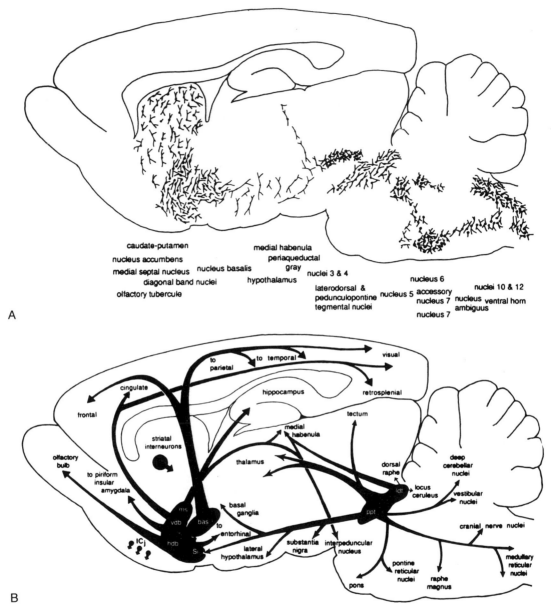

FIG. 1. Schematic representations of parasagittal sections of rat brain. **A**: The distribution of the cholinergic cell bodies and dendrites in the CNS. The various cholinergic subsystems are contiguous throughout the rostrocaudal extent of the brain. **B**: The projections of the cholinergic cell subsystems shown in A. The entire cholinergic mantle is innervated by the basal forebrain subsystem and the subcortical mass is innervated by the pontomesencephic system. Abbreviations: *ms*, medial septal nucleus; *hdb*, nucleus of the horizontal limb of the diagonal band; *vdb*, nucleus of the vertical limb of the diagonal band; *si*, substantia innominata; *bas*, nucleus basalis; *ppt*, pedunculopontine tegmental nucleus; *ldt*, laterodorsal tegmental nucleus. (From ref. 230, with permission.)

The closely grouped basal forebrain cholinergic projection system, on the other hand, is more topographically focused: for example, in rat neocortex, it has been estimated that each cholinergic projection cell innervates a region averaging 1 to 2 mm^2 (14).

Basal Forebrain Cholinergic Subsystems

The basal forebrain projections can be readily divided into three branches. The most rostral branch originates in the medial septal nucleus and the vertical limb of the diagonal band (abbreviated here to MSA). The ChAT-immunopositive fibers climb dorsally into the cingulum and caudally by the fornix to innervate the entire hippocampal formation, and the entorhinal and perirhinal cortex (4). In the hippocampal formation, ChAT-positive afferents exhibit a laminar terminal organization. Fibers are particularly abundant in the hilus and the supragranular band of the dentate gyrus (33); they are densely located in the supra- and infrapyramidal zones throughout hippocampus proper and in the superficial stratum lacunosum moleculare of CA_1 (132). Ultrastructurally, most cholinergic terminals are seen on dendrites, rather than perikarya (33,74).

A second, medial pathway arises from the horizontal limb of the diagonal band and the magnocellular preoptic area to innervate a range of allocortical structures, particularly the olfactory bulb, amygdala, and insular and piriform cortexes (see Fig. 1B). A more extensive set of projections, which make up a collection of mainly laterally coursing pathways innervating the entire neocortex, originate from the ChAT-positive somata of the nucleus basalis, substantia innominata, and nucleus ansa lenticularis (abbreviated here to NBM). The topography of the cholinergic projections from the NBM follows a rostrocaudal gradient, for the most part, in that rostral NBM cells innervate the frontal cortex, and the parietal and temporal cortex are innervated by successively more caudal regions of NBM (14). At all levels of the cortex, as in the hippocampal formation, lamination of ChAT-positive afferent innervation is apparent, with dense terminal and fiber staining in layers 2–3 and 5 (60,128), corresponding to the layers of dense muscarinic and nicotinic receptor immunoreactivity (216).

If we take these three major basal forebrain systems together, the cholinergic neurons appear to be, to a greater or lesser extent, reciprocally linked with the allo- and neocortical regions they innervate: the cortical inputs to NBM being the most topographically focused (189). However, innervation from target structures is generally sparse, with most hippocampal and cortical projections to unspecified dendrites in the vicinity of the cholinergic cells (189). If the corticofugal afferents innervate the cholinergic neurons directly, it is likely to be at distal dendritic junctions, where immunohistochemical detection is difficult (123). Tracer studies have also identified a variety of sparse projections from chemically specific sources in the midbrain and hindbrain, including dopaminergic afferents from the substantia nigra, noradrenergic inputs from locus coeruleus, 5-hydroxytryptaminergic inputs from the dorsal raphe, and a small cholinergic input from the pedunculopontine and laterodorsal tegmental nuclei (107, 108).

Features of Cholinergic Interconnections

From these general principles of distal dendritic cholinergic cell interconnection and sparse, but widespread, afferent innervation from a variety of sources, it is apparent that the output of the cholinergic system operates as a slow integrator of multiple inputs. This contrasts sharply with the highly specific and rapidly activated responsiveness of hierarchical circuitry that characterizes much of the cholinergic system's targets (i.e., within the thalamus and the entire cortical mantle). In a recent synthesis, based on morphologic and hodologic data of the entire cholinergic system, Woolf

(230) has proposed that simultaneous sensory input from target sites, together with modulatory input from several subcortical areas, can enable a coordinated pattern of activity throughout entire networks of cholinergic cells. The activity patterns of cholinergic networks are likely to depend more on local cholinergic cell-to-cell interactions than on afferent inputs, since the former are much richer. A further feature of cholinergic cell assemblies is the presence of γ-aminobutyric acid (GABA)ergic interneurons, the function of which may be to fine-tune the activity of individual cholinergic cells to maintain synchronous activity within the subsystem ensemble (230). The net output of such a synchronized system would thus be coordinated programs of neural activity. Examples of global activity patterns believed to be attributable to the outputs of cholinergic systems include the generation of cerebral rhythms associated with states of arousal (23,182,204); coordinated activity within motor neuron pools producing integrated muscle movements (193); and selective parallel facilitation or inhibition of incoming sensory and association fiber afferents on pyramidal cells in the cortex and hippocampus as a basis for cognitive processing (93) (see later discussion on parallel and inhibitory modulation by ACh, under the section "Cholinergic Physiology and Pharmacology").

Cholinergic Cells and Nerve Growth Factor

One of the most interesting features of cholinergic cells, and of particular relevance to grafting experiments, is the continuing utilization of nerve growth factor (NGF) in these neurons. The use of and responsiveness to growth factors in most CNS cells is developmentally regulated; some growth factors provide the stimulus for, and perhaps the limits to, cell division and migration; others (collectively known as the neurotrophins) furnish the stimulus for morphologic differentiation during neurogenesis. Neuronal responsiveness to growth

factors is normally complete soon after birth. Basal forebrain cholinergic neurons, however, retain NGF receptors throughout adulthood (178) and, following uptake by these receptors, they retrogradely transport exogenous NGF (208). The target areas of these neurons, namely the hippocampus and cortex, contain the highest levels of NGF mRNA in the brain (81). The administration of exogenous NGF is able to promote the growth of cholinergic cells and to prevent their death after axotomy (217). This unique "plasticity" of basal forebrain cholinergic neurons may be responsible for the compensatory hypertrophy of contralateral NBM neurons following unilateral lesions (169), and recent data from our laboratory have demonstrated compensatory increases in AChE-positive terminals in ipsilateral terminals of the medial cholinergic pathway following excitotoxic NBM lesions (M. Caliminici et al., *in preparation*). The presence of NGF receptors or the ability to transport NGF in other cholinergic cells, such as striatal or pedunculopontine cholinergic neurons, is less clearcut (89,231). This variability in NGF uptake may represent a fundamental functional difference between cholinergic cells in different regions and, therefore, may permit us to answer specific questions about the role of NGF in grafted cholinergic cells (see below). Alternatively, it may represent the means by which different cholinergic cells developmentally establish their topography and distribution.

CHOLINERGIC PHYSIOLOGY AND PHARMACOLOGY

Diffuse Versus Hierarchic Neuronal Systems

It is a general principle to divide CNS neuronal systems and their accompanying neurotransmitter actions into two main functional categories. The first of these, often referred to as hierarchic or point-to-point, and best exemplified by direct sensory and major motor pathways, is characterized by rapid information-processing. Excitatory postsynaptic potentials (EPSPs) from the major projection or relay pathways are mediated by excitatory amino acid (EAA) neurotransmitters. Some of these compounds bind to receptors directly coupled to ion channels, with short-lived EPSPs. Local circuit neurons, associated with hierarchic systems through recurrent feedback and feedforward pathways, are generally inhibitory, releasing GABA or glycine as transmitters, and binding to ion–channel-gated receptors to produce a rapid increase of Cl conductance.

The second major category of neuronal systems, the nonspecific or diffuse type, is characterized by fundamentally different organizational principles, typified by projections using the monoamines, norepinephrine (NE), dopamine (DA), or serotonin (5-hydroxytryptamine; 5-HT). In these systems, a relatively few neurons in hindbrain or midbrain nuclei project fine, unmyelinated axons that branch extensively to sparsely populate wide areas of terminal regions, with periodic varicosities containing large numbers of vesicles. This morphologic pattern suggests that the neurotransmitter may be released in a global, diffuse manner. Rather than operating through ligand-gated ion channel receptors and, thereby, allowing rapid postsynaptic response to the transmitter, diffuse neurotransmitter systems generally involve a receptor molecule coupled to G proteins and possibly membrane-bound second messengers (151). The net effect is a longer-term modulation of the membrane potential (by, for example, voltage-dependent ion channels) of the postsynaptic cell, which enhances or depresses activity (126).

Slow Versus Fast Synaptic Activity: Muscarinic and Nicotinic Actions

This hierarchic and diffuse separation is far from rigid. The EAAs may provide not only the basis for fast cell-to-cell excitatory communication in the cortex and hippo-

campus, but *N*-methyl-D-aspartate (NMDA) receptors can mediate a slower, voltage-dependent component of EPSPs (133), which is probably a prerequisite for the occurrence of long-term potentiation (40). The cholinergic system, which is often seen as a diffuse, modulatory system, both on morphologic grounds and in terms of its actions at muscarinic receptors (see below), does have a rapid ion-gated action at nicotinic receptors in the brain, similar to its actions on spinal Renshaw cells (137). As well as showing long-lasting muscarinic responses, thalamic neurons have short-lasting EPSPs (blocked by the nicotinic antagonist, mecamylamine) in response to laterodorsal tegmental cholinergic stimulation (42). However, in spite of receptor-binding, immunohistochemical, and *in situ* hybridization studies that show widespread and dense nicotine receptor reactivity in the cortex (82,206), and demonstrations of reduced nicotine receptor binding in the cortex of Alzheimer's patients (224), evidence for nicotine-like actions of ACh in the terminal areas of the FCPS is lacking. Recent studies of evoked field potentials in cortical slices have shown an enhanced negative wave to iontophoresed nicotine at high concentrations, representing summed excitability in a population of cortical neurons (218). A nicotinic action for ACh in this preparation was seen following large ejection currents in the presence of AChE inhibition (218), suggesting the possibility that muscarinic actions of ACh may desensitize and become nicotinic under strong transmitter stimulation (at least when ACh is delivered exogenously), particularly under conditions in which AChE is reduced, for example, by cholinergic deafferentation.

The predominant modulatory actions of ACh on muscarinic receptors have been extensively studied in cortical and hippocampal pyramidal neurons. Krnjevic et al. (117) were first to demonstrate that iontophoresed ACh *in vivo* increased cortical neuronal activity over long periods, associated with an increase in membrane resistance, by means of a reduction in potassium ion (K^+) conductance. Since then, several patch–clamp studies have identified muscarinic excitation as mainly caused by blockade of voltage-dependent K^+ current (I_M) (91), and by at least three other types of potassium- or calcium-activated K^+ conductances (134). These K^+ conductances normally serve to impede spike generation in response to depolarization, with the calcium-activated K^+ current potentiating the slow after-hyperpolarization that appears following a train of action potentials. Therefore, the effects of these muscarinic receptor-induced membrane changes are to enhance the neuronal response to depolarizing inputs (136).

Parallel Excitatory and Inhibitory Modulation by Acetylcholine: Implications for Cognition

Inhibition of neuronal activity following iontophoretic application of ACh has often been reported at all targets of the cholinergic system. Frequently, this inhibition is an initial hyperpolarization preceding the slow depolarization response (68,71,136). This "cholinergic inhibition" (136) is unlikely to be a direct muscarinic response affecting the membrane conductance of the recorded neuron, since blockade of GABAergic transmission eliminates the early hyperpolarization (87). Hence, muscarinic stimulation of hippocampal and cortical neurons is excitatory, but of two apparently distinct forms: a slow depolarization of pyramidal neurons, and a relatively rapid excitation of presumably GABAergic interneurons, the latter neurons mediating presynaptic inhibition of the pyramidal cell response (135). It remains unclear as to which of the muscarinic receptor subtypes are responsible for the differing muscarinic actions (151).

Much is yet to be learned about the parallel nature of ACh's actions in mediating excitation and inhibition in different hippocampal and cortical circuits. There is evidence that cholinergic agonists can suppress activity in Schaffer collateral (CA_1; 213) and mossy fiber (CA_3; 229) synapses, and can block activity in intrinsic fiber laminae of pyriform cortex slices (94), presumably by a presynaptic mechanism. On the other hand, afferent (particularly sensory) input to many of these circuits is facilitated by iontophoretically applied ACh [e.g., visual input to the cat striate cortex (190, 197); somatic stimuli input to the cat somatosensory cortex (210); and afferent fiber inputs from lateral olfactory tract in rat pyriform cortex slices (94)]. A mix of cholinergic facilitation of strong afferent inputs and presynaptic inhibition of weak inputs and, in some identified circuits, intrinsic fiber inputs, will enhance the signal/noise ratio and provide a rudimentary neurobiologic basis for cortical activation and attention (26).

A more specific role for ACh in learning and memory is now beginning to be explored. A role for basal forebrain neurons in learning tasks is suggested by studies of the activity of NBM neurons correlated with performance in go–no-go learning in primates (179). However, activity of these neurons appeared to be more dependent on anticipation of reinforcement, rather than any specific associative or memory-based process. Nevertheless, the dependence of NBM activity on specific aspects of behavioral tasks, presumably through feedback regulation from a variety of forebrain sources, including cortical, striatopallidal, and amygdalofugal afferents (2), represents a unique feature of the modulatory role of the FCPS, compared with the modulatory afferents from mid- and hindbrain locus coeruleus (NE) and raphe (5-HT). Neurons in these regions respond with a great deal less specificity for the behavior state of the animal (12,104). Moreover, cholinergic enhancement of learning-related neuronal firing has been shown in association cortex *in vivo*. In rat frontal cortex, the (predominantly excitatory) neuronal responses to a discriminative auditory stimulus paired with reinforcing brain stimulation were facilitated by a muscarinic action of ACh (171). The study of cholinergic innervation at the local circuit level is also beginning to demonstrate that ACh's dual excitation—inhibition role may aid learning and memory processing. By taking advantage of the laminar organization of the olfactory cortex, where lateral olfactory tract input and intrinsic fibers synapse at different strata of pyramidal cell dendrites, Hasselmo et al. (93) have recently proposed a model for associative learning and memory of distributed odor patterns in the cortex. Learning is enhanced by cholinergic facilitation of afferent synaptic input; the accompanying cholinergic inhibition (by GABAergic interneurons) of intrinsic fiber activity (94) permits the best learning and memory performance by blocking interference from previously stored patterns. The success of this model in predicting a role for ACh in the fine-tuning of local hierarchic circuits for optimal learning and memory performance suggests (if it can be applied to a range of real experimental situations) an important role for ACh in cognition beyond a simple activational one. The main source of information supporting a role for ACh in cognition comes, however, not from physiologic studies, but from a wide range of lesion and behavior studies.

EFFECTS OF LESIONS TO THE FOREBRAIN CHOLINERGIC PROJECTION SYSTEM

Theoretical Issues: Permissive Versus Directive and Separate Versus Unitary Functions

Because the basal forebrain cholinergic projection system is divided topographically into three major pathways, it is tempting to suppose that any disruption of one or more of these branches will produce behavioral deficits that mimic damage to the tar-

get structures themselves (181). Such a view presupposes an activational or enabling function to the FCPS, and suggests that the cholinergic cells themselves do not play any particular informational role. This view would also hold that the cholinergic cells have a monolithic, unitary function, and it has been recently criticized by Fibiger (69) as conceptually sterile, having led us no farther in our understanding of the functional role of the cholinergic system than some recent equivalents of the "steering" function described 25 years ago by Carlton (28). Furthermore, there are three major lines of evidence against such a strong unitary view. The first is that executive structures in the cortical mantle have a variety of parallel inputs from many so-called diffuse systems and, with the development of selective methods to manipulate these systems, fractionation of their role in the performance of cognitive tasks is at least possible (184). Second, such a view ignores the interconnected anatomic and physiologic nature of the cholinergic system, reviewed above, suggesting the potential for a controlling, rather than merely permissive, function of this system. The final, and perhaps most telling, evidence against this view is that, although loss of cholinergic projection cells to the cortex and hippocampus may reproduce some of the consequences of damage within the target structures (181), there are numerous instances in which it may not (1a,7,37).

The major interest in the basal forebrain cholinergic system has been spurred largely by the global cognitive deficits seen in Alzheimer's disease and the close relation between loss of cholinergic projection cells and neuropathology in these cells' targets (9). Attention has focused extensively on the projection from NBM to the neocortex; surprisingly so, in view of a long tradition of evidence implicating the hippocampal formation in cognitive function, particularly memory (164,174). As we shall see below, evidence from lesion studies suggests that all branches of the FCPS discharge functions that are important to cognition; whether these functions are the same for each branch and whether they are qualitatively similar to or different from damage within the systems' targets remain topics of current research.

Effects of Different Lesioning Agents: Implications for Functions of the Forebrain Cholinergic Projection System

Experimental attack on the functions of the FCPS is rendered difficult by the lack of any method for selective manipulation of the cholinergic projection cells, which are scattered more (MSA) or less (NBM) densely among a rich variety of other neuronal systems (2). Claims for ethylcholine mustard aziridinium ion (or AF64A) as a selective cholinergic neurotoxin by irreversible inhibition of high affinity choline uptake have been made over a number of years (92,130), notwithstanding evidence that this toxin produces a range of nonspecific damage at the site of infusion (3,106,138). Selective lesions of cholinergic systems using immunotoxins have recently been reported to show considerable promise (155a). Thus, the best available lesion method is the local injection of an excitotoxin, such as ibotenate, quisqualate or α-amino-3-hydroxy-4-isoxozole propionic acid (AMPA), destroying neurons rather than other types of cell, and cell bodies rather than fibers (but see 38) or terminals. These different excitotoxins produce varying amounts of ChAT depletion in the neocortex when injected into NBM regions, in the order AMPA > quisqualate > ibotenate (53). Likewise AMPA and quisqualate produce greater loss of ChAT-like immunoreactive structures in the lesioned area than ibotenate, along with less non–ChAT-positive neuronal loss (166, 185). It has been proposed (53) that ibotenate, but not quisqualate or AMPA, lesions nonspecifically disrupt a range of neuronal systems that course throughout the basal forebrain, including corticostriatal, striato-

pallidal, and amygdalofugal projection neurons (2). In addition, several other topographically specific projection neurons are found within the MSA and NBM regions; for example, GABAergic neurons project from MSA and NBM to synapse mostly on GABAergic interneurons in the hippocampus (72) and cortex (73), respectively. The parallel effects of GABAergic innervation on the activity of cholinergic and other synaptic processes in cortical mantle target areas are likely to be of considerable importance to cognitive function. The extent to which the different excitotoxins differentially damage GABAergic neurons is unknown; however, ibotenate, but not quisqualate, lesions of NBM damage a possible neurotensin projection pathway to the cortex (222).

Behavioral Effects of Lesions to the Different Branches of the Forebrain Cholinergic Projection System

In terms of behavioral consequences, bilateral or unilateral ibotenate lesions of NBM produce a wider range of impairments in learning and memory tasks (see 46,172,202, for reviews) than similar-sized lesions using either quisqualate or AMPA (see 53, for review). Hence, it has been proposed (53) that noncholinergic damage is primarily responsible for most learning and memory impairments seen following ibotenate lesions, either because they are unaffected by quisqualate or AMPA lesions, or because they did not respond to cholinergic agonist administration or were not reversed by cholinergic-rich transplants. This list includes: win–shift and win–stay operant memory tasks (49,66), operant conditional visual discriminations (67), operant win–shift/lose–stay and win–stay/lose–shift conditional memory performance (198), and spatial navigation in the water maze (56,166). So far, published studies using AMPA lesions of NBM, which produce near-total frontal cortex ChAT depletion, have shown clearcut deficits in only passive avoidance retention (166), although this toxin has been reported to produce the greatest deficits in serial reaction time of the three excitotoxins (53). We have recently shown that AMPA lesions of NBM, which increased the sensitivity of frontal cortex neurons to iontophoretically applied ACh or carbachol, by a postsynaptic, atropine-sensitive mechanism, produced substantial deficits in a battery of sensorimotor tests (1). These sensorimotor deficits are partially reversible by systemic administration of the cholinergic agonist, arecoline or by cholinergic-rich grafts to the cortex (1, F. A. Abdulla et al., *in preparation*). Hence, current evidence gives support to the view that the primary deficit following damage to the NBM–neocortex cholinergic innervation is in attentional and sensorimotor function (53), implying that the role of ACh through this pathway is a simple activational one on target neurons. In addition, the passive avoidance deficit may involve changes in reactivity to aversive stimuli through the pathway from rostral NBM cholinergic neurons innervating the amygdala (166).

Many studies have investigated the behavioral and cognitive effects of mechanical, radiofrequency, or electrolytic lesions of the MSA (reviewed in 85). Compared with studies of the cognitive effects of NBM lesions, relatively few experiments have examined the effects of excitotoxic lesions of MSA. Indeed, where comparisons have been made between the cognitive effects of lesions to the MSA–hippocampus and NBM–neocortex cholinergic pathways, many experiments have employed fimbria–fornix cuts to damage the former pathway (49,66), lesions that will disrupt almost all subcortical innervation of the hippocampal formation and destroy many hippocampal and retrohippocampal outputs, the latter pathways with some behavioral roles independent of learning and memory function (175). In one report in which ibotenate and electrolytic lesions of MSA were directly compared on extinction in a runway after continuous or partial reinforcement—a be-

havioral task highly sensitive to a wide range of conventional lesions of the septo-hippocampal system—ibotenate lesions did not reproduce the well-known effects of electrolytic lesions (37), paralleling a similar discrepancy in the effects of aspiration and excitotoxic lesions of the hippocampal formation on radial maze spatial memory function (105).

The medial cholinergic projection pathway from the vertical and horizontal limbs of the diagonal band to the cingulate and retrosplenial cortexes has received little attention in cognitive function, given the relative difficulty in selectively targeting these neurons by the excitotoxic method. However, a recent study has shown that restricted knife cuts to this pathway at anterior levels produced radial maze deficits, partially reversible by systemic injection of cholinergic agonists (139).

Combined Lesions of the Forebrain Cholinergic Projection System: Evidence for and Against Unitary Cholinergic Function

From the foregoing discussion of the anatomic integration and overlap of the cholinergic system, it could be argued that the NBM and MSA cholinergic neurons may well be capable of functioning in unison. Although unable to resolve issues about the possibly differing functions of cholinergic interactions with different target areas, combined lesion studies may provide a more representative model of the effects of cholinergic deficiency in Alzheimer's disease. Similar deficits following ibotenate lesions in the two areas have been reported in rewarded alternation in the T-maze (a measure of working memory) tests (95); and for measures in the radial-arm maze test of both reference (long-term) and working memory in both spatial and nonspatial modes (the latter cued by textured inserts into the arms of the maze) (7). Furthermore, combining the two lesions had either effects that were the equivalent of either lesion on its own (95), or additive behavioral effects (7). [These experiments from our own laboratory are discussed in greater detail in later sections]. The results suggest that, at least in some tasks, the FCPS promotes equipotent functional interactions between its multiple target structures, rather than exerting discrete effects specific to the cortex and hippocampus separately.

In contrast, there is evidence that, in some tasks, lesions to the NBM and MSA produce very different cognitive effects. For example, Hagan et al. (88), when using the water maze, found an impairment in spatial navigation after lesions to the MSA, but not after those to the NBM. More strikingly, in an operant temporal discrimination task, rats with ibotenate MSA lesions underestimate, and those with NBM lesions overestimate, the time until they receive reward; and rats with NBM, but not MSA, lesions are unable to perform a divided-attention task (142,165), the only published evidence of a double dissociation between the effects of excitotoxic lesions of NBM and MSA. We know of no published studies that have examined the cognitive effects of quisqualate or AMPA lesions of MSA; our own data suggest that all three excitotoxins produce comparable, albeit limited, ChAT losses in the hippocampus (211 and unpublished data; but see 7), and even total septal ibotenate lesions produced no disruption to ascending catecholaminergic projections (37). Moreover, anatomic overlap with other noncholinergic forebrain projection systems (aside from the GABAergic system) is less obvious in MSA than in NBM.

Taking all these data together, we have suggested (7,86,96) that there is a functional unity of the three branches of the FCPS in many choice-based maze tasks. Whether this means that the FCPS serves a single cognitive function remains open to experimentation and debate. One possibility is that combining damage to separate cholinergic functional systems will increase (or induce, above an unknown threshold) manifestations of cognitive impairment by some

version of the law of mass action. For example, what we call spatial-learning or working-memory tasks may tax a variety of cognitive processes for successful performance and, therefore, may reflect more than simple, unitary cognitive functions. Thus, the greater the damage to the FCPS, the greater the likelihood of deficits occurring. An alternative, and more parsimonious, view (e.g., 50) is that these tasks predominantly rely on a general, unitary cognitive mechanism, such as stimulus processing or attention, to guide correct choices, and loss of cholinergic neurons will disrupt ACh's modulatory alerting or activational action on target circuits in the cortical mantle. Behavioral evidence for the latter view comes from the disruption of performance in the place version of Jarrard's radial maze task in well-trained unlesioned rats when visual cues are restricted; rats with FCPS lesions show no further disruption when cues are so restricted (see discussion in 96 and later in this chapter). Further comparative studies of excitotoxic lesions of NBM and MSA, both separately and combined, using tasks that more easily discriminate between attentional processes and memory—for example, serial reaction time (183) and divided attention (165) versus simple (49) and complex (198) conditional memory tasks—are required to resolve the issue of whether the two branches of the FCPS are concerned with different aspects of cognitive function.

THE FOREBRAIN CHOLINERGIC PROJECTION SYSTEM AND MAZE PERFORMANCE

Strategies to Triangulate the System's Function

The experiments reviewed in the foregoing clearly demonstrate that damage that includes the nuclei of origin of the FCPS causes the kinds of impairments in cognitive function that resemble, at least grossly, those seen in Alzheimer's disease. However, the lack of neurochemical specificity of the excitotoxic technique precludes definite interpretation of these findings in terms of cholinergic dysfunction. Our own major strategy, therefore, has been to assess the effects of different manipulations of the FCPS across a common range of behavioral tasks. We have employed not only excitotoxic lesions, which carry a particular set of interpretative problems, but also prolonged alcohol administration. This latter procedure has important implications for the neurobiology of Korsakoff's psychosis and alcoholic dementia, as well as providing a model for chronic neurodegenerative processes with considerably more face validity than short-term lesion models. From the point of view of understanding the functions of the FCPS, prolonged administration of ethanol in drinking water (20% v/v for 28 weeks) produced declines in hippocampal (15–25%) and cortical (30–40%) ChAT levels (and other cholinergic markers, as well as AChE-positive MSA and NBM structures) that broadly mimic the effects of excitotoxic lesions (7,8,98). The additional damage following alcohol was unlike that seen following the lesions: it involved substantial losses of noradrenergic, serotonergic and, to a lesser degree, dopaminergic markers in a widespread range of forebrain structures (7,98). Thus, an approach that combines two entirely distinct means of damaging the FCPS, together with subsequent cholinergic pharmacologic challenges and transplantation of cholinergic cells, might be capable of triangulating the cholinergic system and separating it out from other systems potentially implicated by each approach on its own.

Effects of Lesions of the Forebrain Cholinergic Projection System on Radial and Water Maze Tasks

The major task we have employed is concurrent training of the place–cue, refer-ence–working memory versions of the radial arm maze, as developed for studies of lesions within the hippocampal formation by Jarrard (105). Since, in early studies with this task, we found similar and additive deficits in all four measures of performance following ibotenate lesions of MSA, or NBM, or both (7), subsequent studies have employed ibotenate (96), quisqualate (211), and AMPA (H. Hodges et al., in preparation) infusions to lesion the origins of both pathways. In all cases, a similar pattern of global working and reference memory deficits was found, which was long-lasting and, provided the animals were not overtrained or left untested for several weeks (211), was remarkably stable. Thus, these tasks provide a good steady-state baseline for investigating drug or transplant effects.

In our hands, ibotenate and quisqualate produced equivalent ChAT loss in the cortex (30–40%) and hippocampus (25%) (96, 211); AMPA had more marked effects on cortical ChAT (75%); whereas hippocampal loss is similar to the other toxins (30–40%) (authors' unpublished data). Making comparisons across many experiments using the different excitotoxins in our laboratory, there is some evidence for the view (53) that cholinergic damage is not entirely responsible for radial maze impairments, in that ibotenic acid produced the greatest impairments with the least terminal ChAT loss and the largest amount of cell loss within the NBM and surrounding substantia innominata and globus pallidus (96). However, a direct comparison of ibotenic and quisqualic acid lesions, which produced equivalent reductions in cortical and hippocampal ChAT activity, also produced quantitatively similar radial maze impairments (211). The consistency of effects overall suggests that, despite incidental damage to other systems that may increase the degree of impairment, radial maze performance is highly sensitive to cholinergic disruption.

Equivalent effects of ibotenate, quisqualate, and AMPA lesions of NBM and MSA on acquisition (but not retention, once learned) of a hidden platform location in the water maze (99, Fletcher et al., *submitted; unpublished data*), particularly when using a difficult training regimen (two trials per day with a 10-minute intertrial interval; 129), suggest that a common cholinergic loss also contributed to these deficits. Acquisition deficits in difficult spatial tasks may represent an important consequence of FCPS cholinergic cell loss. In a recent study from our laboratory, using the T-maze, we found that AMPA lesions of NBM and MSA did not impair performance in a quickly learned win–shift (alternation) version of this task, even with the imposition of a 20-second information choice delay. However, reversal to a win–stay rule, which required extensive training in intact rats to achieve criterion performance, was significantly impaired by the lesion (Bradbury et al., *in preparation*).

Data from experiments with rats following prolonged alcohol consumption are entirely consistent with those using excitotoxic lesions to the FCPS. Alcohol-induced damage to the cholinergic system is progressive, both in terms of duration of exposure (7) and amount of ethanol consumed and retained as blood alcohol levels (98). Whereas prolonged (28 week) alcohol consumption apparently spares noncholinergic structures in the basal forebrain, it damages NE, 5-HT, and DA input to many forebrain structures (7). However, the effects on place–cue, reference–working memory in the radial arm maze, and the effects on cholinergic markers in the FCPS terminal areas were in parallel, and associated with loss of AChE-positive neurons in the NBM and MSA (7,8,10,98).

The cholinergic basis for the radial maze (and, in the lesion cases, water maze) deficits is further supported by the beneficial effects of the cholinergic agonists, arecoline and nicotine, on performance following prolonged alcohol ingestion (98) and lesions by the different excitotoxins (97,99,211; un-

published data) at doses that failed to affect performance in unlesioned controls. In contrast, the noncholinergic stimulant, amphetamine, was ineffective (211).

As will be reviewed later, the reversal of cognitive impairments produced by damage to the FCPS with transplants from fetal brain, rich in, though not confined to, cholinergic cells, but not by transplants poor in such cells, provides complementary evidence for the role of the FCPS in some aspects of cognitive function.

Differential Effects of Cholinergic and Hippocampal Damage on Maze Performance

The foregoing data hint at some of the behavioral differences between lesions of the ascending cholinergic projections and damage to the target neurons of these projections in the cortex and hippocampus. In our laboratory, cerebral ischemia by four-vessel occlusion (173) (see Chapter 14) for periods of 15 and 30 minutes produces substantial damage to hippocampal CA_1 cells. At the longer duration, more extensive cell loss in the hippocampus, as well as cortical and striatal damage, are additionally observed (159). Neither duration of the ischemia produced deficits in the place–cue, reference–working memory task, although both produced substantial impairments in water maze acquisition (160) (see Chapter 14). Thus, we have evidence for dissociation between selective lesions to the cholinergic projection system and selective damage to specific circuits within their target structures. Our own data and those of others (105,147) suggest that spatial navigation in the water maze is far more sensitive to cell loss in the hippocampal formation than is performance on the Jarrard radial maze, whereas our observations over a series of experiments suggest that the converse is true for lesions to the FCPS. This suggests some degree of dissociation between the behavioral consequences of damage to a hierarchic system and its modulatory inputs, and has additional implications for interpretations of the behavioral effects of the vigorous growth of grafts within the hippocampal formation (see later discussion on grafts after MSA lesions in the section on cholinergic grafts and recovery of cognitive function).

CHOLINERGIC-RICH GRAFTS

Neuronal Graft Tissue

There are numerous potential biologic sources of cholinergic-rich tissue for grafting studies, many of which have been successfully exploited at the anatomic, biochemical, physiologic, and behavioral levels to understand patterns of cholinergic regeneration and functional recovery. The major source (and, until recently, the almost universal source for studies of cognitive function) is fetal brain, particularly basal forebrain dissected at a time, which can range (in the rat) from day 14–17 (E14–17) of gestational age, when final differentiation of cholinergic cells is completed, but neurite outgrowth is still limited. Most often tissue is dissociated in trypsin before suspension and injection into target regions. Fetal tissue grafts have the advantage of providing a source of cholinergic neurons, with the potential for organizational and regulatory properties, although they will invariably contain cell types other than neurons and neurons expressing other transmitters. Given the variety of sources of cholinergic neurons in the CNS with different ontogenetic projection targets, fetal cholinergic-rich cell grafts with dissected tissue fragments, ranging throughout the cholinergic system from striatum to spinal cord, have been made into the denervated hippocampus to determine whether graft origin or host environment determines the degree of organotypic cholinergic innervation (5,36,57,80,154).

Alternatives to fetal-derived neuronal tissue have also been studied. The peripheral nervous system contains a rich variety of cholinergic neurons, and recent studies suggest survival of, and AChE-positive structures in, nodosal (103) and myenteric plexus (122) ganglion cells grafted to denervated cortex or hippocampus, respectively. Adrenal chromaffin cells have multipotential neuronal precursor characteristics when deprived of glucocorticoid stimulation *in vitro* (48) and, after a period in culture, display cholinergic features (17,161). When such tissue was transplanted to the cortex of NBM-lesioned rats, enhanced AChE staining was seen around the grafted cells (221). However, in all these peripheral cell grafts, there was no clearcut evidence of graft-derived cholinergic fiber innervation of lesioned host neurons.

Nonneuronal Grafts

There is increasing interest in fibroblast and tumor-derived cell lines as drug- or gene-delivery systems (78). Immortal cell lines have the advantage of providing a readily available source of homogeneous, reproducible cells for grafting. Cultured cell line grafts do not always grow into the circumscribed tissue masses that typify fetal grafts, and identification of graft cells from host will pose continuing problems (115, 131,177). Moreover, cell-line grafts lack many of the regulated neuronal properties of fetal tissue grafts. Interest in the cholinergic system comes from work on implants of cell lines genetically engineered to produce recombinant NGF (65,112,186). Transfected autologous fibroblast cell lines, which are amitotic and will survive in the brain parenchyma at a constant size for up to 8 weeks (110), have provided substantial trophic support to cholinergic neurons by, for example, dramatically enhancing survival of medial septal neurons following fimbria–fornix axotomy (186) and inducing cholinergic axonal growth and terminal synaptic innervation (112). The implanted cells also encourage AChE-positive fibers to grow toward them, indicating that the NGF-secreting cells can induce trophic actions on cholinergic terminals (65). Moreover, NGF-secreting fibroblasts implanted in striatum are able to induce cholinergic axons from host NBM to abnormally sprout and penetrate the graft milieu (111). Tumorigenicity of neuroblastoma or pheochromocytoma cell lines can be avoided by chemical (115,131) or *ras* oncogene (163) differentiation. Furthermore, retroviral infection of a neuroblastoma with a temperature-sensitive conditional immortalizing gene permits the cells to differentiate on implantation. Transplanted, conditionally immortal HT4 cells, which express NGF, were able to rescue medial septal cholinergic neurons following fimbria–fornix lesions (226). In addition, chemically differentiated neuroblastoma cell lines may also express cholinergic (and other neurotransmitter) neuronal features *in vitro* or *in vivo* and thereby, may have the potential for transmitter replacement. Some passages of cultured IMR-32 cells (79) express AChE staining following grafting; LA-N-2, C-1300 (115), and NS20Y (K. M. Marsden et al., *in preparation*) cells expressed ChAT immunoreactivity in culture.

Work on cell lines transfected with a gene for ChAT is in its early stages (71,192), but clearly demonstrates the potential for genetically modified cell delivery systems as grafts. Problems to be resolved include the development of neuronal cell lines that will survive and integrate better than currently available lines—here the prospects appear to be very bright (177)—and the use of vectors that will maintain stable expression of the transfected gene over sufficient time periods to permit long-term tests of cognitive function.

Given the variety of potentially suitable material for grafting in the cholinergically depleted CNS, the mechanisms by which the different grafts may function, if they are able to improve cognitive function, are potentially equally as various. Mechanisms of action of neural grafts have been exten-

sively discussed elsewhere (50,52,77,86, 199). From the foregoing examples, fetal grafts may replace a normal cholinergic synaptic input to a denervated target set of neurons, a property unlikely to be shared by peripheral nervous, fibroblast, or neuroblastoma cells. These latter may operate by paracrine or endocrine neuropharmacologic release of molecules in the grafted region that, for example, have trophic effects on the host (clearly true for NGF-secreting cells) or provide tonic neurotransmitter stimulation to the host. One must be cautious in interpreting diffuse release of ACh from grafts, however, since extrasynaptic ACh will be rapidly hydrolyzed, particularly when grafts may restore AChE levels.

Factors Affecting the Survival and Integration of Cholinergic Grafts

The development of reliable fetal tissue cell suspension techniques in the early 1980s (16) has encouraged uniformity in approach and has permitted surprising consistency of data on survival and integration of grafted tissue from many fetal sources (including cholinergic ones; 15) across a number of different laboratories. In general, grafts derived from cholinergic-rich fetal tissue taken at the optimal stage of embryonic development usually grow into a well-vascularized cellular mass, the boundaries of which are clearly distinct from the host brain (Fig. 2); interfaces between graft and host often show patterns of scar astrocyte reactivity (119). Most experiments place the fetal cholinergic cells ectopically: they are put proximal to the normal targets of the FCPS and so distal to their normal location in the nuclei of origin of this projection. Such procedures are adopted because fetal cells placed in the adult brain are not normally capable of projecting their axons over the large distance separating the projection nucleus from its terminal area. Trophic bridges across fimbria–fornix lesion cavities, using, for example, hippocampal grafts with NGF infusions (212), sciatic

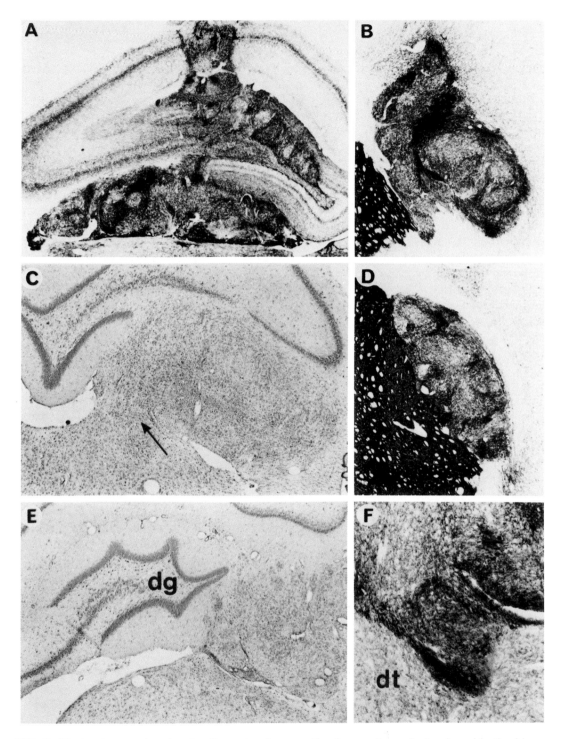

FIG. 2. Photomicrographs showing the extensive growth of some transplants placed in the hippocampus (**A,C,E,F**) and neocortex (**B,D**) in the rat following prolonged alcohol consumption. Some implants into the hippocampus grow prolifically into the ventricles (A), or so close to the dorsal thalamus that bridges are established (C at *large arrow* and F). The intrinsic cytoarchitecture of the hippocampus sometimes seems to be disrupted by the growing transplant (C), or severely displaced (E). Grafts to the neocortex sometimes grow clearly within the cortex (B), or just under the corpus callosum in the striatum, apparently completely detached from cortical tissue (D) (13-wk posttransplant; Coronal cryostat sections: A,B,D,F, AChE reaction; C,E, Nissl staining). *dg,* dentate gyrus; *dt,* dorsal thalamus. Original magnifications: A–E, ×25; F, ×63. (From ref. 7, with permission.)

nerve fragments (143), and Schwann cell suspensions (145), help regenerate the septohippocampal cholinergic projection.

Growth, cholinergic cell numbers, and innervation patterns of cholinergic-rich grafts are dependent on several factors. First, Gage and Björklund (76) estimated that grafts of fetal septum into the hippocampus were more than doubled in volume by a prior fimbria–fornix denervation. Although the density of AChE-positive cells did not vary within the grafts, the number of such cells was more than doubled in the denervated environment, as was the hippocampal ChAT activity. Axotomy of the septohippocampal cholinergic cells probably results in NGF accumulation in the hippocampus (116,120), the effect of which is to enhance growth of, and fiber outgrowth from, cholinergic fetal grafts (64,65).

A second related factor determining cholinergic graft size and outgrowth is the degree of organotypic integration between graft and host environment. In the denervated hippocampus, early studies suggested that cholinergic cells from fetal septum, striatum, and habenula, all produced similar patterns of fiber ingrowth, with the same, essentially normal, laminar specificity (5,80). However, Dunnett et al. (57) reported that, with equivalent initial cell suspensions, septal grafts grew larger in the deafferentated hippocampus than in the cortex, whereas the converse was true for NBM grafts. More recently, Nilsson et al. (154) and Clarke et al. (36) have compared grafts into fimbria–fornix-lesioned hippocampus of the same number of viable cells, but derived from five different cholinergic-rich sources: septum, NBM, striatum, pontomesencephalon, and spinal cord. In the first of these studies (154), graft size varied substantially, with NBM and spinal cord grafts growing considerably larger than septal and pontomesencephalon grafts which, in turn, were much larger than striatal grafts. Outgrowth of AChE-positive fibers, however, followed a different ordering. Large NBM and smaller pontomesencephalon grafts had limited outgrowth and in-

nervation of the host hippocampus compared with septal grafts. Large spinal cord grafts had very poor outgrowth into the hippocampus. In a later ChAT immunohistochemical study, Clarke et al. (36) showed that AChE-positive outgrowth was correlated with the number of ChAT-positive neurons in the different grafts, with septal grafts having the most of both. The forebrain cholinergic grafts (septum, NBM, and striatum) all had qualitatively similar overall fiber growth into the denervated hippocampus, although they varied considerably in efficiency, with striatal grafts surviving poorly. Interestingly, pontomesencephalon and spinal cord grafts, in spite of good survival, showed qualitatively different and abnormal patterns of ingrowth compared with the forebrain grafts. This relative failure in plasticity may be a consequence of the relative inability of hindbrain and spinal cord cholinergic neurons to retain their responsivity to NGF (231).

Combined retrograde tracer injection and ChAT immunohistochemical assay has identified cholinergic neurons in basal forebrain grafts as innervating frontal cortical neurons over some millimeters of distance following NBM lesions (26a). Ultrastructural studies have demonstrated extensive synaptic contacts between the ChAT-immunoreactive graft-derived fibers and vacated host target neurons in both the hippocampus and cortex (5,34,35). Unlike the ontogenetic distribution of synapses, where most terminations were on dendrites and particularly on dendritic shafts (33), graft-derived synapses were most frequently aberrantly located on perikarya. When synaptic innervation of the denervated hippocampus by grafted cells from different fetal cholinergic regions was investigated (36), ChAT-positive synaptic contacts were seen from fibers of all types of graft. However, septal grafts made the most contacts, and striatum and spinal cord made very few. The contacts from septal grafts were mostly onto perikarya; but from the other cholinergic grafts, the contacts were more like normal cholinergic contacts (i.e., located on dendrites). From a functional point of view, there are no data on the relative transplant-derived cholinergic innervation of denervated pyramidal cells and interneurons, which would indicate the extent of restoration of cholinergic excitation–inhibition patterns.

A further major factor determining graft viability is the extent of donor–host genetic immunohistocompatibility. Although tissue transplanted to the brain may be able to enjoy a relatively high degree of immunologic privilege, compared with tissue grafted to the periphery (150,228), recent research suggests that cross-species and even cross-strain established neural transplants are immunologically unstable. There are some reports of survival of mouse-to-rat cholinergic transplants into the denervated hippocampus (44,140), but most reports indicate eventual rejection of xenografts unless host animals are immunosuppressed (228). Allografts may not provoke as vigorous a rejection response, but the site of a graft and type of grafted tissue are important factors determining the rate of rejection. In PVG basal forebrain grafts to NBM-lesioned F344 inbred rat hosts (Patel et al., *submitted*), there was gradient of rejection, with surface grafts showing rapid rejection, probably owing to their proximity to meningeal vessels, but deep grafts remained unrejected. Furthermore, if the host animal is sensitized to antigens from the donor species or strain (e.g., by peripheral skin grafts or injection of cells from the donor), then rapid rejection of the neural graft can ensue (200,201). The rejection of established grafts can be experimentally employed to determine if the continuing presence of the transplant is necessary for graft-induced functional changes (27).

CHOLINERGIC GRAFTS AND RESTORATION OF CHOLINERGIC FUNCTION

Physiology and Pharmacology

Given that cholinergic-rich grafts can reinnervate denervated targets in the host brain in an organotypic and laminarly correct fashion and can make a number of, albeit abnormally sited, synaptic contacts onto target neurons, to what extent can such graft-induced anatomic integration restore cholinergic function? Most of the data addressing this question are behavioral or neurochemical, and we will review these in some detail in the following. There are, however, regrettably few data on the normalization and regulation of physiologic, pharmacologic, and molecular function of grafted cholinergic neurons or their post-synaptic targets, which may be a prerequisite to behavioral restoration.

Muscarinic receptor binding of the putative M_1 and M_2 types has been investigated in fimbria–fornix-lesioned hippocampus and following transplants of solid fetal septal tissue to the lesion cavity (45). Eight months after surgery, laminar-specific increases in CA_{2-3} stratum radiatum M_1 and CA_{2-4} stratum oriens M_2 receptor densities, produced by the lesion, were reduced to control values by the grafts, in confirmation of other reports using less specific muscarinic receptor ligands (109,195).

In vivo dialysis studies in freely moving rats have shown that KCl-stimulated ACh release in the fimbria–fornix-lesioned hippocampus is increased after both solid septal grafts (in the lesion cavity) and cell suspension grafts placed in hippocampal parenchyma, compared with the lesion-alone group. The transmitter release was increased in a manner qualitatively similar to that seen in intact rats by electrical stimulation of the lateral habenula (155) or by behavioral activation through handling, immobilization, and swim stress (152). The data, therefore, suggest some degree of host afferent regulatory control over impulse-dependent ACh release from grafted cholinergic neurons, both when these neurons are in direct contact with forebrain structures (i.e., in the lesion cavity) and when relatively isolated (i.e., as cell suspensions lying deep in hippocampus). The degree of behavioral or stress-related activation of the grafted cholinergic neurons was, however, quite limited compared with unlesioned animals. Moreover, suspension grafts in the hippocampus, which showed weaker activation, demonstrated greater cholinergic fiber innervation of the denervated hippocampus.

A more pronounced difference between solid lesion cavity and intrahippocampal suspension grafts following fimbria–fornix lesions was shown in studies of graft-induced restoration of hippocampal theta rhythm (25). The rhythmic electroencephalographic (EEG) activities of both the cortex and hippocampus partly depend on cholinergic innervation from the FCPS (182,204). Rhythmic slow activity (RSA or theta) in the hippocampal formation and adjacent retrohippocampal areas is believed to be actively paced by neurons in the MSA, since a proportion of MSA neurons fire in phase with hippocampal theta (6), and lesions in this structure and its connections with the hippocampus block theta. Although there is no direct evidence that the pacemaker cells are cholinergic (see 84 for review), coactivation of cholinergic and GABAergic inputs from medial septum appears to have an important role in theta modulation (203). For example, pyramidal theta cells in the hippocampus show a sustained depolarization, oscillating with theta frequency (158), most likely because of cholinergic attenuation of K^+ currents and disinhibition of local GABA interneurons (118). Functions ascribed to the theta rhythm have ranged from control over "voluntary" motor function (215) to facilitation of long-term potentiation (121).

Lesions of the NBM, however, increased the power of slow waves in the neocortex, particularly in the delta range (23). These slow waves are generated in pyramidal cells by calcium-mediated potassium conductances (41), which are attenuated by ACh (see earlier discussion on slow vs fast synaptic activity under "Cholinergic Physiology and Pharmacology"). Slow waves are normally actively suppressed during behavioral arousal by the firing of NBM neurons,

which will, in turn, permit these waves to be displayed by thalamocortical desynchronization (23,47).

Fimbria–fornix lesions abolished hippocampal theta activity, whereas solid transplants of E17 septum (and, in some cases, E17 hippocampus) restored movement-related hippocampal theta (25). In contrast, rats with cell suspension grafts of fetal septum into the hippocampus displayed limited hippocampal theta that was seen only during immobility (i.e., in an incorrect behavioral context, despite the suspension grafts' producing extensive cholinergic reinnervation of hippocampus; 25). The authors argue that the solid grafts may be forming a trophic ("passive") or relay ("active") bridge between the denervated hippocampus and subcortical theta pacemaker neurons; suspension grafts, however, although retaining some pacemaker characteristics, lack subcortical afferent controls. As in the study by Nilsson and Björklund (152), behavioral control of cholinergic hippocampal function was not simply a function of graft-induced cholinergic reinnervation.

In a similar fashion, the suppression of low-voltage, fast electroencephalographic (EEG) activity during awake immobility by slow waves in NBM-lesioned rats was progressively reduced, 2 to 14 weeks after neocortical grafts of E15–16 basal forebrain, compared with rats with control hippocampal grafts (214). Unlike hippocampal theta, however, restoration of normal EEG patterns of electrocortical arousal may not depend on host control over grafts, since muscarinic agonist injection was equally effective (205).

Evidence for functional physiologic synaptic innervation of cholinoceptive host target neurons by grafted cholinergic cells remains somewhat limited. In one early study (194), E17–18 septal cell suspensions were implanted into fimbria–fornix-lesioned hippocampus and intracellular recordings in CA_1 pyramidal cells were made at varying times after grafting, in transverse slice preparations. Electrical stimulation of the graft induced several pyramidal cell responses, indicative of muscarinic receptor stimulation: namely, an initial hyperpolarization followed by a longer-lasting depolarization. The depolarizations were voltage-dependent, and they were blocked by topical application of atropine and mimicked by local ACh application. These data give a clear indication of relatively normal functional cholinergic synaptic innervation of host neurons, but it remains unknown whether graft neurons (particularly the cholinergic ones) retain the physiologic characteristics, regulation, and organization of normal medial septal neurons.

CHOLINERGIC GRAFTS AND RECOVERY OF COGNITIVE FUNCTION

Theoretical Considerations

Given the range of uncertainties from lesion and drug studies about the role of the cholinergic system in cognitive function, studies with transplants of cholinergic-rich tissue may assist in our interpretation of the effects of cholinergic depletion, as well as providing a basis for promoting functional recovery. If functional recovery occurs with cholinergic-rich, but not noncholinergic, grafts, the findings would support the involvement of ACh in the deficit. Furthermore, if the site of grafts is varied, it may be possible to see whether cortical or hippocampal placement differentially affects performance, in line with the hypothesis that the different branches of the FCPS have different cognitive roles. Alternatively, grafts at each site may be equally effective, and their combined effects additive, in line with a hypothesis of unitary function of the FCPS.

When one looks at possible mechanisms of graft action, there is, from the above discussion, clear evidence that fetal cholinergic neurons can (a) innervate denervated host target regions of the FCPS, although the vigor and normality of anatomic integration is dependent on organotypic constraints; (b) form synapses with host pyramidal cells in these target regions, although in denervated targets the topography of these synapses is somewhat abnormal; (c) show restoration of ACh release and recovery of normal EEG patterns within these regions, although the degree of restoration is dependent on host regulation of grafted cells in their ectopic location; and (d) send relatively normal muscarinic excitation to denervated host pyramidal cells, although the degree of autoregulation and host regulation of these responses remains to be determined. An important question, therefore, is which, if any, of the above regeneration capacities of grafted cholinergic neurons play important roles in the abilities of cholinergic grafts to restore cognitive function, or are these capacities redundant to the range of effects of cholinergic grafts on performance of animals in cognitive tasks that have been observed? The answer to this question partly lies in a consideration of the constraints to behavioral recovery seen following fetal grafts, and partly on the determination of whether nonneuronal, but cholinergic-related, grafts are equally as capable of restoring cognitive function as fetal cholinergic grafts. These issues will form a background to the review of the behavioral effects of cholinergic grafts that occupies the remainder of this chapter.

The Effects of Cholinergic Grafts in the Hippocampus

Grafts Following Fimbria–Fornix Lesions

As in the studies examining graft-induced cholinergic innervation, fimbria–fornix lesions have provided the most frequently studied experimental model for transplant-induced recovery of cognitive function. These lesions destroy the major cholinergic, GABAergic, noradrenergic, serotonergic, and other, mainly peptidergic, inputs to the hippocampus and produce deficits in most tasks addressing spatial and temporal learning and memory in the rat (164). Low et al. (127) and Dunnett et al. (54) were first to investigate the effects of fetal solid and cell suspension septal transplants some 7 months postgrafting on recovery in radial maze- and T-maze-rewarded alternation, respectively. In the first of these studies (127), an improvement in radial maze performance was not seen in the grafted, fornix-lesioned rats unless administration of the AChE inhibitor, physostigmine, was made concurrently with behavioral testing. The need for AChE inhibition gives some support to the view that the grafts are effective by extrasynaptic ACh overflow, rather than synaptic innervation. Improvements in T-maze-rewarded alternation, however, were seen without AChE inhibition following septal grafts, but not control grafts of noradrenergic locus coeruleus primordia (54). The success of fetal basal forebrain cell suspension grafts in improving acquisition of T-maze-rewarded alternation in fimbria–fornix-lesioned rats has been confirmed (113); the rate of acquisition that was seen in the grafted group was similar to that of the previous study (54), although posttransplant testing began soon after grafting. Evidence for recovery in normal memory performance was limited, however, since, at the end of posttransplant training, when control and grafted groups did not significantly differ, imposition of a 20-second delay between information and choice phases of the trials reduced the grafted (but not unlesioned) group's performance to no better than that of the ungrafted lesion controls (113). Furthermore, a neuroblastoma cell line (IMR-32)-implant group showed qualitatively similar, if marginally significant, improvements in acquisition to the fetal graft group, suggesting cognitive improvements may be possible in the absence of graft-derived AChE hippocampal innervation.

Partial restoration following solid and suspension septal grafts in fimbria–fornix-lesioned rats was also found in learning and memory of a hidden platform location in the water maze (156). The primary deficit in the lesioned rats was spatial, but, with continued training, lesioned rats were able to compensate partially for this deficit by the adoption of nonspatial strategies to find the platform (156; see also 61). The authors argued that the graft-induced amelioration of performance was due to improvements in spatial ability, since septal grafts, although not giving definitive evidence of improvement in latency measures, always significantly increased searching in the correct platform location in probe trials, similar to control rats. This graft effect was reversed by atropine at doses that had less effect on control rats, suggesting a muscarinic cholinergic mechanism of graft action (156). More clearcut relations between the partial recovery in tests of spatial learning and memory and hippocampal cholinergic function, respectively, following fetal septal grafts in fimbria–fornix-lesioned animals were shown by significant correlations between high-affinity choline uptake in the hippocampus and measures of acquisition and retention of a hidden platform position and a choice-based matching to position task in the water maze (207), although the inclusion of lesion-only and unlesioned animals may well have biased the correlations toward significance.

The more or less 50% improvement seen following fetal septal grafts into rats with fimbria–fornix lesions in these experiments is suggestive of the reinstatement of one among a number of parallel neurochemical systems that normally innervate the hippocampal formation through this pathway; although along with cholinergic input, GABAergic and peptidergic pathways derived from medial septum may also be restored. Evidence that combined grafts of septal and raphe tissues are more effective than septal tissue alone (153,180) supports this view. Balanced against the reports of successful cholinergic-rich grafts in this lesion model, however, are reports, mostly from Will's laboratory, showing either no effects of septal grafts or additional impairments in grafted animals. In the first of these studies (43), rats were given electrolytic lesions targeted to destroy the fornix or the fimbria or the combined pathway. E16–17 fetal basal forebrain cell suspensions were grafted to the hippocampus of groups of rats with the different lesions. Irrespective of lesion locus, rats with cholinergic grafts showed greater impairments than their lesion-only counterparts in both a serial alternation task and standard eight-arm radial maze learning up to 7 months after transplant. The authors argued that extensive graft-induced dorsal hippocampal damage (leading to evidence of cytotoxicity and overt convulsive seizures in some cases) or over-expression of AChE histochemical staining in the grafted hippocampus, which was found in many of the rats, was probably responsible for the graft-induced behavioral impairments (43). In a second study, Cassel et al. (29) showed that similar graft-induced impairments occurred in spite of graft-induced increases in hippocampal ACh concentrations, compared with lesioned controls; furthermore, graft-induced impairments were seen in the cholinergic-rich septal, but not cholinergic-poor hippocampal, graft groups, suggesting that the impairments may be a consequence of over-growth of cholinergic grafts.

In a time-course study, Cassel et al. (31) found that septal grafts were only effective in significantly improving radial maze performance following fimbria–fornix lesions when tested 5 to 6 months postgrafting: shorter (1–2 months) and longer (10–11 months) postgrafting intervals produced null effects. A further recent report from this group (32) has confirmed the overall negative effects of cholinergic-rich grafts on radial maze learning in fimbria–fornix-lesioned rats.

There are a number of reasons why septal grafts that restore cholinergic afferent innervation to the denervated hippocampus may not ameliorate radial maze perfor-mance. First, given the nonspecificity of fimbria–fornix lesions, restoration of cholinergic function may have ameliorative effects on only a subset of the behavioral tasks disrupted by this lesion. There are a few reports in the literature of task-specific recovery in different lesion–graft models (58,198). Second, fimbria–fornix deafferentation may remove inhibitory control over an amplifying reverberating cortical–hippocampal circuit, the effects of which are capable, in pathologic states such as denervating lesions, of generating kindling and seizure activity (22) and, thereby, producing behavioral deficits greater than those found following loss of nearly all hippocampal pyramidal and dentate granule cells (105). It may be that grafts are only effective following fimbria–fornix lesions to the extent that they can tone down the lesion-induced hyperactivity of this circuit (24). This argument, however, would predict that reinnervation by noradrenergic grafts, which reduce epileptic-like EEG activity in the denervated hippocampus (26), would also improve cognitive function, and this has been found not to be true (54). Nevertheless, coinnervation by cholinergic and inhibitory projection fibers (notably GABAergic, since these projection neurons may also be present in basal forebrain grafts) may be a necessary requirement for recovery of cognitive function in rats with fimbria–fornix lesions.

Indirect evidence for this view comes from recent studies of the effects of fetal septal grafts derived at slightly different embryonic stages in fimbria–fornix-lesioned rats. Dunnett et al. (55) compared suspension grafts of E13–14 and approximately E16 septum on both a noncognitive measure (home-cage activity) and cognitive performance (learning of an operant schedule of differential reinforcement of low rates of response; DRL). Early fetal-aged grafts improved learning of the cognitive task, but did not reverse the lesion-induced hyperactivity. Later fetal-aged grafts had the reverse effects. A similar fetal donor age dif-

Further transplant studies with differentiated neuroblastoma cells depended on clear evidence for their continued survival. Hence, we labeled differentiated IMR-32 cells in culture with fluorescent latex microspheres to visualize both cell bodies and processes in culture. Prior treatment with mitomycin and bromodeoxyuridine prevented their reversion to tumors. After survival times up to 12 weeks postimplant, the labeled cells could be clearly identified as dispersed elements within the grafted cortex and hippocampus, and ultrastructurally resembled their *in vitro* appearance (131). In rats with ibotenate lesions of NBM and medial septal area, deficits in place–cue, reference–working memory performance in the radial maze were improved by grafts of both IMR-32 and NS20Y cells. At the end of testing, performance of the neuroblastoma graft groups was not significantly different from that of the unlesioned controls (Fig. 4A,B). Moreover, the time course of recovery was similar to that of fetal basal

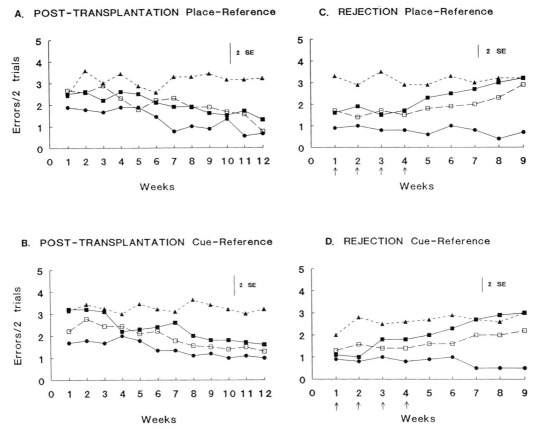

FIG. 4. Effects of grafts of amitotic IMR-32 and NS20Y neuroblastoma cell lines into terminal regions following ibotenate lesions of the FCPS. Mean numbers of place (**A,C**) and cue (**B,D**) errors on the radial arm maze are presented for 12 weeks of postgraft testing (A,B). Both cell lines produced significant recovery of function, similar to the effects of fetal basal forebrain grafts (not shown). The rats were then injected subcutaneously with the irradiated cell lines during maze testing every week for 4 weeks (*arrows* in C and D), and the rats were tested for a further 5 weeks. A gradual diminution in behavioral effectiveness of the grafts was seen, which was consistent with histologic and peripheral mixed lymphocyte response evidence for immune rejection of the grafts. *Open squares,* IMR-32; *solid squares,* NS20Y; *solid circle,* control; *solid triangle,* sham. (Adapted from Marsden et al., in preparation; ref. 199.)

forebrain grafts (data not shown), suggesting a similar mechanism of graft-induced recovery (K. M. Marsden et al., *in preparation*).

The original xenogeneic (human or mouse) source of these cell line grafts provided an opportunity to establish whether or not the grafts were operating through trophic effects on host brain. At the end of 12 weeks of postgraft testing, when asymptotic improvements in radial maze performance were seen in the IMR-32 and NS20Y groups, the appropriate neuroblastoma cells were irradiated and subcutaneously injected to the grafted and control groups. Rats were tested weekly on the radial maze during this time and for a further 5 weeks. The grafted rats' performance declined progressively over the 9 weeks, to the level of the lesioned controls, although performance in the other groups was unchanged (see Fig. 4C,D) (K. M. Marsden et al., in preparation). *Postmortem* investigation showed substantial signs of graft rejection, including an elevated peripheral lymphocyte response and, in the grafted cortical and hippocampal areas, mononuclear cell infiltration and high levels of major histocompatibility complex (MHC) class I and II antibody staining, particularly in the NS20Y graft group. Thus, dysfunction in or destruction of the grafted cells by the immune rejection removed the grafts' behavioral efficacy, indicating that the grafted cells themselves and not changes to host brain were responsible for the efficacy. Since neither grafted cell line affected ChAT activity *in vivo* (K. M. Marsden et al., in preparation), further studies on the *in vivo* neurochemical properties of these cells are required to determine how these grafts produce their effects on cognitive function.

Evidence for a Role of Graft-Derived Glia in Cognitive Recovery

One approach we have taken, in an attempt to unravel the multiplicity of local neurochemical changes at the site of transplants that may mediate the behavioral effects of cholinergic-rich grafts, has been to examine protein changes in the frontal cortex of rats with ibotenate lesions of the FCPS and fetal basal forebrain grafts that produced long-term behavioral recovery versus transplants of fetal hippocampus that were ineffective (223). After two-dimensional gel electrophoresis, 33 proteins were reliably identified on each sample gel and measured by image analysis. The normalized values were related to type of transplant group (cholinergic-rich cholinergic-poor) and individually correlated with performance on the radial maze. Of the 33 proteins, 7 showed differences that depended on type of transplant or were correlated with behavior. Only one identified protein was elevated in the cholinergic-rich, compared with cholinergic-poor, transplants in frontal cortex tissue and was positively correlated with behavior. This protein, glial fibrillary acidic protein, is a glial marker, mostly of astrocytes. On the other hand, some nonspecific neuronal cytoskeletal proteins and neuron-specific enolase were negatively correlated with radial maze performance, but did not differ between transplant groups (223). These data suggest that, even when measured 12 months postlesion and 7 months posttransplant, the trophic support provided by cholinergic-rich transplant-related glia may aid cognitive recovery, whereas high levels of some nonspecific neural elements may inhibit the recovery process.

Experimental support for the role of what may be trophic support from glia as an important factor in behaviorally effective transplants in rats with damage to the FCPS has recently been reported (21), and a similar experiment is underway in our laboratory (Bradbury et al., *in preparation*). In the Brückner and Arendt (21) study, rats treated with prolonged alcohol were implanted into cortex and hippocampus with primary cultures of postnatal day 1 or 2 cortical astrocytes or fetal basal forebrain cell suspension. Postgraft testing on the place version of the Jarrard maze showed that fetal basal forebrain grafts improved performance with a time course consistent with growth of the transplant and outgrowth of cholinergic fibers. Primary astrocyte grafts, however, improved performance soon after grafting and produced an overall behavioral improvement similar to that seen after basal forebrain grafts. Interestingly, the astrocyte, and to a smaller extent the basal forebrain, grafts increased ChAT activity in the basal forebrain region of host rats, confirming earlier observations (7) and suggesting that grafted glia may induce recovery in damaged cholinergic neurons, possibly by providing trophic factors. In a recent study (Bradbury et al., *in preparation*), we have derived primary cultures separately enriched either in postmitotic astrocytes or in neurons or neuronal precursors from E15 basal forebrain, and compared grafts of these cell types with E15 basal forebrain cell suspension grafts in rats with AMPA lesions of the MSA and NBM. The rats were trained 4 months after lesion and grafting on a T-maze win–stay learning task. The astrocyte and fetal basal forebrain graft groups were significantly better at learning the task than the lesion-alone group. Performance of the group with neuronal cell grafts, on the other hand, was significantly poorer than the lesion-alone group at early stages of training. Both whole fetal basal forebrain and neuronal primary cell grafts increased ChAT activity in cortex and hippocampus; grafted astrocytes, however, had no significant effect on terminal area ChAT activity. Unlike whole basal forebrain and neuronal transplants, grafted astrocytes were difficult to identify in histologic preparations beyond a short postgrafting interval (21; Bradbury et al., *in preparation*); this is consistent with labeling studies that have shown that astrocytes migrate considerably after grafting (63).

CONCLUSIONS

Cholinergic innervation of the cortical mantle from networks of interconnected neurons in the basal forebrain promotes potent and long-lasting excitatory and inhibitory effects on target circuit neurons. Lesion studies that have achieved some relative success in confining damage to cholinergic neurons of the NBM, suggest that cholinergic innervation of the neocortex is primarily involved in behavioral activation and stimulus selection, with effects on more complex cognitive processes possibly secondary to a primary attentional deficit. The effects of selective cholinergic deafferentation of allocortical structures, particularly the hippocampus, remain to be fully elucidated. Although a unitary, activational view of the modulatory role of the FCPS in cognitive function has many heuristic merits, it may ignore important aspects of selective cholinergic excitation and inhibition patterns in individual target circuits that, for example, may be selectively involved in enhancing acquisition or retention of specific information (93).

With few exceptions, the tasks used to assess improvements in cognitive function following cholinergic grafts have shown qualitatively similar recovery whether the grafts are fetal neurons or cultured neuroblastoma, glial and peripheral cells that may lack many neuronal physiologic features. Lacking are experiments on more complex cognitive function (e.g., 198), but interpretation of failures or behavioral dissociations in graft-induced recovery is complicated by the lack of lesion specificity in assessing the role of the cholinergic system in cognitive function (53).

Overall, if one compares the effects of transplants of cholinergic cells derived from fetal cholinergic tissue on improvement in cognitive function in cholinergically depleted animals with grafts from a variety of other sources that bear some functional relation to cholinergic cells, a very complex picture emerges. This is undoubtedly due to the variety of mechanisms by which transplants may improve function within a diffuse and widespread modulatory neural system such as the FCPS (52,77). These mechanisms include trophic support to undamaged host cholinergic neurons; bridging regions of undamaged tissue across a lesion cavity; diffuse, paracrine release of ACh or some compound related to it; and synaptic innervation of grafted cholinergic neurons by host afferents or afferent innervation from grafted cholinergic cells onto vacated host synapses. Fetal grafts from organotypic sources appear to be capable of many of these effects; other sources of grafts of only a limited subset. Whether grafted cells need to operate in the same way as normal host neurons or whether the transmitter release needs to be synaptically regulated (graft–host or host–graft) depends partly on the degree of circuit integration required for the control of the given behavior and partly on our understanding (or ignorance) of the neural mechanisms involved in that behavior. A further problem is determining the required number of ectopically grafted cholinergic cells that would provide an appropriate "engraftment" of widely denervated target areas. Even though synaptic connectivity and neuronal regulation may be features of fetal transplants rich in cholinergic neurons, results showing the positive behavioral effects of various cell lines and glial grafts suggest that these features may be unimportant in many cognitive recovery experiments.

ACKNOWLEDGMENTS

The preparation of this review was supported by the U.K. Medical Research Council (MRC). Support for research on cholinergic grafts in our laboratory has been from the U.K. MRC, the Wellcome Trust, the British Council, and the European Community.

REFERENCES

1. Abdulla FA, Calaminisi MR, Stephenson JD, Sinden JD. Unilateral AMPA lesions of nucleus basalis magnocellularis induce a sensorimotor deficit which is differentially altered by arecoline and nicotine. *Behav Brain Res* 1994; 60:161–169.

1a. Aigner TG, Mitchell SJ, Aggleton JP, DeLong MR, Struble RG, Price DL, Wenk GL, Pettigrew KL, Mishkin M. Transient impairment of recognition memory following ibotenic-acid lesions of the basal forebrain in macaques. *Exp Brain Res* 1991;86:18–26.

2. Alheid GF, Heimer L. New perspectives in basal forebrain organization of special relevance for neuropsychiatric disorders: the striatopallidal, amygdaloid, and corticopetal components of substantia innominata. *Neuroscience* 1988;27:1–39.

3. Allen YS, Marchbanks RM, Sinden JD. Nonspecific effects of the putative cholinergic neurotoxin ethylcholine mustard aziridinium ion in the rat brain examined by autoradiography, immunocytochemistry and gel electrophoresis. *Neurosci Lett* 1988;95:69–74.

4. Amaral DG, Kurz J. An analysis of the origins of the cholinergic and noncholinergic septal projections to the hippocampal formation of the rat. *J Comp Neurol* 1985;281:337–361.

5. Anderson KJ, Gibbs RB, Cotman CW. Transmitter phenotype is a major determinant in the specificity of synapses formed by cholinergic neurons transplanted to the hippocampus. *Neuroscience* 1988;25:19–25.

6. Apostol G, Creutzfeldt OD. Cross-correlation between the activity of septal units and hippocampal EEG during arousal. *Brain Res* 1974; 67:65–75.

7. Arendt T, Allen Y, Marchbanks R, Schugens MM, Sinden J, Lantos PL, Gray JA. Cholinergic system and memory in the rat: effects of chronic ethanol, embryonic basal forebrain transplants and excitotoxic lesions of cholinergic basal forebrain projection systems. *Neuroscience* 1989;33:435–462.

8. Arendt T, Allen Y, Sinden J, Schugens MM, Marchbanks RM, Lantos PL, Gray JA. Cholinergic-rich brain transplants reverse alcohol-induced memory deficits. *Nature* 1988;332:448–450.

9. Arendt T, Bigl V, Tennstedt A, Arendt A. Neuronal loss in different parts of the nucleus basalis is related to neuritic plaque formation in cortical target areas in Alzheimer's disease. *Neuroscience* 1985;14:1–14.

10. Arendt T, Hennig D, Gray JA, Marchbanks RM. Loss of neurons in the rat basal forebrain projection system after prolonged intake of ethanol. *Brain Res Bull* 1988;21:563–570.

11. Armstrong DM, Saper CB, Levey AI, Wainer BH, Terry RD. Distribution of cholinergic neurons in the rat brain: demonstrated by the immunocytochemical localization of choline acetyltransferase. *J Comp Neurol* 1983;216:53–68.

12. Aston-Jones G, Bloom FE. Activity of norepinephrine-containing locus coeruleus neurons in behaving rats anticipates fluctuations in the sleep-waking cycle. *J Neurosci* 1981;1:876–886.

13. Bartus RT, Dean RL, Beer B, Lippa AS, The cholinergic hypothesis of geriatric memory dysfunction. *Science* 1982;217:408–417.

14. Bigl V, Woolf NJ, Butcher LL. Cholinergic

projections from the basal forebrain to frontal, parietal, temporal, occipital and cingulate cortices: a combined fluorescent tracer and acetylcholinesterase analysis. *Brain Res Bull* 1982; 8:727–749.

15. Björklund A, Gage FH, Stenevi U, Dunnett SB. Intracerebral grafting of neuronal cell suspensions. IV. Survival and growth of intrahippocampal implants of septal cell suspensions. *Acta Physiol Scand [Suppl]* 1983;522:49–58.

16. Björklund A, Stenevi U, Schmidt RH, Dunnett SB, Gage FH. Intracerebral grafting of neuronal cell suspensions. 1. Introduction and general methods of preparation. *Acta Physiol Scand [Suppl]* 1983;522:1–7.

17. Boksa P. Acetylcholine synthesis by adult bovine adrenal chromaffin cell cultures. *J Neurochem* 1985;45:1254–1261.

18. Bowen DM, Francis PT. Neurochemistry, neuropharmacology and aetiological factors in Alzheimer's disease. *Semin Neurosci* 1990;2:101–108.

19. Bowen DM, Smith CB, White P, Davison AN. Neurotransmitter-related enzymes and indices of hypoxia in senile dementia and other abiotrophies. *Brain* 1976;99:459–496.

20. Brion JP. Molecular pathology of Alzheimer amyloid and neurofibrillary tangles. *Semin Neurosci* 1990;2:89–100.

21. Brückner M, Arendt T. Intracortical grafts of purified astrocytes ameliorate memory deficits in rat induced by chronic treatment with ethanol. *Neurosci Lett* 1992;141:251–254.

22. Buzsaki G. Hippocampal sharp-waves: their origin and significance. *Brain Res* 1986;398:242–252.

23. Buzsaki G, Bickford RG, Ponomareff G, Thal LJ, Mandel R, Gage FH. Nucleus basalis and thalamic control of neocortical activity in the freely moving rat. *J Neurosci* 1988;8:4007–4026.

24. Buzsaki G, Gage FH. Mechanisms of action of neural grafts in the limbic system. *Can J Neurol Sci* 1988;15:99–105.

25. Buzsaki G, Gage FH, Czopf J, Björklund A. Restoration of rhythmic slow activity (theta) in the subcortically denervated hippocampus by fetal CNS transplants. *Brain Res* 1987;400:334–347.

26. Buzsaki G, Ponomareff G, Bayardo F, Shaw T, Gage FH. Suppression and induction of epileptic activity by neuronal grafts. *Proc Natl Acad Sci USA* 1988;85:9327–9330.

26a. Calaminici M, Abdulla FA, Sinden JD, Stephenson JD. Direct evidence for axonal outgrowth from cholinergic grafts to cholinergically-deafferented rat cortex. *Neuroreport* 1993;4:585–587.

27. Carder RK, Snyder-Keller AM, Lund RD. Behavioral and anatomical correlates of immunologically induced rejection of nigral xenografts. *J Comp Neurol* 1988;277:391–402.

28. Carlton PL. Cholinergic mechanisms in the control of behavior by the brain. *Psychol Rev* 1963;70:19–39.

29. Cassel JC, Kelche C, Hornsperger JM, Jackisch R, Hertting G, Will BE. Graft-induced learning impairment despite graft-enhanced cholinergic functions in the hippocampus of rats with septohippocampal lesions. *Brain Res* 1990;534:295–298.

30. Cassel JC, Kelche C, Peterson GM, Ballough GP, Goepp I, Will B. Graft-induced behavioral recovery from subcallosal septohippocampal damage in rats depends on maturity stage of donor tissue. *Neuroscience* 1991;45:571–586.

31. Cassel JC, Kelche C, Will B. Time-dependent effects of intrahippocampal grafts in rats with fimbria–fornix lesions. *Exp Brain Res* 1990; 81:179–190.

32. Cassel JC, Neufang B, Kelche C, Aiple F, Will BE, Hertting G, Jackisch R. Effects of septal and/or raphe cell suspension grafts on hippocampal choline acetyltransferase activity, high affinity synaptosomal uptake of choline and serotonin, and behaviour in rats with extensive septohippocampal lesions. *Brain Res* 1992; 585:243–254.

33. Clarke DJ. Cholinergic innervation of the rat dentate gyrus: an immunocytochemical and electron microscopical study. *Brain Res* 1985; 360:349–354.

34. Clarke DJ, Dunnett SB. Ultrastructural organisation of the choline–acetyltransferase-immunoreactive fibres innervating the neocortex from embryonic ventral forebrain grafts. *J Comp Neurol* 1986;250:192–205.

35. Clarke DJ, Gage FH, Björklund A. Formation of cholinergic synapses by intrahippocampal septal grafts as revealed by choline acetyltransferase immunocytochemistry. *Brain Res* 1986; 369:151–162.

36. Clarke DJ, Nilsson OG, Brundin P, Björklund A. Synaptic connections formed by grafts of different types of cholinergic neurons in the host hippocampus. *Exp Neurol* 1990;107:11–22.

37. Coffey PJ, Feldon J, Mitchell S, Sinden J, Gray JA, Rawlins JNP. Ibotenate-induced total septal lesions reduce resistance to extinction but spare the partial reinforcement extinction effect in the rat. *Exp Brain Res* 1989;77:140–152.

38. Coffey PJ, Perry VH, Allen Y, Sinden J, Rawlins JNP. Ibotenic acid induced demyelination in the central nervous system: a consequence of a local inflammatory response. *Neurosci Lett* 1988;84:178–184.

39. Collerton D. Cholinergic function and intellectual decline in Alzheimer's disease. *Neuroscience* 1986;19:1–28.

40. Collingridge GL, Kehl SJ, McLennan H. Excitatory amino acids in synaptic transmission in the Schaffer collateral–commissural pathway of the rat hippocampus. *J Physiol (Lond)* 1983;334:33–46.

41. Connors B, Gutnick MJ, Prince DA. Electrophysiological properties of neocortical neurons *in vitro*. *J Neurophysiol* 1982;48:1302–1320.

42. Curro Dossi R, Pare D, Steriade M. Short-lasting nicotinic and long-lasting muscarinic depolarizing responses of thalamocortical neurons to stimulation of mesopontine cholinergic nuclei. *J Neurophysiol* 1991;65:394–406.

43. Dalrymple-Alford JC, Kelche C, Cassel JC, Toniolo G, Pallage V, Will BE. Behavioral def-

icits after intrahippocampal fetal septal grafts in rats with selective fimbria–fornix lesions. *Exp Brain Res* 1988;69:545–558.

44. Daniloff JK, Bodony RP, Low WC, Wells J. Cross-species embryonic septal transplants: restoration of conditioned learning behavior. *Brain Res* 1985;346:176–180.

45. Dawson VL, Gage FH, Hunt MA, Wamsley JK. Normalization of subtype-specific muscarinic receptor binding in the denervated hippocampus by septodiagonal band grafts. *Exp Neurol* 1989;106:115–124.

46. Dekker AJAM, Connor DJ, Thal LJ. The role of cholinergic projections from the nucleus basalis in memory. *Neurosci Biobehav Rev* 1991; 15:299–317.

47. Detari I, Vanderwolf CH. Activity of cortically projecting and other basal forebrain neurons during large slow waves and cortical activation in anesthetised cat. *Brain Res* 1987;437:1–8.

48. Doupe AJ, Landis SC, Patterson PH. Environmental influences in the development of neural crest derivatives: glucocorticoids, growth factors, and chromaffin cell plasticity. *J Neurosci* 1985;5:2119–2142.

49. Dunnett SB. Comparative effects of cholinergic drugs and lesions of the nucleus basalis and fimbria–fornix on delayed matching in rats. *Psychopharmacology* 1985;87:357–363.

50. Dunnett SB. Neural transplantation in animal models of dementia. *Eur J Neurosci* 1990;2: 567–587.

51. Dunnett SB, Badman F, Rogers DC, Evenden JL, Iversen SD. Cholinergic grafts in the neocortex or hippocampus of aged rats: reduction of delay-dependent deficits in the delayed nonmatching to position task. *Exp Neurol* 1988; 102:57–64.

52. Dunnett SB, Björklund A. Mechanisms of function of neural grafts in the adult mammalian brain. *J Exp Biol* 1987;132:265–289.

53. Dunnett SB, Everitt BJ, Robbins TW. The basal forebrain–cortical cholinergic system: interpreting the functional consequences of excitotoxic lesions. *Trends Neurosci* 1991;14:494–501.

54. Dunnett SB, Low WC, Iversen SD, Stenevi U, Björklund A. Septal transplants restore maze learning in rats with fornix–fimbria lesions. *Brain Res* 1982;251:335–348.

55. Dunnett SB, Martel FL, Rogers DC, Finger S. Factors affecting septal graft amelioration of differential reinforcement of low rates (DRL) and activity deficits after fimbria-fornix lesions. *Rest Neurol Neurosci* 1989;1:83–92.

56. Dunnett SB, Toniolo G, Fine A, Ryan CN, Björklund A, Iversen SD. Transplantation of embryonic ventral forebrain neurons to the neocortex of rats with lesions of nucleus basalis magnocellularis—II. Sensorimotor and learning impairments. *Neuroscience* 1985;16:787–797.

57. Dunnett SB, Whishaw IQ, Bunch ST, Fine A. Acetylcholine-rich neuronal grafts in the forebrain of rats: effects of environmental enrichment, neonatal noradrenaline depletion, host transplantation site and regional source of em-

bryonic donor cells on graft size and acetylcholinesterase-positive fibre outgrowth. *Brain Res* 1986;378:357–373.

58. Dunnett SB, Whishaw IQ, Rogers DC, Jones GH. Dopamine-rich grafts ameliorate whole body motor asymmetry and sensory neglect but not independent limb use in rats with 6-hydroxydopamine lesions. *Brain Res* 1987;415: 63–78.

59. Eccles JC, Eccles RM, Fatt P. Pharmacological investigations on a central synapse operated by acetylcholine. *J Physiol(Lond)* 1956;131:154–169.

60. Eckenstein FP, Baughman RW, Quinn J. An anatomical study of cholinergic innervation in rat cerebral cortex. *Neuroscience* 1988;25:457–474.

61. Eichenbaum H, Stewart C, Morris RGM. Hippocampal representation in place learning. *J Neurosci* 1991;10:3531–3542.

62. Emerich DF, Black BA, Kesslak JP, Cotman CW, Walsh TJ. Transplantation of fetal cholinergic neurons into the hippocampus attenuates the cognitive and neurochemical deficits induced by AF64A. *Brain Res Bull* 1992;28:219–226.

63. Emmett CJ, Lawrence JM, Seeley PJ. Visualisation of migration of transplanted astrocytes using polystyrene microspheres. *Brain Res* 1988;447:223–233.

64. Eriksdotter-Nilsson M, Skirboll S, Ebendal T, Hersh L, Grassi J, Massoulie J, Olson L. NGF treatment promotes development of basal forebrain tissue grafts in the anterior chamber of the eye. *Exp Brain Res* 1989;74:89–98.

65. Ernfors P, Ebendal T, Olson L, Mouton P, Stromberg I, Persson H. A cell line producing recombinant nerve growth factor evokes growth responses in intrinsic and grafted central cholinergic neurons. *Proc Natl Acad Sci USA* 1989;86:4756–4760.

66. Etherington R, Mittleman G, Robbins TW. Comparative effects of nucleus basalis and fimbria–fornix lesions on delayed matching and alternation tests of memory. *Neurosci Res Commun* 1987;1:135–143.

67. Everitt BJ, Robbins TW, Evenden JL, Marston HM, Jones GH, Sirkia TE. The effects of excitotoxic lesions of the substantia innominata, ventral and dorsal globus pallidus on the acquisition and retention of a conditional visual discrimination: implications for cholinergic hypotheses of learning and memory. *Neuroscience* 1987;22:441–469.

68. Ffrench-Mullen JMH, Nori H, Nakanishi H, Slater NT, Carpenter DO. Assymetric distribution of acetylcholine receptors and M channels on prepyriform neurons. *Cell Mol Neurobiol* 1983;3:163–181.

69. Fibiger HC. Cholinergic mechanisms in learning, memory and dementia: a review of recent evidence. *Trends Neurosci* 1991;14:220–223.

70. Fine A, Dunnett SB, Björklund A, Iversen SD. Cholinergic ventral forebrain grafts into the neocortex improve passive avoidance memory in a rat model of Alzheimer's disease. *Proc Natl Acad Sci USA* 1985;82:5227–5230.

71. Fisher LJ, Schinstine M, Dekker A, Thal L, Gage FH. *in vivo* microdialysis of primary fibroblasts genetically modified to produce acetylcholine after implantation in the rat hippocampus. *Restor Neurol Neurosci* 1992;4:192.

72. Freund TF, Antal M. GABA-containing neurons in the septum control inhibitory interneurons in the hippocampus. *Nature* 1988;336:170–173.

73. Freund TF, Meskenaite V. γ-Aminobutyric acid-containing basal forebrain neurons innervate inhibitory interneurons in the neocortex. *Proc Natl Acad Sci USA* 1992;89:738–742.

74. Frotscher M, Leranth C. Cholinergic innervation of the rat hippocampus as revealed by choline acetyltransferase immunocytochemistry: a combined light and electron microscopic study. *J Comp Neurol* 1985;239:237–246.

75. Gaffan D, Gaffan EA, Harrison S. Effects of fornix transection on spontaneous and trained non-matching by monkeys. *Q J Exp Psychol* 1984;36B:285–303.

76. Gage FH, Björklund A. Enhanced graft survival in the hippocampus following selective denervation. *Neuroscience* 1986;17:89–98.

77. Gage FH, Fisher LJ. Intracerebral grafting: a tool for the neurobiologist. *Neuron* 1991;6:1–12.

78. Gage FH, Kawaja MD, Fisher LJ. Genetically modified cells: applications for intracerebral grafting. *Trends Neurosci* 1991;14:328–333.

79. Gash DM, Notter MFD, Okawara SH, Kraus AL, Joynt RJ. Amitotic neuroblastoma cells used for neural implants in monkeys. *Science* 1986;233:1420–1422.

80. Gibbs RB, Anderson K, Cotman CW. Factors affecting innervation in the CNS: comparison of three cholinergic cell types transplanted to the hippocampus of adult rats. *Brain Res* 1986;383:362–366.

81. Goedert M, Fine A, Hunt SP, Ullrich A. Nerve growth factor mRNA in peripheral and central rat tissues and in the human central nervous system. Lesion effects in the rat brain and levels in Alzheimer's disease. *Mol Brain Res* 1986;1:85–92.

82. Goldman D, Deneris E, Luyten W, Kochhar A, Patrick A, Patrick J, Heinemann S. Members of a nicotine acetylcholine receptor gene family are expressed in different regions of the mammalian central nervous system. *Cell* 1987;48:965–973.

83. Gould E, Woolf NJ, Butcher LL. Cholinergic projections to the substantia nigra from the pedunculopontine and laterodorsal tegmental nuclei. *Neuroscience* 1989;28:611–623.

84. Gray, JA. *The neuropsychology of anxiety: an enquiry into the function of the septo-hippocampal system.* Oxford: Oxford University Press; 1982.

85. Gray JA, McNaughton N. Comparison between the behavioural effects of septal and hippocampal lesions: a review. *Neurosci Biobehav Rev* 1983;7:119–188.

86. Gray JA, Sinden JD, Hodges H. Cognitive function: neural degeneration and transplantation. *Semin Neurosci* 1990;2:133–142.

87. Haas HL. Cholinergic disinhibition in hippocampal slices of the rat. *Brain Res* 1982;233:200–204.

88. Hagan JJ, Salamone JD, Simpson J, Iversen SD, Morris RGM. Place navigation in rats is impaired by lesions of the medial septum and diagonal band but not nucleus basalis magnocellularis. *Behav Brain Res* 1988;27:9–20.

89. Hagg T, Hagg F, Vahlsing HL, Manthorpe M, Varon S. Nerve growth factor effects on cholinergic neurons of neostriatum and nucleus accumbens in the adult rat. *Neuroscience* 1989;30:95–103.

90. Hallanger AE, Levey AI, Lee HJ, Wainer BH. The origin of cholinergic and other subcortical afferents to the thalamus in the rat. *J Comp Neurol* 1987;262:105–124.

91. Halliwell JV, Adams PR. Voltage-clamp analysis of muscarinic excitation in hippocampal neurons. *Brain Res* 1982;250:71–92.

92. Hanin I. AF64A-induced cholinergic hypofunction. *Prog Brain Res* 1990;84:289–299.

93. Hasselmo ME, Anderson BP, Bower JM. Cholinergic modulation of cortical associative memory function. *J Neurophysiol* 1992;67:1230–1246.

94. Hasselmo ME, Bower JM. Cholinergic suppression specific to intrinsic not afferent fiber synapses in rat piriform (olfactory) cortex. *J Neurophysiol* 1992;67:1222–1229.

95. Hepler DJ, Olton DS, Wenk GL, Coyle JT. Lesions in nucleus basalis magnocellularis and medial septal area of rats produce qualitative similar memory impairments. *J Neurosci* 1985;5:866–873.

96. Hodges H, Allen Y, Kershaw T, Lantos PL, Gray JA, Sinden J. Effects of cholinergic-rich neural grafts on radial maze performance of rats after excitotoxic lesions of the forebrain cholinergic projection system. 1. Amelioration of cognitive deficits by transplants into cortex and hippocampus but not into basal forebrain. *Neuroscience* 1991;45:587–607.

97. Hodges H, Allen Y, Sinden J, Lantos PL, Gray JA. The effects of cholinergic-rich neural grafts on radial maze performance of rats after excitotoxic lesions of the forebrain cholinergic projection system. 2. Cholinergic drugs as probes to investigate lesion-induced deficits and transplant-induced functional recovery. *Neuroscience* 1991;45:609–623.

98. Hodges H, Allen Y, Sinden J, Mitchell SN, Lantos PL, Gray JA. The effects of cholinergic drugs and cholinergic-rich foetal neural transplants on alcohol-induced deficits in radial-maze performance in rats. *Behav Brain Res* 1991;43:7–28.

99. Hodges H, Sinden J, Turner JJ, Netto CA, Sowinski P, Gray JA. Nicotine as a tool to characterise the role of forebrain cholinergic projection system in cognition. In: Collins AC, Gray JA, Robinson JH, Lipiello PM, eds. *The biology of nicotine.* New York: Raven Press; 1992:157–180.

100. Houser CR, Crawford DG, Salvaterra PM, Vaughn JE. Immunocytochemical localization of choline acetyltransferase in rat cerebral cor-

tex: a study of cholinergic neurons and synapses. *J Comp Neurol* 1985;234:17–34.

101. Ikegami S, Nihonmatsu I, Hatanaka H, Takei N, Kawamura H. Transplantation of septal cholinergic neurons to the hippocampus improves memory impairments of spatial learning in rats treated with AF64A. *Brain Res* 1989; 496:321–326.

102. Ikegami S, Nihonmatsu I, Kawamura H. Transplantation of ventral forebrain cholinergic neurons to the hippocampus ameliorates impairment of radial-arm maze learning in rats with AF64A treatment. *Brain Res* 1991;548:187–195.

103. Itakura T, Yokote H, Yukawa S, Nakai M, Komai N, Unemento M. Transplantation of peripheral cholinergic neurons into Alzheimer model rat brain. *Stereotact Funct Neurosurg* 1990;54:368–372.

104. Jacobs BL, Wilkinson LO, Fornal CA. The role of brain serotonin. A neurophysiologic perspective. *Neuropsychopharmacology* 1990;3: 473–479.

105. Jarrard LE. Selective hippocampal lesions and behavior: implications for current research and theorizing. In: Isaacson R, Pribram K, eds. *The hippocampus*, vol. 4. New York: Plenum Press; 1986.

106. Jarrard L, Kant G, Meyerhoff J, Levy A. Behavioral and neurochemical effects of intraventricular administration of AF64A in rats. *Pharmacol Biochem Behav* 1984;21:273–280.

107. Jones BE, Cuello AC. Afferents to the basal forebrain cholinergic area from pontomesencephalic-catecholamine, serotonin and acetylcholine-neurons. *Neuroscience* 1989;31:37–61.

108. Jones BE, Yang TZ. Efferent projections from the reticular formation and the locus coeruleus studied by anterograde and retrograde axonal transport in the rat. *J Comp Neurol* 1985; 242:56–92.

109. Kaseda Y, Simon JR, Low WC. Restoration of high affinity choline uptake in the hippocampal formation following septal cell suspension transplants in rats with fimbria–fornix lesions. *J Neurochem* 1989;53:482–488.

110. Kawaja MD, Fagan AM, Firestein BL, Gage FH. Intracerebral grafting of cultured autologous skin fibroblasts into the rat striatum: assessment of graft size and ultrastructure. *J Comp Neurol* 1991;307:695–706.

111. Kawaja MD, Gage FH. Reactive astrocytes are substrates for the growth of adult CNS axons in the presence of elevated levels of nerve growth factor. *Neuron* 1991;7:1019–1030.

112. Kawaja MD, Rosenberg MB, Yoshida K, Gage FH. Somatic gene transfer of nerve growth factor promotes the survival of axotomized septal neurons and the regeneration of their axons in adult rats. *J Neurosci* 1992;12:2849–2864.

113. Kershaw TR, Sinden JD, Allen YS, Gray JA, Lantos PL. Behavioural recovery following transplantation of the neuroblastoma cell line IMR-32. *Prog Brain Res* 1990;82:47–53.

114. Kimura H, McGeer PL, Peng JH, McGeer EG. The central cholinergic system studied by choline acetyltransferase immunohistochemistry in the cat. *J Comp Neurol* 1981;200:151–201.

114a. Kleschevnikov AM, Marchbanks RM. Behavioral parameters of the spatial memory correlate with the potentiation of the population spike, but not with the population excitatory postsynaptic potential, of the CA_1 region in rat hippocampal slices. *Neurosci Lett* 1993;152: 125–128.

115. Kordower JH, Notter MFD, Gash DM. Neuroblastoma cells in neural transplants: a neuroanatomical and behavioral analysis. *Brain Res* 1987;417:85–98.

116. Korsching S, Heumann R, Thoenen H, Hefti F. Cholinergic denervation of the rat hippocampus by fimbrial transection leads to a transient accumulation of nerve growth factor (NGF) without change in mRNA NGF content. *Neurosci Lett* 1986;66:175–180.

117. Krnjevic K, Pumain P, Renaud L. The mechanism of excitation by acetylcholine in the cerebral cortex. *J Physiol(Lond)* 1971;215:247–268.

118. Krnjevic K, Ropert N. Electrophysiological and pharmacological characteristics of facilitation of hippocampal population spikes by stimulation of the medial septum. *Neuroscience* 1982;7:2165–2183.

119. Kruger S, Sievers J, Hansen C, Sadler M, Berry M. Three morphologically distinct types of interface develop between adult host and fetal brain transplants: implications for scar formation in the adult central nervous system. *J Comp Neurol* 1986;249:103–116.

120. Larkfors L, Stromberg I, Ebendal T, Olson L. Nerve growth factor protein level increases in the adult rat hippocampus after a specific cholinergic lesion. *J Neurosci Res* 1987;18:525–531.

121. Larson J, Wong D, Lynch G. Patterned stimulation at the theta frequency is optimal for the induction of hippocampal long-term potentiation. *Brain Res* 1986;368:347–350.

122. Lawrence JM, Raisman G, Mirsky R, Jessen KR. Transplantation of postnatal rat enteric ganglia into denervated adult rat hippocampus. *Neuroscience* 1991;44:371–379.

123. Lemann W, Saper CB. Evidence for a cortical projection to the magnocellular basal nucleus in the rat: an electron microscopic axonal transport study. *Brain Res* 1985;334:339–343.

124. Levey AI, Wainer BH, Rye DB, Mufson EJ, Mesulam MM. Choline acetyltransferase-immunoreactive neurons intrinsic to rodent cortex and distinction from acetylcholinesterase-positive neurons. *Neuroscience* 1984;13:341–353.

125. Li YJ, Simon JR, Low WC. Intrahippocampal grafts of cholinergic-rich striatal tissue ameliorate spatial memory deficits in rats with fornix lesions. *Brain Res Bull* 1992;29:147–155.

126. Llinas RR. The intrinsic electrophysiological properties of mammalian neurons: insights into central nervous system function. *Science* 1988;242:1654–1664.

127. Low WC, Lewis PR, Bunch ST, Dunnett SB, Thomas SR, Iversen SD, Björklund A, Stenevi U. Functional recovery following neural transplantation of embryonic septal nuclei in adult

rats with septohippocampal lesions. *Nature* 1982;300:260–262.

128. Lysakowski A, Wainer BH, Bruce G, Hersh LB. An atlas of the regional and laminar distribution of choline acetyltransferase immunoreactivity in rat cerebral cortex. *Neuroscience* 1989;28:291–336.

129. Mandel RJ, Gage FH, Thal LJ. Enhanced detection of nucleus basalis magnocellularis lesion-induced spatial learning deficit in rats by modification of training regimen. *Behav Brain Res* 1989;31:221–229.

130. Mantione CR, Fisher A, Hanin I. The AF64A-treated mouse: possible model for central cholinergic hypofunction. *Science* 1981;213:579–580.

131. Marsden KM, Kershaw TR, Sinden JD, Lantos PL. Survival and distribution of transplanted human IMR-32 neuroblastoma cells. *Brain Res* 1991;568:76–84.

132. Matthews DA, Salvaterra PM, Crawford GD, Houser CR, Vaughn JE. An immunocytochemical study of choline acetyltransferase-containing neurons and axon terminals in normal and partially deafferented hippocampal formation. *Brain Res* 1987;402:30–43.

133. Mayer ML, Westbrook GL. The physiology of excitatory amino acids in the vertebrate central nervous system. *Prog Neurobiol* 1987;28:197–276.

134. McCormick DA. Neurotransmitter actions in the thalamus and cerebral cortex and their role in neuromodulation of thalamocortical activity. *Prog Neurobiol* 1992;39:337–388.

135. McCormick DA, Connors BW, Lighthall J, Prince DA. Comparative electrophysiology of pyramidal and sparsely spiny stellatc neurones of the neocortex. *J Neurophysiol* 1985;54:782–806.

136. McCormick DA, Prince DA. Mechanisms of action of acetylcholine in the guinea-pig cerebral cortex *in vitro*. *J Physiol(Lond)* 1986;375:169–194.

137. McCormick DA, Prince DA. Acetylcholine causes rapid nicotinic excitation in the medial habenular nucleus of guinea pig *in vitro*. *J Neurosci* 1987;7:742–752.

138. McGurk SR, Hartgraves SL, Kelly PH, Gordon MN, Butcher LL. Is ethylcholine aziridinium ion a specific cholinergic neurotoxin? *Neuroscience* 1987;22:215–224.

139. McGurk SR, Levin ED, Butcher LL. Impairment of radial-arm maze performance in rats following lesions of the cholinergic medial pathway: reversal by arecoline and differential effects of muscarinic and nicotinic antagonists. *Neuroscience* 1991;44:137–147.

140. McKeon RJ, Vietje BP, Wells J. Interactions between donor and host tissue following cross-species septohippocampal transplants. *Exp Neurol* 1989;103:213–221.

141. McKhann G, Drachman D, Folstein M, Katzman R, Price D, Stadlan EM. Clinical diagnosis of Alzheimer's disease: report on the NINCDS-ADRA work group under the auspices of Department of Health and Human Services task force on Alzheimer's disease. *Neurology* 1984;34:939–944.

142. Meck WH, Church RM, Wenk GL, Olton DS. Nucleus basalis magnocellularis and medial septal area lesions differently impair temporal memory. *J Neurosci* 1987;7:3505–3511.

143. Messersmith DJ, Fabrazzo M, Mochetti I, Kromer LF. Effects of sciatic nerve transplants after fimbria–fornix lesion: examination of the role of nerve growth factor. *Brain Res* 1991;557:293–297.

144. Mesulam MM, Mufson EJ, Wainer BH, Levey AJ. Central cholinergic pathways in the rat. An overview based on an alternative nomenclature. *Neuroscience* 1983;10:1185–1201.

145. Montero-Menei CN, Pouplard-Barthelaix A, Gumpel M, Van Evercooren AB. Pure Schwann cell suspension grafts promote regeneration of the lesioned septo-hippocampal cholinergic pathway. *Brain Res* 1992;570:198–208.

146. Morris RG, Kopelman MD. The memory deficits in Alzheimer-type dementia: a review. *Q J Exp Psychol* 1986;38A:575–602.

147. Morris RGM, Schenk F, Tweedie F, Jarrard LE. Ibotenate lesions of the hippocampus and/or subiculum: dissociating components of allocentric spatial learning. *Eur J Neurosci* 1990;2:1016–1028.

148. Muir JL, Dunnett SB, Robbins TW, Everitt BJ. Attentional functions of the forebrain cholinergic systems: effects of intraventricular hemicholinium, physostigmine, basal forebrain lesions and intacortical grafts on a multiple-choice serial reaction time task. *Exp Brain Res* 1992;89:611–622.

149. Neary D, Snowden JS. The differential diagnosis of dementias caused by neurodegenerative disease. *Semin Neurosci* 1990;2:81–88.

150. Nicholas MK, Arnason BGW. Immunological considerations in transplantation to the central nervous system. In: Seil FJ, ed. *Neural regeneration and transplantation*. New York, Alan R Liss; 1989:239–284.

151. Nicoll RA, Malenka RC, Kauer JA. Functional comparison of neurotransmitter receptor subtypes in mammalian central nervous system. *Physiol Rev* 1990;70:513–565.

152. Nilsson OG, Björklund A. Behaviour-dependent changes in acetylcholine release in normal and graft-reinnervated hippocampus: evidence for host regulation of grafted cholinergic neurons. *Neuroscience* 1992;49:33–44.

153. Nilsson OG, Brundin P, Björklund A. Amelioration of spatial memory impairment by intrahippocampal grafts of mixed septal and raphe tissue in rats with combined cholinergic and serotonergic denervation of the forebrain. *Brain Res* 1990;515:193–206.

154. Nilsson OG, Clarke DJ, Brundin P, Björklund A. Comparison of growth and reinnervation properties of cholinergic neurons from different brain regions grafted to the hippocampus. *J Comp Neurol* 1988;268:204–222.

155. Nilsson OG, Kalen P, Rosengren E, Björklund A. Acetylcholine release from intrahippocampal septal grafts is under control of the host

brain. *Proc Natl Acad Sci USA* 1990;87:2647–2651.

155a. Nilsson OG, Leanza G, Rosenblad C, Lippa DA, Wiley RG, Björklund A. Spatial learning impairments in rats with selective immunolesion of the forebrain cholinergic system. *Neuroreport* 1992;3:1005–1008.

156. Nilsson OG, Shapiro ML, Gage FH, Olton DS, Björklund A. Spatial learning and memory following fimbria–fornix transection and grafting of fetal septal neurons to the hippocampus. *Exp Brain Res* 1987;67:195–215.

157. Nishino H, Koide K, Aihara N, Mitzukawa K, Nagai H. Striatal grafts in infarct striatum after occlusion of the middle cerebral artery improve passive avoidance/water maze learning, GABA release and GABA_A receptor deficits in the rat. *Restor Neurol Neurosci* 1992;4:178.

158. Nunez A, Garcia-Austt E, Buno W Jr. Intracellular theta rhythm generation in identified hippocampal pyramids. *Brain Res* 1987;416:289–300.

159. Nunn JA, Le Peillet E, Netto CA, Sowinski P, Hodges H, Gray JA, Meldrum BS. CA_1 cell loss produces deficits in learning and memory in the water maze regardless of additional intra- and extra-hippocampal damage. *J Cereb Blood Flow Metab* 1991;11(suppl 2):338.

160. Nunn JA, Le Peillet E, Netto CA, Sowinski P, Hodges H, Meldrum BS, Gray JA. CA_1 cell loss produces deficits in the water maze but not in the radial maze. *Soc Neurosci Abstr* 1991;17:108.

161. Ogawa M, Ishikawa T, Irimajiri A. Adrenal chromaffin cells form functional cholinergic synapses in culture. *Nature* 1984;307:66–68.

162. Oh JD, Woolf NJ, Roghani A, Edwards RH, Butcher LL. Cholinergic neurons in the rat central nervous system demonstrated by *in situ* hybridization of choline acetyltransferase mRNA. *Neuroscience* 1992;47:807–822.

163. Okuda O, Bressler J, Chang L, Brightman M. Viral Kirsten *ras* infection differentiates PC12 cells and enhances their survival upon implantation into brain. *Exp Neurol* 1991;113:330–337.

164. Olton DS, Becker JT, Handelman GE. Hippocampus, space and memory. *Behav Brain Sci* 1979;2:315–365.

165. Olton DS, Wenk GL, Church RM, Meck WH. Attention and the frontal cortex as examined by simultaneous temporal processing. *Neuropsychologia* 1988;26:307–318.

166. Page KJ, Everitt BJ, Robbins TW, Marston HM, Wilkinson LS. Dissociable effects on spatial maze and passive avoidance acquisition and retantion following AMPA- and ibotenic acid-induced excitotoxic lesions of the basal forebrain in rats: differential dependence on cholinergic neuronal loss. *Neuroscience* 1991;43:457–472.

167. Pallage V, Orenstein D, Will B. Nerve growth factor and septal grafts: a study of behavioral recovery following partial damage to the septum in rats. *Behav Brain Res* 1992;47:1–12.

168. Pare D, Smith Y, Parent A, Steriade M. Projec-

tions of upper brainstem cholinergic and noncholinergic neurons of cat to intralaminar and reticular thalamic nuclei. *Neuroscience* 1988;25:69–86.

169. Pearson RCA, Neal JW, Powell TPS. Hypertrophy of cholinergic neurones of the basal nucleus in the rat following damage of the contralateral nucleus. *Brain Res* 1986;382:149–152.

170. Perry EK, Perry RH, Blessed G, Tomlinson BE. Necropsy evidence of central cholinergic deficits in senile dementia. *Lancet* 1977;1:189–189.

171. Pirch JH, Turco K, Rucker HK. A role for acetylcholine in conditioning-related responses of rat frontal cortex neurons: microiontophoretic evidence. *Brain Res* 1992;586:19–26.

172. Price DL. New perspectives on Alzheimer's disease. *Annu Rev Neurosci* 1986;9:489–512.

173. Pulsinelli WA, Brierley MD, Plum F. Temporal profile of neuronal damage in a model of transient forebrain ischemia. *Ann Neurol* 1982;11:491–498.

174. Rawlins JNP. Associations across time: the hippocampus as a temporary memory store. *Behav Brain Sci* 1985;8:479–528.

175. Rawlins JNP, Feldon J, Tonkiss J, Coffey PJ. The role of subicular output in the development of the partial reinforcement extinction effect. *Exp Brain Res* 1989;77:153–160.

176. Rawlins JNP, Maxwell TJ, Sinden JD. The effects of fornix section on win–stay/lose–shift and win–shift/lose–stay performance in the rat. *Behav Brain Res* 1988;31:17–28.

177. Renfranz PJ, Cunningham MG, McKay RDG. Region-specific differentiation of the hippocampal stem cell line HiB5 upon implantation into the developing mammalian brain. *Cell* 1991;66:713–729.

178. Richardson PM, Verge Issa VMK, Riopelle R. Distribution of neuronal receptors for nerve growth factor in the rat. *J Neurosci* 1986;6:2312–2321.

179. Richardson RT, DeLong MR. Context-dependent responses of primate nucleus basalis neurons in a go/no-go task. *J Neurosci* 1990;10:2528–2540.

180. Richter-Levin G, Segal M. Raphe cells grafted into the hippocampus can ameliorate spatial memory deficits in rats with combined serotonergic/cholinergic deficiencies. *Brain Res* 1989;478:184–186.

181. Ridley RM, Baker HF. A critical evaluation of monkey models of amnesia and dementia. *Brain Res Rev* 1991;16:15–37.

182. Riekkinen P, Buzsaki G, Riekkinen P Jr, Soininen H, Partanen J. The cholinergic system and EEG slow waves. *Electroencephalogr Clin Neurophysiol* 1991;78:89–96.

183. Robbins TW, Everitt BJ, Marston HM, Wilkinson J, Jones GH, Page KJ. Comparative effects of ibotenic acid- and quisqualic acid-induced lesions of the substantia innominata on attentional function in the rat: further implications for the role of the cholinergic neurons of the nucleus basalis in cognitive processes. *Behav Brain Res* 1989;35:221–241.

184. Robbins TW, Everitt BJ, Muir JL, Harrison A. Understanding the behavioural functions of neurochemically defined arousal systems. *IBRO News* 1992;20(3):7.

185. Robbins TW, Everitt BJ, Ryan CN, Marston HM, Jones GH, Page KJ. Comparative effects of quisqualic and ibotenic acid-induced lesions of the substantia innominata and globus pallidus on the acquisition of a conditional visual discrimination: differential effects on cholinergic mechanisms. *Neuroscience* 1989;28:337–352.

186. Rosenberg MB, Friedmann T, Robinson RC, Tuszynski M, Wolff JA, Breakefield XO, Gage FH. Grafting of genetically modified cells to the damaged brain: restorative effects of NGF expression. *Science* 1988;242:1575–1578.

187. Russell RW. Behavioral aspects of cholinergic transmission. *Fed Proc* 1969;28:121–131.

188. Rye DB, Wainer BH, Mesulam MM, Mufson EJ, Saper CB. Cortical projections arising from the basal forebrain: a study of cholinergic and non-cholinergic components employing combined retrograde tracing and immunohistochemical localization of choline acetyltransferase. *Neuroscience* 1984;13:627–643.

189. Saper CB. Organization of cerebral cortical afferent systems in the rat. II. Magnocellular basal nucleus. *J Comp Neurol* 1984;222:313–342.

190. Sato H, Hata Y, Masui H, Tsumoto T. A functional role of cholinergic innervation to neurons in the cat visual cortex. *J Neurophysiol* 1987;58:765–780.

191. Satoh K, Fibiger HC. Distribution of central cholinergic neurons in the baboon (*Papio papio*). 1. General morphology. *J Comp Neurol* 1985;236:197–214.

192. Schinstine M, Rosenberg MB, Routledge C, Friedmann T, Gage FH. Effects of choline and quiescence on drosophila choline acetyltransferase expression and acetylcholine production by transduced rat fibroblasts. *J Neurochem* 1992;58:2019–2029.

193. Schoenen J. Dendritic organization of the human spinal cord: the motorneurons. *J Comp Neurol* 1982;211:226–247.

194. Segal M, Björklund A, Gage FH. Transplanted septal neurons make viable cholinergic synapses with a host hippocampus. *Brain Res* 1985;336:302–307.

195. Segal M, Greenberger V, Pearl E. Septal transplants ameliorate spatial deficits and restore cholinergic functions in rats with a damaged septo-hippocampal connection. *Brain Res* 1989;500:139–148.

196. Shute CCD, Lewis PR. The ascending cholinergic reticular system: neocortical, olfactory and subcortical projections. *Brain* 1967;90:497–520.

197. Sillito AM, Kemp JA. Cholinergic modulation of the functional organization of the cat visual cortex. *Brain Res* 1983;289:143–155.

198. Sinden JD, Allen YS, Rawlins JNP, Gray JA. The effects of ibotenic acid lesions of the nucleus basalis and cholinergic-rich neural transplants on win–stay/lose–shift and win–shift/lose–stay performance in the rat. *Behav Brain Res* 1990;36:229–249.

199. Sinden JD, Marsden KM, Hodges H. Neural transplantation and recovery of function. Animal studies. In: Rose FD, Johnson DA, eds. *Recovery from brain damage: reflections and directions*. New York: Plenum Press; 1992.

200. Sloan DJ, Baker BJ, Puklavec M, Charlton HM. The effect of site of transplantation and histocompatibility differences on the survival of neural tissue transplanted to the CNS of defined inbred rat strains. *Prog Brain Res* 1990;82:141–152.

201. Sloan DJ, Wood MJ, Charlton HM. The immune response to intracerebral neural grafts. *Trends Neurosci* 1991;14:341–346.

202. Smith G. Animal models of Alzheimer's disease: experimental cholinergic denervation. *Brain Res Rev* 1988;13:103–118.

203. Smythe JW, Colom LV, Bland BH. The extrinsic modulation of hippocampal theta depends on the coactivation of cholinergic and GABAergic medial septal inputs. *Neurosci Biobehav Rev* 1992;16:289–308.

204. Steriade M, Gloor P, Llinas RR, Lopes da Silva FH, Mesulam MM. Basic mechanisms of cerebral rhythmic activities. *Electroencephalogr Clin Neurophysiol* 1990;76:481–508.

205. Stewart DJ, MacFabe DG, Vanderwolf CH. Cholinergic activation of the electrocorticogram: role of the substantia innominata and effects of atropine and quinuclidinyl benzilate. *Brain Res* 1984;322:219–232.

206. Swanson LW, Simmons DH, Whiting PJ, Lindstrom J. Immunohistochemical localization of neuronal nicotinic receptors in rodent central nervous system. *J Neurosci* 1987;7:3334–3342.

207. Tarricone BJ, Keim SR, Simon JR, Low WC. Intrahippocampal transplants of septal cholinergic neurons: high affinity choline uptake and spatial memory function. *Brain Res* 1991;548:55–62.

208. Thoenen H, Edgar D. Neurotrophic factors. *Science* 1985;229:238–242.

209. Tomlinson BE, Blessed G, Roth M. Observations on the brains of demented old people. *J Neurol Sci* 1970;11:205–242.

210. Tremblay N, Warren RA, Dykes RW. Electrophysiological studies of acetylcholine and the role of the basal forebrain in the somatosensory cortex of the cat. II. Cortical neurons excited by somatic stimuli. *J Neurophysiol* 1990;64:1212–1222.

211. Turner JJ, Hodges H, Sinden JD, Gray JA. Comparison of radial maze performance of rats after ibotenate and quisqualate lesions of the forebrain cholinergic projection system: effects of pharmacological challenge and changes in training regimen. *Behav Pharmacol* 1992;3:359–374.

212. Tuszynski MH, Buzsaki G, Gage FH. Nerve growth factor infusions combined with fetal hippocampal grafts enhance reconstruction of the lesioned septohippocampal projection. *Neuroscience* 1990;36:33–44.

213. Valentino RJ, Dingledine R. Presynaptic inhibitory effect of acetylcholine in the hippocampus. *J Neurosci* 1981;1:784–792.

214. Vanderwolf CH, Fine A, Cooley RK. Intracortical grafts of embryonic basal forebrain tissue restore low voltage fast activity in rats with basal forebrain lesions. *Exp Brain Res* 1990; 81:426–432.

215. Vanderwolf CH, Robinson TH. Reticulocortical activity and behavior: a critique of the arousal theory and a new synthesis. *Behav Brain Sci* 1981;4:459–514.

216. van der Zee EA, Streefland C, Strosberg AD, Schroder H, Luiten PGM. Visualization of cholinoceptive neurons in the rat neocortex: colocalization of muscarinic and nicotinic acetylcholine receptors. *Mol Brain Res* 1992; 14:326–336.

217. Varon S, Hagg T, Manthorpe M. Neuronal growth factors. In: Seil FJ, ed. *Neural regeneration and transplantation*. New York: Alan R Liss; 1989:101–121.

218. Vidal C, Changeux JP. Pharmacological profile of nicotinic acetylcholine receptors in the rat prefrontal cortex: an electrophysiological study in a slice preparation. *Neuroscience* 1989; 29:261–270.

219. Vilaro MT, Wiederhold KH, Palacios JM, Mengod G. Muscarinic M$_2$ receptor mRNA expression and receptor binding in cholinergic and non-cholinergic cells in the rat brain: a correlative study using *in situ* hybridization histochemistry and receptor autoradiography. *Neuroscience* 1992;47:367–393.

220. Welner SA, Dunnett SB, Salamone JD, MacLean B, Iversen SD. Transplantation of embryonic ventral forebrain grafts to the neocortex of rats with bilateral lesions of nucleus basalis magnocellularis ameliorates a lesion-induced deficit in spatial memory. *Brain Res* 1988; 463:192–197.

221. Welner SA, Koty ZC, Boksa P. Chromaffin cell grafts to rat cerebral cortex reverse lesion-induced memory deficits. *Brain Res* 1990;527: 163–166.

222. Wenk GL, Markowska AL, Olton DS. Basal forebrain lesions and memory: alterations in neurotensin, not acetylcholine, may cause amnesia. *Behav Neurosci* 1989;103:765–769.

223. Wets KM, Sinden J, Hodges H, Allen Y, Marchbanks RM. Specific brain protein changes correlated with behaviourally effective brain transplants. *J Neurochem* 1991;57:1661–1670.

224. Whitehouse PJ, Martino AH, Antuono PG, Lowenstein PR, Coyle J, Price DL, Kellar KJ. Nicotinic acetylcholine binding sites in Alzheimer's disease. *Brain Res* 1986;371:146–151.

225. Whitehouse PJ, Price DL, Struble RG, Clark AW, Coyle JT, DeLong MR. Alzheimer's disease and senile dementia: loss of neurons in the basal forebrain. *Science* 1982;215:1237–1239.

226. Whittemore SR, Holets VR, Keane RW, Levy DJ, McKay RDG. Transplantation of a temperature-sensitive, nerve growth factor-secreting, neuroblastoma cell line into adult rats with fimbria–fornix lesions rescues cholinergic septal neurons. *J Neurosci* 1991;28:156–170.

227. Wictorin K. Anatomy and connectivity of intrastriatal striatal transplants. *Prog Neurobiol* 1992;38:611–639.

228. Widner H, Brundin P. Immunological aspects of grafting in the mammalian central nervous system. A review and speculative synthesis. *Brain Res Rev* 1988;13:287–324.

229. Williams S, Johnston D. Muscarinic depression of long-term potentiation in CA$_3$ hippocampal neurons. *Science* 1988;242:84–87.

230. Woolf NJ. Cholinergic systems in mammalian brain and spinal cord. *Prog Neurobiol* 1991; 37:475–524.

231. Woolf NJ, Gould E, Butcher LL. Nerve growth factor receptor is associated with cholinergic neurons of the basal forebrain but not the pontomesencephalon. *Neuroscience* 1989;30:143–152.

Functional Neural Transplantation,
edited by S. B. Dunnett and A. Björklund.
Raven Press, Ltd., New York © 1994.

11

Transplantation, Aging, and Memory

Karen S. Chen and *Fred H. Gage

Department of Neurosciences, Genentech, Inc., South San Francisco, California 94080;
*Department of Neurosciences, University of California, San Diego, La Jolla, California 92093

Neural transplantation can be used both as a tool to understand basic mechanisms of brain function and dysfunction and as a potential therapeutic intervention for injury and disease. Specifically, neural transplantation can help elucidate the biologic mechanisms underlying the functional consequences of aging. Associations between cognitive deficits observed during aging and postmortem indices of neurotransmitter function or neuropathology are correlational and not causal. In contrast, demonstration of functional recovery after implantation of specific neural tissue or cells would support the hypothesis that dysfunction of the cells or neural systems that are specifically affected by the implants may underlie some of the age-related cognitive impairments.

Neural transplantation has been used to investigate mechanisms underlying age-related learning and memory impairments in experimental models of neurodegenerative diseases. The neural grafting technique has been used to examine the efficacy of "neuronal replacement" (89) therapies in the lesioned brain. For example, grafts of fetal dopamine-rich tissue to the striatum of rats with 6-hydroxydopamine lesions of the nigrostriatal pathway—a model for Parkinson's disease—and grafts of fetal cholinergic-rich tissue to animals with hippocampal or neocortical lesions—a model for Alzheimer's disease (AD)—can serve as re-placements for cells in the host brain that have degenerated. The amelioration of behavioral deficits after the implantation of specific types of cells demonstrates that those cells may either directly or indirectly mediate the behavior of interest.

The present chapter first reviews studies that have examined the role of the central cholinergic neurotransmitter system in aging and memory function. Then, studies that have examined two animal models of age-related changes in the cholinergic system—lesions of the septohippocampal or nucleus basalis magnocellularis (NBM)–cortical pathway—as well as in aged animals themselves, are presented. In particular, studies that examined the cognitive effects of grafts implanted into aged animals are discussed in detail. Finally, several studies that have used neural transplantation to examine the process of neurodegeneration are presented.

CENTRAL CHOLINERGIC SYSTEMS AND AGING

Aging and the Cholinergic System

This review focuses primarily on the cholinergic neurotransmitter system. The cholinergic system has received much attention in studies of aging and AD. Evidence of the role of the cholinergic system in age-related cognitive deficits has been obtained from studies in patients with AD. Alzheimer's disease is characterized by a progressive deterioration of cognitive functions, especially learning and memory, and is associated with distinctive patterns of degeneration in the central nervous system (CNS). A severe functional deterioration of the cholinergic system is one of the most consistent, as well as one of the earliest, pathologic changes in AD (reviewed in 22, 42). Choline acetyltransferase (ChAT) is an enzyme involved in the synthesis of acetylcholine (ACh) and serves as a marker for cholinergic neurons. In the CNS, a significant reduction in ChAT activity was found to accompany normal aging and dementia (30,38,50,146,169,171,232). Recent studies have indicated that, in addition to reduced cortical ChAT activity, atrophy of basal forebrain cholinergic neurons may be correlated with the degree of cognitive impairment and the presence of neuropathologic markers, such as senile plaques in AD (38,79,120,172). This cholinergic deficit appears to be mainly a presynaptic dysfunction, because the level of postsynaptic muscarinic receptors appears unchanged or only slightly decreased (51,186,232).

Neuroanatomically, a dramatic degeneration of cholinergic cells in the nucleus basalis of Meynert, which provides the major cholinergic input to the neocortex, was observed in patients with AD (42,52,167,233). The cholinergic projection neurons in the basal forebrain provide the major cholinergic afferent input to the hippocampal formation, amygdala, and neocortex as well as olfactory bulb in a widespread and topographic pattern in humans, nonhuman primates, and rodents (149,194,224,238). The cholinergic neurons are located in a band-like structure divided into the medial septum (MS), the vertical limb of the diagonal band (VDB), the horizontal limb of the diagonal band, substantia inominata, and NBM regions. Neurons of the MS and VDB project dorsally to the hippocampus mainly through the fimbria–fornix, supracallosal

stria, and a ventral pathway (83,135). About 50% of the MS/VDB neurons sending fibers through the fimbria–fornix are cholinergic (6,225), and provide the hippocampus with about 90% of its total cholinergic innervation (209). Neurons of the NBM provide the major source of cholinergic input to the neocortex via a medial pathway from the medial NBM over the genu of the corpus callosum through the cingulate bundle to the medial and frontal cortices, and a lateral pathway from the lateral NBM through the external capsule to lateral cortical areas, including the temporal cortex (148,191). Approximately 80% to 90% of the neurons in the NBM are cholinergic. Lesions of the NBM with neurotoxins deplete cortical cholinergic levels by up to 70% (229). Cholinergic neurons, axons, and terminals can be visualized by immunocytochemistry for ChAT (13) and the degradative enzyme, acetylcholinesterase (AChE) (33). Terminal fields within the hippocampal formation and the neocortex can be quantified biochemically by measuring extracted ChAT activity (77,78).

Another reason to focus on the cholinergic system to elucidate the biologic mechanisms underlying age-related learning and memory deficits is the well documented involvement of the hippocampus in learning and memory function. Lesion and psychopharmacology studies have demonstrated that the cholinergic system is involved in learning and memory function (54,55). Lesions in the hippocampal system of humans (223,242), monkeys (154,243), and rats (25, 63) resulted in memory deficits (for a recent review, see 205), especially spatial memory deficits (164,165,212). Drugs that selectively alter central cholinergic neurotransmission have been administered to normal subjects to determine its role in learning and memory function. Low doses of scopolamine, a cholinergic antagonist that blocks central muscarinic receptors, produced a loss of recent memory and working memory in humans and nonhuman primates (24,55). The effects of scopolamine were reversed by physostigmine, a cholinergic agonist that increases ACh levels by inhibiting AChE (2,21,55,150). In rodents and primates, lesions of the NBM resulted in learning and memory impairments that were partially reversed by cholinergic agonists, such as physostigmine, oxotremorine, and arecholine (156,158,159,183, 218).

This evidence of the involvement of the cholinergic system in aging and AD, as well as in learning and memory function, led to formation of the "cholinergic hypothesis of age-related memory dysfunction" (22,42). The cholinergic hypothesis asserts that 1) significant, functional disturbances in cholinergic activity occur in the brains of aged, especially demented patients; 2) these disturbances play an important role in the memory loss and other cognitive problems related to aging and dementia; and 3) enhancement or restoration of cholinergic function may significantly reduce the severity of the cognitive loss (23).

It should be stressed that the cholinergic hypothesis does not exclude the involvement of other neurotransmitter systems in age-related cognitive dysfunctions. In addition to deficiencies in the cholinergic system, AD affects other transmitter and peptide systems, including noradrenergic (1,29, 43,170), serotonergic (7,46,79,239), and somatostatin-containing neuron systems (49, 188).

There also are morphologic changes that occur in aging, AD, or both. For example, there is a significant shrinkage of neocortical neurons (215) and a reduction in hippocampal cell number (17). Masliah and colleagues (142) immunohistochemically quantified presynaptic nerve terminal populations in healthy subjects and patients with AD using an antibody against synaptophysin. These investigators showed significant synaptic loss in the neocortex and in the molecular layer of the hippocampus. These changes in synaptophysin immunoreactivity may be more highly correlated with cognitive deficits in AD than the presence of plaques and tangles (216). Other investigators have found dendritic degeneration in dentate gyrus granule cells (53) and a regression in dendritic branching in parahippocampal pyramidal neurons (32) in patients with AD.

Consequently, some investigators have shifted their focus away from the cholinergic system; however, results indicating that therapeutic interventions that can supplement or increase cholinergic function can ameliorate some of the cognitive deficits associated with aging in experimental animals support the idea that increasing cholinergic function *alone* may be adequate for the reversal of some age-related deficits. Therefore, although there may be numerous changes in various transmitter systems during aging, reversal of the cholinergic deficit may be sufficient for significant functional recovery.

Lesion Models of Age-Related Changes

A standard approach used by many investigators to model deficits, especially cognitive deficits associated with aging, has been to damage specific regions of the brains of young rats selectively in order to mimic certain age-related alterations. These include surgical lesions of the septohippocampal or NBM–neocortical cholinergic pathways, the MS or NBM region, and the hippocampus or cerebral cortex. Complete transection of the fimbria–fornix pathway in young adult rats resulted in a rapid and consistent retrograde degeneration and death of many of the MS/VDB neurons (including the cholinergic ones) that originally contributed axons through this pathway (45,99,106,129). Markers of cell survival (Nissl stains) (91), transmitter enzyme expression (AChE, ChAT) (14), and nerve growth factor receptor (NGFr) expressed in cells of the MS (157) demonstrated a loss of 70% to 90% of the cells in this region. One study has suggested that some of these cells may persist for extended periods in a dysfunctional state after fimbria–fornix lesions (102), although other studies using retrograde fluorescent markers suggested that most of these cells actually die (12,157,163,220). Thus, lesions of the septohippocampal pathway have been used frequently as an analogous animal model of aging, especially in modeling age-related cognitive declines.

Lesions of the NBM also have been used to investigate age-related cognitive declines. NBM lesions have resulted in neocortical morphologic changes (192,226), as well as producing significant behavioral deficits. Cognitive deficits have been demonstrated on a variety of learning and memory tasks, including passive avoidance (5,26,76,81,104,134,155), active avoidance (76,134), Morris water maze (144), radial arm maze (107,155,239), and T-maze (107, 125).

Lesion models do not usually reproduce all the changes associated with aging. Instead, a few of the morphologic changes may be induced, so that the correlation between these morphologic changes and specific behavioral, biochemical, or electrophysiologic consequences can be examined. Another objective in using this type of model is to observe the effectiveness of various therapeutic manipulations in reversing the induced changes. It should be emphasized, however, that this approach does not reproduce normal aging and thus cannot be used to investigate the mechanisms underlying the cognitive dysfunction observed during aging.

Aging in Rodents

Parallel to this work, studies have used the aged rodent to investigate age-dependent impairments in brain function and behavior, as well as morphologic alterations. In this approach, the natural development of changes during aging is studied to determine the correlation between the functional and neuropathologic deficits in the aged rat. Unlike lesioned animals, aged animals can be used to investigate the underlying mechanisms and etiology of various age-related alterations such as cognitive impairments.

Aged animals show many of the neurochemical changes characteristic of aged humans. There are marked decreases in cholinergic function as measured by decreased ACh synthesis and release, ChAT activity, high-affinity choline uptake, and receptor binding (28,93,94,101,136,140,145,151,196, 197,203,211,230). Aged rats and primates also exhibit declines in levels of dopamine, noradrenaline, and their metabolites (70, 96,147,166,175).

Neuronal cell loss in subcortical and cortical areas of aged rodents also has been observed in some studies (31,132,133), but not others (80,173). Specifically, morphometric analyses have demonstrated shrinkage or loss of ChAT-immunoreactive basal forebrain neurons in the MS, VDB, and NBM of aged rats (4,28,74,75,94,112,140). Some investigators report a significant shrinkage and not a loss of cholinergic neurons (149). These differing results may be due to the use of different histologic markers (AChE, ChAT, or NGFr) or strains of rats.

Rodents also show age-related behavioral impairments on a variety of tasks that assess learning and memory, motivation, and motoric and sensory function. Among the variety of cognitive deficits exhibited by aged rats, deficits in complex maze learning and spatial discrimination have been most thoroughly characterized (19, 74,85,97,98,100,116,139,141,152,176,222, 244). Aged rats also were impaired on operant delayed response (delayed nonmatching to position) (57), passive avoidance (31,95,136,141), shuttle-box avoidance (190), temporal discrimination (34), and complex nonspatial tasks, such as the 14-unit Stone maze (115). Aged rodents also exhibited impaired memory for a spatial environment as assessed by habituation (141).

Aged rats, as a group, were significantly impaired compared to young rats on the Morris water maze task, a test of spatial learning ability (74,75,85,141). Several studies have found a significant correlation between cholinergic cell loss and atrophy; cognitive impairments in aged rats have been noted on the water maze task (72, 74,75,126). In addition, these age-related deficits have been found to correlate with metabolic and cholinergic activity in the hippocampus (74,90).

Aged animals also showed reduced motor coordination, locomotor activity, and exploration. Several studies have indicated that aged rats are impaired on a variety of motoric tasks (34,116,141,217). In tests of activity and exploration in automated open-field boxes, aged rats showed significantly reduced levels of locomotor activity and exploration compared to young animals (3,97, 141,204,217,231). Furthermore, the unconditioned startle response to somatosensory stimulation of aged rats was significantly longer than that of the young group (141).

Aged rats, like aged humans, display considerable variability in the pattern and extent of age-related changes that they exhibit. This heterogeneity is manifested by the wide range in the degree of impairments observed on a variety of behavioral tests (18,19,75,85,86,176). Analysis of individual animal scores indicated that not all animals exhibited age-related deficits. The performances of some of the aged rats did not differ from those of the control rats, whereas other animals were severely impaired. In the water maze task, only a subgroup (approximately 30%) of the aged animals demonstrated a marked impairment, accounting for all the impairment in the aged group (74,75,85).

In addition, the decline in performance was not necessarily correlated across different behavioral tests (85,86,141). Multivariate analyses indicated that age-related impairments on a battery of different tests of cognitive function and motor coordination occur independently (86). This heterogeneity has also been observed by other investigators (74,75,82,84,90). Lamour and coworkers (131) examined the performance of aged rats on two different cognitive tasks, passive avoidance and spontaneous alternation. Subpopulations of aged ani-

mals were impaired on both tasks; however, most of the impaired animals were not impaired on both tasks. Markowska and colleagues (141) also tested aged rats on a battery of cognitive and sensorimotor tasks. In general, they found that sensorimotor performance was not correlated with cognitive performance. Also, the performances of individual aged rats on the different cognitive tasks were not correlated, even though the tasks supposedly measured the same cognitive processes (e.g., spatial memory was tested in the Morris water maze and the Barnes circular maze).

Therefore, age-related declines in different neuroanatomic systems, such as the limbic system and the basal ganglia, may progress independently of each other. This suggests that different anatomic systems may degenerate or become dysfunctional at different rates during aging, and that age-related degenerative changes are not likely to be controlled by a common underlying mechanism. Furthermore, correlations between behavioral, anatomic, biochemical, and electrophysiologic changes have helped elucidate the neurobiologic factors underlying functional impairments during senescence in rats.

GRAFTING INTO THE LESIONED BRAIN

Grafts and the Septohippocampal System

Investigators have transplanted various types of tissue into animals with fimbria–fornix lesions or lesions of the hippocampus to reverse some of the observed cognitive deficits. In one of the first studies, Dunnett and coworkers (59) grafted septal and locus coeruleus cells into the hippocampus of fimbria–fornix-lesioned rats, and then examined the functional effects of these grafts on the T-maze alternation task and the eight-arm radial maze. The septal, but not the locus coeruleus grafts restored the animals' ability to learn the T-maze task, demonstrating the specificity of the behavioral amelioration. The degree of recovery correlated with the extent of AChE fiber ingrowth from the septal grafts. Several other investigators also have shown recovery on the T-maze and radial arm maze tasks in rats that received fetal septal grafts after fimbria–fornix lesions (47,108,138); the recovery was correlated with the restoration of cholinergic activity, as measured by high-affinity choline uptake (214). The performance of the rats with grafts on the radial arm maze task was affected more by the administration of both cholinergic agonists and antagonists than the performance of control, nonlesioned rats (109). In a study using the Morris water maze task, septal grafts resulted in impairments, as well as improvements (58), but another study demonstrated that a substantial number of rats with septal grafts showed recovery on this task (161). This recovery was sensitive to atropine, a cholinergic antagonist, and thus presumably involved the cholinergic system. Fimbria–fornix and aspirative hippocampal lesions also produced deficits on an operant differential reinforcement of low rates task that could be reversed by fetal septal (60) and fetal hippocampal grafts implanted into the hippocampus (235). Woodruff and colleagues have also used the neurotoxin trimethyltin to lesion the hippocampus. The memory deficits observed on the passive avoidance but not the water maze task were ameliorated by fetal hippocampal grafts (236,237). Hippocampal grafts also reversed the deficits in the passive avoidance task that resulted from x-irradiation lesions of the dentate granule cells (153).

Recovery in fimbria–fornix lesioned rats after the implantation of cholinergic-rich fetal cells is not very robust, perhaps because of the additional disruption of noradrenergic, γ-aminobutyric acid–ergic, and serotonergic afferents and other subcortical efferents of the hippocampus. Therefore, Segal and colleagues (195) compared the effects of septal grafts in rats after either fimbria–fornix lesions or electrolytic lesions of

the MS, which are more specific. Both lesions disrupted performance on the water maze task. The septal grafts did not result in recovery in the rats with fimbria–fornix lesions, but were able significantly to ameliorate the deficits in the rats with MS lesions. Similarly, intrahippocampal septal grafts also were able to ameliorate behavioral deficits on the radial arm maze task after MS lesions (168). Similar recovery has been reported on spatial maze learning after aspirative hippocampal lesions (124). Fetal hippocampal tissue grafted into the hippocampus of rats with colchicine lesions, which specifically destroyed dentate gyrus granule cells and mossy fibers, ameliorated the lesion-induced spatial learning deficits observed on the radial arm maze and water maze tasks (20,213). The ability of septal grafts to induce recovery on the T-maze and radial arm maze tasks after damage to the hippocampus also has been observed in other studies using AF64A (ethylcholine aziridium ion), a cholinergic neurotoxin (113,114). The recovery on the radial arm maze task also was associated with restoration of high-affinity choline uptake levels in animals with septal grafts (64).

Most studies that attempt to model age-related alterations in animals have used rodents. Although rodents have been very useful, an alternative model for examining potential therapeutic interventions in humans is the nonhuman primate. Two recent studies by Ridley and colleagues (184,185) examined the effects of grafting fetal basal forebrain neurons into fornix-lesioned hippocampus of nonhuman primates (see Chapter 13). Animals that received grafts showed complete recovery from severe age-related deficits in visual learning, visuospatial conditional discriminations, visual conditional discrimination, and nonconditional spatial response tasks. In addition, dense AChE-positive fiber outgrowth was observed extending from the graft into the surrounding host tissue. Therefore, fetal cholinergic grafts are effective in reversing behavioral and morphologic alterations in lesioned nonhuman primates, as well as in lesioned rodents.

Most studies also have focused on lesions in only one neurotransmitter system, even though many neurotransmitter systems undergo age-related changes. Several studies did examine the result of more than one type of lesion and graft. Serotonergic raphe neurons, which send projections to the hippocampus, also exhibit age-related degeneration. To examine the contribution of other neurotransmitter systems besides the cholinergic system, Nilsson and colleagues (160) lesioned both the serotonergic and cholinergic systems in adult rats to reflect the multisystemic character of the aging process or AD. Combined cholinergic and serotonergic lesions of the hippocampus in rats resulted in more severe deficits in the water maze than either lesion alone (162). In a subsequent study (160), rats received either bilateral fetal septal, mesencephalic raphe, or mixed septal and raphe cell suspension grafts into the hippocampus, and were then tested in the Morris water maze. Only rats with combined cholinergic and serotonergic grafts were significantly improved on the water maze task. Similarly, Richter-Levin and Segal (180) depleted the forebrain serotonergic system with 5,7-dihydroxytryptamine (5,7-DHT) and then implanted raphe grafts. No deficits were observed on the water maze task. When animals were given atropine injections before testing, however, the lesion group demonstrated an impairment, whereas the raphe-grafted group did not, suggesting an interaction between the cholinergic and serotonergic systems. In a subsequent study, these investigators combined septal lesions with the 5,7-DHT lesions and observed a deficit on the water maze task that was ameliorated after intrahippocampal raphe grafts (181), and to a lesser extent by septal grafts (182).

Another issue that has been addressed in grafting studies is whether the administration of neurotrophic factors in addition to fetal grafting may augment the effect of fetal grafts alone, perhaps either by increasing the survival of the fetal grafts, by indirectly affecting the host, or by having an independent, additive effect on the host directly. In a recent study, Tuszynski and co-workers (221) combined chronic NGF infusions with fetal hippocampal grafts to reconstruct the cholinergic component of the septohippocampal pathway after fimbria–fornix lesion in the rat more completely than with grafting alone. Lesioned rats that received a 2-week infusion of NGF in addition to the fetal grafts had significantly greater long-term (8 months) savings of ChAT-positive cells in the MS compared to the group that received only a graft. There also was more extensive cholinergic reinnervation of the hippocampus in the combined NGF infusion and graft group. Even a short duration of NGF administration appeared able to augment the protective effect of fetal grafts in the lesioned rat model.

Barone and colleagues (20) assessed the effects of chronic NGF infusion alone or in combination with fetal hippocampal grafts on the recovery of spatial learning after damage to hippocampal dentate granule cells by the administration of colchicine. Lesioned rats were impaired compared to nonlesioned controls on the water maze task. At 4 weeks postgrafting, NGF, but not the transplant alone, ameliorated the deficit. The NGF-plus-transplant group performed better than the lesion-alone or the transplant-alone group. By 10 weeks, the colchicine-induced deficits could not be ameliorated by NGF, transplants, or the combination. In addition, NGF has been shown to promote survival and growth of transplanted septal and basal forebrain neurons (67,202,219), and enhance ChAT activity in septal grafts implanted into the hippocampus (219).

Almost all types of neural and nonneural cells have been implanted into the brain to ameliorate the behavioral deficits induced in lesion models. Differentiated neuroblastoma cells from human- and rat-derived cell lines also have been transplanted into the hippocampus of rats with MS lesions (128). These grafts were able to ameliorate deficits on a delayed nonmatching to sample task in a T-maze. Thus peripheral cholinergic cells, adrenal chromaffin cells, and differentiated neuroblastoma cells may provide viable alternatives to the use of fetal cholinergic cells.

Recently, transplantation of cells that have been genetically modified to express various neurotransmitters and neurotrophic factors has been used as a potentially powerful therapeutic approach in models of neuropathologic conditions such as AD, as well as in investigations of development, function, and repair in the CNS (89,92). Grafts of genetically modified cells can, in localized areas of the brain, secrete trophic factors that may directly or indirectly support survival and function of damaged or dying neurons, secrete neurotransmitters or hormones to replace missing or deficient ones, act as functioning neurons by making synaptic contacts on appropriate postsynaptic receptors, or act as bridges for cut or sprouting axons heading toward their target sites. Potentially, these "biologic pumps" can express specific functional proteins stably for a long time. Until recently, the use of neuronal cells for this purpose was limited owing to lack of cell culture techniques available to induce replication of neuronal cells. The lack of availability of genetically modifiable neuronal cells led to the use of nonneuronal cells for grafting in the brain, which precludes the establishment of specific neuronal connections with target cells. The grafted nonneuronal cells can act by secreting required gene products, thereby affecting the target cells.

Several investigators have used genetically modified cells that secrete NGF to determine whether these cells can save MS cholinergic neurons after fimbria–fornix lesions. Rosenberg and colleagues (187) and Stromberg and colleagues (210) have been able to rescue basal forebrain cholinergic neurons after the implantation of geneti-

cally modified fibroblasts that produce recombinant NGF. Both allografts of 208F cells and xenografts of 3T3 cells resulted in over 90% savings of MS cells 2 and 6 weeks after grafting. Whittemore and coworkers (234) grafted temperature-sensitive, NGF-secreting cells (HT4 cells), obtained from a mouse neuroblastoma cell line, and also found significant savings of MS cholinergic cells after fimbria–fornix lesions. In a related study, Kawaja and colleagues (121) grafted primary rat skin fibroblasts genetically modified using retroviral vectors containing the cDNA for NGF and observed significantly greater survival of NGF receptor-positive cells in the MS of animals that received grafts of NGF-producing fibroblasts (over 60%). These studies all demonstrated that genetically modified, NGF-secreting cells can have a beneficial morphologic effect in animal models of AD.

Grafts and the Nucleus Basalis Magnocellularis–Cortical System

In addition to the role of the septohippocampal system in learning and memory function, cholinergic projections from the NBM to the neocortex also may play a role in mnemonic function, and degeneration of NBM cholinergic neurons may underlie some of the cognitive deficits associated with aging, dementia, or both.

Basal forebrain grafts into the neocortex of animals with kainic acid or ibotenic acid lesions of the NBM attenuated deficits in simple active and passive avoidance learning tests (8,9,62,71,198). In addition, either septal or hippocampal grafts implanted into the neocortex were able to reverse the passive avoidance task deficits, but neither type of graft had any effect on deficits in operant win-stay/lose-shift and win-shift/lose-stay tasks (198). The inability to reverse the operant task deficit was perhaps the result of additional noncholinergic damage induced by the lesions, which may have been responsible for the deficit. Adrenal chromaffin cells transplanted into the cortex of animals with bilateral quisqualic acid lesions of the NBM also were able to reverse the memory deficit on spatial alternation in the T-maze (227).

Cholinergic cells of the NBM atrophy after the loss of its cortical targets (200,201). Fetal cortical cell suspensions implanted into the excitotoxically lesioned neocortex can prevent the retrograde degeneration of the host NBM neurons (199); the grafts also were heavily innervated by host cholinergic fibers from the NBM. This finding supports the hypothesis that target-derived trophic factors are necessary for the maintenance of some projection neurons, and can be replaced by neural transplants.

Grafts implanted into the cortex can also functionally replace the lost cortical cells. Fetal frontal cortex grafts placed into the lesioned prefrontal or medial frontal cortex significantly improved performance of rats on a spatial alternation task in the T-maze (61,122,130,208). Homotypic transplants of fetal neocortex grafts into the lesioned gustatory cortex resulted in recovery of conditioned taste aversion (27,68,69,137,241). Similar recoveries have been reported on a variety of tasks after cortical grafting, such as spatial memory in the water maze after prefrontal cortex lesions (127), visual brightness and pattern discrimination after occipital cortex lesions (105,206), and spatial maze learning after hippocampal lesions (124).

Because of the rapid time course of behavioral recovery seen after implantation of these cortical grafts, it is unlikely that synaptic connections between the graft and the host brain are responsible for the observed functional improvements. Therefore, these cortical grafts may stimulate or secrete neurotrophic substances that promote functional recovery in the host brain (61, 123,206,208). Implants of purified cultured astrocytes or adult glia were found to be as effective as transplants of fetal cortical tissue in reducing deficits in a delayed alternation task (122,123). Stein and Mufson

(207) demonstrated that graft removal before testing on the water maze task did not abolish recovery from the deficits induced by prefrontal lesions in rats with cortical grafts, a finding that lent support to the trophic hypothesis of graft-induced recovery.

Itakura and coworkers (117) examined the effects of grafting peripheral cholinergic neurons from the nodosal ganglion into the parietal cortex of NBM-lesioned rats that were tested on two different memory tests, a passive avoidance and a maze task. The transplanted rats exhibited fewer errors on these memory tasks than the lesioned rats without grafts. In addition, AChE-positive cells were seen in the grafts, but no sprouting of cholinergic fibers into the cortex was observed. In another study, Welner and colleagues (228) grafted adrenal chromaffin cells obtained from adult rats to the cerebral cortex of bilateral NBM lesioned rats. The chromaffin cell grafts enhanced cortical AChE staining and completely reversed the spatial memory deficits seen in NBM-lesioned animals on a T-maze alternation task.

The effects of combined grafts into both the septohippocampal and the NBM–neocortical cholinergic pathways also have been examined by some investigators. On the radial maze, combined grafts into both target regions produced additive ameliorative effects compared to grafts into hippocampus or cortex alone (10,11,108,109).

GRAFTING INTO THE AGED BRAIN

Morphologic Analysis

Although grafting studies have primarily used young adult animals as the hosts, one study examined the survival and growth of fetal cortical tissue in rats from 5 to 180 days of age. Neuronal survival within the grafts was found to be comparable in the young (10-day) and adult (180-day) hosts (103). Therefore, it appears that graft survival and outgrowth are not significantly affected by host age until the recipient is quite old.

Gage and colleagues (84,85,87) found fetal septal or substantia nigra graft survival in aged hosts (21 to 23 months old). Dense outgrowth of AChE-positive fibers was seen up to about 2 mm from the septal implants. Examination of the ingrowing cholinergic fibers using ChAT immunocytochemistry at the electron microscopic level (37) revealed that the cholinergic grafts were capable of forming mature synaptic contacts with neurons in the aged host hippocampi. The distribution of AChE-positive fibers from the septal implants in the aged hippocampi appeared more diffuse than the pattern observed in the young adult hippocampi in other studies. Another study also demonstrated the survival and growth of cholinergic grafts in the aged hippocampus and neocortex (56). Grafts of different cell types implanted into a number of brain regions also have exhibited good survival and growth. Serotonergic grafts into the aged hippocampus (15,16) and dopaminergic, cholinergic, and noradrenergic grafts into lateral or third ventricles (39, 40,41,143) and caudate–putamen (48,83,87, 174) all demonstrate the aged brain can support the survival and growth of embryonic neural grafts. The survival of grafts into the aged brain may be decreased, however, because these studies did not directly compare graft survival in aged compared to young, adult hosts.

Another illustration of graft survival in the aged brain was done by Azmitia and colleagues (16), who implanted female raphe grafts into the intact hippocampus of adult (4 to 6 months old) versus aged (24 months old) mice. The grafts to both groups of hosts survived, contained serotonin-immunoreactive neurons, and gave rise to appropriate innervation of the hippocampus. The extent of the serotonergic innervation into the hippocampus from the grafts may have been slightly less in the aged hosts compared to adult hosts. Kaplan and colleagues (119) found no detectable differences in size

of the graft or in the length or branching frequency of neuronal dendrites within hypothalamic grafts implanted in the third ventricle of young compared to aged hosts.

The most detailed comparisons and the effects of host age on graft survival have been in the *in oculo* model. Grafts of embryonic cortical tissue implanted in the anterior eye chamber of 1.5-month-old rats were larger than grafts to 3- to 7.5-month-old hosts (65). There was a greater decrease in graft survival for cortical, septal, cerebellar, and hippocampal grafts, but not locus coeruleus grafts, implanted into 17-month-old hosts (66). In contrast, the internal structure of the grafts was not influenced by host age.

Recently, Crutcher (44) compared the survival of superior cervical ganglia grafted into the hippocampi of aged (23 to 25 months old) and young (3 to 4 months old) hosts. Ganglia obtained from both the aged and young donors survived equally well in young hosts; however, within aged hosts, neuronal survival within the grafts dropped by 50%. Further, although grafts within aged hosts showed extensive fiber growth within the grafts, the outgrowth into the host brain was poor. These results indicate that sympathetic outgrowth from the graft to the host is decreased in aging, primarily owing to decreased receptivity of the host hippocampal target tissue, which may be the result of reduced trophic support or increased inhibition of growth. Thus, there may be changes within the aged brain that limit neuronal plasticity. Whether these changes involve an increase in nonpermissive factors or a decrease in essential trophic or tropic molecules remains to be clarified.

Functional Analysis

The first studies of the functional effects of grafts in aged animals focused on the motoric impairments associated with aging. Gage and colleagues (87) demonstrated amelioration of motor coordination deficits

3 months after implantation of fetal nigral cells into the aged caudate–putamen. The recovery was specific to the coordination impairments, because there was no effect on global locomotor activity or muscular strength.

Subsequent studies sought to determine whether and to what extent the grafts could ameliorate any of the learning deficits seen in impaired aged animals before grafting. If these deficits are related to cholinergic deficiencies, then treatments enhancing cholinergic activity should be beneficial. Therefore, a logical approach is to alleviate these deficits with fetal septal grafts that contain cholinergic neurons. Fetal septal grafts implanted into the hippocampi of aged rats were able to improve the performance of these rats on the Morris water maze (84). These results demonstrate the ability of intracerebral grafts to ameliorate age-related impairments in complex cognitive behaviors. To what extent this effect depends on the cholinergic neurons in the septal grafts is not clear at present. Intrahippocampal septal grafts have no effect on age-related deficits in motor coordination, whereas fetal substantia nigra implanted into the striatum is effective in reducing the motor deficits but not the cognitive deficits (87). This finding suggests that different types of cell suspension grafts specifically affect different neuroanatomic systems, and thus have an effect on different behavioral deficits. The specificity of the cholinergic cells on the behavioral effects in the Morris water maze task was demonstrated by the ability of the muscarinic receptor antagonist atropine completely to abolish the improvement in performance observed in the grafted rats, as well as in behaviorally nonimpaired aged rats without grafts. In contrast, atropine had no significant effect on the aged, impaired rats that did not receive grafts, and only marginal effects on young control rats (82). Therefore, graft-mediated improvements in water maze performance appear to depend on intact cholinergic neurotransmission.

In a similar study, Schenk and colleagues (193) grafted fetal septal–diagonal band cells into the hippocampus of aged rats. The rats were tested on two different memory tests, the radial maze and a place-learning task. Considerable improvement was observed in the aged rats that received fetal basal forebrain grafts compared to the aged rats that did not receive fetal grafts.

Dunnell has used an alternative test paradigm, involving an operant delayed response task (delayed matching to position) to obtain a more specific evaluation of memory function in aged rats. Similar to the observation on the water maze, aged rats have a specific delay-dependent deficit in short-term memory (57) that is partially ameliorated by septal implants into either the hippocampus or neocortex (56). Thus, it appears that both hippocampal and medial prefrontal circuits are implicated in short-term memory functions measured in such delayed response tasks.

Grafts of basal forebrain cells also have been implanted into the "homotypic site," the region of the cholinergic cell bodies, namely, the NBM (35). Previous studies have attempted to reverse age-related functional and morphologic deficits by implanting fetal basal forebrain cells into their target areas (hippocampus or cortex). The natural source of these cells, however, is the basal forebrain. If the cells were grafted to their normal area of growth and innervation, perhaps a more naturally regulated control of growth and function could be established. The grafted cells may replace the aged, dysfunctional cells, or have a trophic effect on these intrinsic neurons. To examine these possibilities, fetal basal forebrain grafts were implanted into the NBM of aged impaired rats. The fetal basal forebrain grafts were able to ameliorate the performance of the aged, initially impaired rats on the water maze task. In addition, a significant hypertrophy of basal forebrain cholinergic cells was observed in the animals that received grafts. Thus, the grafts were able partially to replace compromised host cholinergic neurons in the NBM or have a trophic effect on the remaining intrinsic cells.

In another study, primary fibroblasts that had been genetically modified to express NGF were transplanted into the aged brain (36). The grafts were implanted in the region of the NBM in aged, initially impaired rats that had been pretested on the water maze task. After transplantation, the aged rats that received NGF-producing grafts performed significantly better than aged rats that received non–NGF-producing fibroblast grafts. Morphologically, low-affinity (P75) NGF receptor-positive cholinergic neurons in the basal forebrain were hypertrophied in the rats that received NGF-producing grafts. In addition, NGF receptor-positive fibers from the host were observed in the NGF-producing grafts and not in the control grafts. In contrast, grafts of NGF-producing fibroblasts implanted into the region of the NBM in young adult animals caused a transient deficit on the water maze task. This behavioral deficit was associated with hypertrophy of basal forebrain cholinergic neurons. Therefore, a balance of cholinergic function may be required for normal memory function, and disruption of this balance may impair cognitive performance.

Collier and colleagues (40,41) implanted embryonic locus coeruleus grafts into the ventricles of aged rats and demonstrated an amelioration of passive avoidance learning. The noradrenergic specificity of these graft effects was confirmed by demonstrating that cerebellar grafts did not have an effect, that chronic intraventricular infusions of noradrenaline could mimic the effect, and that treatment with the β-blocker propranolol could reverse the effect in the grafted rats.

These studies demonstrate the effectiveness of the grafting paradigm in ameliorating behavioral deficits on specific tasks, as well as the potential of grafting in elucidating the structures and systems in the brain that underlie performance on specific tasks. For example, manipulations of the cholinergic system had significant effects on the cognitive deficits observed in the aged rat. Further experiments on this model of age-related deficits and the ameliorative effects of specific transplants are required to determine more concretely the transmitter specificity of these transplants on specific behaviors, but clearly the transplant paradigm can be a useful tool in localizing regionally important cell populations for different age-related deficits.

GRAFTING INTO THE TRISOMY 16 BRAIN

The transplantation technique itself also can provide more adequate models of the primary pathology in AD, such as in recent studies of trisomy 16 mouse hippocampal grafts. In this approach, pathologic tissue was implanted in normal hosts to monitor the pathogenic processes in the grafts or in the host brain. Accumulation of β-amyloid protein is a characteristic feature of brains from people with Down's syndrome (trisomy 21), as well as in AD. People with trisomy 21 are at high risk for development of AD. Amyloid was deposited in the brains of people with trisomy 21 at an earlier age than is typical in the normal population (189). The gene encoding APP has been mapped on human chromosome 21 (118), which is equivalent to mouse chromosome 16. Therefore, it is interesting to examine whether overexpression of chromosome 16 genes, which include the amyloid precursor protein (APP) gene, in trisomy 16 (Ts 16) mice would produce neuropathologic changes similar to those observed in AD. Since Ts 16 is lethal *in utero,* transplantation of selected brain regions permitted the study of the development of Ts 16 tissue in a normal host. This allowed differentiation of the effect of intrinsic properties of the transplanted cells from the effects of the host environment. Two papers by Richards and colleagues (178,179) examined the neuropathologic changes in Ts 16 neocortical and hippocampal tissue transplanted into normal mice. Numerous cells located within the hippocampal Ts 16 grafts, but not within control grafts from littermates, were densely stained with antibodies against synthetic APP, β-amyloid, the serine protease inhibitor α_1-antichymotrypsin protein (which is associated with amyloid deposits), and antibodies against components of neurofibrillary tangles.

In a related study, Holtzman and colleagues (110) grafted cells from the basal forebrain region of embryonic Ts 16 and control littermates into the hippocampus of normal adult mice. Six months after grafting, cholinergic neurons in the transplants from Ts 16 mice were significantly shrunken compared to those in the control grafts. Fimbria–fornix transections, which can increase NGF levels in the denervated hippocampus, significantly increased the size of cholinergic cells from both Ts 16 and control embryos. Therefore, although cholinergic neurons from Ts 16 animals were intrinsically atrophied, they can still be influenced by the host environment. In a subsequent study, the atrophy of the grafted cholinergic neurons could be reversed by chronic infusions of NGF into the host brain (111). These studies demonstrated that neural grafting techniques could be a useful paradigm with which to study the etiology of the neurodegeneration.

CONCLUSIONS

To conclude, although neural transplantation into aged animals to investigate cognitive function is quite useful, there are a few caveats. First, the studies discussed earlier, as well as many others, demonstrate that transplants of fetal tissue can survive in the adult and aged mammalian brain and modify the function and behavior of the host in a positive manner, although neural transplantation may not always be beneficial. This was demonstrated by the induction of behavioral deficits in intact adult animals after the transplantation of NGF-producing fibroblast grafts (36). Restoration of function, as well as the induction of dysfunction, may both be useful in elucidating the biologic mechanisms underlying cognitive functions.

Second, the heterogeneity of the aged population requires the categorization of individuals into different subgroups based on behavioral performance to understand the biologic basis of those behavioral deficits. Otherwise, subtle differences between aged versus young adult groups may be overlooked owing to the variability within the aged group. In addition, screening the aged animals to eliminate noncognitive impairments is very important when examining the correlation between age-related biologic changes and cognitive deficits.

In summary, the changes that occur during aging are complex, and creation of a suitable animal model has been difficult. There is a need to distinguish the brain structures responsible for the observed cognitive dysfunctions from those that display age-related alterations but are unrelated to the cognitive dysfunction. Neural transplantation is a tool that can be used to answer this question. Transplants also can provide alternative strategies for brain repair that may provide localized and cell-specific effects.

REFERENCES

1. Adolfsson R, Gottfries GC, Roos BE, Winblad B. Changes in brain catecholamines in patients with dementia of Alzheimer-type. *Br J Psychiatr* 1979;135:216–223.
2. Aigner TG, Mitchell SJ, Aggleton MR, et al. Effects of scopolamine and physostigmine on recognition memory in monkeys with ibotenic-acid lesions in the nucleus basalis of Meynert. *Psychopharmacology* 1987;92:292–300.
3. Alleva E, Castellano C, Oliverio A. Ontogeny of behavioral development, arousal and stereotypes in two strains of mice. *Exp Aging Res* 1979;5:335–350.
4. Altavista MC, Bentivoglio AR, Crociani P, Rossi P, Albanese A. Age-dependent loss of cholinergic neurons in the basal ganglia in rats. *Brain Res* 1988;455:177–181.

5. Altman RT, Crosland RD, Jenden DJ, Berman RF. Further characterizations of the nature of the behavioral and neurochemical effects of lesions to the nucleus basalis of Meynert in the rat. *Neurobiol Aging* 1985;6:125–130.

6. Amaral DG, Kurz J. An analysis of the origins of the cholinergic and noncholinergic septal projections to the hippocampal formation of the rat. *J Comp Neurol* 1985;240:37–59.

7. Arai H, Kosaka K, Iizuka R. Changes of bigenic amines and their metabolites in postmortem brains from patients with Alzheimer-type dementia. *J Neurochem* 1984;43:388–393.

8. Arendash GW, Mouton PR. Transplantation of nucleus basalis magnocellularis cholinergic neurons into the cholinergic-depleted cerebral cortex: morphological and behavioral effects. *Ann NY Acad Sci* 1987;495:431–443.

9. Arendash GW, Strong PN, Mouton PR. Intracerebral transplantation of cholinergic neurons in a new animal model for Alzheimer's disease. In: Hutton JT, Kenny AD, eds. *Senile dementia of the Alzheimer type*. New York: Alan R. Liss; 1985:351–376.

10. Arendt T, Allen Y, Marchbanks RM, et al. Cholinergic system and memory in the rat: effects of chronic ethanol, embryonic basal forebrain brain transplants and excitotoxic lesions of cholinergic basal forebrain projection system. *Neuroscience* 1989;33:435–462.

11. Arendt T, Allen Y, Sinden J, et al. Cholinergic-rich brain transplants reverse alcohol-induced memory deficits. *Nature* 1988;332:448–450.

12. Arimatsu Y, Miyamoto M, Tsukui H, Hatanaka H. Nerve growth factor enhances survival of identified projection neurons in the rat septal and diagonal band regions *in vitro*. *Soc Neurosci Abstr* 1988;14:1114.

13. Armstrong DM, Saper CB, Levey AI, Wainer BH, Terry RD. Distribution of cholinergic neurons in rat brain: demonstrated by the immunocytochemical localization of choline acetyltransferase. *J Comp Neurol* 1983;216:53–68.

14. Armstrong DM, Terry RD, Deteresa RM, Bruce G, Hersh LB, Gage FH. Response of septal cholinergic neurons to axotomy. *J Comp Neurol* 1987;264:421–436.

15. Azmitia EC. A serotonin–hippocampal model indicates adult neurons survive transplantation and aged target may be deficient in a soluble serotonergic growth factor. *Ann NY Acad Sci* 1987;495:362–377.

16. Azmitia EC, Perlow MJ, Brennan MJ, Lauder JM. Fetal raphe and hippocampal transplants into adult and aged C57B/6N mice: a preliminary immunocytochemical study. *Brain Res Bull* 1981;7:703–710.

17. Ball MJ. Neuronal loss, neurofibrillary tangles and granulovacuolar degeneration in the hippocampus with aging and dementia: a quantitative study. *Acta Neuropathol* 1977;37:111–118.

18. Barnes CA. Memory deficits associated with senescence: a neurophysiological and behavioral study in the rat. *J Comp Physiol Psychol* 1979;93:74–104.

19. Barnes CA, Nadel L, Honig WK. Spatial memory deficits in senescent rats. *Can J Psychol* 1980;34:29–39.

20. Barone S Jr, Tandon P, McGinty JF, Tilson HA. The effects of NGF and fetal cell transplants on spatial learning after intradentate administration of colchicine. *Exp Neurol* 1991;114:351–363.

21. Bartus RT. Evidence for a direct cholinergic involvement in the scopolamine-induced amnesia in monkeys: effects of concurrent administration of physostigmine and methylphenidate with scopolamine. *Pharmacol Biochem Behav* 1978;9:833–836.

22. Bartus RT, Dean RL, Beer B, Lippa AS. The cholinergic hypothesis of geriatric memory dysfunction. *Science* 1982;217:408–417.

23. Bartus RT, Dean RL, Flicker C. Cholinergic psychopharmacology: an integration of human and animal research on memory. In: Meltzer HY, ed. *Psychopharmacology: the third generation of progress*. New York: Raven Press; 1987.

24. Bartus RT, Johnson HR. Short term memory in the rhesus monkey: disruption from the anticholinergic scopolamine. *Pharmacol Biochem Behav* 1976;5:39–46.

25. Becker JT, Walker JA, Olton DS. Neuroanatomical bases of spatial memory. *Brain Res* 1980;200:307–320.

26. Berman RF, Crosland RD, Jenden DJ, Altman HJ. Persisting behavioral and neurochemical deficits in rats following lesions of the basal forebrain. *Pharmacol Biochem Behav* 1988;29:581–586.

27. Bermudez-Rattoni F, Fernandez J, Sanchez MA, Aguilar-Roblero R, Drucker-Colin R. Fetal brain transplants induce recuperation of taste aversion learning. *Brain Res* 1987;416:147–152.

28. Biegon A, Greenberger V, Segal M. Quantitative histochemistry of brain acetylcholinesterase and learning rate in the aged rat. *Neurobiol Aging* 1986;7:215–217.

29. Bondareff W, Mountjoy CQ, Roth M. Loss of neurons of origin of the adrenergic projection to cerebral cortex (nucleus locus ceruleus) in senile dementia. *Neurology* 1982;32:164–168.

30. Bowen DM, Smith CB, White P, Davison AN. Neurotransmitter-related enzymes and indices of hypoxia in senile dementia and other abiotrophies. *Brain* 1976;99:459–496.

31. Brizzee KR, Ordy JM. Age pigments, cell loss and hippocampal function. *Mech Aging Dev* 1979;9:143–162.

32. Buell SJ, Coleman PD. Dendritic growth in the aged human brain and failure of growth in senile dementia. *Science* 1979;206:854–856.

33. Butcher LL. Acetylcholinesterase histochemistry. In: *Handbook of chemical neuroanatomy*. Amsterdam: Elsevier; 1983:1–49.

34. Campbell BA, Haroutunian V. Effects of age on long-term memory: retention of fixed interval responding. *J Gerontol* 1981;36:338–341.

35. Chen KS, Buzsaki G, Benoualid M, Gage FH. Fetal cholinergic grafts to the basal forebrain in the aged rat. *Soc Neurosci Abstr* 1989;19:1095.

36. Chen KS, Gage FH. Intracerebral grafts of genetically modified cells: ameliorative and detrimental effects of NGF in aged and adult rats. (*Submitted for publication.*)

37. Clarke DJ, Gage FH, Nilsson OG, Björklund A. Grafted septal neurons form cholinergic synaptic connections in the dentate gyrus of behaviorally impaired aged rats. *J Comp Neurol* 1986;252:483–492.

38. Collerton D. Cholinergic function and intellectual decline in Alzheimer's disease. *Neuroscience* 1986;19:1–28.

39. Collier TJ, Gash DM, Sladek JR Jr. Norepinephrine deficiency and behavioral senescence in aged rats: transplanted locus coeruleus neurons as an experimental replacement therapy. *Ann NY Acad Sci* 1987;495:396–403.

40. Collier TJ, Gash DM, Sladek JR Jr. Transplantation of norepinephrine neurons into aged rats improves performance of a learned task. *Brain Res* 1988;448:77–87.

41. Collier TJ, Gash DM, Bruemmer V, Sladek JR. Impaired regulation of arousal in old age and the consequences for learning and memory: replacement of brain norepinephrine via neuron transplants improves memory performance in aged F344 rats. In: Davies BB, Wood WG, eds. *Homeostatic function and aging.* New York: Raven Press; 1985:99–110.

42. Coyle JT, Price PH, Delong MR. Alzheimer's disease: a disorder of cortical cholinergic innervation. *Science* 1983;219:1184–1189.

43. Cross AJ, Crow TJ, Perry EK, Blessed G. Reduced dopamine-B-hydroxylase activity in Alzheimer's disease. *Br Med J* 1981;282:93–94.

44. Crutcher KA. Age-related decrease in sympathetic sprouting is primarily due to decreased target receptivity: implications for understanding brain aging. *Neurobiol Aging* 1990;11:175–183.

45. Cunningham TJ. Naturally occuring neuron death and its regulation by developing neural pathways. *Int Rev Cytol* 1982;74:163–186.

46. Curcio CA, Kemper T. Nucleus raphe dorsalis in dementia of the Alzheimer type: neurofibrillary changes and neuronal packing density. *J Neuropathol Exp Neurol* 1984;143:359–368.

47. Daniloff JK, Bodony RP, Low WC, Wells J. Cross-species embryonic septal transplants: restoration of conditioned learning behavior. *Brain Res* 1985;346:176–180.

48. Date I, Feltin SY, Feltin DL. The effect of adrenal medullary grafts in MPTP treated aging mouse brain. *Soc Neurosci Abstr* 1989;15:1356.

49. Davies P, Katzman R, Terry RD. Reduced somatostatin-like immunoreactivity in cerebral cortex from cases of Alzheimer disease and Alzheimer senile dementia. *Nature* 1980;288:279–280.

50. Davies P, Maloney AJF. Selective loss of central cholinergic neurons in Alzheimer's disease. *Lancet* 1976;2:1403.

51. Davies P, Verth AH. Regional distribution of muscarinic acetylcholine receptors in normal and Alzheimer's type dementia brains. *Brain Res* 1978;138:385–392.

52. Davison AN. Pathophysiology of ageing brain. *Gerontology* 1987;33:129–135.

53. de Ruiter JP, Uylings HB. Morphometric and dendritic analysis of fascia dentata granule cells in human aging and senile dementia. *Brain Res* 1987;402:217–229.

54. Deutsch JA. The cholinergic synapse and the site of memory. *Science* 1971;174:788–794.

55. Drachman DA. Memory and cognitive function in man: does the cholinergic system have a specific role? *Neurology* 1974;27:783–790.

56. Dunnett SB, Badman F, Rogers DC, Evenden JL, Iversen SD. Cholinergic grafts in the neocortex or hippocampus of aged rats: reduction of delay-dependent deficits in the delayed nonmatching to position task. *Exp Neurol* 1988;102:57–64.

57. Dunnett SB, Evenden JL, Iversen SD. Delay-dependent short-term memory deficits in aged rats. *Psychopharmacology (Berlin)* 1988;96:174–180.

58. Dunnett SB, Gage FH, Björklund A, Stenevi U, Low WC, Iversen SD. Hippocampal deafferentation: transplant-derived reinnervation and functional recovery. *Scand J Psychol* 1982;(Suppl 1):104–111.

59. Dunnett SB, Low WC, Iversen SD, Stenevi U, Björklund A. Septal transplants restore maze learning in rats with fornix–fimbria lesions. *Brain Res* 1982;251:335–348.

60. Dunnett SB, Martel FL, Rogers DC, Finger S. Factors affecting septal graft amelioration of differential reinforcement of low rates (DRL) and activity deficits after fimbria-fornix lesions. *Rest Neurol Neurosci* 1989;1:83–92.

61. Dunnett SB, Ryan CN, Levin PD, Reynolds M, Bunch ST. Functional consequences of embryonic neocortex transplanted to rats with prefrontal cortex lesions. *Behav Neurosci* 1987;101:489–503.

62. Dunnett SB, Toniolo G, Fine A, Ryan CN, Björklund A, Iversen SD. Transplantation of embryonic ventral forebrain neurons to the neocortex of rats with lesions of nucleus basalis magnocellularis: II. sensorimotor and learning impairments. *Neuroscience* 1985;16:787–797.

63. Eichenbaum H, Fagan A, Cohen NJ. Normal olfactory discrimination learning set and facilitation of reversal learning after medial-temporal damage in rats: implications for an account of preserved learning abilities in amnesia. *J Neurosci* 1986;6:1876–1884.

64. Emerich DF, Black BA, Kesslak JP, Cotman CW, Walsh TJ. Transplantation of fetal cholinergic neurons into the hippocampus attenuates the cognitive and neurochemical deficits induced by AF64A. *Brain Res Bull* 1992;28:219–226.

65. Eriksdotter-Nilsson M, Björklund H, Dahl D, Olson L. Growth and development of intraocular fetal cortex cerebri grafts in rats of different ages. *Brain Res* 1986;393:75–84.

66. Eriksdotter-Nilsson M, Olson L. Growth of brain tissue grafts is dependent upon host age. *Mech Ageing Dev* 1989;49:1–22.

67. Eriksdotter-Nilsson M, Skirboll S, Ebendal T, Olson L. Nerve growth factor can influence growth of cortex cerebri and hippocampus: evidence from intraocular grafts. *Neuroscience* 1989;30:755–766.

68. Escobar M, Fernandez J, Guevara-Aguilar R, Bermudez-Rattoni F. Fetal brain grafts induce recovery of learning deficits and connectivity in rats with gustatory neocortex lesion. *Brain Res* 1989;478:368–374.

69. Fernandez-Ruiz J, Escobar ML, Pina AL, Diaz-Cintra S, Cintra-McGlone FL, Bermudez-Rattoni F. Time-dependent recovery of taste aversion learning by fetal brain transplants in gustatory neocortex-lesioned rats. *Behav Neural Biol* 1991;55:179–193.

70. Finch CE. Catecholamine metabolism in the brains of ageing male mice. *Brain Res* 1973; 52:261–276.

71. Fine A, Dunnett SB, Björklund A, Iversen SD. Cholinergic ventral forebrain grafts into the neocortex improve passive avoidance memory in a rat model of Alzheimer disease. *Proc Natl Acad Sci USA* 1985;82:5227–5230.

72. Fischer W, Björklund A, Chen K, Gage FH. NGF improves spatial memory in aged rodents as a function of age. *J Neurosci* 1991;11:1889–1906.

73. Fischer W, Chen KS, Gage FH, Björklund A. Progressive decline in spatial learning and integrity of forebrain cholinergic neurons in rats during aging. *Neurobiol Aging* 1992;13:9–23.

74. Fischer W, Gage FH, Björklund A. Degenerative changes in forebrain cholinergic nuclei correlate with cognitive impairments in aged rats. *Eur J Neurosci* 1989;1:34–45.

75. Fischer W, Wictorin K, Björklund A, Williams LR, Varon S, Gage FH. Amelioration of cholinergic neuron atrophy and spatial memory impairment in aged rats by nerve growth factor. *Nature* 1987;329:65–68.

76. Flicker C, Dean RL, Watkins DL, Fisher SK, Bartus RT. Behavioral and neurochemical effects following neurotoxic lesions of a major cholinergic input to the cerebral cortex in the rat. *Pharmacol Biochem Behav* 1983;18:973–981.

77. Fonnum F. Radiochemical micro assays for the determination of choline acetyltransferase and acetylcholinesterase activities. *J Biochem* 1969; 115:465–472.

78. Fonnum F. Topographical and subcellular localization of choline acetyltransferase in the rat hippocampal region. *J Neurochem* 1984;24: 407–409.

79. Francis PT, Palmer AM, Sims NR, et al. Neurochemical studies of early-onset Alzheimer's disease: possible influence on treatment. *N Engl J Med* 1985;313:7–11.

80. Freund G. Cholinergic receptor loss in brains of aging mice. *Life Sci* 1980;26:371–375.

81. Friedman E, Lerer B, Kuster J. Loss of cholinergic neurons in the rat neocortex produces deficits in passive avoidance learning. *Pharmacol Biochem Behav* 1983;19:309–312.

82. Gage FH, Björklund A. Cholinergic septal grafts into the hippocampal formation improve spatial learning and memory in aged rats by an atropine sensitive mechanism. *J Neurosci* 1986; 2837–2847.

83. Gage FH, Björklund A, Stenevi U, Dunnett SB. Functional correlates of compensatory collateral sprouting by aminergic and cholinergic afferents in the hippocampal formation. *Brain Res* 1983;268:39–47.

84. Gage FH, Björklund A, Stenevi U, Dunnett SB, Kelly PAT. Intra-hippocampal septal grafts ameliorate learning impairments in aged rats. *Science* 1984;225:533–536.

85. Gage FH, Dunnett SB, Björklund A. Spatial learning and motor deficits in aged rats. *Neurobiol Aging* 1984;5:43–48.

86. Gage FH, Dunnett SB, Björklund A. Age-related impairments in spatial memory are independent of those in sensorimotor skills. *Neurobiol Aging* 1989;10:347–352.

87. Gage FH, Dunnett SB, Stenevi U, Björklund A. Aged rats: recovery of motor impairments by intrastriatal nigral grafts. *Science* 1983; 221:966–969.

88. Gage FH, Dunnett SB, Stenevi U, Björklund A. Intracerebral grafting of neuronal cell suspensions: VIII. survival and growth of implants of nigral and septal cell suspensions in intact brains of aged rats. *Acta Physiol Scand* 1983; (Suppl 522):67–75.

89. Gage FH, Kawaja MD, Fisher LJ. Genetically modified cells: applications for intracerebral grafting. *TINS* 1991;14:328–333.

90. Gage FH, Kelly PAT, Björklund A. Regional changes in brain glucose metabolism reflect cognitive impairments in aged rats. *J Neurosci* 1984;4:2856–2865.

91. Gage FH, Wictorin K, Ficher W, Williams LR, Varon S, Björklund A. Life and death of cholinergic neurons: in the septal and diagonal band region following fimbria–fornix transection. *Neuroscience* 1986;19:241–255.

92. Gage FH, Wolff JA, Rosenberg MB, et al. Grafting genetically modified cells to the brain: possibilities for the future. *Neuroscience* 1987; 23:795–807.

93. Gibson GE, Peterson C, Jenden DJ. Brain acetylcholine synthesis declines with senescence. *Science* 1981;213:674–676.

94. Gilad GM, Rabey IM, Tizabi Y, Gilad VH. Age-dependent loss and compensatory changes of septohippocampal cholinergic neurons in two rat strains differing in longevity and response to stress. *Brain Res* 1987;436:311–322.

95. Gold PE, McGaugh JL. Changes in learning and memory during aging. In: Ordy JM, Brizzee KR, eds. *Neurobiology of aging.* New York: Plenum Press; 1975:145–158.

96. Goldman-Rakic PS, Brown RM. Regional changes of monoamines in cerebral cortex and subcortical structures of aging rhesus monkeys. *Neuroscience* 1981;6:177–187.

97. Goodrick CL. Exploration of nondeprived male Sprague-Dawley rats as a function of age. *Psychol Rep* 1967;20:159–163.

98. Goodrick CL. Learning, retention and extinc-

tion of a complex maze habit for mature-young and senescent Wistar albino rats. *J Gerontol* 1968;23:298–304.

99. Grady S, Reeves T, Steward O. Time course of retrograde degeneration of the cells of origin of the septohippocampal pathway after fimbria–fornix transections. *Dev Brain Res* 1984;9:45–52.

100. Greene E, Naranjo JN. Degeneration of hippocampal fibers and spatial memory deficit in the aged rat. *Neurobiol Aging* 1987;8:35–43.

101. Gurwitz D, Egozi Y, Henis YL, Kloog Y, Sokolowsky M. Agonist and antagonist binding to rat brain muscarinic receptors: influence of aging. *Neurobiol Aging* 1987;8:115–122.

102. Hagg T, Manthorpe M, Vahlsing HL, Varon S. Delayed treatment with nerve growth factor reverses the apparent loss of cholinergic neurons after acute brain damage. *Exp Neurol* 1988; 101:303–312.

103. Hallas BH, Das GD, Das KG. Transplantation of brain tissue in the brain of rat: II. growth characteristics of neocortical transplants in hosts of different ages. *Am J Anat* 1980; 158:147–159.

104. Haroutunian V, Kanof P, Davis KL. Pharmacological alleviation of cholinergic lesion induced memory deficits in rats. *Life Sci* 1985; 37:945–952.

105. Haun F, Rothblat LA, Cunningham TJ. Visual cortex transplants in rats restore normal learning of a difficult visual pattern discrimination. *Invest Opthalmol Vis Sci* 1985;26(Suppl 3):288.

106. Hefti F. Nerve growth factor promotes survival of septal cholinergic neurons after fimbrial transections. *J Neurosci* 1986;14:2155–2162.

107. Hepler DJ, Wenk GL, Cribbs B, Olton DS, Coyle JT. Memory impairments following basal forebrain lesions. *Brain Res* 1985;346:8–14.

108. Hodges H, Allen Y, Kershaw T, Lantos PL, Gray JA, Sinden J. Effects of cholinergic-rich neural grafts on radial maze performance of rats after excitotoxic lesions of the forebrain cholinergic projection system: I. amelioration of cognitive deficits by transplants into cortex and hippocampus but not into basal forebrain. *Neuroscience* 1991;45:587–607.

109. Hodges H, Allen Y, Sinden J, et al. The effects of cholinergic drugs and cholinergic-rich foetal neural transplants on alcohol-induced deficits in radial maze performance in rats. *Behav Brain Res* 1991;43:7–28.

110. Holtzman DM, Li YW, DeArmond SJ, et al. Mouse model of neurodegeneration: atrophy of basal forebrain cholinergic neurons in trisomy 16 transplants. *Proc Natl Acad Sci USA* 1992; 89:1383–1387.

111. Holtzman DM, Li Y, Chen KS, Gage FH, Epstein CJ, Mobley WC. Nerve growth factor reverses neuronal atrophy in a Down syndrome model of age-related neurodegeneration *(submitted for publication)*.

112. Hornberger JC, Buell SJ, Flood DG, McNeill TH, Coleman PD. Stability of numbers but not size of mouse forebrain cholinergic neurons to 53 months. *Neurobiol Aging* 1985;6:269–275.

113. Ikcgami S, Nihonmatsu I, Hatanaka H, Takei N, Kawamura H. Transplantation of septal cholinergic neurons to the hippocampus improves memory impairments of spatial learning in rats treated with AF64A. *Brain Res* 1989; 496:321–326.

114. Ikegami S, Nihonmatsu I, Kawamura H. Transplantation of ventral forebrain cholinergic neurons to the hippocampus ameliorates impairment of radial-arm maze learning in rats with AF64A treatment. *Brain Res* 1991;548:187–195.

115. Ingram DK. Analysis of age-related impairments in learning and memory in rodent models. *Ann NY Acad Sci* 1985;444:312–331.

116. Ingram DK, London ED, Reynolds MA, Waller SB. Goodrick CL. Differential effects of age on motor performance in two mouse strains. *Neurobiol Aging* 1981;2:221–227.

117. Itakura T, Yokote H, Yukawa S, Nakai M, Komai N, Umemoto M. Transplantation of peripheral cholinergic neurons into Alzheimer model rat brain. *Stereotact Funct Neurosurg* 1990;54–55:368–372.

118. Kang J, Lemaire HG, Unterbeck A, et al. The precursor of Alzheimer's disease amyloid protein resembles a cell-surface receptor. *Nature* 1987;325:733–736.

119. Kaplan AS, Gash DM, Flood DG, Coleman PD. A Golgi study of hypothalamic transplants in young and old host rats. *Neurobiol Aging* 1985;6:205–211.

120. Katzman R. Alzheimer's disease. *N Engl J Med* 1986;314:964–973.

121. Kawaja MD, Rosenberg MB, Yoshida K, Gage FH. Somatic gene transfer of nerve growth factor promotes the survival of axotomized septal neurons and the regeneration of their axons in adult rats. *J Neurosci* 1992;12:2849–2864.

122. Kesslak JP, Brown L, Steichen C, Cotman CW. Adult and embryonic frontal cortex transplants after frontal cortex ablation enhance recovery on a reinforced alternation task. *Exp Neurol* 1986;94:615–626.

123. Kesslak JP, Nieto-Sampedro M, Globus J, Cotman CW. Transplants of purified astrocytes promote behavioral recovery after frontal cortex ablation. *Exp Neurol* 1986;92:377–390.

124. Kimble DP, Bremiller R, Stickrod G. Fetal brain implants improve maze performance in hippocampal lesioned rats. *Brain Res* 1986; 363:358–363.

125. Knowlton BJ, Wenk GL, Olton DS, Coyle JT. Basal forebrain lesions produce a dissociation of trial-dependent and trial-independent memory performance. *Brain Res* 1985;345:315–321.

126. Koh S, Chang P, Collier TJ, Loy R. Loss of NGF receptor immunoreactivity in basal forebrain neurons of aged rats: correlation with spatial memory impairment. *Brain Res* 1989; 498:397–404.

127. Kolb B, Reynolds B, Fantie B. Frontal cortex grafts have opposite effects at different postoperative recovery times. *Behav Neural Biol* 1988;50:193–206.

128. Kordower JH, Notter MF, Gash DM. Neuroblastoma cells in neural transplants: a neuroan-

atomical and behavioral analysis. *Brain Res* 1987;417:85–98.

129. Kromer LF. Nerve growth factor treatment after brain injury prevents neuronal death. *Science* 1987;235:214–216.

130. Labbe R, Firl A Jr, Mufson EJ, Stein DG. Fetal brain transplant: reduction of cognitive deficits in rats with frontal cortex lesions. *Science* 1983;221:470–472.

131. Lamour Y, Bassant MH, Jobert A, Joly M. Septo-hippocampal neurons in the aged rat: relation between their electrophysiological and pharmácological properties and behavioral performances. *Neurobiol Aging* 1989;10:181–186.

132. Landfield PW, Rose G, Sandles L, Wohlstadter TC, Lynch G. Patterns of astroglial hypertrophy and neuronal degeneration in the hippocampus of aged, memory-deficient rats. *J Gerontol* 1977;32:3–12.

133. Landfield SJ, Braun LD, Pitler TA, Lindsey JD, Lynch G. Hippocampal aging in rats: a morphometric study of multiple variables in semithin sections. *Neurobiol Aging* 1981;2: 265–275.

134. Lerer B, Warner J, Friedman E, Vincent G, Gamzu E. Cortical cholinergic impairment and behavioral deficits produced by kainic acid lesions of rat magnocellular basal forebrain. *Behav Neurosci* 1985;99:661–667.

135. Lewis PR, Shute CCD, Silver A. Confirmation from cholineacetylase of a massive cholinergic innervation to the rat hippocampus. *J Physiol* 1967;191:215–224.

136. Lippa AS, Pelham RW, Beer B, Critchett DJ, Dean RL, Bartus RT. Brain cholinergic dysfunction and memory in aged rats. *Neurobiol Aging* 1980;1:13–19.

137. Lopez-Garcia JC, Fernandez-Ruiz J, Bermudez-Rattoni F, Tapia R. Correlation between acetylcholine release and recovery of conditioned taste aversion induced by fetal neocortex grafts. *Brain Res* 1990;523:105–110.

138. Low W, Lewis P, Bunch S, et al. Function recovery following neural transplantation of embryonic septal nuclei in adult rats with septo-hippocampal lesions. *Nature* 1982;300:260–262.

139. Lowy AM, Ingram DK, Olton DS, Waller SB, Reynolds MA, London ED. Discrimination learning requiring different memory components in rats: age and neurochemical comparisons. *Behav Neurosci* 1985;99:638–651.

140. Luine VN, Renner KJ, Heady S, Jones KJ. Age and sex-dependent decreases in ChAT in basal forebrain nuclei. *Neurobiol Aging* 1986;7:193–198.

141. Markowska AL, Stone WS, Ingram DK, et al. Individual differences in aging: behavioral and neurobiological correlates. *Neurobiol Aging* 1989;10:31–43.

142. Masliah E, Terry RD, DeTeresa R, Hansen LA. Immunohistochemical quantification of the synapse related protein synaptophysin in Alzheimer's disease. *Neurosci Lett* 1989;103:234–239.

143. Matsumoto A, Murakami S, Arai Y, Nagatsu I. Ultrastructural and immunohistochemical analysis of fetal mediobasal hypothalamic tissue transplanted into the aged rat brain. *Ann NY Acad Sci* 1987;495:404–414.

144. Mayo W, Kharouby M, Le Moal M, Simon H. Memory disturbances following ibotenic acid injections in the nucleus basalis magnocellularis of the rat. *Brain Res* 1988;455:213–222.

145. McGeer EG, Fibiger HC, McGeer PL, Wickson V. Aging and brain enzymes. *Exp Gerontol* 1971;6:391–396.

146. McGeer EG, McGeer PL. Neurotransmitter metabolism in the aging brain. In: Terry RD, Gershon S, eds. *Neurobiology of aging.* vol. 2. New York: Raven Press; 1976:389–403.

147. McIntosh MH, Westfall TC. Influence of aging on catecholamine levels, accumulation, and release in F-344 rats. *Neurobiol Aging* 1987;3: 233–239.

148. Mesulam MM, Mufson EJ, Levey AI, Wainer BH. Cholinergic innervation of cortex by the basal forebrain: cytochemistry and cortical connections of the septal area, diagonal band nuclei, nucleus basalis (substantia innominata), and hypothalamus in the rhesus monkey. *J Comp Neurol* 1983;214:170–197.

149. Mesulam MM, Mufson EJ, Rogers J. Age-related shrinkage of cortically projecting cholinergic neurons: a selective effect. *Ann Neurol* 1987;22:31–36.

150. Mewaldt SP, Ghoneim MM. The effects and interactions of scopolamine, physostigmine and methamphetamine on human memory. *Pharmacol Biochem Behav* 1978;10:205–210.

151. Meyer EM, Otero E, Crews FT. Effects of aging on rat cortical presynaptic cholinergic processes. *Neurobiol Aging* 1984;5:315–317.

152. Michel ME, Klein AW. Performance differences in a complex maze between young and aged rats. *Age* 1978;1:13–16.

153. Mickley GA, Ferguson JL, Mulvihill MA, Nemeth TJ. Early neural grafts transiently reduce the behavioral effects of radiation-induced fascia dentata granule cell hypoplasia. *Brain Res* 1991;550:24–34.

154. Mishkin M. Memory in monkeys severely impaired by combined but not by separate removal of amygdala and hippocampus. *Nature* 1978;273:297–298.

155. Miyamoto M, Kato J, Narumi S, Nagoaka A. Characteristics of memory impairment following lesioning of the basal forebrain and medical septal nucleus in rats. *Brain Res* 1987;419:19–31.

156. Miyamoto M, Narumi S, Nagaoka A, Coyle JT. Effects of continuous infusion of cholinergic drugs on memory impairment in rats with basal forebrain lesions. *J Pharmacol Exp Ther* 1989; 248:825–835.

157. Montero CN, Hefti F. Rescue of lesioned septal cholinergic neurons by nerve growth factor: specificity and requirement for chronic treatment. *J Neurosci* 1988;8:2986–2999.

158. Murray CL, Fibiger HC. Learning and memory deficits after lesions of the nucleus basalis magnocellularis: reversal by physostigmine. *Neurosci* 1985;14:1025–1032.

159. Murray CL, Fibiger HC. Pilocarpine and physostigmine attenuate spatial memory impairments produced by lesions of the nucleus basalis magnocellularis. *Behav Neurosci* 1986; 100:23–32.
160. Nilsson OG, Brundin P, Björklund A. Amelioration of spatial memory impairment by intrahippocampal grafts of mixed septal and raphe tissue in rats with combined cholinergic and serotonergic denervation of the forebrain. *Brain Res* 1990;515:193–206.
161. Nilsson OG, Shapiro ML, Gage FH, Olton DS, Björklund A. Spatial learning and memory following fimbria–fornix transection and grafting of fetal septal neurons to the hippocampus. *Exp Brain Res* 1987;67:195–215.
162. Nilsson OG, Strecker RE, Daszuta A, Björklund A. Combined cholinergic and serotonergic denervation of the forebrain produces severe deficits in a spatial learning task in the rat. *Brain Res* 1988;453:235–246.
163. O'Brien TS, Svendsen CN, Isacson O, Sofroniew MV. Loss of true blue labelling from the medial septum following transection of the fimbria–fornix: evidence for the death of cholinergic and non-cholinergic neurons. *Brain Res* 1990;508:249–256.
164. Olton DS, Becker JT, Handelman GE. Hippocampus, space and memory. *Behav Brain Sci* 1979;2:313–365.
165. Olton DS, Walker JA, Gage FH. Hippocampal connections and spatial discrimination. *Brain Res* 1978;139:295–308.
166. Osterburg HH, Donahue HG, Severson JA, Finch CE. Catecholamine levels and turnover during aging in brain regions of male C57BL/6J mice. *Brain Res* 1981;224:337–352.
167. Oyanagi K, Takahashi H, Wakabayashi K, Ikuta F. Correlative decrease of large neurons in the neostriatum and basal nucleus of Meynert in Alzheimer's disease. *Brain Res* 1989; 504:354–357.
168. Pallage V, Toniolo G, Will B, Hefti F. Long-term effects of nerve growth factor and neural transplantation on behavior of rats with medial septal lesions. *Brain Res* 1986;386:197–208.
169. Perry EK. The cholinergic hypothesis in old age and Alzheimer's disease. *Ageing* 1980;9:1–8.
170. Perry EK, Blessed G, Tomlinson BE, et al. Neurochemical activities in the human temporal lobe related to aging and Alzheimer-type changes. *Neurobiol Aging* 1981;2:251–256.
171. Perry EK, Perry RH, Blessed G, Tomlinson BE. Necropsy evidence of central cholinergic deficits in senile dementia. *Lancet* 1977;2:143.
172. Perry EK, Tomlinson BE, Blessed G, Bergmann K, Gibson PH, Perry RH. Correlation of cholinergic abnormalities with senile plaques and mental test scores in senile dementia. *Br Med J* 1978;2:1457–1459.
173. Peters A, Feldman ML, Vaughan DW. The effect of aging on the neuronal population within area 17 of adult rat cerebral cortex. *Neurobiol Aging* 1983;4:273–282.
174. Pezzoli G, Fahn S, Dwork A, et al. Non-chro-
175. Ponzio F, Calderini G, Lomuscio G, Vantini G, Toffano G, Algeri S. Changes in monoamines and their metabolite levels in some brain regions of aged rats. *Neurobiol Aging* 1982;3:23–29.
176. Rapp PR, Rosenberg A, Gallagher M. An evaluation of spatial information processing in aged rats. *Behav Neurosci* 1987;101:3–12.
177. Renfranz PJ, Cunningham MG, McKay RD. Region-specific differentiation of the hippocampal stem cell line HiB5 upon implantation into the developing mammalian brain. *Cell* 1991;66:713–729.
178. Richards SJ, Waters JJ, Beyreuther K, et al. Transplants of mouse trisomy 16 hippocampus provide a model of Alzheimer's disease neuropathology. *EMBO J* 1991;10:297–303.
179. Richards SJ, Waters JJ, Rogers DC, et al. Hippocampal grafts derived from embryonic trisomy 16 mice exhibit amyloid (A4) and neurofibrillary pathology. *Prog Brain Res* 1990; 82:215–223.
180. Richter-Levin G, Segal M. Raphe cells grafted into the hippocampus can ameliorate spatial memory deficits in rats with combined serotonergic/cholinergic deficiencies. *Brain Res* 1989; 478:184–186.
181. Richter-Levin G, Segal M. The effects of serotonin depletion and raphe grafts on hippocampal electrophysiology and behavior. *J Neurosci* 1991;11:1585–1596.
182. Richter-Levin G, Segal M. Restoration of serotonergic innervation underlies the behavioral effects of raphe grafts. *Brain Res* 1991;566:21–25.
183. Ridley RM, Murray TK, Johnson JA, Baker HF. Learning impairment following lesion of the basal nucleus of Meynert in the marmoset: modification of cholinergic drugs. *Brain Res* 1986;376:108–116.
184. Ridley RM, Thornley HD, Baker HF, Fine A. Cholinergic neural transplants into hippocampus restore learning ability in monkeys with fornix transections. *Exp Brain Res* 1991;83: 533–538.
185. Ridley RM, Gribble S, Clark B, Baker HF, Fine A. Restoration of learning ability in fornix-transected monkeys after fetal basal forebrain but not fetal hippocampal tissue transplantation. *Neuroscience* 1992;48:779–792.
186. Rinne JO, Laakso K, Lonnberg P, et al. Brain muscarinic receptors in senile dementia. *Brain Res* 1985;336:19–25.
187. Rosenberg MB, Friedmann T, Robertson RC, et al. Grafting genetically modified cells to the damaged brain: restorative effects of NGF expression. *Science* 1988;242:1575–1578.
188. Rossor MN, Emson PC, Mountjoy CQ, Roth M, Iverson LL. Reduced amounts of immunoreactive somatostatin in the temporal cortex in senile dementia of Alzheimer type. *Neurosci Lett* 1980;20:373–377.
189. Rumble B, Retallack R, Hilbich C, et al. Amy-

loid A4 protein and its precursor in Down's syndrome and Alzheimer's disease [see comments]. *N Engl J Med* 1989;320:1446–1452.

190. Ruthrich H-L, Wetzel W, Matthies H. Acquisition and retention of different learning tasks in old rats. *Behav Neural Biol* 1982;35:139–146.

191. Saper CB. Organization of cerebral cortical afferent systems in the rat: I. magnocellular basal nucleus. *J Comp Neurol* 1984;222:313–342.

192. Sarter M, Dudchenko P. Dissociative effects of ibotenic and quisqualic acid-induced basal forebrain lesions on cortical acetylcholinesterase-positive fiber density and cytochrome oxidase activity. *Neuroscience* 1991;41:729–738.

193. Schenk F, Contant B, Werffeli P. Intrahippocampal cholinergic grafts in aged rats compensate impairments in a radial maze and in a place learning task. *Exp Brain Res* 1990;82:641–650.

194. Schwaber JS, Rogers WT, Satoh K, Fibiger HC. Distribution and organization of cholinergic neurons in the rat forebrain demonstrated by computer-aided data acquisition and three-dimensional reconstruction. *J Comp Neurol* 1987;263:309–325.

195. Segal M, Greenberger V, Milgram NW. A functional analysis of connections between grafted septal neurons and host hippocampus. *Prog Brain Res* 1987;71:349–357.

196. Sherman KA, Kuster JE, Dean RL, Bartus RT, Friedman E. Presynaptic cholinergic mechanisms in brains of aged rats with memory impairments. *Neurobiol Aging* 1981;2:99–104.

197. Sims NR, Marek KL, Bowen DM, Davison AN. Production of [¹⁴C] acetylcholine and [¹⁴C] carbon dioxide from [U-¹⁴C] glucose in tissue prisms from aging rat brain. *J Neurochem* 1982;38:488–492.

198. Sinden JD, Allen YS, Rawlins JN, Gray JA. The effects of ibotenic acid lesions of the nucleus basalis and cholinergic-rich neural transplants on win-stay/lose-shift and win-shift/lose-stay performance in the rat. *Behav Brain Res* 1990;36:229–249.

199. Sofroniew MV, Isacson O, Björklund A. Cortical grafts prevent atrophy of cholinergic basal nucleus neurons induced by excitotoxic cortical damage. *Brain Res* 1986;378:409–415.

200. Sofroniew MV, Pearson RCA. Degeneration of cholinergic neurons in the basal nucleus following kainic acid or N-methyl-D-aspartic acid application to the cerebral cortex in the rat. *Brain Res* 1985;339:186–190.

201. Sofroniew MV, Pearson RCA, Eckenstein F, Cuello AC, Powell TPS. Retrograde changes in cholinergic neurons in the basal forebrain of the rat following cortical damage. *Brain Res* 1983;289:370–374.

202. Springer JE, Collier TJ, Sladek JR Jr, Loy R. Transplantation of male mouse submaxillary gland increases survival of axotomized basal forebrain neurons. *J Neurosci Res* 1988;19:291–296.

203. Springer JE, Tairien MW, Loy R. Regional analysis of age related changes in the cholinergic system of the hippocampal formation and basal forebrain of the rat. *Brain Res* 1987;407:180–184.

204. Sprott RL, Eleftheriou S. Open-field behavior in aging inbred mice. *Gerontology* 1974;20:155–162.

205. Squire LR. Memory and the hippocampus: a synthesis from findings with rats, monkeys, and humans. *Psychol Rev* 1992;99:195–231.

206. Stein DG, Labbe R, Attella MJ, Rakowsky HA. Fetal brain tissue transplants reduce visual deficits in adult rats with bilateral lesions of the occipital cortex. *Behav Neural Biol* 1985;44:266–277.

207. Stein DG, Mufson EJ. Morphological and behavioral characteristics of embryonic brain tissue transplants in adults, brain-damaged subjects. *Ann NY Acad Sci* 1987;495:444–464.

208. Stein DG, Palatucci C, Kahn D, Labbe R. Temporal factors influence recovery of function after embryonic brain tissue transplants in adult rats with frontal cortex lesions. *Behav Neurosci* 1988;102:260–267, 325–326.

209. Storm-Mathisen J. Choline acetyltransferase and acetylcholinesterase in fascia dentata following lesions of the entorhinal afferent. *J Brain Res* 1974;80:119–181.

210. Stromberg I, Wetmore CJ, Ebendal T, Ernfors P, Persson H, Olson L. Rescue of basal forebrain cholinergic neurons after implantation of genetically modified cells producing recombinant NGF. *J Neurosci Res* 1990;25:405–411.

211. Strong R, Hicks P, Hsu L, Bartus RT, Enna SJ. Age-related alterations in the rodent brain cholinergic system and behavior. *Neurobiol Aging* 1980;1:59–63.

212. Sutherland RJ, Whishaw IQ, Regehr JC. Cholinergic receptor blockade impairs spatial localization using distal cues in the rat. *J Comp Physiol Psychol* 1982;96:563–573.

213. Tandon P, McLamb RL, Novicki D, Shuey DL, Tilson HA. Fetal hippocampal cell suspensions ameliorate behavioral effects of intradentate colchicine in the rat. *Brain Res* 1988;473:241–248.

214. Tarricone BJ, Keim SR, Simon JR, Low WC. Intrahippocampal transplants of septal cholinergic neurons: high-affinity choline uptake and spatial memory function. *Brain Res* 1991;548:55–62.

215. Terry RD, DeTeresa R, Hansen LA. Neocortical cell counts in normal human adult aging. *Ann Neurol* 1987;21:530–539.

216. Terry RD, Masliah E, Salmon DP, et al. Physical basis of cognitive alterations in Alzheimer's disease: synapse loss is the major correlate of cognitive impairment. *Ann Neurol* 1991;30:572–580.

217. Thompson CI, Fitzsimmons TR. Latency to leave an elevated platform, activity in a dark chamber, and weight in aging Sprague-Dawley rats. *Psychol Rep* 1975;36:231–236.

218. Tilson HA, McLamb RL, Shaw S, Rogers BC, Pediaditakis P, Cook L. Radial-maze deficits produced by colchicine administered into the area of the nucleus basalis are ameliorated by cholinergic agents. *Brain Res* 1988;438:83–94.

219. Toniolo G, Dunnett SB, Hefti F, Will B. Acetylcholine-rich transplants in the hippocampus: influence of intrinsic growth factors and application of nerve growth factor on choline acetyltransferase activity. *Brain Res* 1985;345:141–146.

220. Tuszynski MH, Armstrong DA, Gage FH. Basal forebrain cell loss following fimbria/fornix transection. *Brain Res* 1989;508:241–248.

221. Tuszynski MH, Buzsaki G, Gage FH. Nerve growth factor infusions combined with fetal hippocampal grafts enhance reconstruction of the lesioned septo-hippocampal projection. *Neuroscience* 1990;36:33–44.

222. van der Staay FJ, Raaijmakers WGM, Sakkee AN, van Beezooijen CFA. Spatial working and reference memory in senescent rats after thiopental anaesthesia. *Neurosci Res Comm* 1988;3:55–61.

223. Victor M, Agamanolis J. Amnesia due to lesions confined to the hippocampus: a clinical–pathological study. *J Cog Neurosci* 1990;2:246–257.

224. Wainer BH, Levey AI, Mufson EF, Mesulam MM. Cholinergic systems in mammalian brain identified with antibodies against choline acetyltransferase. *Neurosci Int* 1984;6:163–182.

225. Wainer BH, Levey AI, Rye DB, Mesulam M, Mufson EJ. Cholinergic and non-cholinergic septohippocampal pathways. *Neurosci Lett* 1985;54:45–52.

226. Wellman CL, Sengelaub DR. Cortical neuroanatomical correlates of behavioral deficits produced by lesion of the basal forebrain in rats. *Behav Neural Biol* 1991;56:1–24.

227. Welner SA, Dunnett SB, Salamone JD, MacLean B, Iversen SD. Transplantation of embryonic ventral forebrain grafts to the neocortex of rats with bilateral lesions of nucleus basalis magnocellularis ameliorates a lesion-induced deficit in spatial memory. *Brain Res* 1988;463:192–197.

228. Welner SA, Koty ZC, Boksa P. Chromaffin cell grafts to rat cerebral cortex reverse lesion-induced memory deficits. *Brain Res* 1990;527:163–166.

229. Wenk GL, Olton DS. Recovery of neocortical choline acetyltransferase activity following ibotenic acid injection into the nucleus basalis of Meynert in rats. *Brain Res* 1990;293:184–186.

230. Wenk GL, Pierce DJ, Struble RG, Price DL, Cork LC. Age-related changes in multiple neurotransmitter systems in the monkey brain. *Neurobiol Aging* 1989;10:11–19.

231. Werboff J, Havlena J. Effects of aging on open field behavior. *Psychol Rep* 1962;10:395–398.

232. White P, Goodhardt MJ, Keet JK, Hiley CR, Carrasio LH, Williams IEI. Neocortical cholinergic neurons in elderly people. *Lancet* 1977; 1:668–671.

233. Whitehouse PJ, Price DJ, Clark A, Coyle JT, DeLong M. Alzheimer's disease: evidence for selective loss of cholinergic neurons in the nucleus basalis. *Ann Neurol* 1981;10:122–126.

234. Whittemore SR, Holets VR, Keane RW, Levy DJ, McKay RD. Transplantation of a temperature-sensitive, nerve growth factor-secreting, neuroblastoma cell line into adult rats with fimbria–fornix lesions rescues cholinergic septal neurons. *J Neurosci Res* 1991;28:156–170.

235. Woodruff ML, Baisden RH, Whittington DL, Benson AE. Embryonic hippocampal grafts ameliorate the deficit in DRL acquisition produced by hippocampectomy. *Brain Res* 1987; 408:97–117.

236. Woodruff ML, Baisden RH, Whittington DL, Shelton NL, Wray S. Grafts containing fetal hippocampal tissue reduce activity and improve passive avoidance in hippocampectomized or trimethyltin-exposed rats. *Exp Neurol* 1988;102:130–143.

237. Woodruff ML, Baisden RH, Nonneman AJ. Anatomical and behavioral sequelae of fetal brain transplants in rats with trimethyltin-induced neurodegeneration. *Neurotoxicity* 1991; 12:427–444.

238. Woolf NJ, Wckenstein F, Butcher LL. Cholinergic systems in the rat brain: I. projections to the limbic telecephalon. *Brain Res Bull* 1984; 13:751–784.

239. Wozniak DF, Stewart GR, Finger S, Olney JW, Cozzari C. Basal forebrain lesions impair tactile discrimination and working memory. *Neurobiol Aging* 1989;10:173–179.

240. Yamamoto T, Hirano A. Nucleus raphe dorsalis in Alzheimer's disease: neurofibrillary tangles and loss of large neurons. *Ann Neurol* 1985; 17:573–577.

241. Yirmiya R, Zhou FC, Holder MD, Deems DA, Garcia J. Partial recovery of gustatory function after neural tissue transplantation to the lesioned gustatory neocortex. *Brain Res Bull* 1988;20:619–625.

242. Zola-Morgan S, Squire LR, Amaral DG. Human amnesia and the medial temporal region: enduring memory impairment following a bilateral lesion limited to the field CA1 of the hippocampus. *J Neurosci* 1986;6:2950–2967.

243. Zola-Morgan S, Squire LR, Amaral DG. Lesions of the hippocampal formation but not lesions of the fornix or the mammilary nuclei produce long-lasting memory impairment in monkeys. *J Neurosci* 1989;9:898–913.

244. Zornetzer SF, Thompson R, Rogers J. Rapid forgetting in aged rats. *Behav Neural Biol* 1982;36:49–60.

Functional Neural Transplantation,
edited by S. B. Dunnett and A. Björklund.
Raven Press, Ltd., New York © 1994.

12

Electrophysiologic Analysis of Grafts in the Hippocampus

Menahem Segal and Gal Richter-Levin

Department of Neurobiology, The Weizmann Institute, Rehovot 76100, Israel

The original exciting observations, demonstrating that embryonic neurons grafted into an adult host brain can survive, send axons into the host brain, and innervate specific target tissue there (36), led to a series of studies directed at the analysis of restoration of behavioral functions by a transplant. The general scheme used in those studies was to create a lesion in an adult rat, assess the degree of impaired behavioral function, graft specific embryonic tissue, and measure the restoration of this function. As predicted, the initial wave of studies came out with an enthusiastically clear messege: Grafts restore impaired functions of the brain (20). These initial observations made intuitive sense; if one removes cholinergic neurons and replaces them with a cholinergic graft, one can expect to find restoration of functions associated with cholinergic neurons. Later studies demonstrated that the real brain is more complex than viewed in these preliminary studies, and that grafts do not always restore "normality" to the brain (e.g., 7,34). The following is a review of studies using physiologic methods to assess functions of the hippocampus and tissue grafted into or next to it. Studies of the physiology of a graft in a host hippocampus can be classified along several dimensions (37). These include the type of damage inflicted on the host brain, the source of tissue and the form

and placement of the graft, and the methods of assessment.

METHODOLOGICAL CONSIDERATIONS

Types of Damage

A typical kind of damage to the hippocampal system involves aspiration of the midline cortex, the corpus callosum, and the fornix–fimbria. This is considered by some to constitute a method for removal of the cholinergic septohippocampal pathway (e.g., 8,37,39). Whereas this is certainly true (although about 20% of the cholinergic innervation of the hippocampus comes from the ventral route, not affected by this lesion), this method produces much more than a selective cholinergic deficit; it ablates all brain stem afferents to the dorsal hippocampus as well as the major descending connection between the hippocampus and brain stem nuclei. As a result, the hippocampus shrinks and may express abnormal, epileptic activity.

More gentle procedures involve ischemic damage to CA1 neurons of the dorsal hippocampus, which follows a temporary occlusion of the arteries to the brain (21), colchicine-induced granular cell death in the dentate gyrus (14a), and kainic acid-induced cell death in CA3 region of the hippocampus, as well as selective lesions of specific hippocampal afferents, such as colchicine lesions of the medial septum, 5,7-dihydroxytryptamine (5,7-DHT) lesions of the serotonergic system, and 6-OHDA lesions of noradrenergic fibers innervating the hippocampus (6,25). These lesions are rather specific and much less traumatic to the brain than the aspiration/knife cut/electrolytic type lesions.

The type of lesion and the production of a specific cavity for the future alien tissue certainly determine the possible physiologic recovery of the hippocampus; the more selective the damage, the more likely a recovery of the impaired function, both spontaneously and after grafting. Likewise, the more selective the lesion, the easier it is to assess the damage and recovery.

Procedural Effects

The physiologic "normality" of the host hippocampus as well as that of the graft depends heavily on the mechanical damage produced by the presence of a piece of alien tissue. The size of this tissue depends on the age of the donor and the size of the original graft, the placement near a rich blood supply, and the possible interruption of the host circulation (1,37). The postlesion delay before grafting may determine the presence of growth factors, and hence the success of the graft and its eventual size. Although some of these factors may not have an obvious effect in a behavioral analysis of the graft, they may contribute to the physiologic properties of the graft–host interaction.

Source of the Grafted Tissue

The source of the grafted tissue is the major object of interest in the physiologic analysis of graft–host interaction. In studies of the hippocampus, the grafted tissue comes from one of four main sources: embryonic hippocampus, an afferent nucleus to the

hippocampus, an alien neuronal tissue (cortex, cerebellum, cholinergic nuclei) that does not innervate the hippocampus normally, and genetically-engineered nonneuronal cells. The results to be discussed in the following paragraphs are clustered on the basis of this parameter.

Methods of Assessment

The selection of the method of assessment of the physiologic recovery of the tissue and graft viability is important to be able to detect certain physiologic properties in the tissue. Two main methods are commonly used: extracellular recording of single cells and populations of cells in the intact brain (e.g., 7–12,24,25), and intracellular recording of cellular activity in the *in vitro* slice (e.g., 18,21). The former method has the advantage of being able to assess the activity of the entire graft *in situ,* but measures a small array of variables, whereas the latter method allows a more comprehensive study of a small subset of grafted neurons. Obviously, the slicing itself disrupts fiber pathways, restricting the ability to assess graft–host interactions.

PHYSIOLOGIC ASSESSMENT OF GRAFTS

Hippocampal Grafts in the Hippocampus

Initial experiments used the grafted hippocampus as a bridge between the severed septohippocampal neurons and their target, the host hippocampus. Earlier studies demonstrated that the cholinergic neurons grow into the bridge, and across it into the host target area. Physiologic experiments in the intact brain showed that the graft indeed contains spontaneously active cells, that stimulation of the host septum can evoke responses of grafted cells, and that an EEG pattern akin to that seen in the normal brain is generated in the graft, and in adjacent areas of the host hippocampus (30,35).

Later experiments by Buszaki et al. (9) indicated that "activity of some graft neurons was regulated in a near normal manner" and that "at least a portion of the graft neurons had come under control of the host hippocampus." Furthermore, physiologically identified complex spike and theta cells were recorded in the graft, and some of these cells were phase locked to a theta rhythm recorded in the intact hemisphere, seen during walking and running (9). Later studies added that the graft can even express long-term potentiation (LTP) in response to tetanic stimulation of the host or even the grafted tissue. Unlike normal LTP, this one was associated with an enhancement of spontaneous spike discharge (12). These studies indicated that the graft is also nearly normal in that it possesses the "mechanisms required for plastic changes in synaptic efficacy" (12).

The bridge graft promotes the extension of cholinergic fibers from the septum into the host hippocampus. This is enhanced by a transient infusion of nerve growth factor into the host brain, resulting in restoration of near-normal theta rhythm (39). This rhythm, however, was blocked by scopolamine, indicating that it misses the noncholinergic component seen in normal theta rhythm. Indications that the graft is not all that normal were already noticed by Hounsgaard and Yarom in 1985 (18), who noticed a lack of inhibition in grafted tissue, and by Buszaki and associates in 1987 (8,9), who recorded a spread of epileptic spikes from the graft to the host. Only in later studies did these authors admit that the grafted hippocampus is actually an "epileptic focus" (7,10). Interestingly, the interictal transitions in the graft occurred when the rat arose from sleep, indicating that some control by host brain of graft epilepsy does take place (7).

The abnormal influence of the graft on host activity is not restricted to a "bridge" of a grafted piece of tissue in a cavity made in the fornix; a graft of dissociated tissue injected directly into the host hippocampus (11, and see below) also can affect host activity. Experiments designed to examine more closely the relations between grafted and host hippocampus were conducted in slices taken from rats that underwent a prior ischemic episode resulting in degeneration of CA1 neurons, and then were grafted with dissociated hippocampal neurons (21). In these studies, grafted neurons appeared quite normal, receiving and extending fibers into the adjacent host hippocampus. Both pyramidal neurons and interneurons were found in the graft. In studying the properties of grafted neurons, it was found that they appear to possess normal-appearing conductances (18,21). One peculiar property of these cells was the total lack of inhibitory postsynaptic potentials, which normally follow a fast excitatory post-synaptic potential (EPSP), in response to afferent stimulation. Although the size of the EPSP appeared normal, its duration was six to eight times longer than that of a normal EPSP, a response seen when inhibitory potentials are blocked by γ-aminobutyric acid (GABA) antagonists (21). This lack of inhibition, in the obvious presence of interneurons, may underlie the epileptic properties of the graft. Interestingly, a morphologic study of similar grafts revealed the absence of chandelier-type inhibitory interneurons, which normally make axoaxonic connections on pyramidal neurons (15). Local inhibition is not totally absent in the graft, because the extracellular response recorded from populations of cells does not consist of multiple population spikes, which can be seen in such slices on blockade of inhibition with bicuculline (14a). The relative lack of inhibition led Mudrick et al. (21) to propose that the graft remains in a juvenile state, which is typically associated with less GABA inhibition, and does not mature in the host brain. Alternately, the absence of strategically located interneurons may lead to apparent abnormal behavior of an otherwise normal set of grafted neurons. The alteration by the graft of host excitability can undoubtedly modify the be-

stimulation of the graft. Indeed, a complex pattern of reactivity to graft stimulation can be seen, and the cholinergic component of this can be sorted out only by using pharmacologic tools (33).

Noradrenergic Cells Grafted into the Hippocampus

Whereas the main effect of noradrenaline, studied over the past decade in brain slices, is mediated by activation of a β-adrenergic receptor and involves excitation (i.e., blockade of accommodation and of a slow calcium-gated potassium current), the main effect of removal of the noradrenergic innervation of the forebrain is to enhance excitability and susceptibility to epileptogenic stimuli (5,14). Grafting of cells from the noradrenergic nucleus locus coeruleus causes a near-complete restoration of normal excitability of the hippocampus. There is a clear correlation between the amount of reinnervation by the grafted noradrenergic fibers and the restoration of normality (2,5,14).

Stimulation of a noradrenergic graft in the intact hippocampus produces a long-lasting inhibition of spontaneous activity of host pyramidal neurons (6), akin to the effect of stimulation of the innate nucleus locus coeruleus. In a slice, stimulation of a graft produces a reduction of slow after-hyperpolarization, much like the effect of topical application of noradrenaline (32). As mentioned with regard to septal neurons, the graft of the locus coeruleus contains much more than just noradrenergic cells, and so electrical stimulation of the graft may not be all that specific.

Raphe Grafts in the Hippocampus

Perhaps the most studied graft is the serotonin-containing raphe implanted into the hippocampus. As with noradrenergic innervation of the hippocampus, serotonergic innervation can be selectively depleted with a neurotoxin, 5,7-DHT. This drug causes degeneration of serotonergic fibers throughout the forebrain. Embryonic raphe neurons grafted into the serotonin-deprived hippocampus send axons into the host and innervate it in a dense network akin to the pattern of innervation seen in the normal brain (1). Intracellular recording from grafted neurons in a hippocampal slice revealed that grafted neurons, recorded at least a month after grafting, possess electrophysiologic properties similar to those of normal adult raphe neurons; these include a high input resistance, lack of inward rectification, presence of a large, transient outward current, relative lack of accommodation in response to a long depolarizing current pulse, and a slow component of an action potential. These properties are seen in normal adult serotonergic cells (28,31). The graft sends axons to innervate the host hippocampus, and these appear to have a slow conduction velocity, but they leave the graft to innervate host neurons. Stimulation of the graft produces a slow hyperpolarization that is potentiated by the serotonin precursor 5-hydroxytryptophan (5-HT) (28, 29). This effect is similar to the primary effect of serotonin acting at a 5-HT1a receptor. Stimulation of the host hippocampus, on the other hand, could evoke an excitatory response in grafted neurons, recorded intracellularly (32).

Release of serotonin from its terminals, using known releasers (e.g., fenfluramine), was found to cause an enhancement of reactivity of the hippocampal dentate gyrus to stimulation of the perforant path (25,26). This enhanced reactivity is not likely to be caused by an enhanced release of the excitatory neurotransmitter from the perforant path terminals, because the slope of the EPSP, indicative of an effect on the synapse, was not changed in these studies. Several lines of evidence indicated that serotonin released from the terminals interacts with the local inhibitory network to enhance reactivity of the dentate granular cells to the stimulation. These effects of serotonin releasers were not seen in 5,7-DHT-treated rats (Fig. 2).

Experiments using grafts in the intact hippocampus were done to test some aspects of this hypothesis. It was found, for example, that a raphe graft in the hippocampus, but not in the entorhinal cortex or the septum, can restore the effect of fenfluramine. Furthermore, this effect depended on the presence of a dense network of graft-originated serotonin fibers in the host hippocampus (27).

As seen with the noradrenergic innervation of the hippocampus, the lack of serotonin causes hyperexcitability of the depleted hippocampus and enhanced reactivity to afferent stimulation. Here, too, the raphe graft restored the normal excitability of the tissue (27). These studies indicate that the graft regulates host brain activity continuously, either under host brain control or independent of the host brain. The reduced susceptibility to seizure with raphe

transplants has also been seen in other brain areas (13).

The possibility that the host brain regulates graft activity was examined in intact animals. Cellular activity recorded from tentatively identified serotonergic cells in the freely moving animal showed a regular pattern of firing, and was not affected much by sleep–wake cycles, unlike the behavior of cells in the normal brain (38). These results led Trulson et al. (38) to conclude that grafted neurons are not under the control of the host brain, yet some hormonal effects still are seen in these cells. This is actually not a surprising conclusion, because the normal afferents to the native raphe come from brain stem structures, which are remote from the graft. Other studies using *in vivo* dialysis of neurotransmitter substances released from the graft do suggest that the graft is under some host brain control, in that some afferents that affect normal cell activity also affect grafted cells (36).

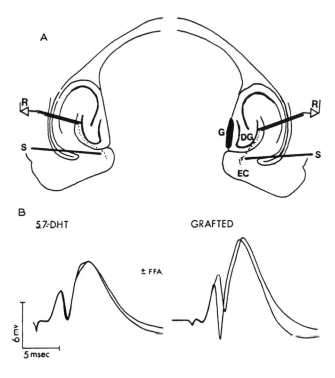

FIG. 2. Serotonin released from a raphe graft can potentiate reactivation of the hippocampus to afferent stimulation. **A**: Schematic drawing of the location of the graft and the stimulation and recording electrodes. A graft is positioned unilaterally near the host dentate gyrus, where responses to perforant path stimulation are recorded. **B**: Averaged population response recorded in the two hemispheres before and after parenteral injection of fenfluramine (*FFA*). Although the response is markedly enhanced in the grafted hemisphere, it is not affected by FFA in the nongrafted hemisphere. The animal was treated with 5,7-dihydroxytryptamine (5,7-DHT) before grafting. Further details are presented elsewhere (24).

Double Lesions and Double Graft Functions

One of the interesting open questions in graft physiology is the organization of cellular connectivity within the graft. Some observations indicate that within a graft there is some segregation of cell types, such that serotonergic neurons are localized in the periphery of the graft, making them more likely to be in contact with the host. This of course depends on the graft shape and size, because large grafts tend to have few viable neurons in the center anyway. One type of graft that has been explored behaviorally but not yet physiologically is a double graft, that is, a graft containing serotonergic and cholinergic neurons (23). An interaction between the cholinergic and serotonergic afferents to the hippocampus has been suggested to have a major impact on hippocampal activity (25,26), and the double graft may provide a unique system for analysis, which has yet to be conducted.

OUTSTANDING ISSUES IN THE PHYSIOLOGIC ANALYSIS OF GRAFT–HOST INTERACTION

Although the results summarized to date demonstrate that the graft contains viable neurons that possess normal-appearing properties and interact with the host brain, several questions remain open and await extensive analysis in both *in vivo* and *in vitro* systems. Among these are 1) the comparison between normal and graft-derived innervation. This is particularly relevant in cases of hyperinnervation by serotonergic or noradrenergic fibers of the host hippocampus. In most cases studied, there is a gradient of innervation, with the highest density near the graft. Will this pattern create a larger-than-normal physiologic effect near the graft, or will it be associated with desensitization? 2) The properties of individual synaptic potentials of central biogenic amine-containing neurons have never been studied. In fact, it is not clear whether these amines do produce conventional synaptic potentials, because there is a number of morphologic studies suggesting that they do not have the typical synaptic specializations seen in conventional synapses. This is of particular interest because there are many assumed modulators of release of biogenic amines, as well as many types of presynaptic receptors on them. Although this question has no direct bearing on graft–host interaction, the graft does provide a unique test system that allows the study of central connections that are remote *in vivo,* in a convenient *in vitro* test system.

COMPLEMENTARY METHODS

Although electrophysiologic methods are irreplaceable when it comes to studying properties of individual cells and synaptic connections, there are alternative methods for assessment of functional recovery of grafts and their interactions with the host brain. Among the most powerful ones is *in vivo* dialysis, which can be conducted in the awake, freely moving rat, and can give an estimate of the behaviorally relevant release of neurotransmitter substances associated with the graft in comparison to the normal pattern of release (4,22,36).

Another method, serving similar purposes, is *in situ* electrochemistry, which also can give a more localized estimate of release of neurotransmitter substances and their metabolites (17). These two methods have been used in the past, but certainly can add to the much-needed database on graft–host interaction.

A third method of potential interest involves imaging of voltage/calcium/pH/sodium from an array of adjacent sites in a slice containing host and graft tissue. Preliminary data indicate the feasibility of this method and its potential usefulness for the accurate delineation of the boundries of interactions between the two types of tissues (*authors' unpublished observations*). More has to be done to explore the potential of these methods.

CONCLUSIONS

The neuronal graft has been used extensively over the past decade as (1) a means of replacing lost neurons in experimental models of neurodegenerative diseases, and (2) as a research tool for analysis of simplified, reconstructed neuronal circuits. The demands from a physiologic analysis of recovered functions are modest; if indeed we are interested in replacement therapy, we need not be too concerned with the question of what is actually happening, as long as the function is restored. On the other hand, the graft has not been explored much as a research tool for the study of neuronal connections, probably because of technical difficulties associated with the *in vitro* analysis of graft–host interactions. Although physiologic studies to date indicate that the graft becomes incorporated into host brain circuitry, this is by no means a simple replacement of lost connections. Minute changes in graft circuitry compared to the normal innervation pattern can generate epileptic activity, which may spread into the host brain. Also, the fact that the graft is not under tight host brain control may cause unpredictable behavior of the graft in its interactions with the host. One possible complication in the physiologic analysis of the graft is the fact that it is quite heterogenous, and the proportion of cells carrying the "right" neurotransmitter substance is rather low. Progress will be made if a procedure for implantation of a more homogenous population of cells can be devised. One possible move in this direction may be the grafting of genetically engineered cells that will behave like normal ones and make synaptic interactions with the host (16,19). Research in this direction is still in its infancy, but the prospects are promising.

REFERENCES

1. Azmitia EC, Perlow MJ, Brennan MJ, Lauder JM. Fetal raphe and hippocampal transplants into adult and aged C57B1/6M mice: a preliminary immunohistochemical study. *Brain Res Bull* 1981;7:703–710.
2. Barry DI, Kikvadze I, Brundin P, Bolwig TG, Björklund A, Lindvall O. Grafted noradrenergic neurons suppress seizure development in kindling induced epilepsy. *Proc Natl Acad Sci USA* 1987;84:8712–8715.
3. Bassant MH, Joly M, Nilsson OG, Björklund A, Lamour Y. Electrophysiological and pharmacological properties of neurons within solid basal forebrain transplants in the rat brain. *Brain Res* 1988;460:8–16.
4. Bengzon J, Brundin P, Kalen P, Kokaia M, Lindvall O. Host regulation of noradrenaline release from grafts of seizure-suppressant locus coeruleus neurons. *Exp Neurol* 1991;111:49–54.
5. Bengzon J, Kokaia M, Brundin P, Lindvall O. Seizure suppression in kindling epilepsy by intrahippocampal locus coeruleus grafts: evidence for an alpha 2-adrenoreceptor mediated mechanism. *Exp Brain Res* 1990;81:433–437.
6. Björklund A, Segal M, Stenevi U. Functional reinnervation of rat hippocampus by locus coeruleus implants. *Brain Res* 1979;170:409–426.
7. Buszaki G, Bayardo F, Miles R, Wong RKS, Gage FH. The grafted hippocampus: an epileptic focus. *Exp Neurol* 1989;105:10–22.
8. Buzsaki G, Gage FH, Czopf J, Björklund A. Restoration of rhythmic slow activity in the subcortically denervated hippocampus by fetal CNS transplants. *Brain Res* 1987;400:334–347.
9. Buzsaki G, Gage FH, Kelleny L. Björklund A. Behavioral dependence of the electrical activity of intracerebrally transplanted fetal hippocampus. *Brain Res* 1987;400:321–333.
10. Buzsaki G, Masliah E, Chen LS, Horvath Z, Terry R, Gage FH. Hippocampal grafts into the intact brain induce epileptic patterns. *Brain Res* 1991;554:30–37.
11. Buzsaki G, Ponomareff G, Bayardo F, Shaw T, Gage FH. Suppression and induction of epileptic activity by neuronal grafts. *Proc Natl Acad Sci USA* 1988;85:9327–9330.
12. Buzsaki G, Wiesner J, Henriksen SJ, Gage FH. Long term potentiation of evoked and spontaneous neuronal activity in the grafted hippocampus. *Exp Brain Res* 1989;76:401–408.
13. Camu W, Marlier L, Lerner-Natoli M, Rondouin G, Privat A. Transplantation of serotonergic neurons into the 5,7-DHT-lesioned rat olfactory bulb restores the parameters of kindling. *Brain Res* 1990;518:23–30.
14. Clough RW, Browning RA, Maring ML, Jobe PC. Intracerebral grafting of fetal dorsal pons in genetically epilepsy-prone rats: effects on audiogenic-induced seizures. *Exp Neurol* 1991;112:195–199.
14a. Dawe GS, Gray JA, Sinden JD, Stephenson JD, and Segal M. Extracellular recording in the colchicine-treated rat dentate gyrus and CA1 hippocampal subfield tissue. *Brain Res* 1993;625:63–74.
15. Freund TF, Buzsaki G. Alternations in excitatory and GABAergic inhibitory connections in hippocampal transplants. *Neuroscience* 1988;27:373–385.

16. Gage FH, Wolff TA, Rosenberg MB, et al. Grafting genetically modified cells to the brain: possibilities for the future. *Neuroscience* 1987;23:795–807.
17. Hoffer B, Rose G, Gerhardt G, Strömberg I, Olson L. Demonstration of monoamine release from transplant-reinnervated caudate nucleus by in vivo electrochemical detection. In: Björklund A, Stenevi U, eds. *Neural grafting in the mammalian CNS*. New York: Elsevier; 1985:437–447.
18. Hounsgaard J, Yarom Y. Cellular physiology of transplanted neurons. In: Björklund A, Stenevi U, eds. *Neural grafting in the mammalian CNS*. New York: Elsevier; 1985:401–408.
19. Kordower JH, Notter MFD, Gash DM. Neuroblastoma cells in neural transplants: a neuroanatomical and behavioral analysis. *Brain Res* 1987;417:85–98.
20. Low WC, Lewis PR, Bunch ST, et al. Functional recovery following neural transplantation of embryonic septal nuclei in adult rats with septohippocampal lesions. *Nature* 1982;300:260–262.
21. Mudrick LA, Baimbridge KG, Peet MJ. Hippocampal neurons transplanted into ischemically lesioned hippocampus: electroresponsiveness and reestablishment of circuitries. *Exp Brain Res* 1988;76:333–342.
22. Nilsson OG, Kalén P, Rosengren E, Björklund A. Acetylcholine release from intrahippocampal septal graft is under control of host brain. *Proc Natl Acad Sci USA* 1990;87:2647–2651.
23. Nilsson OG, Brundin P, Björklund A. Amelioration of spatial memory impairment by intrahippocampal grafts of mixed septal and raphe tissue in rats with combined cholinergic and serotonergic denervation of the forebrain. *Brain Res* 1990;515:193–206.
24. Olton DS, Shapiro ML. Electrophysiological correlates of recovery of function. *Acta Neurobiol Exp* 1990;50:125–133.
25. Richter-Levin G, Segal M. Grafting of midbrain neurons into the hippocampus restores serotonergic modulation of hippocampal activity in the rat. *Brain Res* 1990;521:1–6.
26. Richter-Levin G, Segal M. The effects of serotonin depletion and raphe grafts on hippocampal electrophysiology and behavior. *J Neurosci* 1991;11:1585–1596.
27. Richter-Levin G, Segal M. Raphe grafts in the hippocampus but not in the entorhinal cortex reverse hyperexcitability in serotonin depleted rats and their responsiveness to serotonin releasing drugs. *Dev Neurosci* 1992;14:166–172.
28. Segal M. Interaction between grafted neurons and adult host rat hippocampus. *Ann NY Acad Sci* 1987;495:284–295.
29. Segal M. An analysis of interactions between grafted serotonin neurons and an adult host hippocampus. In: Vernadakis A, ed. *Model systems of development and aging of the nervous system*. Boston: Martinus Nijhoff; 1987:75–84.
30. Segal M. Neural grafts in the study of brain plasticity. In: Milgram NW, Petitt T, eds. *Neuroplasticity, learning and memory*. New York: Alan R. Liss; 1987:265–278.
31. Segal M, Azmitia EC. Fetal raphe neurons grafted into the hippocampus develop normal adult physiological properties. *Brain Res* 1986;364:162–166.
32. Segal M, Azmitia EC, Björklund A, Greenberger V, Richter-Levin G. Physiology of graft–host interactions in the rat hippocampus. *Prog Brain Res* 1988;78:95–101.
33. Segal M, Björklund A, Gage FH. Transplanted septal neurons make viable cholinergic synapses with a host hippocampus. *Brain Res* 1985;336:302–307.
34. Segal M, Greenberger V, Pearl E. Septal transplants ameliorate spatial deficits and restore cholinergic functions in rats with a damaged septo-hippocampal connection. *Brain Res* 1989;500:139–148.
35. Segal M, Stenevi U, Björklund A. Reformation in adult rats of functional septo-hippocampal connections by septal neurons regenerating across an embryonic hippocampal tissue bridge. *Neurosci Lett* 1981;27:7–12.
36. Sharp T, Foster GA. In vivo measurement using microdialysis of the release and metabolism of 5-hydroxytryptamine in raphe neurons grafted to the rat hippocampus. *J Neurochem* 1989;53:303–306.
37. Stenevi U, Björklund A, Svendgaard NA. Transplantation of central and peripheral monoamine neurons to the adult rat brain: techniques and conditions for survival. *Brain Res* 1976;114:1–20.
38. Trulson ME, Hosseini A, Trulson TJ. Serotonin neuron transplants: electrophysiological unit activity of intrahippocampal raphe grafts in freely moving cats. *Brain Res Bull* 1986;17:461–468.
39. Tuszynski MH, Buzsaki G, Gage FH. Nerve growth factor infusions combined with fetal hippocampal grafts enhance reconstruction of the lesioned septohippocampal projection. *Neuroscience* 1990;36:33–44.
40. Vinogradova OS, Bragin AG, Kitchigina VF. Spontaneous and evoked activity of neurons in the intrabrain allo- and xenografts of the hippocampus and septum. In: Björklund A, Stenevi U, eds. *Neural grafting in the mammalian CNS*. New York: Elsevier; 1985:409–419.

Functional Neural Transplantation,
edited by S. B. Dunnett and A. Björklund.
Raven Press, Ltd., New York © 1994.

13

Cognitive Function after Intracerebral Grafting in Monkeys

R. M. Ridley and H. F. Baker

Division of Psychiatry, Clinical Research Centre, Harrow HA1 3UJ, United Kingdom

The use of monkeys has been of crucial importance in the development of the technique of transplantation of dopamine-rich fetal ventral mesencephalic tissue into animals with neurotoxic lesions within dopamine projection systems (for review, see 9,23). This technique is now being assessed as an experimental treatment for the motor symptoms of Parkinson's disease in a variety of neurologic centers worldwide (69). Although, overall, clinical improvements are modest, substantial restitution of motor function has been seen in some patients (52,53). This has encouraged the hope that neural tissue transplantation may have a clinical application in the treatment of complex neurologic disease and offers the possibility that cognitive disorders also may be amenable to such treatment.

Monkeys have been used to a lesser extent so far in the assessment of the restitution of cognitive rather than motor function after neural tissue transplantation, but the development of several rat models of cognitive dysfunction, in which the effects of neural grafts have been assessed (see 22), suggests that these techniques could be carried forward in monkeys and, it is to be hoped, ultimately into human application. In addition to the assessment of the effects of transplanting acetylcholine-rich fetal basal forebrain (ACh-rich) tissue into the hippocampus of monkeys with fornix transection, which already has been undertaken

(76,79), there are other aspects of transplantation that have been investigated in rats and which could be investigated in monkeys. These include the transplanting of ACh-rich neural tissue into cortex in rats with *cortical* cholinergic dysfunction resulting from neurotoxic lesions of the basal nucleus of Meynert (NBM) or as a consequence of normal aging (20,24), the transplantation of cortical tissue into rats with cortical lesions (28,51), and the transplantation of hippocampal cells into rats with ischemic damage to the CA1 cells of the hippocampus (63). Grafting of neural tissue into the basal ganglia in monkey models of Parkinson's disease (2,89) and Huntington's disease (45) also has been undertaken, and these systems are therefore available for assessment of the effects on cognition as well as on motor aspects, which have been studied in more detail so far.

The use of monkeys is warranted partly because the neuroanatomy and physiology (e.g., the immune system) of monkeys more closely resemble those of humans than those of rats, but mainly because of the greater sophistication and resemblance to human performance of monkey cognitive ability. Unlike drug treatments, a transplant cannot easily be stopped or removed. Procedures that could affect mental activity and have adverse as well as beneficial effects require the most stringent preclinical testing. For a radical treatment such as neural tissue transplantation to be used routinely, it must be established not only that the treatment works but that it does so consistently. Extensive experimentation therefore is required to understand all aspects of the procedure and to develop the optimum techniques.

MEASURING COGNITIVE ABILITY IN MONKEYS

There are various ways of measuring cognitive ability in monkeys, and most involve the use of either the manual Wisconsin General Test Apparatus (WGTA; Fig. 1), which was first developed in the 1930s (43), or automated, computerized versions of the apparatus (e.g., 84). In the manual apparatus, the monkey is presented with a series of discrete trials in which it must choose and displace one of (usually) two objects to find a food reward that is hidden consistently under one of the objects. Learning ability is measured as the number of trials required to reach a predetermined criterion (for example, 27 correct responses in 30 consecutive trials, 27/30). This technique therefore assesses the ability of the monkey to perceive the difference between two objects (or patterns), and acquire a stimulus–reward, or, in some cases (see later), a stimulus–response association. Because the relationships between stimulus, response, and reward is constant from trial to trial, these tasks are called *trial-independent* tasks.

Perceptual ability can be assessed differentially by making the stimulus objects or patterns more similar to each other, whereas learning ability can be specifically taxed by requiring the animal to learn to discriminate between several pairs of objects in the same test period (concurrent

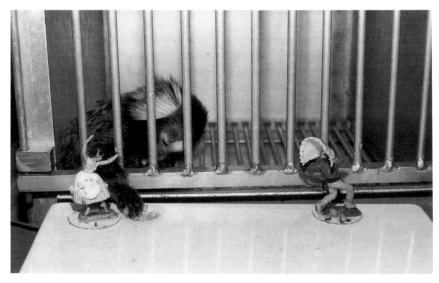

FIG. 1. Marmoset learning a simple visual discrimination in the Wisconsin General Test Apparatus. In this task, the left/right position of the two stimuli varies from trial to trial but the food reward is always placed under one stimulus. The monkey must learn that one stimulus has positive reward *value,* whereas the other stimulus does not. This task therefore requires *evaluative memory. (Nonevaluative memory* is required to acquire information other than reward value; for example, in visuospatial discrimination the monkey must learn to go left when one pair of identical stimuli is presented and to go right when an alternative identical pair is presented. Both pairs of stimuli have equal reward value, but a particular response to each pair must be remembered.)

discrimination). Provided the animal is sufficiently motivated to make responses (by mild food deprivation and the use of a much-preferred food as reward), this form of testing is not contaminated by fluctuations in motivation, arousal, or motor activity, all of which may affect the animal's speed of responding but have little influence on which of the two objects is chosen. The ability of a monkey to relinquish or "unlearn" an association can be tested by reversal learning, where the reward contingencies are reversed and the previously unrewarded object becomes the rewarded one.

Memory, as distinct from learning ability, can be assessed in two main ways. Long-term memory can be measured by retesting an animal on a discrimination learned days, weeks, or months earlier and measuring the improvement or "savings" from the original learning. Short-term memory or working memory can be tested by requiring the animal to make a choice between two objects based on information from the previous trial. This is trial-dependent or trial-unique testing. In *trial-dependent* tasks, the monkey may be required, for example, to alternate from one trial to the next between two objects or two spatial positions. In *trial-unique* tasks, the monkey may be shown one object on a "sample" trial and then be required to choose that object when it is presented again together with another object on a "choice" trial a few seconds or minutes later. New objects are used for each pair of trials to prevent interference across trials. Memory can be assessed by measuring the decline in correct performance as the delay between sample and choice trials is increased. There is also a *trial-dependent* version of this task where the same two objects are used throughout. In this case, either object can be the "sample" on each pair of trials.

Fifty years of neuropsychological testing in monkeys has defined the patterns of impairment seen after circumscribed cortical and subcortical ablations and, taking species differences into account, these impairments can be related to the neuropsychological localization of human conditions such as agnosia and amnesia. This process of comparative psychology generates many interesting questions. For example, it is debatable whether trial-independent visual discrimination learning, which is impaired in monkeys with various cortical ablations, assesses the acquisition of semantic knowledge, as we have suggested (71), or whether it requires habit formation—that is, procedural skill learning (87)—as has been argued by Mishkin (58,60). Procedural skills can be demonstrated only by the quality of an action (e.g., being able to walk a tightrope), whereas semantic knowledge implies the existence of a databased information storage system that can be used to answer questions either verbally or by choosing between stimuli. We have argued (71) that choice behavior in a WGTA does not depend on motor skill because different movements are required on different trials but the same overall movements are required across all trials. Nor does it depend on a perceptual skill, because the objects used are easily discriminable by monkeys on the first presentation (39,59,74). Rather, it would seem that when a monkey has learned a discrimination, he *knows* which object to choose.

One advantage of using discrete trial testing methods is that, with small concessions to species differences, the same tasks also can be used in patients. Although most such tests in humans have used trial-unique paradigms, trial-independent tasks also have been used (e.g., 1,36,64,65,88), and have been found to be sensitive to cognitive defects found in a variety of groups of patients with neurologic deficits.

The type of cognitive ability required to perform trial-unique, delayed, (non)-matching tasks also is open to question. This form of testing requires recognition of previously presented objects, but whether this recognition operates at the level of episodic memory (conscious recollection of events), which is lost in human amnesia (15), or whether it depends on relatively transient working memory, and is therefore not related to human amnesia (7), depends on the delay interval and other parameters of testing. Despite these difficulties (discussed in more detail in 71), sufficient is known about the cortical and subcortical localization of function in monkeys and humans to be able to design tests in monkeys that assess the functional integrity of different brain areas in ways that can predict the effects of grafting tissue into human brain.

ROLE OF ACETYLCHOLINE
IN COGNITION

Several lines of evidence suggest that the central cholinergic system is involved in learning and memory in rats, monkeys, and humans. Demonstrating that different parts of the central cholinergic system are specifically involved in different cognitive functions has, however, proved problematic and controversial. Work in monkeys may be particularly important here because the larger monkey brain, with its more discretely organized rising cholinergic projections, may make anatomic fractionation of the cholinergic system more feasible than in rats. The greater variety of neuropsychological abilities in monkeys, whose cerebral localization is known from ablation studies, may make demonstration of separate functions easier.

Blockade of the central (and peripheral) cholinergic muscarinic receptors with scopolamine or atropine results in impaired acquisition of new information in monkeys (75) and humans (18). Where tests are devised such that acquisition and retention are separable in time, drug can be administered during one but not the other. It is then clear that it is the process of acquisition rather than storage and retrieval that is affected (75). Caution is required in interpreting the nature of the impairment when cholinergic drugs are given during trial-unique

"recognition" tests in monkeys because drug treatment is present during acquisition and retention phases. What may appear to be a memory loss (i.e., forgetting) may in fact be a failure to acquire information in an appropriate form for subsequent recollection (i.e., an encoding problem). There are grounds for believing that poor acquisition is a more important feature than faster forgetting in amnesia (34,44) and dementia (35,50).

In the most common form of dementia, Alzheimer's disease, there is a marked loss of cholinergic markers in the cortex and hippocampus (12,67) and degeneration of cholinergic neurons in the NBM and the vertical limb of the diagonal band of Broca (VDB) (6,90). Although there are many other neurotransmitter and structural alterations in Alzheimer's disease, the correlation between mental test scores premortem and cholinergic loss measured postmortem (68), together with the effects of cholinergic drugs on learning in animals and young people already cited, strongly implies that the cholinergic dysfunction in Alzheimer's disease contributes to the mental impairment. Kopelman (50) has argued that it is the information encoding failure that is specifically related to the cholinergic loss in both Alzheimer's disease and Korsakoff's syndrome. The cholinergic system also is affected in a number of other dementing illnesses, including Parkinson's disease with dementia (66) and Creutzfeldt-Jakob disease (5). Thus, the cholinergic system is in need of and, it is to be hoped, will be amenable to, therapeutic strategies in dementia.

WHERE SHOULD CHOLINERGIC
GRAFTS BE PLACED?

Although cholinergic drugs that cross the blood–brain barrier can be expected to affect the whole central cholinergic system, ACh-rich grafts would have to be placed strategically to affect the required cognitive function. This requires a precise understanding of the contribution of different brain areas to cognition, but has the advantage over drug treatment that certain central and peripheral cholinergic systems that contribute to sleep, arousal, endocrine function, and autonomic responses can be avoided.

In rats, lesions of the basal forebrain, which contains the NBM, using the neurotoxins ibotenic acid or kainic acid, lead to severe impairments on many tasks, including active avoidance, passive avoidance, spatial alternation, spatial delayed matching, and water maze navigation, as well as to sensorimotor and attentional deficits (see 26). Subsequent work using the neurotoxin quisqualic acid, which produced cortical cholinergic losses as great as those produced by ibotenic acid infusion, showed that these animals were as impaired as the ibotenic acid-treated animals only on passive avoidance tests (30). This suggests that many of the effects of ibotenic acid lesions in rats may have resulted from neuronal damage outside the NBM (e.g., in the overlying globus pallidus), and may have been motor rather than cognitive in nature. Quisqualic acid lesions of the NBM did, however, produce severe impairments on acquisition of delayed nonmatching to position and reversal to nonmatching after matching (27), and on visual discrimination reversal (82), that is, on difficult tasks that put considerable demand on learning processes. Impairment also was seen on performance of a demanding attentional task after quisqualic acid lesions of the NBM (80,82), and on acquisition of the spatial water maze, conditional discrimination learning, and delayed matching to position after quisqualic acid lesions of the septum/VDB area, from which cholinergic neurons project to the medial cortical and hippocampal regions in the rat (21,29,42,81).

Looking at the anatomy of the cholinergic projections, it can be proposed that these projections play a role in sustaining the function of these target areas in which they terminate. Viewed in this way, the functions of the rising cholinergic projections will be as diverse as the functions of the neocortical mantle, the amygdala, and the hippocampus. In so far as these target areas are involved in learning and memory processes, particularly in those tasks that can be described as "difficult" or "demanding," then the cholinergic system also can be said to be involved in learning and memory. But the cortex also has other important functions in perception, attention, and motor activity to which the cholinergic projections may be said to contribute. Demonstrating the contribution of different parts of the cholinergic projection systems to the processes of learning and memory in rats is limited, however, by a lack of consensus on precisely which tasks should be impaired by specific cortical or limbic ablations and therefore by lesions within the associated components of the cholinergic basal forebrain projections.

In monkeys, impairment in visual discrimination learning (i.e., visual agnosia) results from lesions of the inferotemporal cortex (46), whereas impairment in reversal learning (i.e., perseveration) occurs after frontal cortical removals (41). Neurotoxic lesions of the NBM, which produced the greatest reductions of the cholinergic marker choline acetyltransferase (ChAT) in the inferotemporal and frontal cortex, resulted in similar impairments in visual discrimination (77) and reversal learning (73). By contrast, lesions of the fornix or hippocampus in monkeys produce severe spatial impairments (55,56). Neurotoxic lesions of the VDB in monkeys result in ChAT depletions limited to the hippocampus and entorhinal cortex and learning impairments limited, so far, mainly to visuospatial tasks (70,78). These results emphasize the extreme importance of choosing appropriate tests based on the effects of ablation of the target areas, to demonstrate the contribution of the cholinergic projections to cognition. To show that ACh-rich neural tissue grafts restore cognitive abilities by direct interaction with host tissue, it also is necessary to show that they specifically restore the function of these areas in which they are placed and in which they establish cholinergic reinnervation.

GRAFTS OF ACh-RICH NEURAL TISSUE IN MONKEYS WITH FORNIX TRANSECTIONS

Work in rats already has demonstrated that when ACh-rich neural tissue taken from the fetal septal area is transplanted into the cortex or hippocampus of animals whose cholinergic projections to these areas have been damaged by excitotoxin infusion, fimbria–fornix transection, or alcoholic poisoning, there is improved perfor-

mance in learning and memory (4,32,54, 62). It seemed appropriate, therefore, to determine whether similar ACh-rich septal grafts from fetal monkeys could restore cognitive abilities in monkeys with learning impairments resulting from transection of the fornix. Fornix transection was achieved by inserting a small hook between the hemispheres, through the corpus callosum, around each limb of the fornix in turn, and then retracting (Fig. 2; and see 79). Transection of the fornix cuts the cholinergic projection from the VDB to the hippocampus (Fig. 3A,B). The common marmoset *(Callithrix jacchus)* was used because this small primate can be tested in the WGTA (8) and has a rapid and reliable reproductive rate in captivity, with a gestation period of

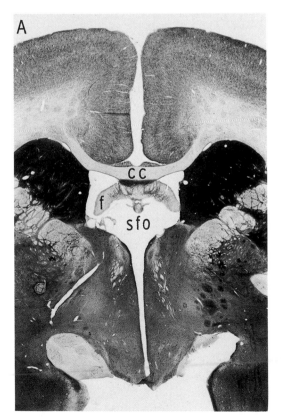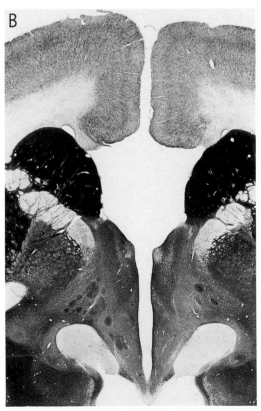

FIG. 2. AChE stained marmoset brain. **A**: Normal. **B**: After fornix transection. Note absence of fornix (*f*), subfornical organ (*sfo*), and part of corpus callosum (*cc*), but lack of damage to surrounding brain areas.

147 days (3,19). Ovulation occurs every 12 days and conception usually occurs on the first ovulation postpartum. A good breeding female therefore has two pregnancies per year, yielding two or three offspring per pregnancy (although only rarely are more than two offspring reared per pregnancy). The stage of pregnancy can be assessed accurately by transabdominal palpation (see 3 for details). Fetuses were collected by hysterotomy at 78 to 81 days' gestation, calculated as 90 to 93 days after previous parturition. (Donor females subsequently go on to further breeding.) According to the Carnegie staging of fetal development (14), this is equivalent to embryonic days 15 to 16 in the rat, which is the preferred time for ACh-rich neural tissue collection in rats (25). Tissue was dissected, prepared, and injected using methods originally established in rat experiments and modified for use in monkeys (33).

Two experiments using fetal ACh-rich neural tissue transplants have been undertaken so far in our laboratory. In the first (79), the learning ability of four marmosets with fornix transections and intrahippocampal grafts of ACh-rich fetal neural tissue was compared with that of five marmosets with fornix transection alone and seven control marmosets with either no surgery or with small control ablations of the corpus callosum (which also is damaged during the fornix transection procedure). In experiment 2 (76), which was designed to confirm and extend the results of experiment 1, there were five unoperated control animals, five with fornix transection alone, four with fornix transection and intrahippocampal ACh-rich transplants, and four with intrahippocampal grafts of ACh-poor neural tissue taken from fetal hippocampus.

In both experiments, marmosets were first trained on several tasks and then divided into groups matched for performance on these tasks. All animals, except those in the control groups, were then given bilateral fornix transections. Testing restarted 1 to 2 weeks after surgery to demonstrate the impairments resulting from the fornix transections, and on the basis of these tests the fornix-transected animals were divided into two matched groups (in experiment 1) or three matched groups (in experiment 2). In experiment 1, one group was given ACh-rich transplants bilaterally into each hippocampus, whereas the other group received no further treatment. In experiment 2, one group was given ACh-rich transplants bilaterally into each hippocampus, one group was given ACh-poor transplants into each hippocampus, and a third group received no further treatment. All animals then rested for 3 months to allow the transplants to grow and became established. Testing was then restarted and continued for approximately 8 months. At the end of the experiment, the animals were perfused for histologic study, and brain sections were stained for acetylcholinesterase (AChE) activity (Fig. 3C,D) and/or with cresyl violet. Some sections were immunostained with antibodies raised to nerve growth factor receptors, which are found on cholinergic neurons (Fig. 4).

Behavioral tests were all conducted in the WGTA, and consisted of two classes of tasks: "control" tasks on which the fornix-transected animals were not expected to be impaired, and "experimental" tasks on which impairment was anticipated for theoretical reasons. "Control" tasks consisted of visual discriminations on which reward always was to be found under the same one of the two stimulus objects (i.e., stimulus–reward association tasks). "Experimental" tasks consisted of visuospatial discriminations in which the animal must choose the stimulus on the left if one pair of identical objects is presented and the stimulus on the right if a second pair of identical objects is presented. Each task uses new sets of objects. Other "experimental" tasks included conditional discriminations, visuospatial reversal, and spatial tasks. All these "experimental" tasks require stimulus–response associations to be formed. The theoretical difference between these two classes of

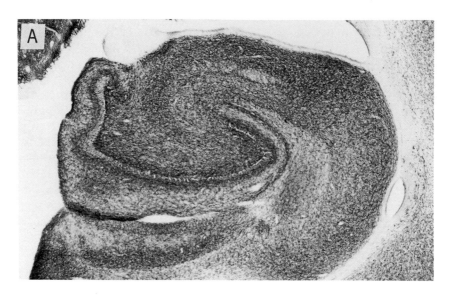

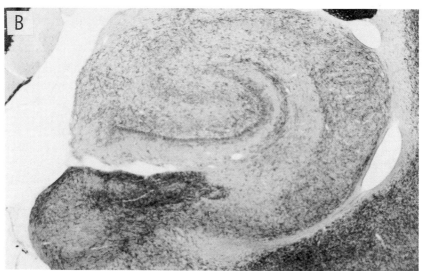

FIG. 3. AChE-stained marmoset temporal lobe. **A**: Normal. **B**: After fornix transection. **C**: After fornix transection and subsequent transplantation of ACh-rich tissue into hippocampus. **D**: After fornix transection and subsequent transplantation of ACh-poor tissue into hippocampus. Transplants at more caudal and rostral levels to that shown. Note severe depletion of AChE in (B), restitution to near-normal levels of AChE in (C), and abnormal AChE staining in (D). This abnormal staining may represent a host response to hippocampal trophic factors present in large quantities in embryonic hippocampal graft tissue.

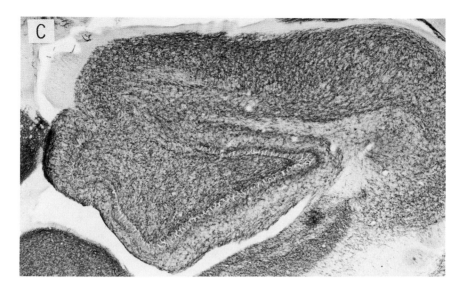

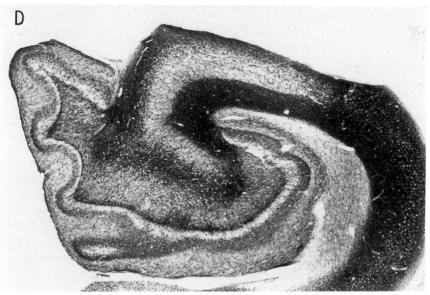

FIG. 3. *Continued.*

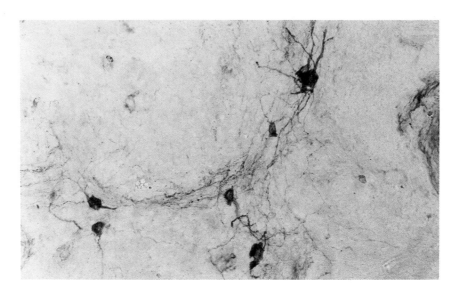

FIG. 4. Nerve growth factor receptor-positive neurons in ACh-rich transplants. Such neurons were not seen in ACh-poor transplants.

tasks and the dependence of only the latter class on the functional integrity of the hippocampal system are discussed in Ridley and Baker (71). The complete details of these tasks and other experimental details of experiment 1 are published in Ridley et al. (79) and of experiment 2 in Ridley et al. (76).

Figure 5 shows that the groups of animals were well matched for learning ability on both "control" and "experimental" tasks before surgery, but that after surgery groups of animals with fornix transections all were significantly impaired relative to control animals on "experimental" but not "control" tasks. This demonstrates the specificity of the fornix transection on learning ability. In both experiments, the fornix-transected groups did not differ from each other before transplantation. After transplantation, the groups did not differ on learning "control" tasks, demonstrating that the space-occupying grafts had not produced functional disruption of the adjacent temporal neocortex, which is involved in visual perception. Monkeys with ACh-rich transplants in both experiments showed complete restitution of learning ability on "experimental" tasks,

whereas monkeys with ACh-poor transplants showed no improvement in learning ability. Analysis of the time course of the effects of transplantation showed that the beneficial effects of grafting ACh-rich tissue were present when behavioral testing recommenced 3 months after surgery and persisted throughout the remainder of the experiments, which lasted approximately a further 8 months. Monkeys grafted with ACh-poor tissue showed no improvement across time relative to monkeys with fornix transection alone. Figure 6 shows ACh-rich and ACh-poor grafts in monkeys assessed histologically after behavioral testing had finished.

CRITICAL APPRAISAL OF EFFICACY OF CHOLINERGIC GRAFTS IN MONKEYS

To argue that ACh-rich neural tissue grafts really do restore function, it is necessary to be convinced that (1) the behavioral measure used does test some aspect of cognition; (2) the lesion significantly disrupts the cholinergic system; (3) the result-

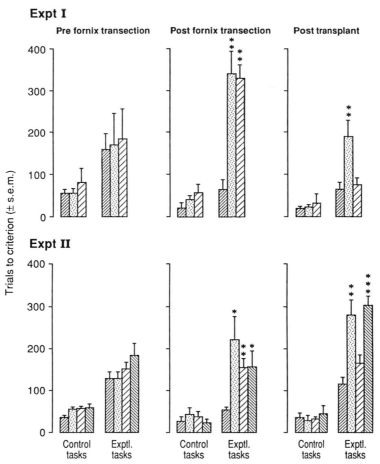

FIG. 5. Mean number of trials required to reach criterion (usually 27/30 for each task) on "control," stimulus–reward association or evaluative tasks, and "experimental," stimulus–response association or nonevaluative tasks, before and after fornix transection and after transplantation. ▨, fornix-intact animals; ▨, animals with fornix transections alone; ▨, animals with fornix transection and ACh-rich grafts into hippocampus; ▨, animals with fornix transection and ACh-poor grafts into hippocampus. $*p < 0.05$; $**p < 0.01$, $***p < 0.001$ compared to control, fornix-intact animals.

ing behavioral impairment is a consequence of the lesion within the cholinergic system rather than of other extraneous damage; (4) the ACh-rich graft produces substantial improvement only in those functions disturbed by the cholinergic lesion; and (5) an equivalent improvement is not produced by transplantation of ACh-poor tissue or (6) by the ameliorative effects of practice or spontaneous recovery. Finally, having established that restitution of function has occurred, it is important to understand the mechanisms underlying this restitution.

The next sections address these issues, with particular reference to the two experiments outlined above.

Does the Behavioral Measure Assess Some Aspect of Cognition?

Transection of the fornix produced impairment on learning a specific subset of tasks, principally visuospatial discriminations. The difference between those tasks on which fornix-transected monkeys are

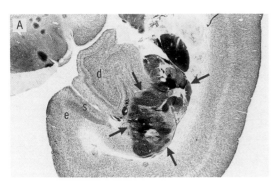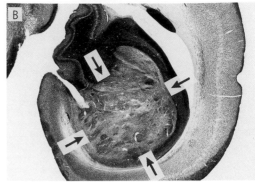

FIG. 6. AChE-stained marmoset temporal lobe. **A**: After fornix transection and subsequent transplantation of ACh-rich tissue into hippocampus. Transplant stains densely for AChE, and surrounding tissue shows near-normal levels of AChE stain. **B**: After fornix transection and subsequent transplantation of ACh-poor tissue into hippocampus. Transplant stains poorly for AChE and surrounding tissue shows abnormal AChE staining (see text). Arrows indicate transplanted tissue. *d,* Dentate gyrus; *e,* entorhinal cortex; *s,* subiculum.

or are not impaired in terms of evaluative and nonevaluative memory systems is discussed in Ridley and Baker (71), but for the current discussion the important point is that monkeys with fornix transections are impaired only on one class of task in the WGTA. Thus, we can exclude the possibility that fornix transection produced a nonspecific performance decrement consequent on some noncognitive impairment such as poor motivation (which would have resulted in nonresponding), poor motor ability (which would have resulted in slow or clumsy performance but not in inappropriate choice of stimuli), or impaired perception (which would have resulted in impaired performance in all tasks, including simple visual discriminations, that used stimuli of comparable complexity).

Having excluded these nonspecific variables, there is a clear *prima facie* case for regarding acquisition of a discrimination to a fixed criterion as requiring learning. As we argued earlier, we regard this form of learning as the acquisition of semantic knowledge. In the case of visuospatial tasks (which can be described as nonevaluative because each pair of stimuli is of equal reward-value), the information that has to be encoded into a semantic memory store

comprises the response to be made (choose the left object, choose the right object) according to which pair of objects has been presented. This type of task cannot be solved by attaching secondary reinforcing properties (reward-value) to the "correct" object, but requires that a specific piece of information (go left, go right), which is not present in the environment, be stored in memory. That this form of memory also has at least a partially separate neural substrate in humans is demonstrated by the single case study of Frith et al. (38), in which the patient, who suffered from mild Korsakoff's amnesia, was able to learn visual discriminations with differential reward, but not visuospatial discriminations.

Does Fornix Transection Severely Disrupt the Cholinergic Projection to the Hippocampus?

The depletion of AChE in fornix-transected monkeys was equal or greater to that seen in monkeys with neurotoxic lesions of the VDB (78). This depletion is confined to the dentate, posterior hippocampus and entorhinal cortex, and is not seen in the neocortex and all other subcortical areas, including the subiculum. Acetylcholinesterase occurs in cholinergic terminals and is therefore a marker of cholinergic activity. In addition to the cholinergic projection from the VDB to the hippocampus via the fornix (57), there is also a ventrofugal projection from the NBM to the anterior portion of the hippocampus (48). Acetylcholinesterase staining was spared in the anterior hippocampus of fornix-transected animals.

Does the Learning Impairment Result from the Effect of the Fornix Transection on the Cholinergic Projection to the Hippocampus?

In addition to the cholinergic projections from the VDB to the hippocampus, the fornix carries other, mainly γ-aminobutyric acid-ergic, afferents (49) and, mainly glutamatergic, efferents (91), which also must be severed by fornix transection and which could contribute to cognitive function.

It is unlikely that impaired performance on visuospatial tasks after fornix transection is caused by severance of the hippocampal efferents because neurotoxic lesions of the VDB in marmosets that damage cholinergic afferents but spare the hippocampal efferents produce the same impairments on visuospatial performance as does fornix transection (78; see Fig. 7). Furthermore, impairment after either a VDB lesion or fornix transection could be substantially ameliorated with intramuscular injections of directly acting cholinergic agonists such as arecoline or pilocarpine (78,79). It is, however, possible to argue that this implicates the cholinergic system in the original impairment only if it can be demonstrated that cholinergic agonists have a therapeutic

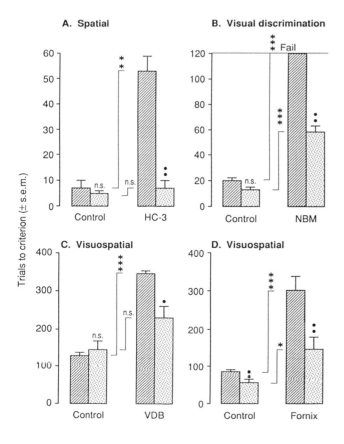

FIG. 7. Effects of cholinergic agonist treatment on learning ability in marmosets with cholinergic dysfunction. **A**: 1.0 mg/kg pilocarpine i.m. in marmosets pretreated with intracerebroventricular hemicholinium-3 (HC-3) on simple spatial learning (72). **B**: ~1.0 mg/kg arecoline i.m. in marmosets with NBM lesions on visual discrimination learning (77). **C**: ~0.5 mg/kg pilocarpine i.m. in marmosets with VDB lesions on visuospatial discrimination learning (78). **D**: ~0.5 mg/kg pilocarpine i.m. in marmosets with fornix transections on visuospatial discrimination learning (79). ▨, Saline; ▧, cholinergic agonist. *$p < 0.05$; **$p < 0.01$ comparing animals with and without drug (matched-pair t test) **$p < 0.01$, ***$p < 0.001$ comparing lesioned with unlesioned animals (unmatched t test).

effect *only* in circumstances of cholinergic dysfunction. Marmosets with neurotoxic lesions of the NBM, which deplete the neocortex and amygdala of up to 40% of its ChAT, are impaired in learning simple visual discriminations, and this impairment also is ameliorated by cholinergic agonist treatment (77). Marmosets whose entire central cholinergic system has been disrupted by intracerebroventricular injections of hemicholinium-3, which blocks choline reuptake and therefore gradually decreases levels of ACh (37), are impaired on simple spatial learning, and this impairment can be completely overcome by cholinergic agonist treatment (72). The unlesioned control marmosets showed no significant improvement in performance when treated with cholinergic agonists [except in Ridley et al. (79)]. Furthermore, unoperated marmosets and those that had shown substantial recovery of learning ability over time after neurotoxic lesioning of the NBM did not show an improvement in performance when treated with pilocarpine, even when tested on a visual discrimination that had been made as difficult to learn (by making the stimulus objects more similar than usual) as the tests performed by the NBM-lesioned monkeys immediately after surgery. Thus, when matched for task difficulty, the cholinergic agonist was effective only in monkeys with lesion-induced impairments. This argues against the effect of the cholinergic agonist being nonspecific, and suggests that the cognitive impairment resulting from fornix transection is caused by cholinergic dysfunction comparable to that produced by the other procedures that disrupt cholinergic activity.

Does the Cholinergic Graft Affect only Those Aspects of Function that Are Disturbed by the Cholinergic Lesion?

In experiments 1 and 2, performance by animals with ACh-rich transplants was substantially improved relative to that of fornix-transected animals on those tasks in which fornix-transected animals were impaired ("experimental" tasks), but was neither improved nor impaired on those tasks in which fornix-transected animals were not impaired ("control" tasks). Transplantation of ACh-rich tissue did not produce any detectable impairment despite comprising a space-occupying intracranial mass, nor did it produce learning scores lower than those seen in control animals, even on difficult tasks where there was scope for improvement. Thus, transplantation does not produce a global or nonspecific improvement or impairment in learning ability.

At the present time, we know of no way of producing a specific learning impairment in marmosets of the same magnitude as that produced in experiments 1 and 2 by procedures other than those that damage the cholinergic system. Thus, we cannot assess whether transplants of ACh-rich tissue would improve learning ability in animals with impairments resulting from noncholinergic damage. It may be possible at a later time to determine whether ACh-rich tissue transplanted into an "inappropriate" site (e.g., in cortex in fornix-transected animals or in hippocampus in animals with neurotoxic lesions of NBM) has an effect on learning ability. This would provide a degree of spatial specificity to the graft procedure.

Is an Equivalent Level of Improvement Produced by Transplantation of ACh-Poor Tissue?

This question is essentially answered by experiment 2. No improvement was seen after transplantation of hippocampal tissue, which in marmosets contains no cholinergic cell bodies (31), into the hippocampus in fornix-transected animals. Indeed, the worst performance was seen in animals with this transplant, suggesting that transplantation of inappropriate tissue might actually impair performance. This makes it unlikely that the ACh-rich transplants exerted their effects on hippocampal function by a nonspecific mechanism such as stimulating regenerative processes in the host, or secreting chemicals or neurotransmitters that are ubiquitous in brain. It remains possible that the ACh-rich tissue contained another population of neurons secreting a specific chemical or neurotransmitter that the ACh-poor tissue did not secrete, and that had a beneficial effect comparable to the effect of cholinergic agonist treatment on learning only in those tasks in which fornix-transected animals were impaired, but such an argument is extremely unparsimonious. At the present time there are no data to suggest the action of a neurotransmitter other than ACh.

Another way of addressing this issue is to ask whether there is a relationship between the size of the transplant and/or the extent of restitution of AChE staining in the surrounding tissue, which we take to indicate reinnervation of host tissue by outgrowth from the transplant (c.f. rats, 11,16,17), and the degree of improvement in learning ability. This analysis is constrained by the fact that all animals with ACh-rich tissue grafts showed substantial restitution of function and, therefore, very similar levels of performance. Nevertheless, in experiment 1 the animal with the most extensive hippocampal reinnervation learned the posttransplantation tasks with the fewest errors, whereas the animal with the least extensive reinnervation committed the most errors. In experiment 2, all the animals were ranked according to a score denoting the normality of their hippocampal structure and AChE staining, and this was found to correlate significantly with learning ability (Spearman rank correlation coefficient $r_s = 0.8411$, $p < 0.01$, n = 18).

Is the Improvement in Transplanted Animals Due to Practice or Spontaneous Recovery?

All the animals in experiments 1 and 2 were subjected to extensive training over the course of about 12 months. They all improved with practice, but to compensate for this we gave the animals intrinsically more difficult tasks toward the end of the test period. For this reason, performance by the transplanted animals always was compared to performance by the other groups on the same task given at the same time after surgery. Because the animals with fornix transection alone took more trials to learn most tasks, they actually had more training than the transplanted and control animals, who rested between tasks.

In experiment 1, performance on the last task (a very difficult visuospatial reversal using black objects) by the control animals was not different from their performance on the visuospatial task given immediately before surgery. The fornix-transected monkeys were, however, significantly impaired relative to their preoperative performance ($p < 0.01$), whereas the transplanted animals did not differ from their preoperative performance (i.e., they had regained their original learning ability). The fornix-transected animals' performance did not differ at the end of the experiment from that on the first visuospatial task after fornix transection, indicating that they maintained their impairment throughout, whereas transplanted animals showed significant improvement ($p < 0.02$) compared to postfornix transection, pretransplantation performance. In experiment 2, the increasing task difficulty that occurred across testing as we explored more aspects of learning ability was not so neatly compensated for by the beneficial effects of practice in the control animals, so it was not so easy to make comparisons across time. Nonetheless, the persistent difference between the abilities of fornix-transected animals with ACh-rich transplants and those with ACh-poor transplants tested at the same time indicates that the improvements seen in these experiments were not due to practice.

WHAT IS THE MECHANISM OF ACTION OF ACh-RICH TRANSPLANTS?

Once a beneficial effect of transplantation has been demonstrated, it is pertinent to ask by what mechanism this effect is achieved. Various studies (reviewed in 10) have suggested that surgical trauma and the transplantation of tissue that does not survive can, by the release of trophic factors, stimulate host responses, including the sprouting of host neuronal processes, that could result in behavioral recovery. Surgical trauma, and the transplantation of foreign tissue cannot account for the results of experiment 2 because transplantation of hippocampal tissue did not produce functional recovery. It remains possible, however, that the ACh-rich tissue stimulated host tissue recovery via some trophic mechanism that was not exerted by the ACh-poor tissue. It has not yet been possible to demonstrate in monkeys that the near-normal pattern of AChE staining in the dentate gyrus and hippocampus of fornix-transected animals with ACh-rich grafts comprises outgrowth from the graft, but very long AChE-containing fibers running along the needle track suggest that graft-derived axonal processes can travel over at least several millimeters. This would be sufficient to reinnervate the greater part of the hippocampus in the marmoset. In rats with fornix transections, it has been shown by ultrastructural studies that grafted basal forebrain neurons make cholinergic synaptic connections with host neurons (16,17), that such transplants can restore normal levels of ACh release in host hippocampus, and that this release is under host control (61). The comparable near-normal AChE staining in hippocampus of rats and monkeys with ACh-rich tissue grafts suggests that the interaction between graft and host demonstrated in rats also occurs in monkeys.

In cholinergic synapses, ACh is broken down rapidly on release into the synaptic cleft into choline and acetate by the action of AChE. If ACh were released from transplanted neurons into extracellular space rather than within synapses, it probably would be broken down before it could influence postsynaptic receptors. Thus, if cognitive recovery is mediated by ACh release from the transplant, it seems that such mediation must take place via functional synaptic connections between transplant and host.

The demonstration that systemic injections of muscarinic agonists can restore learning ability in fornix-transected monkeys indicates that the role of cholinergic projections in hippocampal function is tonic or permissive. This is comparable to the action of dopamine in permitting movements that are programmed in nondopaminergic neurons, and suggests that information that is to be acquired is not encoded in the pattern of neuronal firing in the cholinergic projections within the fornix. In the nonlesioned animal, the levels of electrical activity in the fornix and ACh release in the hippocampus probably are modulated by sensory input and levels of arousal or motivation, which may contribute to determining what is learned in the natural environment. In the absence of the intrinsic cholinergic innervation, an ACh-secreting transplant may function well enough in most circumstances. By analogy, a running tap can supply water for most purposes, although one that can be turned off and on may have other advantages in the long term.

CONCLUSION

The experiments described in this chapter demonstrate that ACh-rich neural tissue transplants but not ACh-poor neural tissue transplants into the hippocampus of fornix-transected monkeys can restore learning ability on those tasks that are impaired by fornix transection. This restoration is complete and appears to be permanent. This raises the issue of whether a similar treatment could have therapeutic value in human diseases in which there is degeneration of the cholinergic projections. These include Alzheimer's disease (12), Parkinson's disease with dementia (66), and Korsakoff's syndrome (6). Degeneration of the cholinergic projection to the hippocampus may be particularly important in producing the amnesia found in dementing illnesses. Reasons for believing this include the involvement of the hippocampus in ischemic amnesia (92) and the hippocampus and fornix in iatrogenic amnesia (40,86), and because memory impairment is less marked in olivopontocerebellar atrophy where hippocampal ACh levels are less affected than in Alzheimer's disease (47). In some cases of dementia, cholinergic loss may be confined to the hippocampus (13,85). Cholinergic transplantation into the hippocampus may have a role in treating the memory symptoms in some of these cases, particularly those rare cases that are traumatic or surgical in origin and in which the disease process is not itself progressive. It must be recognized, however, that neurodegenerative diseases are progressive and ultimately fatal and, in the later stages at least, involve massive cell loss and the accumulation of abnormal brain proteins. Neurotransmitter-secreting transplants will not arrest or reverse this process. On the other hand, in so far as much of the amnesia of dementia may result from loss of the cholinergic projections to the hippocampus, any treatment aimed at either the symptoms or the disease process that does not address the relationship between amnesia and cholinergic loss is unlikely to be fully effective. In this context, cholinergic tissue grafts may have a role in ameliorating the suffering of those afflicted with neurodegenerative disease later in life.

REFERENCES

1. Aggleton JP, Nicol RM, Huston AE, Fairbarn AF. The performance of amnesic subjects on tests of experimental amnesia: delayed matching-to-sample and concurrent learning. *Neuropsychologia* 1988;26:265–272.
2. Annett LE, Dunnett SB, Martel FL, et al. A functional assessment of embryonic dopaminergic grafts in the marmoset. *Prog Brain Res* 1990;82:535–542.
3. Annett LE, Ridley RM. Neural transplantation in primates. In: Dunnett SB, Björklund A, eds. *Neural transplantation: a practical approach.* Oxford: Oxford University Press; 1992:123–138.
4. Arendt T, Allen Y, Marchbanks RM, et al. Cholinergic system and memory in the rat: effects of chronic ethanol, embryonic basal forebrain brain transplants and excitotoxic lesions of cholinergic basal forebrain projection systems. *Neuroscience* 1989;33:435–462.
5. Arendt T, Bigl V, Arendt A. Neurone loss in the nucleus basalis of Meynert in Creutzfeldt-Jakob disease. *Acta Neuropathol (Berlin)* 1984;65:85–88.
6. Arendt T, Bigl V, Arendt A, Tennstedt A. Loss of neurons in the nucleus basalis of Meynert in Alzheimer's disease, paralysis agitans and Korsakoff's disease. *Acta Neuropathol (Berlin)* 1983;61:101–108.
7. Baddeley AD, Warrington EK. Amnesia and the distinction between short-term and long-term memory. *Journal of Verbal Learning and Verbal Behavior* 1970;9:176–189.
8. Baker HF, Ridley RM. Use of the common marmoset *(Callithrix jacchus)* in psychopharmacological research. In: Joseph MH, Waddington JL, eds. *Working methods in neuropsychopharmacology.* Manchester, UK: Manchester University Press; 1986:41–73.
9. Baker HF, Ridley RM. Neural transplantation in primates: towards brain repair in humans. *Rev Neurosci* 1992;3:175–190.
10. Björklund A, Lindvall O, Isacson O, et al. Mechanisms of action of intracerebral neural implants. *Trends Neurosci* 1987;10:509–516.
11. Björklund A, Stenevi U. Reformation of the severed septohippocampal pathway in the adult rat by transplanted septal neurones. *Cell Tissue Res* 1977;185:289–302.
12. Bowen DM, Smith CB, White P, Davison AN. Neurotransmitter-related enzymes and indices of hypoxia in senile dementia and other abiotrophies. *Brain* 1976;99:459–496.
13. Bowen DM, White P, Spillane JA, et al. Accelerated ageing or selective neuronal loss as an important cause of dementia? *Lancet* 1979;1:11–14.
14. Butler H, Juurlink BHJ. An atlas for staging mammalian and chick embryos. Boca Raton, FL: *CRC Press;* 1987.
15. Butters N. The clinical aspects of memory disorders: contributions from experimental studies of amnesia and dementia. *J Clin Neuropsychol* 1984;6:17–36.
16. Clarke DJ, Gage FH, Björklund A. Formation of cholinergic synapses by intrahippocampal septal grafts as revealed by choline acetyltransferase immunocytochemistry. *Brain Res* 1986;369:151–162.
17. Clarke DJ, Nilsson OG, Brundin P, Björklund A. Synaptic connections formed by grafts of different types of cholinergic neurons in the host hippocampus. *Exp Neurol* 1990;107:11–22.
18. Crow TJ, Grove-White IG. An analysis of the learning deficit following hyoscine administration to man. *Br J Pharmacol* 1973;49:322–327.
19. Dixson AF, Lunn SF. Post-partum changes in

hormones and sexual behaviour in captive groups of marmosets *(Callithrix jacchus)*. *Physiol Behav* 1987;41:577–583.

20. Dunnett SB. Anatomical and behavioural consequences of cholinergic-rich grafts to the neocortex of rats with lesions of the nucleus basalis magnocellularis. *Ann NY Acad Sci* 1987;495:415–429.

21. Dunnett SB. Role of pre-frontal cortex and striatal output systems in short-term memory deficits associated with ageing, basal forebrain lesions, and cholinergic-rich grafts. *Can J Psychol* 1990;44:210–232.

22. Dunnett SB. Neural transplantation in animal models of dementia. *Eur J Neurosci* 1990;2:567–587.

23. Dunnett SB, Annett LE. Nigral transplants in primate models of parkinsonism. In: Lindvall O, Björklund A, Widner H, eds. *Intracerebral transplantation in movement disorders*. B.V.: Elsevier Science Publishers; 1991:27–51.

24. Dunnett SB, Badman F, Rogers DC, Evenden JL, Iversen SD. Cholinergic grafts in the neocortex or hippocampus of aged rats: reduction of delay dependent deficits in delayed non-matching to position tasks. *Exp Neurol* 1988;102:57–64.

25. Dunnett SB, Björklund A. Staging and dissection of rat embryos. In: Dunnett SB, Björklund A, eds. *Neural transplantation: a practical approach*. Oxford: Oxford University Press; 1992:1–19.

26. Dunnett SB, Everitt BJ, Robbins TW. The basal forebrain–cortical cholinergic system: interpreting the functional consequences of excitotoxic lesions. *Trends Neurosci* 1991;14:494–501.

27. Dunnett SB, Rogers DC, Jones GH. Effects of nucleus basalis magnocellularis lesions in rats on delayed matching and non-matching to position tasks. *Eur J Neurosci* 1989;1:395–406.

28. Dunnett SB, Ryan CN, Levin PD, Reynolds M, Bunch ST. Functional consequences of embryonic neocortex transplanted to rats with prefrontal cortex lesions. *Behav Neurosci* 1987;101:489–503.

29. Dunnett SB, Wareham AT, Torres EM. Cholinergic blockade in prefrontal cortex and hippocampus disrupts short-term memory in rats. *Neuro Report* 1990;1:61–64.

30. Dunnett SB, Whishaw IQ, Jones GH, Bunch ST. Behavioural, biochemical and histochemical effects of different neurotoxic amino acids injected into nucleus basalis magnocellularis of rats. *Neuroscience* 1987;20:653–669.

31. Everitt BJ, Sirkia TE, Roberts AC, Jones GH, Robbins TW. Distribution and some projections of cholinergic neurones in the brain of the common marmoset, *Callithrix jacchus. J Comp Neurol* 1988;271:533–558.

32. Fine A, Dunnett SB, Björklund A, Iversen SD. Cholinergic ventral forebrain grafts into the neocortex improve passive avoidance memory in a rat model of Alzheimer's disease. *Proc Natl Acad Sci USA* 1985;82:5227–5230.

33. Fine A, Hunt SP, Oertel WH, et al. Transplan-

tation of embryonic marmoset dopaminergic neurons to the corpus striatum of marmosets rendered parkinsonian by 1-methyl-4-phenyl-1,2,3,6-tetrahydropyridine. *Prog Brain Res* 1988;78:479–489.

34. Freed DM, Corkin S, Cohen NJ. Forgetting in H.M.: a second look. *Neuropsychologia* 1987;25:461–471.

35. Freed DM, Corkin S, Growdon JH, Nissen MJ. Selective attention in Alzheimer's disease: characterising cognitive subgroups of patients. *Neuropsychologia* 1989;27:325–339.

36. Freedman M, Oscar-Berman M. Spatial and visual learning deficits in Alzheimer's and Parkinson's disease. *Brain Cogn* 1989;11:114–126.

37. Freeman JJ, Macri JR, Choi RL, Jenden DJ. Studies on the behavioural and biochemical effects of hemicholinium in vivo. *J Pharmacol Exp Ther* 1979;210:91–97.

38. Frith CD, Cahill C, Ridley RM, Baker HF. Memory for what it is and memory for what it means: a single case of Korsakoff's amnesia. *Cortex* 1992;28:53–67.

39. Gaffan D. Recognition impaired and association intact in the memory of monkeys after transection of the fornix. *J Comp Physiol Psychol* 1974;86:1100–1109.

40. Gaffan EA, Gaffan D, Hodges JR. Amnesia following damage to the left fornix and to other sites. *Brain* 1991;114:1297–1313.

41. Gross CG. Comparison of the effects of partial and total lateral frontal lesions on test performance by monkeys. *J Comp Physiol Psychol* 1963;56:41–47.

42. Hagan JJ, Salamone JD, Simpson J, Iversen SD, Morris RGM. Place navigation in rats is impaired by lesions of medial septum and diagonal band but not nucleus basalis magnocellularis. *Behav Brain Res* 1988;27:9–20.

43. Harlow HF, Bromer JA. A test-apparatus for monkeys. *Psychol Rec* 1938;2:434–436.

44. Huppert FA, Piercy M. Normal and abnormal forgetting in organic amnesia: effect of locus of lesion. *Cortex* 1979;15:385–390.

45. Isacson O, Hantraye P, Maziere M, Sofroniew MV, Riche D. Apomorphine-induced dyskinesias after excitotoxic caudate–putamen lesions and the effects of neural transplantation in nonhuman primates. *Prog Brain Res* 1990;82:523–533.

46. Iversen SD, Weiskrantz L. An investigation of a possible memory defect produced by inferotemporal lesions in the baboon. *Neuropsychologia* 1970;8:21–36.

47. Kish SJ, Robitaille Y, el-Awar M, et al. Non-Alzheimer-type pattern of brain cholineacetyltransferase reduction in dominantly inherited olivopontocerebellar atrophy. *Ann Neurol* 1989;26:362–367.

48. Kitt CA, Mitchell SJ, DeLong MK, Wainer BH, Price DL. Fiber pathways of basal forebrain cholinergic neurons in monkeys. *Brain Res* 1987;406:192–206.

49. Köhler C, Chan-Palay V, Wu J-Y. Septal neurons containing glutamic acid decarboxylase im-

munoreactivity project to the hippocampal region in the rat brain. *Anat Embryol* 1984;169:41–44.

50. Kopelman MD. Rates of forgetting in Alzheimer-type dementia and Korsakoff's syndrome. *Neuropsychologia* 1985;23:623–638.

51. Labbe R, Firl A, Mufson EJ, Stein DG. Fetal brain transplants: reduction of cognitive deficits in rats with frontal cortex lesions. *Science* 1983;221:470–472.

52. Lindvall O, Brundin P, Widner H, et al. Grafts of fetal dopamine neurons survive and improve motor function in Parkinson's disease. *Science* 1990;247:574–577.

53. Lindvall O, Rehncrona S, Brundin P, et al. Human fetal dopamine neurons grafted into the striatum in two patients with severe Parkinson's disease. *Arch Neurol* 1989;46:615–631.

54. Low WC, Lewis PR, Bunch ST, et al. Function recovery following neural transplantation of embryonic septal nuclei in adult rats with septohippocampal lesions. *Nature* 1982;300:260–262.

55. Mahut H. Spatial and object reversal learning in monkeys with partial temporal lobe ablations. *Neuropsychologia* 1971;9:409–424.

56. Mahut H. A selective spatial deficit in monkeys after transection of the fornix. *Neuropsychologia* 1972;10:65–74.

57. Mesulam M-M, Mufson EJ, Levey AI, Wainer BH. Cholinergic innervation of cortex by the basal forebrain: cytochemistry and cortical connections of the septal area, diagonal band nuclei, nucleus basalis (substantia innominata) and hypothalamus in the rhesus monkey. *J Comp Neurol* 1983;214:170–197.

58. Mishkin M, Appenzeller T. The anatomy of memory. *Sci Am* 1987;256:62–71.

59. Mishkin M, Delacour J. An analysis of short term visual memory in the monkey. *J Exp Psychol [Anim Behav]* 1975;1:326–334.

60. Mishkin M, Petri HL. Memories and habits: some implications for the analysis of learning and retention. In: Squire LR, Butters N, eds. *Neuropsychology of memory*. New York: Guilford Press; 1984;287–296.

61. Nilsson OG, Kalen P, Rosengren E, Björklund A. Acetylcholine release from intrahippocampal septal grafts is under control of the host brain. *Proc Natl Acad Sci USA* 1990;87:2647–2651.

62. Nilsson OG, Shapiro ML, Gage FH, Olton DS, Björklund A. Spatial learning and memory following fimbria–fornix transection and grafting of fetal septal neurones to the hippocampus. *Exp Brain Res* 1987;67:195–215.

63. Onifer SM, Low WC. Spatial memory deficit resulting from ischaemia-induced damage to the hippocampus is ameliorated by intra-hippocampal transplants of fetal hippocampal neurons. *Prog Brain Res* 1990;82:359–376.

64. Oscar-Berman M, Zola-Morgan SM. Comparative neuropsychology and Korsakoff's syndrome: I. spatial and visual reversal learning. *Neuropsychologia* 1980;18:499–512.

65. Oscar-Berman M, Zola-Morgan SM. Comparative neuropsychology and Korsakoff's syndrome: II. two choice visual discrimination learning. *Neuropsychologia* 1980;18:513–525.

66. Perry EK, Curtis M, Dick DJ, et al. Cholinergic correlates of cognitive impairment in Parkinson's disease: comparison with Alzheimer's disease. *J Neurol Neurosurg Psychiatry* 1985;48:413–421.

67. Perry EK, Gibson PH, Blessed G, Perry RH, Tomlinson BE. Neurotransmitter enzyme abnormalities in senile dementia. *J Neurol Sci* 1977;34:247–265.

68. Perry EK, Tomlinson BE, Blessed G, Bergmann K, Gibson PH, Perry RH. Correlation of cholinergic abnormalities with senile plaques and mental test scores in senile dementia. *Br Med J* 1978;2:1457–1459.

69. Quinn NP. The clinical application of cell grafting techniques in patients with Parkinson's disease. *Prog Brain Res* 1990;82:619–625.

70. Ridley RM, Aitken DM, Baker HF. Learning about rules but not about reward is impaired following lesions of the cholinergic projections to the hippocampus. *Brain Res* 1989;502:306–318.

71. Ridley RM, Baker HF. A critical evaluation of monkey models of amnesia and dementia. *Brain Res Rev* 1991;16:15–37.

72. Ridley RM, Baker HF, Drewett B. Effects of arecoline and pilocarpine on learning ability in marmosets pretreated with hemicholinium-3. *Psychopharmacology* 1987;91:512–514.

73. Ridley RM, Baker HF, Drewett B, Johnson JA. Effects of ibotenic acid lesions of the basal forebrain on serial reversal learning in marmosets. *Psychopharmacology* 1985;86:438–443.

74. Ridley RM, Baker HF, Murray TK. Basal nucleus lesions in monkeys: recognition memory impairment or visual agnosia? *Psychopharmacology* 1988;95:289–290.

75. Ridley RM, Bowes PM, Baker HF, Crow TJ. An involvement of acetylcholine in object discrimination learning and memory in the mamoset. *Neuropsychologia* 1984;22:253–263.

76. Ridley RM, Gribble S, Clark B, Baker HF, Fine A. Restoration of learning ability in fornix-transected monkeys after fetal basal forebrain but not fetal hippocampal tissue transplantation. *Neuroscience* 1992;48:779–792.

77. Ridley RM, Murray TK, Johnson JA, Baker HF. Learning impairment following lesion of the basal nucleus of Meynert in the marmoset: modification by cholinergic drugs. *Brain Res* 1986;376:108–116.

78. Ridley RM, Samson NA, Baker HF, Johnson JA. Visuospatial learning impairment following lesion of the cholinergic projection to the hippocampus. *Brain Res* 1988;456:71–87.

79. Ridley RM, Thornley HD, Baker HF, Fine A. Cholinergic neural transplants into hippocampus restore learning ability in monkeys with fornix transections. *Exp Brain Res* 1991;83:533–538.

80. Robbins TW, Everitt BJ, Marston H, Wilkinson J, Jones GH, Page KJ. Comparative effects of ibotenic acid and quisqualic acid induced lesions of the substantia innominata on attentional functions in the rat: further implications for the role

of the cholinergic neurons of the nucleus basalis in cognitive processes. *Behav Brain Res* 1990; 35:321–340.

81. Robbins TW, Marston HM, Wilkinson LS, Everitt BJ. A comparison of the effects of excitotoxic lesions to septal nuclei and the hippocampal formation on the acquisition of decision rules. *Soc Neurosci Abstr* 1990;16:605.

82. Robbins TW, Roberts AC, Muir J, Parker R, Gore M, Everitt BJ. Quisqualate-induced lesions of the substantia innominata and ventral pallidum (SI/VP) in the rat: effects on acquisition and serial reversal of a visual discrimination. *Soc Neurosci Abstr* 1989;15:1104.

83. Roberts AC, Robbins TW, Everitt BJ, et al. The effects of excitotoxic lesions of the basal forebrain on the acquisition, retention and serial reversal of visual discriminations in marmosets. *Neuroscience* 1990;34:311–329.

84. Roberts AC, Robbins TW, Everitt BJ. The effects of intradimensional and extradimensional shifts on visual discrimination learning in humans and non-human primates. *Q J Exp Psychol* 1988;40:321–341.

85. Rossor MN, Iversen LL, Reynolds GP, Mountjoy CQ, Roth M. Neurochemical characteristics of early and late onset types of Alzheimer's disease. *Br Med J* 1984;288:961–964.

86. Scoville WB, Milner B. Loss of recent memory after bilateral hippocampal lesions. *J Neurol Neurosurg Psychiatry* 1957;20:11–21.

87. Squire LR. Mechanisms of memory. *Science* 1986;232:1612–1619.

88. Squire LR, Zola-Morgan S, Chen KS. Human amnesia and animal models of amnesia: performance of amnesic patients on tests designed for the monkey. *Behav Neurosci* 1988;102:210–221.

89. Taylor JR, Elsworth JD, Roth RH, Collier TJ, Sladek JR, Redmond DE. Improvements in MPTP-induced object retrieval deficits and behavioural deficits after fetal nigral grafting in monkeys. *Prog Brain Res* 1990;82:543–559.

90. Whitehouse PJ, Price DL, Struble RG, Clark AW, Coyle JT, DeLong MR. Alzheimer's disease and senile dementia: loss of neurones in the basal forebrain. *Science* 1982;215:1237–1238.

91. Zaczek R, Hedreen JL, Coyle JT. Evidence for a hippocampal–septal glutamatergic pathway in the rat. *Exp Neurol* 1979;65:145–156.

92. Zola-Morgan S, Squire LR, Amaral DG. Human amnesia and the medial temporal region: memory impairment following a bilateral lesion limited to field CA1 of the hippocampus. *J Neurosci* 1986;6:2950–2967.

Functional Neural Transplantation,
edited by S. B. Dunnett and A. Björklund.
Raven Press, Ltd., New York © 1994.

14

Cerebral Transplantation in Animal Models of Ischemia

Helen Hodges, John Sinden, *Brian Meldrum, and Jeffrey Gray

*Departments of Psychology and *Neurology, Institute of Psychiatry,
London SE5 8AF, United Kingdom*

The normal adult human brain receives 15% of the total output of blood from the heart to manufacture the energy (via glucose oxidation) necessary to sustain electrical activity and other functions. Because neither glucose nor oxygen are stored in the brain, it is highly vulnerable to interruptions of cerebral blood flow (CBF); irreversible damage can occur within minutes. Although there are many patterns of damage associated with different types of arterial or cardiac malfunction (54), two basic types are distinguishable: those arising from the abrupt and near total interruption of CBF, as in cardiac arrest or coronary artery occlusion, in which discrete populations of neurons are selectively vulnerable; and those arising from major cerebral artery occlusion, as in stroke, where infarcts of total tissue loss occur in the core region supplied by the artery, surrounded by a penumbra of variable and partially reversible damage (97,101). Animal models of ischemia have therefore focused on one of these two major types: models of "global" cerebral ischemia seek to replicate the consequences of heart attack, whereas models of "focal" cerebral ischemia reproduce the effects of stroke. These models provide valid systems in which to investigate the pathologic and behavioral effects of cerebral ischemia, and possible therapeutic strategies, because regardless of the inducing circumstances reduced content of oxygen in the blood or reduced CBF represent the final common determinants of ischemic brain damage. Moreover, induction of ischemia can be carefully controlled in animal models; body/head temperature and blood glucose levels, which affect the magnitude of ischemic lesions (25,104), can be standardized; and physiologic variables (blood pressure, blood gas exchange) can be monitored and controlled. Thus, it is possible to develop highly reproducible patterns of brain damage against which to evaluate experimental manipulations and behavioral outcomes. In humans, both stroke and heart attack can result in long-lasting impairments. After stroke, neurologic movement disorders are prominent, ranging from lack of fine digit control to contralateral hemiplegia, and articulatory disturbance with left-sided strokes. There also may be cognitive impairments featuring confusion and global amnesia. After heart attack, one of the most persistent impairments, seen in about 20% of survivors, is moderate to profound anterograde amnesia (13,28). Postmortem studies of patients showing loss of memory after anoxic incidents have consistently revealed bilateral hippocampal pathology, together with variable damage in other brain regions (13,28,132,177,197). Animals have similarly shown neurologic deficits and impaired learning after arterial occlusion (118) and a more restricted pattern of learning and memory deficits, together with cell loss largely confined to the hippocampus, particularly the CA1 field, after global ischemia (32). Therefore, in terms of mechanisms, pathology, and behavioral outcome, focal and global ischemia offer apt models for the effects of stroke and heart attack in humans.

This chapter describes the main methods for inducing ischemia in animals, and their effects, in terms both of gross histologic damage and mechanisms for selective and delayed neuronal death, in relation to the excitotoxic hypothesis of ischemic cell loss and possibilities for pharmacologic protection. The behavioral effects of focal and global ischemia are discussed, focusing on the relationship between cognitive deficits and CA1 cell loss after transient global ischemia. Therapeutic approaches can be divided into "vascular" and "parenchymal" (86), and although grafting techniques to repair damaged peripheral blood vessels and heart defects are well developed, neural grafting in the CNS to repair ischemic brain damage has only recently begun to be investigated in animal models. Strategies for cerebral transplantation, the main findings to date in global and focal ischemic models, and implications for therapy in humans, are evaluated. It is our contention that graft-induced functional recovery after focal ischemia will be unpredictable, and will involve a number of factors such as support and guidance for ingrowing host neurons, and/or their rescue by delivery of trophic factors. The lack of lamination and limited outgrowth from grafts within large infarct regions does not indicate reestablishment of normal patterns of innervation. Moreover, it is not known whether grafts will complement or conflict with the normal stages of functional cerebral reorganization that have been identified by imaging techniques after stroke damage in humans. In contrast, graft-induced recovery of cognitive function after the limited hippocampal damage induced by transitory global ische-

mia appears to be a more promising target for eventual therapeutic application in humans. Behavioral effects of global ischemia have been more thoroughly investigated than those induced by focal ischemia, and fetal hippocampal grafts have been shown to reestablish normal patterns of structural and electrophysiologic connectivity in ischemic host hippocampus, and to promote functional recovery. Recent demonstrations that grafts from fetal CA1, but not CA3 or dentate gryrus fields, alleviate ischemic deficits in spatial learning suggest that these grafts exert a remarkable degree of functional specificity. Further studies are in progress to show whether there is commensurate histologic evidence for point-to-point reconstruction of the host circuit.

METHODS OF INDUCING CEREBRAL ISCHEMIA AND THEIR PATHOLOGIC EFFECTS

Many different methods have been used for inducing ischemic damage, including arterial ligation, cauterization, or blockade by clots (platelet aggregators, microspheres, or intraluminal threads). Currently, the Rose Begal technique (thrombosis induced by a photolabile dye;112) is being developed as a noninvasive method of producing cortical infarcts. Focal arterial occlusion in stroke models usually involves either the permanent occlusion of the middle cerebral artery (MCAO) by cauterization or ligation intracranially through a route above the cheek bone (or transorbitally in cats or primates), or reversible occlusion through the insertion of a fiber into the arterial lumen (97). More complex reversible models (15) involve tandem unilateral occlusion of both the carotid and MCA for periods of 1 to 4 hr. Focal ischemia, because it is most commonly irreversible, results in more severe damage than transitory global ischemia, related to the territory served by the occluded artery, but the extent of damage varies according to the degree of compensatory inflow from the anterior (ACA) and posterior (PCA) cerebral arteries (54), and shows strain and species differences (97, 99). With MCAO the striatum is most vulnerable to infarction, but there is almost invariably damage to large areas of frontal and parietal cortex, so that total infarct volumes of approximately 150 mm³ are commonly found in the rat (154). Subsequent retrograde degeneration of large areas (e.g., thalamic damage after loss of cortical projections; 68) also have been reported. In humans, hypertension is a risk factor for stroke, and several animal models (50,51) use spontaneously hypertensive rats (SHR) as a more appropriate model, in which the bed vasculature is compromised. In SHR, the extent of infarction is both larger and more standardized than in normotensive animals. The size of infarction bears a general relationship to the extent of reduction in CBF. In the rat, where CBF is reduced to below 10% of control level for 5 min or more, infarction invariably occurs. However, where CBF is reduced to 12% in the first 5 min, the extent of infarction is variable, and hence CBF does not appear to be a reliable predictor of areas committed to infarction, nor local CBF to correlate with neuronal loss (167). Moreover, transitory stroke models have shown that the spread of infarction to penumbral regions appears to be relatively gradual and reversible after reperfusion (97,101), so that permanent damage may not occur for 2 to 3 hr after reduction of CBF to 10% to 20% of control level in the rodent (15).

The two-vessel occlusion (2-VO) model of transitory global ischemia in rats involves ligation of the common carotids in paralyzed and ventilated animals, with blood pressure reduced (pharmacologically or by exsanguination). The most consistent loss is in dorsal hippocampus, where up to 50% to 60% of CA1 cells die within 3 to 4 days after ischemia (97,149). The 4-VO method, developed by Pulsinelli and colleagues (134), is a two-stage procedure in which the vertebral arteries are electrocoa-

gulated and the carotids loosely snared under anesthesia, and 24 hr later the snares are tightened for a specified period. Rats lose righting reflex within 2 min, or are excluded, so that the extent of brain damage is standardized. Cerebral blood flow is reduced by approximately 95% in this model, so that it is possible to increase the duration of ischemia to 30 min without risk of seizures that occur after about 12 min in the 2-VO model, where reduction in CBF is partial. The extent of cell loss is related to the duration of 4-VO (134). With occlusion for 15 min, loss of neurons is largely confined to the CA1 area of the hippocampus, where cell loss in dorsal CA1 field is near total (80%–90%), whereas after 30 min damage within the hippocampus is more extensive, and there also is loss of cells in cortex and striatum (120,122), so that is possible to compare effects of discrete and widespread lesions with precision. Primate models of global ischemia include cardiac arrest or use of a pediatric blood pressure cuff around the neck, with pharmacologically induced hypotension (115,198). Primate models of focal ischemia include MCAO (transcranial or transorbital in monkey or baboon; 97), or surgical bilateral occlusion of the PCA (8), which supplies the posterior hippocampus.

SELECTIVE VULNERABILITY TO ISCHEMIC BRAIN DAMAGE, AND DELAYED NEURONAL DEATH

The hippocampus is an area of predilection for ischemic and epileptic damage, and within the hippocampus CA1 pyramidal and hilar cells are more vulnerable to reduced cerebral blood flow than cells in the CA2, CA3, and dentate gyrus fields. This pattern of "selective vulnerability" holds across several mammalian species, including humans (145), so that animal models may provide homologous neuronal mechanisms. Studies with limited periods of global ischemia in animals (5–30 min) suggest that several processes contribute to discrete neuronal damage. Postischemic changes follow two broad stages: an acute phase of reactive changes lasting 1 to 2 days, and a delayed phase where changes are selective to vulnerable cells, and irreversible (97,145). Early effects are common to all hippocampal regions, and center around the massive release of glutamate triggered by ischemia (see later), which leads to influx of calcium into postsynaptic cells, the activation of many enzymes, and modification of gene expression. This phase is marked by swelling of dendrites, mitochondria loaded with calcium, and disaggregation of polyribosomes. The delayed phase of neuronal death is marked by multiple vacuoles in the cell body, and proliferating glia in the region of the doomed cells (97,149). Considerable effort has been spent in trying to find out why some types of neuron in the hippocampus proceed to this second stage and not others, because potentially lethal changes (e.g., changes in energy metabolism; activation of phospholipase A2 that releases free fatty acids, including arachidonic acid; and activation of proteases that increase the production of free radicals, or calpain proteases that attack neurofilaments and microtubules) occur across the hippocampus (97,145). Some markers during the acute reactive phase appear to distinguish vulnerable CA1 cells from those in other fields. For instance, heat shock protein 70, expressed after 10 min of ischemia in gerbil hippocampus, striatum, and some neocortical areas, is seen after 12 to 16 hr in dentate gyrus, after 24 to 48 hr in CA3 area, and is minimally expressed in the CA1 area, where cells are in the process of dying (174), and thus appears to be a marker for cell survival. In contrast, microtubule-associated protein-2, located on postsynaptic dendrites and cell bodies, appears after only 3 min of occlusion, starting at the subiculum–CA1 junction, and seems to be a sensitive marker of vulnerability to ischemia (83). However, it

is difficult to determine whether these protein changes contribute to, or merely reflect, delayed neuronal death. Findings that less vulnerable CA2 neurons contain higher expression of the calcium-binding proteins parvalbumin and calbindin (89), whereas the calcium/calmodulin-dependent protein kinase II and neurofilament protein NF 68 are decreased in vulnerable but not resistant cells after 4-VO (22,113), suggest that vulnerable cells may be both more structurally fragile and less well endowed with calcium-binding proteins to maintain homeostasis in the face of calpain-mediated cytoskeletal destruction. Differential distribution of types of glutamate receptors may play a fundamental role in selective vulnerability, given the evidence for an excitotoxic mechanism (see section on the excitotoxic hypothesis, below) in ischemic cell death. Ionotropic glutamate receptors are classified as N-methyl-D-aspartate (NMDA)-, kainate (KA)-, and α-amino-3-hydroxy-4-izoxazole propionic acid (AMPA)-preferring, on the basis of selective agonist and antagonist effects (45). Metabotropic receptors enhance phosphoinositide hydrolysis or decrease cyclic adenosine monophosphate formation. Glutamate can produce excitotoxic effects through all three types of ionotropic receptor, although studies to date have emphasized treatments that reduce glutamate transmission via the NMDA receptor, partly because of the availability of potent selective antagonists (97,99). Within the hippocampus, NMDA and AMPA receptors are most densely located on CA1 neurons, whereas the more resistant CA3 region has a greater number of KA receptors. Kainate receptors also are dense in the hilar region, which is relatively vulnerable, so that receptor type cannot be the sole determinant of selective vulnerability. Finally, the trisynaptic circuit culminates in the CA1 field, so that it is exposed to a build-up of excitatory transmission, in particular to the burst firing of Schaffer collaterals. This normal bombardment might prove pathogenic in cells with compromised receptor membrane function after ischemia (145).

THE CONTRIBUTION OF NONGLUTAMATERGIC SYSTEMS TO ISCHEMIC BRAIN DAMAGE

Ischemia induces abrupt changes in several neurotransmitter systems, which may lead to long-lasting modifications in transmission that affect the selective loss of CA1 cells with transitory global ischemia, the extent of infarction after focal ischemia, and degree of secondary degeneration from areas of damage. Excitatory amino acid (EAA) transmission within the hippocampus, striatum, and cortex interacts with γ-aminobutyric acid (GABA)ergic, noradrenergic (NA), serotonergic (5-HT), dopaminergic (DA), and peptidergic systems. Several studies have shown that there are increases in extracellular levels of monoamines during cerebral ischemia, including DA in the striatum, and NA and 5-HT in cortex and hippocampus (29,47,48,57,114) which may exacerbate ischemic lesions. Drugs that modify monoaminergic activity have been found to alter the extent of ischemic brain damage, although effects are inconsistent. Depletion of NA through treatment with α-methyl paratyrosine has been found both to reduce (16) and to increase (186) ischemic damage, whereas reduction in 5-HT transmission has more consistently afforded protection (10,98). Lesions to ascending monoaminergic systems indicate that DA lesions provide powerful protection against KA toxicity, whereas lesions of 5-HT and NA inputs to hippocampus are ineffective (99). Like monoamines, GABA is released during ischemia, but GABAergic interneurons are not damaged (47). Facilitation of GABA through indirect agonists (e.g., pentobarbital and benzodiazepines) has been found to reduce ischemic cell loss and to reduce epileptic seizure activity (96).

There is a temporary fall in hippocampal levels of acetylcholine (ACh) during ischemia and some loss of receptors in the CA1 area (127), but cholinergic input to hippocampus appears resistant to ischemic insult. In contrast, there is substantial loss of cortical choline acetyltransferase (ChAT) activity after focal MCAO infarction of the striatum, via damage to fibers of passage (75), whereas devascularizing cortical lesions (91) destroy basal forebrain cholinergic cell bodies, via retrograde degeneration. Cholinergic damage could contribute significantly to confusional states and dementia symptoms that have been reported after stroke in humans (54; see section on focal ischemia). Adenosine has been proposed as an endogenous protectant against ischemic damage (11), which reduces the number of A1 receptors (127). These widespread effects of ischemia on many neuronal systems carry implications for the use of transplants to promote recovery from ischemic brain damage. Such effects must influence the strategy employed, for instance whether to replace focal loss of tissue, or to boost systems affected by secondary degeneration. The extent of graft-induced recovery from ischemic brain damage also may be profoundly affected by the interactions of ischemic damage with other systems.

THE EXCITOTOXIC HYPOTHESIS OF ISCHEMIC BRAIN DAMAGE

The appearance of neurons damaged by global and focal ischemia resembles the cytopathology induced by EAAs injected directly into the brain (124). Damage is postsynaptic, whereas axons of passage and presynaptic terminals are spared. Dendrites exhibit acute focal swelling, mitochondria are loaded with calcium, and multiple vacuoles appear within cells (149,45). This similarity in appearance has led to the suggestion that reduced CBF (and also anoxia and epilepsy) trigger excessive release of glutamate and other EAAs, which concentrate in extracellular space, activate postsynaptic receptors, and increase membrane permeability to calcium, with lethal intracellular consequences. The hypothesis is based on several pieces of evidence. First, enhanced levels of extracellular glutamate are found after ischemia. In rat hippocampus and striatum, glutamate concentrations rise seven- to eightfold after global ischemia (47), whereas 20- to 30-fold increases in striatal and cortical (62) glutamate have been reported after MCAO. Second, vulnerable brain regions are rich in glutamate receptors, and, as we have seen, within the hippocampus the concentration of NMDA receptors in the CA1 region may contribute to the particular vulnerability of this area. However, a preferential link between excitotoxic cell death and NMDA receptor distribution is not consistent across different brain regions or conditions. Within the cortex, NMDA receptors are most dense in layers 1 and 2, and KA receptors in layers 5 and 6; however, in epileptic models, cell loss is focused in layers 3, 5, and 6 (96), whereas in 4-VO ischemic models (88, 120,122) damage is more marked in layers 3 and 4. Third, findings that EAA receptor antagonists potently protect against ischemia-, anoxia-, or epilepsy-induced cell loss (150,45) provide strong support for the proposal that activity at both NMDA and non-NMDA receptors contributes to ischemic cell death. Finally, lesions to interrupt the glutamatergic relay of transmission around the trisynaptic hippocampal circuit have been shown to reduce the delayed loss of CA1 cells after ischemia. For example, lesions of the perforant path, the mossy fiber projections from CA3 to CA1, Schaffer collaterals, and the hippocampal commisure all have been found to reduce ischemic CA1 damage (72,73,126). Some of these lines of evidence are open to question, so that the initial form of the hypothesis, emphasizing excessive firing of gutamatergic neurons in response to enhanced transmitter release as

the key mechanism, may require modification (145). For instance, microdialysis studies (3,47) have shown that levels of glutamate, although increasing immediately after reperfusion, decline to control levels shortly after ischemia (15–40 min), although functional and morphologic damage in CA1 cells is not detected until several days after the ischemic episode. The firing rate of CA1 cells has not shown sustained elevations, or the burst firing characteristic of excitotoxic lesioning agents, but persistent impairment during and after ischemia with subnormal excitability 4 hr after ischemia, while calcium uptake is in progress (1). Finally, cerebroprotective studies have shown discrepancies between profiles of efficacy of various EAA receptor antagonists, which suggests that a combination of many influences (e.g., receptor subtype and distribution, method and duration of ischemia, species of animal, and variations in vasculature, temperature, blood glucose levels), rather than any unitary hypothesis, will be required to explain in detail the mechanisms of delayed and selective neuronal death. Nevertheless, as a unifying concept, the excitotoxic hypothesis has provided a powerful explanatory framework, and strong impetus to research. Schmidt-Kastner and Freund (145) have proposed that two different excitotoxic mechanisms are involved in the two phases of reactive and neurodegenerative response. In the first phase, which is mediated by NMDA receptor activation, calcium channel opening is nonselective and reversible. Calcium entry triggers a large number of biochemical processes (see above), notably calpain-mediated breakdown of cytoskeletal proteins, predominantly in the CA1 region (147). Several of these plastic changes are NMDA dependent and may be blocked by early modification of glutamate transmission. The second phase, characterized by excitotoxic degeneration and death of biochemically predisposed cells, is independent of NMDA receptor activation and not reversible. If this hypothesis is valid, then pharmacologic interventions to reduce ischemic cell loss may be effective only when given within the acute reactive phase, that is, optimally within 1 hr after reperfusion.

CEREBROPROTECTIVE STRATEGIES

Because of the delayed nature of neuronal death after ischemia, substantial research effort has gone into the identification of compounds that could protect against selective cell loss in global models, or rescue regions from infarction in focal models. Six basic types of approach have been adopted:

1. Postsynaptic blockade of EAAs by NMDA and non-NMDA receptor antagonists. Both direct NMDA antagonists (e.g., 2APV, CPP, and 2APH) and noncompetitive antagonists such as MK 801, which blocks the agonist-gated ion channel, have been shown to protect against focal and global ischemia (99). Alternatively, antagonists at the non-NMDA KA and AMPA receptors have been used (e.g., NBQX and GYKI 52466). These recently have been found to be protective against cortical and, to a lesser extent, hippocampal cell loss when given after ischemia, and GYKI 52466 blocks the extracellular glutamate increase in the striatum after 4-VO ischemia (3,88).
2. Reduction in the release of EAAs induced by ischemia (e.g., the anticonvulsants, phenytoin and lamotrigine, and kappa opioid agonists).
3. Prevention of calcium entry via calcium channel blockers acting on voltage-gated channels (e.g., nimodipine). Rod and Auer (141) found that joint treatment with both agonist- and voltage-gated channel blockers was more effective than either treatment alone.
4. Modification of the intracellular effects of calcium by use of protein kinase C inhibitors to reduce production of free radicals, or reduction in nitric oxide for-

mation by inhibitors of nitric oxide synthase (e.g., nitroarginine;105).
5. Modification of physiologic conditions that increase glutamate toxicity, such as hyperglycemia via insulin treatment (175), or hyperthermia (181).
6. Modification of nonglutamatergic transmitter systems that might contribute to ischemic damage, such as increases in adenosine, GABA agonists, dopamine, and 5-HT antagonists (see section on contribution of nonglutamatergic systems).

This brief list suffices to show that very many different manipulations can affect ischemic outcome, by modification of EAA transmission, by altering calcium entry and its intracellular effects, by controlling physiologic variables, or by changing the modulatory input of other neurotransmitters. The extent of cerebroprotective efficacy relates to the particular ischemic models used. With focal ischemia, penumbral damage develops relatively slowly, and NMDA antagonists have been particularly successful in this model, notably against cortical damage (99). However, in the 4-VO model of global ischemia, NMDA antagonists usually are ineffective (14), possibly because CBF is severely restricted. The evaluation of cerebroprotective treatment efficacy against the cognitive and motor deficits induced by ischemia is far less advanced than histologic assessment of neuropathology. There have been some reports of behavioral improvement, for instance in spatial learning after insulin counteraction of effects of 2-VO (175), but these are the exception rather than the rule, so that behavioral outcome studies merit far more attention. The most serious problem encountered by cerebroprotective strategies is that the therapeutic window of time for intervention appears to be very limited. This varies according to the ischemic model and the tissue involved. In global ischemia, it is inevitably short for striatal neurons (these die within 4–6 hr), but it is longer for CA1 pyramidal neurons (97). Magnesium has been claimed to be effective when injected into the CA1 region as long as 24 hr after ischemia (169), possibly because it blocks calcium channels and inhibits mitochondrial uptake of calcium. With reversible focal ischemia, the development of penumbral damage may proceed relatively slowly (15). However, most studies of cerebroprotection in MCAO in rodents find a marked falling off in efficiency when drug treatments are delayed beyond 60 to 90 min (97). Thus, a serious limitation of pharmacologic treatments is that they will be likely to require administration very shortly after the development of an ischemic emergency in humans. This means that in many cases help will arrive too late. Cerebroprotective treatments have not, to date, demonstrated the capacity to rescue neurons once damage has occurred. However, the postsynaptic nature of immediate excitotoxic ischemic damage means that presynaptic neurons are available in the host for transplants to attract and sustain. Thus, neural transplantation may be able to make an important new contribution to the treatment strategies available for ischemic brain damage.

BEHAVIORAL AND COGNITIVE EFFECTS OF ISCHEMIA

Focal Ischemia

Behavioral and cognitive effects of focal ischemia induced by MCAO in animals have not been extensively investigated, and findings are limited chiefly to rodents. This model has been used primarily to investigate cerebroprotective drug effects, with animals killed 24 hr to 7 days after occlusion. Fairly detailed neurologic measures are generally taken, at specified periods after ischemia, to monitor possible deficits in turning, righting reflex, paw placement, grasping, balance on rotarod or inclined plane, locomotor activity, and normal behaviors such as feeding and grooming (25). In general, after permanent MCAO, resulting in large cortical ($100–150$ cm^3) and striatal ($50–100$ mm^3) infarcts (50,180), neurologic deficits persist throughout the recovery period, whereas with smaller lesions initial deficits decline within a few days. The most common neurologic deficits range from sensorimotor impairment (lack of orientation to light touches on limbs and flanks) on the side contralateral to occlusion, and an increase in amphetamine-induced rotation to the ipsilateral side (50), to hemiplegia with large infarcts. In SHR, where infarcts are uniformly large within cortex and lateral caudate–putamen, Grabowski et al. (50), comparing left and right MCAO, found that sensorimotor and rotation, but not motor, deficits were correlated with lesion size in the right, but not the left hemisphere. Interestingly, in the right hemisphere sensorimotor correlations were found in different brain sections for the different limbs and trunk areas, suggesting both a rostral–caudal somatotopical representation and lateralization of sensory/spatial processes. Grabowski et al. (53) also have shown that contralateral paw-reaching after MCAO shows stable impairment over 3 months of testing, which is highly correlated with extent of infarction, whereas sensorimotor deficits decline over this period, so paw-reaching may provide a suitable method for assessing long-term effects of focal ischemia, in relation to effects of grafts.

Cognitive deficits have been reported with both permanent and reversible MCAO. Wahl et al. (180) found that 4 days after permanent MCAO, which produced large cortical and striatal infarcts, rats showed impairment in retention of passive avoidance, but normal exploratory behavior in the open field, and no deficits in alternation in the Y maze, a measure of working memory. This selective pattern of deficit argues against generalized postoperative confusion. After reversible MCAO for 1 hr, which also induced substantial lateral cortical and striatal damage, Nishino et al. (118) found long-lasting impairments in passive avoidance and deficits in acquisition of radial maze and water maze tasks. In rats pretrained on the radial maze to enter all arms to retrieve food, reentries (working memory errors) were increased after 90 min of MCAO, but this effect lasted for only 3 weeks, so that impairment was only transient in this task (143). Deficits in acquisition of both passive and active avoidance assessed for up to 8 weeks after MCAO also have been reported by Tamura et al. (162). Interestingly, only active avoidance impairment correlated with cortical atrophic ratio (a measure of infarct size in relation to the inact hemisphere) in this study.

Recently, Kataoka et al. (75) have shown that MCAO with lateral striatal infarction leads to substantial deafferentation of cortical cholinergic neurons, shown by reduced ChAT activity and acetylcholinesterase (AChE)-positive neurons, through interruption of cholinergic projections coursing laterally through the striatum. Damage to cholinergic neurons also may occur through retrograde degeneration from ischemic cortical lesions (91). Animals with lesions to the forebrain cholinergic projection system (FCPS) exhibit widespread impairments in passive avoidance, radial maze and water maze tasks, and operant tasks (63,151,170), resembling the pattern of deficits reported after MCAO by Nishino et al., whereas animals with discrete hippocampal lesions after 4-VO show more circumscribed deficits in spatial acquisition and working memory tasks (4,32,120,121,122,179; see section on effects of global ischemia). We have recently confirmed (Smith, Abdulla, and Calaminici, in preparation) that rats subjected to MCAO showed substantial impairment in spatial learning and memory in the water maze, resembling deficits shown by animals with large unilateral S-AMPA lesions to cholinergic cell bodies in the basal forebrain, which were tested as a comparison

group. Both groups showed a substantial reduction in cortical cholinesterase activity, and increased sensitivity to iontophoretic ACh. However, in MCAO animals, where both water maze latency scores and levels of AChE activity were more variable and less deficient than in lesioned rats, a significant correlation was found between behavioral scores and enzyme activity. A floor effect prevented detection of this correlation in lesioned rats. These results imply that there is a relationship between behavioral deficit and impaired cholinergic function in rats with cortical infarcts after MCAO. This relationship also is suggested by recent findings (193) that the selective muscarinic M1 receptor agonist YM796, given orally to rats for 7 days starting a week after MCAO, dose dependently increased retention of passive avoidance without altering locomotor activity or neurologic symptoms, or reducing infarct size. This effect was blocked by intracerebroventricular administration of the muscarinic antagonist pirenzepine. In humans, memory deficits have been reported after anterior communicating artery rupture, which produces either bilateral or unilateral infarction of the basal forebrain, and destroys cholinergic neurons in the nucleus basalis of Meynert (69,133). Decline in the FCPS is a reliable correlate of Alzheimer's disease pathology (131), and cognitive deficits also have been associated with cholinergic deficiency by many pharmacologic and lesion studies (34). Therefore, although there is current debate about lesion specificity and the types of deficit associated with damage to different branches of the FCPS (170), there is little doubt that cholinergic damage is associated with cognitive impairments in animal models and in a variety of neurodegenerative or vascular conditions in humans. Dementia-like symptoms and confusional states are commonly found in stroke victims, particularly the elderly (54,96). It is therefore a possibility meriting investigation that ischemia-induced damage to cholinergic pathways contributes to these deficits after MCAO or anterior communicating artery rupture. In other cases, such as occlusion of the posterior cerebral artery, the anterior choroid artery (AChA), or thalamic penetrating arteries, "amnesic stroke" (129) is more likely to be associated with hippocampal or diencephalic infarction (see section on global ischemia, the hippocampus, and memory loss, later).

Defective glutamate transmission also is fundamental to Alzheimer pathology, because neurofibrillary tangles are associated with glutamatergic cortical and pyramidal cells. Recent findings suggest that amyloid peptides may make these neurons prone to develop tangle-like changes in response to glutamate, because β-amyloid peptides in culture enhance the excitotoxic effects of glutamate, NMDA, and KA (95). A relative loss of NMDA receptors has been detected in brains of patients with Alzheimer's disease, although with considerable individual variation (171), and in brains of aged rats, monkeys, and humans (55,182,35). Excitotoxic brain damage after disruption of glutamatergic neurotransmission may bear other relationships to acute and chronic neurodegenerative conditions (96,100). For instance, HIV infection is associated with dementia and diffuse loss of cortical and other neurons. One contributory factor may be the substantial increase in quinolinic acid detected in the CSF of patients with AIDS, which correlates with degree of dementia, and leads to downregulation of NMDA receptors or to excitotoxic cell death (61). In view of these links with conditions associated with dementia in humans, it is surprising that cognitive deficits after focal ischemia have been so little investigated. Effects of global ischemia have received far more extensive research, largely because it is possible to produce small lesions limited to discrete hippocampal fields, so that global ischemia has been seen as a tool to investigate hippocampal function, as well as a model for the effects of human heart attack.

Global Ischemia, the Hippocampus, and Memory Loss in Animals and Humans

In humans, interruption of blood flow to the brain through heart attack frequently results in anterograde memory deficits and difficulties in learning. These are found in up to 20% of patients surviving a severe heart attack and constitute one of the most frequent and enduring disabilities (13,28, 105,177,197). The pattern of selective loss of memory, in the absence of intellectual impairment, resembles the temporal lobe amnesic syndrome (157). The pattern of memory deficits after cortical ablation in H.M., and other patients with amnesia, led Scoville and Milner (146) to argue that hippocampal damage, common to all cases, was responsible for the selective anterograde loss of memory. Damage to the temporal stem (67), or combined hippocampal and amygdaloid destruction (103), which also have been proposed to underlie amnesia, have appeared, with accumulating postmortem evidence, not to show as consistent a relationship to memory dysfunction (157, 197). Postmortem examination of heart attack victims displaying memory deficits also has identified discrete hippocampal lesions, together with variable damage in other brain regions. A striking example (197) has been provided by patient R.B., who manifested anterograde amnesia after an ischemic episode induced by massive loss of blood (5,000 ml) after heart bypass surgery. During 5 years of testing before death, R.B.'s memory for events (public and autobiographical) before surgery did not differ from those of controls, and he exhibited no signs of cognitive impairment other than an inability to retain new information of all kinds, including recall of complex figures, word lists, paired associates, and stories. Postmortem histologic examination revealed a bilateral hippocampal lesion limited to the CA1 fields, with only minor damage elsewhere, for example in the left globus pallidus and internal capsule, and right postcentral gyrus. This finding suggested not only that hippocampal pathology may be related to memory loss, but also that circumscribed bilateral damage within the hippocampus may be sufficient to produce significant loss of memory.

In addition to general failure of CBF, associated with bilateral hippocampal damage, memory deficits also have been found with unilateral infarction in the territory of the PCA (supplying the middle and posterior hippocampus, and hippocampal gyrus), the AChA (supplying the amygdala and anterior hippocampus), and the penetrating thalamic arteries, which supply the thalamus, or infarction in the area of the genu of the internal capsule, which may isolate the thalamus from its cortical connections (129). Unilateral amnesic stroke is relatively rare, but findings to date implicate damage to 1) limbic structures, including the hippocampus (PCA and AChA occlusion); 2) to the thalamus and its connections; and 3) to the basal forebrain via ACA rupture (see section on focal ischemia). On the basis of memory performance after well defined limbic or diencephalic lesions, Squire and coworkers have discriminated between "declarative memory" (semantic and episodic memory: "knowing that...") and "procedural memory" (skilled performance: "knowing how..."), the former mediated by temporal lobe structures, notably the hippocampus, the latter by diencephalic regions, chiefly the thalamus (157). Vascular territories do not respect our conceptual functional boundaries, so that multiple impairments may occur: PCA stroke victims also may show hemianopsia (via posterior cortical damage), and paramedian artery occlusion (damaging the thalamus) also may produce hemiparesis or hemiataxia. Moreover, infarction may compromise both hippocampal and thalamic regions. However, imaging techniques now enable us to attempt to discriminate between profiles of memory and learning deficits shown by patients with identified regions of limbic or diencephalic infarction (158), and preliminary results tend to support a distinction in

memory performance of patients with medial temporal (including hippocampal) as opposed to diencephalic damage.

In the rat, global cerebral ischemia, like heart attack in humans, induces cell loss primarily in the CA1 region, but with the extent varying according to the duration of the occlusion (134). Global ischemia therefore provides a method of examining hippocampal function, and comparing effects of intrahippocampal and extrahippocampal damage, that is of relevance to clinical pathology in humans. Studies of large hippocampal lesions in animals were initiated to see if they would reproduce the pattern of anterograde amnesia that had been linked to hippocampal damage in humans by Scoville and Milner's evidence (146). Animals were not found to demonstrate profound difficulties in learning and memory; for instance, discrimination learning, object–reward relationships, and retention of passive avoidance were relatively unimpaired by hippocampal lesions (139). Rather, hippocampal deficits were shown in tasks that require use of trial-unique, recent, and relational (including spatial) or conditional information. These include 1) "working memory" tasks, such as delayed nonmatching to sample or position (DNMTS/P), where increasing delays can be imposed between information and choice stages, delayed alternation in the T or Y maze, and avoidance of recently visited arms in the radial maze; 2) spatial learning of rewarded or safe locations in the radial and water maze; 3) tasks that require integration of information across modalities (e.g., visual and auditory cues); and 4) conditional responding as in go–no-go discriminations or negative patterning. This selective pattern of disabilities shown by lesioned animals has fostered the development of several theories of hippocampal function, in particular that it mediates working memory (125), that it processes spatial information (123), that it acts as a temporary store to integrate discontiguous information (135), or that it is adapted to process relational or configural information (38,160). Although none of these theories maps closely onto the generalized anterograde memory loss displayed by humans with hippocampal damage, the identification of reliable clusters of deficits in animals with hippocampal lesions provides a reasonable analogue for some of the effects of human amnesia, bearing in mind that the lack of mediational verbal systems in animals rules out the possibility of developing a fully homologous animal model for processes of learning and memory. Indeed, several tasks, particularly those of delayed nonmatching, are sensitive both to human amnesia and to hippocampal damage in animals. Thus there are several points of similarity between anterograde amnesia in humans and hippocampal damage in animals. For example, animals have been shown to retain tasks learned before lesioning, just as previous memories are preserved in humans with amnesia; and, given sufficient training, lesioned animals can master many tasks, just as humans with amnesia can learn skills (5).

Effects of Global Ischemia in the Rat

Behavioral deficits in ischemic animals have been found largely to conform to patterns of deficits shown by animals with hippocampal lesions, although the reported effects vary in different laboratories. In an extensive series of studies (see 32 for an overview), Volpe's laboratory has shown that rats subjected to 30 min of 4-VO show deficits in learning in the radial maze, where five of eight arms were rewarded, in both reference memory (entry into never-rewarded arms) and working memory (reentry into rewarded arms already visited on a given trial), but their extent depended on the length of training and type of memory. With extensive training after ischemia (95 trials, as opposed to 70 trials; 30,176), reference memory errors declined to control level, whereas working memory remained moderately impaired. Pretraining for 70 trials before ischemia (31) also eliminated both reference and working memory errors, apart from a transient working memory impairment. In a more difficult working memory task, with all eight arms baited, ischemia produced a relatively stable working memory impairment, although here, too, performance improved to control level with extensive pretraining (178). The difference between mild reference memory impairment and more marked working memory deficits found by Volpe's group in the radial maze was confirmed using a split-stem T maze, in which the choice of left or right stem sections (cued either by position or by floor texture) was invariant, whereas the rewarded goal arm alternated according to the choice on the previous trial. Ischemic rats showed deficits in goal, but not stem choices (179). An identical pattern has been reported by Hagan and Beaughard (58), who found that ischemic rats (15 min of 4-VO) were more impaired on forced choice T-maze alternation than on learning to find a platform in the water maze, which is arguably more of a reference memory task, because the position remains constant from trial to trial. Kiyota et al. (84) also found both working and reference memory deficits during acquisition in the eight-arm radial maze after 5 and 20 min of 4-VO, but no impairment of learning in the water maze. The three-door runway, in which rats have to choose one of three correct (opening) doors at four choice points to reach food at the end, also has provided a spatial working memory task sensitive to ischemia- or NMDA-induced CA1 cell loss (159). We have used Jarrard's (70) place and cue radial maze tasks with four of eight arms consistently rewarded in the place task, as in Volpe's experiments, and four of eight textured inserts rewarded on the cue task, with the inserts being moved to different arms on each trial. Jarrard (70) had found that large lesions of the hippocampal formation selectively impaired acquisition of the place, but not the cue task, whereas small intrahippocampal lesions did not impair learning of either task. Because ische-mic damage is largely confined to the CA1 field with 15 min of 4-VO, whereas it is more extensive intrahippocampally and ex-trahippocampally with the 30 min of 4-VO used by Volpe, we compared these two du-rations to see if circumscribed ischemic damage is sufficient to impair learning, or whether more extensive damage is re-quired, as Jarrard's results would suggest. In fact, we found no deficits in either ische-mic group in acquisition, relative to con-trols, over 60 training trials, even though both groups had near total (>90%) cell loss in dorsal CA1 (121,122), were not pre-trained, and showed substantial impairment in water-maze learning. It is possible that the slightly greater load on working mem-ory with five (Volpe's group) as opposed to four (our group) arms baited, or the retar-dation of learning in control animals im-posed by learning two tasks, may account for the discrepancies between our results and those of Volpe's group.

Spatial navigation in the water maze pro-vides another example of a task that is sen-sitive to hippocampal damage (106) but is not invariably impaired after global ische-mia. Auer et al. (4) found that rats sub-jected to 2-VO showed no deficits on the standard task of learning to locate a hidden platform over several days with the plat-form in the same location. However, in a complex "learning set" task, in which rats were given 12 trials/day with a different platform position on each of 6 days, ische-mic animals showed significant impair-ment. Kiyota et al. (88) also found no defi-cits in the standard water-maze procedure in 4-VO rats that exhibited deficits in the radial maze. Jaspers et al. (71), in contrast, found impairment in the standard water-maze acquisition in rats subjected to both 2-VO and 4-VO, despite lack of visible hip-pocampal damage in the 2-VO group. Our results differ from those both of Auer et al., and Kiyota et al. in that we found no defi-cits in either the standard or the learning set task in rats subjected to 2-VO (122),

whereas in rats subjected to 4-VO we have found highly significant and reproducible impairments in water-maze learning in ani-mals occluded for periods of 5 to 30 min (120,122a,122b). Indeed, our results show the reverse pattern to those of Kiyota et al. (85), because we found substantial deficits for water-maze learning in the same 4-VO animals that failed to demonstrate radial-maze impairment. This is not likely to be an order effect, because water-maze deficits were found both before and after radial-maze training (121). To elucidate the nature of this navigational impairment we have ex-amined the performance of ischemic rats in the water maze over a 6-month period after 15 min of 4-VO (116). Impairment is most evident in a novel pool; with repeated test-ing rats are able to find a platform in a novel position as efficiently as controls, but are substantially impaired when switched to a different pool. Ischemic rats, apart from the first training period, do not show significant decrease in spatial bias for the training quadrant on probe trials, indicating that they remember the general position of the platform, but are less accurate in re-tention of its precise position, as shown by reduced time in the "counter" area, twice the platform diameter. Ischemic rats also are more impaired than controls with a dif-ficult training regime (two trials/day with a 10-min intertrial interval [ITI], as opposed to four trials/day with a 5-min ITI), and when tested in a working memory task (four trials/day, a 30-sec ITI, and a different position on each day; a variant of the learn-ing set task).

These results, like those of Volpe's group for radial-maze reference memory errors (32), suggest that ischemic rats are able to acquire and use a long-term spatial repre-sentation, but do not do so as quickly and efficiently as controls. The results are broadly consistent with the suggestion of Eichenbaum et al. (38) or Sutherland and McDonald (160) that animals with hippo-campal damage have difficulty in process-ing relational or configural information, but do not suffer from long-term memory deficits. Eichenbaum et al. suggested that rats with hippocampal damage may use a simple guidance strategy, rather than forming a relational spatial map of their environment. If so, this may explain why, in our hands, the water maze may be more sensitive to ischemic deficits than the radial maze. Slow learning in controls, together with the fact that rats were always started in the center of the maze, might permit ischemic rats to learn the radial maze as a series of discrete rewarded locations, without disadvantage. Moreover, because rats simply had to go down the arm for food, localization deficits would not be detected in the radial maze. Despite some discrepancies, the frequency of impairment in tasks with a spatial or working memory component, or both, but not in simple retention (e.g., passive avoidance; 11), suggests that rodents with global ischemic damage share features of impairment found in animals with hippocampal lesions. However, behavioral parameters affected by ischemia still are relatively unexplored; one consequence of the great emphasis on pharmacologic studies with neuropathologically evaluated cerebroprotection has been a lack of interest in the behavioral consequences of ischemia. For investigation of effects of transplants it is important to validate tasks that can be used repeatedly, such as delayed or continuous nonmatching to sample or spatial working memory tasks, rather than acquisition in the water maze, which is heavily influenced by experience.

Correlations between Behavioral Deficits and Ischemic Hippocampal Cell Loss

Reproducible patterns of ischemic cell loss, particularly in the 4-VO model, encourage attempts to look for relationships between extent and site of brain damage and behavioral impairment. As a basis for transplantation, positive correlations be-

tween behavioral deficits and damage to particular brain regions or types of cell would provide an extremely useful pointer to the optimum type of graft. Conversely, if clear-cut correlations between deficits and regional brain damage are not forthcoming, it is possible that neural transplantation might help to determine whether damage in a given region is critical to the manifestation of deficits, by showing functional recovery with specific types or sites of graft. A general relationship between CA1 cell loss and behavioral deficits is evident from findings that this is the major and most consistent area of damage in animals showing deficits. Thus, findings that animals with localized CA1 cell loss after 15 min of 4-VO, and those with more extensive intrahippocampal and extrahippocampal damage after 30 min of 4-VO, showed almost identical deficits in water-maze learning (120,122), suggested that the common loss of CA1 cells was responsible for the deficits. Similarly, Davis and Volpe (32) have compared effects of 30 min of 4-VO with those of large and small excitotoxic hippocampal lesions, to suggest that CA1 cell loss is critical for radial-maze deficits. Attempts to establish quantitative correlational relationships have, however, met with mixed results. There are a few reports of positive correlations between water-maze (140), radial-maze (85), and T-maze (179) deficits and CA1 cell loss, although Jaspers et al. (71) reported water-maze learning deficits after 2-VO in the absence of any histologic evidence for cell loss. We have examined correlations between several indices of water-maze learning and extent of ischemic cell loss, in groups subjected to 5 to 30 min of 4-VO (122a,122b). Although there was a highly significant linear relationship between extent of cell loss in the CA1 region and duration of ischemia (together with increasing damage in other brain regions with increasing durations), the correlation between CA1 cell loss (and other regional damage) and behavioral measures was essentially zero. In part, the discrepancy may arise because some studies reporting positive correlations include nonischemic controls, which biases the results. Rod et al. (140), for example, report a significant correlation between mean latency in a learning set task and histologic damage in rats subjected to 2-VO. However, if the nonischemic controls are removed, these data yield a nonsignificant correlation (122a). It also is possible that correlations are evident only with certain tasks. As learning in the standard water-maze procedure does not provide a steady-state measure of behavioral deficit, and proceeds in a fast "all-or-none" manner in normal rats, one would not intuitively expect it to provide a stable baseline for assessing the extent of brain damage. Performance on discrete trial tasks, such as the radial-maze or T-maze alternation, may prove more appropriate for correlational studies; indeed, Volpe et al. (179) have recently reported a correlation between T-maze working memory errors and CA1 cell loss, after 30 min of 4-VO, whereas Patel et al. (*personal communication*) have found that radial-maze working memory errors, although transient, correlated with CA1 cell loss after 2-VO.

Primate Models of Ischemia with Hippocampal Damage

Primate studies of behavioral deficits induced by ischemia are relatively rare, and involve two different approaches—extracranial transient occlusion of ascending arteries by pressure cuff, with pharmacologic reduction of blood pressure (198), and intracranial permanent bilateral occlusion of the PCA supplying the hippocampus (8). Zola-Morgan et al. (198) compared effects of 15 min of global ischemia in four cynomolgus monkeys with those of animals with lesions restricted to the hippocampal formation and parahippocampal gyrus (H^+), or more extensive temporal lobe lesions including the amygdala, hippocampus, and overlying

cortex (H^+A^+). Performance was assessed on three tasks sensitive to hippocampal damage in animals and amnesia in humans: trial-unique DNMTS, delayed object discrimination, and eight-pair concurrent discrimination; and two tasks that people with amnesia perform normally: pattern discrimination and a test of motor skill. The ischemic group was not impaired on these two latter tasks, nor on delayed object and concurrent discrimination, in which both the lesioned groups showed deficits. However, the ischemic animals showed significant impairment, equivalent to that of the H^+ group on DNMTS, at a retention interval of 10 min, but not at shorter delays. The H^+A^+ group was impaired at all delays. Histologic examination revealed cell loss largely confined to the CA1 and CA2 hippocampal fields; there was reduction in somatostatin staining in hilar neurons and some patchy loss of cerebellar Purkinje cells, but no other evident damage. These results are consistent with the rodent studies of ischemia-induced deficits in hippocampal lesion-sensitive tasks, linked to restricted intrahippocampal damage, although the behavioral impairment was modest. However, effects of ischemia produced by the cuff technique appear to have a sharp threshold for the manifestation of behavioral deficits, and a steep "dose–response" curve. Nemoto et al. (115) (who first developed the procedure) suggested that 15 min was the threshold for neurologic deficits, with a duration of 16 min these deficits were severe, and after 20 min of occlusion the monkeys would die within 7 days. Lanier et al. (86) also quantified neurologic deficits arising from 17 min of occlusion within the first 96 hr in pigtail monkeys, and correlated these with hippocampal pathology (but not damage elsewhere in the brain). There was a significant relationship ($r = 0.82$) between graded neurologic and histopathologic scores in fields CA2 to 4, but a less marked correlation with the CA1 field ($r = 0.61$). Recently, Scheller et al. (144) reported that cynomolgus monkeys subjected to 3 and 9 min of global ischemia were neurologically normal, and showed no deficits in DNMTS, nor signs of CA1 cell loss; monkeys occluded for 12 min showed substantial neurologic deficits, some of which persisted for 30 days, but no impairment in DNMTS, and moderate cell loss in the CA1 area. These findings suggest that the cuff occlusion model is highly sensitive to slight differences in duration, and requires strict standardization. Moreover, interpretation of cognitive deficits may be clouded by the emergence of neurologic deficits at about the same duration of occlusion, which is likely to impair the motor performance of some tasks.

The PCA occlusion model also encounters difficulties. Bechevalier and Mishkin (8) found that damage was variable, ranging from almost none to a large unilateral infarct of the ventromedial and occiptotemporal cortex. However, in four of the macaques in which damage was confined to 20% to 55% of the hippocampal formation, deficits in DNMTS were related to the presence and bilaterality of hippocampal damage. Moreover, the only common damage in animals that showed such deficits lay in fields CA1 and 2, in agreement with Zola-Morgan et al.'s findings (198). Deficits in the Bechevalier and Mishkin study were more marked than in Zola-Morgan et al.'s study, being evident at delays of only 60 to 120 sec and manifest also with increasing list length (presentation of three to ten objects successively in the sample phase, before presentation of one novel and one of the familiar items at the choice stage). As in the Zola-Morgan study, no deficits were found in a concurrent discrimination task. The two studies therefore present a fairly consistent picture of impairment in the "amnesia-sensitive" DNMTS task, in the absence of discrimination failure, and linked to CA1 to 2 cell loss. One puzzling feature of the Bechevalier and Mishkin work was that monkeys with partial hippocampal infarction were more impaired in DNMTS than those with total ablation of the hippo-

campus. This may have resulted from the greater disorganizing effect of damage to a component area, as compared to removal of the entire structure, or from the presence of more extensive functional damage than was detected by the histologic methods used. The finding, however, runs counter to evidence that more extensive hippocampal lesions produce larger deficits in both monkey (198) and rodent (32) models.

STRATEGIES FOR NEURAL TRANSPLANTATION IN ISCHEMIC MODELS

Neural transplantation has been developed in animal models as a promising technique to promote functional recovery after a variety of types of brain damage. Two main strategies have been employed using fetal grafting material: first, to implant cells selected to release particular neurotransmitters for conditions in which damage in these systems is thought to play a critical causal role in impairments; second, to implant grafts from particular brain regions in an attempt to repair local areas of damage within the host. A third strategy aims to rescue or promote sprouting in host neurons by delivery of neurotrophic growth factors to the sites of injury.

There are several examples of the relatively successful use of transmitter-biased grafts in nonischemic models. Fetal nigral grafts provided the earliest evidence for improved aspects of performance in rodents and monkeys with unilateral 6-hydroxydopamine lesions of the nigrostriatal dopamine system as a model of dopamine deficiency in Parkinson's disease (37,130). Cholinergic-rich grafts, implanted in the terminal regions of the FCPS, have similarly proved effective in aged (43), alcohol-treated (2), or lesioned (63) animals showing behavioral impairment and reduced cortical or hippocampal levels of ChAT activity. In these cases, the primary aim has been to replace the lost neurotransmitter thought to be critically involved in the expression of behavioral impairment. The placement of such grafts has been within the terminal regions to which the systems normally project, rather than at the location of the cell bodies where cell loss occurs, because grafts do not normally extend long axons in the host brain. Thus, fetal nigral grafts have been placed ectopically in the host caudate and/or putamen, and cholinergic-rich basal forebrain or septal tissue in the cortex and/or hippocampus. The ectopic placement of these grafts has meant that they cannot achieve normal integration into the brain, although they may grow well and develop normal cell morphology and protein expression in their alien location (152). They also have been shown by histologic, electrophysiologic, and dialysis techniques (117) to achieve a degree of synaptic contact with host neurons. However, several problems are associated with the use of transmitter-biased grafts. In particular, many elements other than cells expressing the substances of interest are included in the graft, making it difficult to ascertain their mechanisms of action. For example, the case of cholinergic-rich grafts thought to promote recovery by release of ACh, intragraft glial fibrillary acidic protein has been found to correlate as highly as ChAT with scores of behavioral improvement in the radial maze in rats with lesions to the FCPS (183). Primary glial cultures (devoid of ChAT activity) were subsequently found to promote behavioral recovery as potently as the parent basal forebrain ChAT-positive tissue itself, whereas primary neuronal cultures (also ChAT positive) were ineffective (12), so that if cholinergic neurons play a role, it may well be in cooperation with glia or other elements in the grafts [see Sinden et al.,(*this volume*)]. Functional recovery has been linked more securely to the presence of DA cells in unilateral striatal lesion models, but it has been difficult to achieve extensive outgrowth from these grafts, so that they generally restore only about 10% of the normal host innervation. Neverthe-

less, changes in early gene and protein expression throughout the denervated striatum (21) suggest that these grafts influence host function beyond the region of direct host–graft neuronal connections. This may explain why grafts of such limited extent can have quite large behavioral effects in animal models, but it also means that there is still much to learn about their mechanisms of action.

Alternative transplant models have sought to repair localized chemical or traumatic damage by grafting tissue of the appropriate type within the lesioned area. The aim of such grafts is to promote functional recovery by repairing a damaged circuit or structure. Because these grafts are homotypic, the expectation would be that they become integrated into the host brain, possibly in a point-to-point manner, which cannot occur with ectopic transmitter-biased grafts. Recent examples of cortical and hippocampal grafts placed within these same regions of host brain have shown, in some cases, promotion of functional recovery, but there has been no convincing evidence for point-to-point restoration of host circuitry. Stein's group, for instance, showed that grafts of cortical tissue improved aspects of visual discrimination in animals with cortical lesions, even if inappropriate frontal cortex grafts were used in rats with visual cortex lesions, and that cortical grafts, although showing features similar to those of host frontal cortex, did not develop a comparable laminar organization (110), suggesting that such grafts function in a nonspecific manner (90). Recent evidence also suggests that whereas host neurons may extensively reinnervate the graft, projections from graft to host are strictly limited. For example, in rats with aspiration lesions of the frontal cortex, neurites cross the corpus callosum, but rarely enter the adjacent cortex and penetrate the caudate–putamen only to a distance of 0.5 to 0.8 mm, insufficient to restore striatal glutamate uptake (60). Fetal sensorimotor cortex, grafted into excitotoxic somatosensory cortical lesion sites, has been shown by retrograde and antero-grade tracers to receive extensive innervation from host regions that normally project to this cortical area (including ipsilateral cortex, thalamus, hypothalamus, nucleus basalis, dorsal raphe, and locus coeruleus), but to extend outgrowth only to the adjacent region of host cortex (20). Grafts of tissue from the hippocampal formation sited in regions of hippocampal damage, like cortical grafts, have had mixed effects on functional recovery, depending on factors such as extent of damage, the behavioral complexity of the task, and graft growth and survival. Several workers have reported improvements in spatial maze tasks (82, 156,163), whereas others have found no amelioration (46), or even exacerbation (190) of spatial deficits. As with Mufson et al.'s (110) findings for cortical grafts, neither solid nor suspension grafts from the whole hippocampus have been found to develop an appropriate laminar organization. The mechanisms of action of homotypic grafts, therefore, may be as difficult to elucidate as those of grafts chosen to express neurotransmitters, and although homotypic grafts appear to be linked into the neural network of the host, outgrowth from grafts is limited, and the grafts generally have not been found to develop appropriate cytoarchitecture.

A third possible strategy for application to ischemic models is to supply growth factors to rescue damaged neurons and promote outgrowth from grafts. Nerve growth factor (NGF), critical to the survival and neurite outgrowth of cells during development, is particularly associated with the terminal regions of the FCPS, so that cortex and hippocampus contain the highest levels of NGF mRNA in the brain (49). Since the demonstrations that exogenous NGF can prevent the death of cholinergic cells after axotomy, reduce cholinergic cell atrophy, and improve spatial memory in aged rats (41,172,184), there has been much experimental effort to identify different growth factors (e.g., brain-derived nerve

factor [BDNF]; basic fibroblast growth factor [bFGF]; epidermal growth factor [EGF]) and to assess their efficacy in promoting outgrowth from various types of cell *in vitro* (152). Considerable ingenuity also has been devoted to the delivery of growth factors *in vivo,* including local infusion (6,184), co-grafts of sciatic nerve (173), and transfection of cells for direct (78) or encapsulated (188) grafting of cells that release growth factors. There are relatively few reports on the behavioral effects of growth factor grafts, but findings to date suggest that these, too, are variable. Kesslak et al. (79) found improvement in T-maze alternation both with cultured astrocytes and gelfoam soaked in wound extract after cortical lesions, but not with astrocyte grafts in rats with hippocampal lesions (80), where fetal hippocampal grafts were efficacious. Conversely, Barone et al. (6) found improvement in water-maze learning in rats with dentate gyrus lesions with infusions of NGF, but not with fetal hippocampal grafts. Despite the paucity of information about the functional efficacy of growth factors, this strategy is potentially of great importance for the amelioration of ischemic deficits. Delayed cell death and the relatively slow spread of infarction in the penumbral regions may promote enhanced susceptibility to the effects of growth factors, particularly in the hippocampus, where endogenous expression of NGF is high. Ischemia also produces enhanced levels of the neurite-promoting protein nexin (66), which might magnify the effects of exogenous growth factors. Evidence is rapidly accumulating to show that expression of growth factors is altered after ischemia (161) and traumatic brain injury (194). Activation of glutamate receptors enhances synthesis of growth factors so that, after both global and focal ischemia, mRNA expression of NGF, BDNF, bFGF, neurotrophin-3 (NT-3), and other neurotrophins is increased in a region-specific manner (111,142,161,168). Thus, the time course and distribution of changes in the expression of trophic factors may be associated with cell survival or death, and with remodeling of neuronal circuitry after ischemia or focal injury. For example, Kar et al. (74) suggest that increased receptors for insulin-like growth factor 1 (IGF-1) in ipsilateral dentate gyrus contribute to the sprouting and synaptogenesis that occur in this region after unilateral entorhinal cortex lesions, whereas bilateral increases in receptors for insulin and IGF-2 are associated with the widespread activation of astrocyte, macrophage, and microglial response to neuronal injury. Expression of bFGF in cortex adjacent to infarct areas after MCAO is sufficiently enriched for extracts of periinfarct tissue to support the growth of embryonic cortical and thalamic neurons *in vitro* (192), whereas the increasing gradient in density of BDNF mRNA and its receptor TrkB outward from the region of cortical photochemical infarct suggests that this factor confers compensatory resistance to ischemia. (26). However, Murase et al. (111) did not find evidence to relate expression of NGF to the "tolerance" conveyed by a short ischemic episode for a subsequent severe episode in gerbils. In addition to possible trophic or protective effects, direct application of bFGF has been found to increase *in vivo* CBF (136), so that a number of mechanisms may contribute to the restorative effects of growth factors. *In vitro* studies have also shown that bFGF, EGF, and other peptide growth factors in the medium protect primary cultures of embryonic rat or chick forebrain neurons from the toxic effects of anoxia, glutamate, and nitric oxide (85, 92,93,148).

TRANSPLANTS IN FOCAL MODELS OF ISCHEMIA

The choice of the type of transplants likely to be effective in promoting functional recovery from focal ischemic brain damage is not easy to make. This is primarily because areas of infarction can be very large, particularly after irreversible MCAO, including both lateral caudate–putamen and lateral cortex. This argues against use of transmitter-biased tissue, but, if homotypic grafts are to be used, decisions are required as to whether to attempt to restore cortical or striatal function. Moreover, with permanent occlusion, or use of hypertensive rats, the blood supply is compromised, which may limit the chances of graft growth across large areas of infarction; early studies emphasize the importance of grafting to a well vascularized region (9). Solid grafts, typically used for homotypic placement in large lesion sites, may be particularly vulnerable to reduced blood flow, because the normal cortex, striatum, and hippocampus are susceptible to hypoglycemia. Kiessling et al. (81) have shown that cerebellar grafts, from a region that is resistant to reduction in CBF, retain the ability to extract glucose efficiently in conditions of low blood glucose levels, even when sited in the vulnerable caudate–putamen of host rats, so that certain resistant ectopic grafts may prove more viable than vulnerable homotypic transplants in conditions of reduced CBF. The extent of vascular reorganization after MCAO in SHR rats, and of incorporation of grafts into the host's blood supply, has recently been directly assessed by Grabowsky et al. (52), using casts obtained by perfusion with latex, from which surface brain tissue was corroded to expose the filigree network of vessels and capillaries to scanning electron microscopy. Casting on both sides of the occlusion showed that connections had been reestablished between the two segments of the MCA, which also had found alternative connections to the PCA and ACA. Infarct cavities were covered with a rich vascular network, in which leptomeningeal vessels and capillaries were intertwined, in contrast to normal cortex, where capillaries are not found on the surface. This infarct network adequately supplied fetal neocortical grafts (implanted in infarct cavities 5 days after MCAO), although vasculature in the 3-

month-old grafts did not form a typical laminar pattern, and grafts were not penetrated by arterioles and venules that normally course downward form the cortex. Grafts also had a lower density of capillaries than typically found in cortex, but the morphology of capillaries was normal. These results suggest that the host vascular system is capable of substantial reorganization after arterial occlusion, and of supplying blood to sustain graft growth, although a reduction in microvascular capacity within the grafts might lead to reduced metabolic activity.

Use of grafts in focal models of ischemia to date is very rare, despite the potential importance of developing good models, given the prevalence of stroke and the often permanent motor and cognitive disabilities that result. There is preliminary evidence that grafts of both cortical and striatal fetal tissue not only survive in ischemic brain but exert ameliorative effects on behavior. An early study (94) investigated embryonic (E) day 16 to 17 cortical solid grafts implanted into the parietal cortex of rats subjected to intraluminal MCAO for 3 hr. This produced variable infarcts in lateral cortex and caudate putamen, some of which were very large. All rats exhibited transient contralateral hemiparesis, marked by turning and falling over after occlusion, but this diminished within 1 to 2 days. Grafting of tissue, suctioned from fetal cortex and transferred directly to the host brain by pipette, was performed 2 to 15 days after ischemia, and nine transplants survived for examination after 1 month. The three grafts that failed to grow were sited in large glial-lined infarct cavities. Some grafts filled the ischemic cavity, and others displaced ischemic but not infarcted tissue. These results showed that cortical grafts can survive in regions of infarct, provided that they are not so large as to prevent access to the host's blood supply, and that, as in lesioned rats, a normal pyramidal cell population was present, although cholinergic cell density in grafts was increased and laminar organization was not preserved. Connectivity between graft and host varied with the relationship to infarction. In some cases there was a gap between graft and host, or a glial boundary, which reduced the number of connecting fibers, but in all cases some fibers were found to cross between graft to host, although the direction of innervation was not determined. Graft survival has been assessed in more stringent conditions using SH rats, where infarction is larger than in normotensive animals. Grabowski et al. (51) compared cortical cell suspension grafts from younger (E12–14) and older (E15–18) donors over a time course of 10 days to 23 weeks after transplantation to regions of host cortical infarct. The older embryonic donor tissue contained larger numbers of normal cells than the younger grafts, and fibers positive for AChE, dopamine-B-hydroxylase, and 5-HT staining increased in density over time. Fluorogold retrograde tracing of host projections to the grafts revealed labeled cells in the host nucleus basalis, ventral pallidum, dorsal raphe, locus coeruleus, and in ipsilateral and contralateral neocortex, indicating substantial innervation from the host. Grafts survived well, forming lobules within or filling areas of infarction, and attracted reinnervation from distal regions of host brain, suggesting substantial integration into the host network, although lack of laminar arrangement in the graft would make the establishment of point-to-point connections unlikely. Grafts did not appear to have exerted a neuroprotective function, because there was evidence for thalamic atrophy, despite extension of thalamic host fibers to the grafts. Behavioral effects of cortical grafts after MCAO have not yet been reported.

Grafts of embryonic striatal tissue into infarcted caudate–putamen of rats subjected to MCAO also recently have come under investigation. Nishino et al. (118) examined the effects of striatal cell suspension grafts sited in striatum of rats after reversible intraluminal MCAO for 1 hr, which resulted in infarcts in both the lateral cortex and striatum, and deficits in retention of passive avoidance, and in the learning of radial- and water-maze tasks. Grafted animals showed improvements in passive avoidance and water-maze learning, but were as impaired as ischemic rats on the radial-maze task. Histologic analysis showed that grafts, which survived well in the regions of infarct, contained both ChAT-positive and GABA-positive cells, whereas autoradiographic binding studies with ^{3}H-labeled antagonists showed that grafts contained the types of receptor normally expressed in the striatum (cholinergic muscarinic, DA D1 and D2, and GABA-A). Moderate recovery of GABA levels, which were reduced by 50% in the damaged striatum, also was found in the grafts. Thus, grafting of striatal tissue not only restored neuronal elements in the striatum, but improved aspects of behavior, despite the presence of cortical damage.

There has been very little work done to evaluate grafts biased to express neurotransmitters or growth factors in models related to focal ischemia. Nishino et al.'s (118) findings suggested that functional recovery after grafting of striatal tissue in rats with striatal infarcts after MCAO may have involved graft-induced recovery of GABAergic function. Decrease in GABAergic inhibitory control has been related to induction of epileptic seizures (96), which shares common excitotoxic mechanisms with ischemia and is facilitated by lesions of the caudate–putamen, a region vulnerable to infarction after MCAO. Fine et al. (40) showed that transplantation of both GABA-rich E16 fetal tissue from the striatal eminence and control sciatic nerve tissue (including Schwann cells expressing trophic factors) bilaterally into the substantia nigra, reduced the severity of pilocarpine-induced seizures in caudate–putamen-lesioned rats. These findings suggest that both neuronal and trophic factors may contribute to resistance to epileptogenic activity, a potentially adverse consequence of striatal infarction. In both rodents and primates there is pre-liminary evidence for protective effects of growth factors in conditions of reduced CBF or excitotoxicity. The expression of IGF-1 is increased in rat brain after ischemia, and intraventricular injection of IGF-1 2 hr after hypoxic–ischemic trauma has been found to reduce cortical and striatal infarction substantially (56,187). Basic fibroblast growth factor also has been found to protect against ischemic infarcts and NMDA-induced striatal lesions in neonatal rats when injected 30 min before, or up to 1 hr after, infusion of toxin, repeated doses being more effective than a single treatment (119). Efficacy of NGF recently has been shown in the monkey, where treatment with recombinant human nerve growth factor alone or together with the monosialganglioside GM1 substantially reduced retrograde degeneration of cholinergic basal forebrain neurons after devascularizing cortical lesions (91). Recombinant human NGF alone prevented decrease in ChAT activity, whereas joint treatment with GM1 also prevented shrinkage of ChAT-IR neurons. Thus, growth factors, in contrast to fetal cortical grafts, may have the potential not only to reduce the initial spread of infarction, but to prevent secondary retrograde degeneration from areas where damage has occurred. However, after ablation of the left forelimb projection area in sensorimotor cortex, which causes retrograde degeneration to ventroposterior lateral (VPL) thalamic neurons, Kataoka et al. (76) found that the reduction in degenerative changes in rats treated with bFGF was not sufficient to elevate firing rates of VPL neurons above the low levels found in untreated lesioned rats. Thus, morphologic improvement is not necessarily associated with functional recovery.

TRANSPLANTS IN GLOBAL MODELS OF ISCHEMIA

The selective loss of hippocampal CA1 cells with brief (10–15 min) episodes of global ischemia in the rat (134; see section on methods of inducing cerebral ischemia) provides the opportunity to look at effects of grafting to a localized area of damage within a well defined circuit. Within the hippocampus, the particular neuronal pathways follow identified laminar routes. Entorhinal cortical fibers synapse within the outer two thirds of the dentate granule dendritic field, whereas mossy fibers from the dentate gyrus project selectively to the juxtacellular area of CA3 pyramidal cells. With tracing techniques it is possible to assess the accuracy with which grafted neurons project along normal routes and receive appropriate afferents from the host. Grafts of homotypic hippocampal tissue therefore have been the method of choice to examine effects of grafting in global models of ischemic damage, where in principle it is possible to look with precision for evidence of point-to-point circuit reconstruction.

Grafts from Whole Hippocampus in Global Ischemic Models

There have been several studies assessing the growth, integration, electrical activity, and behavioral effects of grafts derived from whole fetal hippocampi in the ischemic rodent brain. Mudrick et al. (108) made intracellular recordings from grafts in hippocampal slices 2 to 9 months after implantation of E18 hippocampal cell suspensions in the hippocampi of host rats subjected to 2-VO 1 week earlier. Firing patterns resembling those of normal pyramidal and interneuron cells were identified in the grafts, and potentials evoked by stimulation in the host stratum radiatum and stratum oriens indicated that afferent contacts had been established. Evidence for projections from the graft to host was supplied by evoking antidromic spikes via shocks to the stratum oriens. However, prolonged excitatory postsynaptic potentials (ESPs) within the graft suggested that local inhibitory circuits were absent. In a parallel histologic exami-

nation (109), grafts were shown to contain cells resembling CA1 pyramids, to express neuron-specific proteins (calbindin-D and parvalbumin) found in normal CA1 cells, and to send projections to the host septal area, visualized by retrograde fluorogold labeling, from which cholinesterase-positive host fibers were seen to penetrate the grafts. Similarly, Tønder et al. (164) found that in rats subjected to 4-VO, hippocampal grafts survived well and showed near-normal levels of GFAP reactivity. The grafts contained cells similar to those of normal adult CA1, CA3, and CA4 pyramids, and were richly innervated by host cholinergic fibers from the medial septum. Grafts sent appropriate efferent projections to the posterior levels of host CA1 and subicular regions, and also some abnormal connections to the dentate gyrus molecular layer. Zheng et al. (195) also have shown that expression of inositol triphosphate and forskolin receptors is normal in E19 hippocampal fields, and can be used to distinguish between grafted cells from CA1 and CA3/dentate granule (DG) fields. Findings of Katayama et al. (79) suggested that there may be a limited time window for optimum survival of hippocampal grafts in ischemic brain after 2-VO. Embryonic day 17 to 18 cell suspension grafts showed better survival and more extensive outgrowth if implanted 1 rather than 4 weeks after ischemia, particularly if ischemic cell loss in the host was extensive. Dendrites of grafted cells were aligned parallel to the apical dendrites of normal CA1 pyramidal cells, suggesting that, unlike cortical grafts, hippocampal tissue may achieve a degree of laminar organization. Katayama et al. suggest that this occurs through the release of trophic factors shortly after ischemia, which promotes contact between afferent fibers, disconnected from ischemic CA1 cells, and grafted neurons. Confirmation that this evidence for survival and functional efficacy of fetal hippocampal grafts in ischemic brain might have positive effects on behavior was provided by Onifer and Low (128). Mongolian gerbils were subjected to 2-VO ischemia and trained 10 or 38 days later to find a submerged platform in the water maze. Groups equated for performance received vehicle or hippocampal cell suspension grafts, and were tested 47 days later. Performance on the spatial probe test indicated that grafted animals remembered the platform position as well as controls, and were significantly superior to the ischemic group and to their own pretransplant performance. Even though these animals received transplants some 3 or 7 weeks after ischemia, outside the optimum period suggested by Katayama et al. (77), bilateral survival was 100%. Grafts were sited largely in the corpus callosum above the ischemic dorsal CA1 region, but host-derived AChE-positive fibers penetrated the alveus and reached into the grafts, which contained cells morphologically resembling normal CA1, CA2, and CA3 pyramidal cells.

Grafts from Hippocampal Fields: Connectivity Studies

Efficacy of grafts derived from the whole fetal hippocampus strongly suggested that homotypic grafts are integrated into the host brain, form some laminar organization, and can promote functional recovery, even though they may lack local inhibitory circuits and made some aberrant connections. Workers in Raisman's and Zimmer's laboratories recently have shown that it is possible to microdissect and selectively implant tissue from fetal hippocampal fields, from around E18, when the subfields are clearly distinguishable, and to trace the specificity of graft–host connections with these selective grafts, using a variety of cell stains, monoclonal antibodies, genetic markers, and tracing techniques. Selective labeling of grafts from different hippocampal fields also is under development (195). Tønder et al. (165) implanted E18 to 20 fetal hippocampal CA3 suspension grafts into a host CA3 field lesioned a week earlier with

ibotenic acid to destroy the pyramidal cell bodies while leaving intact the host mossy fiber projections to the area. Six or more weeks later, histologic examination showed that 90% of grafts survived, contained normal CA3 neurons (pyramidal cells, and those reactive to peptidergic, cholecystokinin, and somatostatin immunostaining), and were innervated by host septal AChE-positive and dentate gyrus Timm-positive neurons. Anterograde and retrograde tracing showed that grafts projected to the host CA1 area, and that there were two-way commissural connections between host and graft. The detailed synaptic pattern of connections between host mossy fibers and grafted E20 CA3 neurons was examined by Field et al. (39) using the monoclonal antibody Py to label CA3 cells, and Timm staining for mossy fiber projections. Host dentate granule cells projected exclusively to the normal juxtacellular region of the grafted dendritic field, and were seen at the electron microscopic level to reach 20% of normal synaptic density. CA3 grafts implanted distally in the host septum showed no mossy fiber synapses, whereas grafted CA1 cells implanted in the mossy fiber pathway also received an insignificant number of host projections, with only a few mossy fiber terminals. These findings indicated that grafts of hippocampal fields not only become integrated in the host neural network, but do so in a highly specific manner; host innervation proceeded along normal laminar routes, and faltered when presented with the "wrong" pyramidal cells. A similar specificity has been shown by grafts of entorhinal fetal tissue implanted after lesions to the host entorhinal cortex. Using solid grafts within the lesioned entorhinal cortex and Thy 1.1/Thy 1.2 allelic markers to distinguish between donor and host mouse brain, Zhou et al. (196) showed that grafts projected to the normal terminal regions in the stratum moleculare of the host. Woodhams et al. (189) used the monoclonal antibodies OM 1–4 to provide evidence for an intrinsic signaling system directing fetal entorhinal fibers along appropriate routes. OM 1–4 label the dendritic zones (the outer two thirds) along which fibers from the entorhinal cortex to the dentate gyrus normally project in the rat. Both solid fragments and cell suspension grafts of entorhinal tissue in the denervated dentate gyrus restored staining in this outer band, with OM 2–4 throughout its width, and OM 1 in a narrower inner band.

Transplant Strategy Using Hippocampal Field Grafts

Findings detailed in the previous section provide evidence for an astonishing precision in the patterns of reinnervation after implantation of grafts from discrete hippocampal fields into the appropriate host region. This means that a powerful strategy is available to investigate mechanisms of graft action in rats (or primates) with relatively discrete lesions to the CA1 field after global ischemia. One can ask whether grafts of

CA1 cells are more successful in improving behavioral deficits in ischemic animals, and form richer, more normal connections within ischemic host brain, than grafts from other regions, including other hippocampal fields. Because cells from the major fields (CA1, CA3, and DG) all release glutamate, findings that CA1 grafts are more behaviorally effective and structurally integrated than DG or CA3 grafts would suggest that release of the appropriate neurotransmitter is not a key factor in promoting functional recovery. This in turn would suggest that homotypic field grafts do not function via pharmacologic transmitter replacement, as suggested for dopamine-rich and cholinergic-rich grafts in lesion models (see section on strategies for neural transplantation). Field specificity of functional recovery would indicate that homotypic replacement of cells is important, and this would be consistent with a true point-to-point mechanism of graft action. Initial findings from our laboratory (64,65,116) have suggested that in male Wistar rats sub-

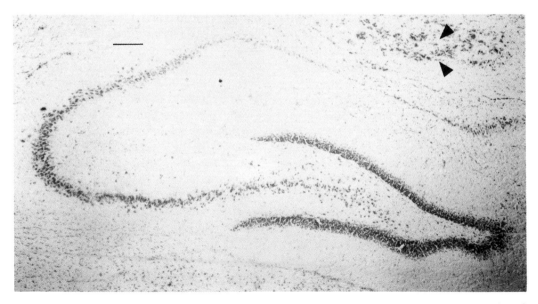

FIG. 1. Nissl-stained coronal section showing a CA1 pyramidal cell graft (*arrows*), 8 months after transplantation, sited above the area of ischemic cell loss in the dorsal CA1 hippocampal field of the host. Scale bar represents 500 μm.

jected to 15 min of 4-VO, grafts from CA1 are indeed more behaviorally effective than grafts from other hippocampal fields.

Comparison of CA1 and Dentate Granule Grafts after Global Ischemia

Our first study (116) compared effects of E18 to 19 CA1 and DG cell suspension grafts, microdissected according to the method of Field et al. (39). Embryonic day 15, cholinergic-rich grafts, which we previously had found to be effective in cholinergic-deficient animals (2,63), were used for nonhippocampal control tissue. Transplantation took place 3 to 4 weeks after 15 min of 4-VO using the method of Pulsinelli (134). For behavioral testing, we used acquisition in the water maze, testing animals after ischemia and from 4 weeks to 6 months after transplantation using retention, reversal, and novel platform positions, with either four trials/day and a 5-min ITI, or the more difficult procedure of two trials/day and a 10-min ITI. We also used a working memory test with four trials/day, a 30-sec ITI, and different platform positions on each of 6 days. When first tested, ischemic rats showed substantial impairment of ac-

a: **Experiment 1**

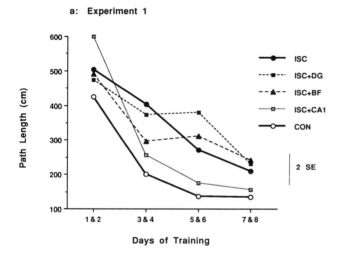

b: **Experiment 2**

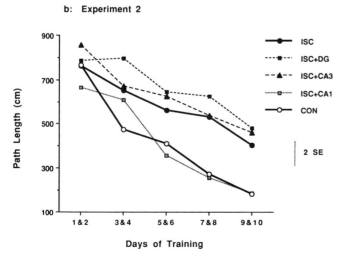

FIG. 2. Distance swum before locating the submerged platform in a novel pool by ischemic rats with hippocampal field grafts (ISC + CA1, ISC + CA3, ISC + DG) or basal forebrain (BF) grafts, in comparison to ischemic (ISC) and nonischemic (CON) controls. Experiment 1 shows the mean path length of CA1-, DG-, and BF-grafted groups (**a**). Experiment 2 shows the path length of rats with grafts from fields CA1 and CA3 (**b**). No survival was found in DG grafts dissected 2 days later (i.e., at postnatal day 1, rather than E18–19) than grafts in experiment 1. Hence this "DG" group must be regarded as a second ischemic control group. All rats were tested 6 months after grafting, but the greater water-maze experience of rats in experiment 1, which had been tested on six previous occasions in a different pool [see Netto et al. (116)], is reflected by shorter path lengths relative to rats in experiment 2, which had been tested only once before. In both experiments, rats with CA1 grafts performed at the nonischemic control level, and learned significantly more rapidly than ischemic rats or the other grafted groups. Rats with CA3 (experiment 2), or DG or BF grafts (experiment 1) were as impaired as the ischemic group relative to nonischemic controls.

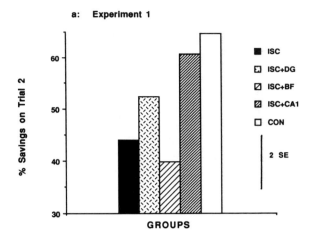

a: **Experiment 1**

GROUPS

■ ISC
▢ ISC+DG
▨ ISC+BF
▨ ISC+CA1
▢ CON

2 SE

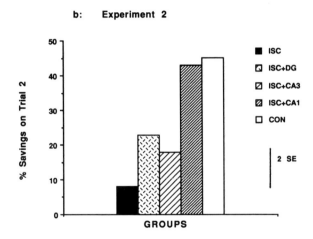

b: **Experiment 2**

GROUPS

■ ISC
▨ ISC+DG
▨ ISC+CA3
▨ ISC+CA1
▢ CON

2 SE

FIG. 3. Water-maze working memory performance in ischemic rats with hippocampal field grafts (ISC + CA1, ISC + CA3, ISC + DG) or basal forebrain (BF) grafts, compared to ischemic (ISC) and nonischemic (CON) controls. Experimental groups (**a,b**) were as in Fig. 2; note that the "DG" group in experiment 2, with no surviving grafts, performed comparably to the ischemic control group. Rats were tested 3 months (experiment 1: data from ref. 116) or 7 months (experiment 2) after grafting, in blocks of four (experiment 1) or three (experiment 2) trials, with a 30-sec ITI, and a different platform position for each block of trials. On trial 1, latency to locate the novel platform position was at chance level, and similar in all groups. Subsequent trials required matching to position, and the difference in latency on trial 2, relative to trial 1, shown as a percentage of trial 1 latency (percent savings), provides a measure of working memory across blocks. Despite the superior performance of the more maze-experienced animals in experiment 1 (also see Fig. 2), the pattern of savings was comparable in the two experiments. Rats with CA1 grafts found the platform as rapidly on trial 2 as controls, and their performance was significantly better than that of the ischemic or other grafted groups (apart from the DG group in experiment 1), whereas the groups with other types of graft or rejected grafts remained as impaired as the ischemic controls.

quisition in terms of latency, path length, and a reduced percentage of time in the training quadrant, and impaired memory for the platform location also was evident on the probe trial. However, on subsequent testing in a familiar pool, all ischemic groups showed improvement, although rats with CA1 grafts showed consistently better performance than the other ischemic groups. Ischemic deficits were most apparent with the sparse training regime, and were seen both in long-term acquisition and the working memory task, indicative of a rather general impairment in spatial learn-

ing. When rats were transferred to a new pool (see Fig. 2a), ischemic rats, and those with DG and basal forebrain grafts again showed substantial deficits, whereas rats with CA1 grafts performed at the nonischemic control level.

These findings showed that deficits in spatial learning can be detected by appropriate testing in a novel environment 7 months after ischemic injury and, also, that ischemic animals are able to form long-term spatial representations, because they performed relatively well in the familiar pool. The findings provided the first indication that CA1 grafts are more effective than those from another hippocampal field in alleviating ischemic deficits in spatial navigation. Histologic examination with Nissl and Timm staining and AChE histochemistry revealed that transplants survived in all the animals examined, sited in the alveus, above the area of maximum ischemic dorsal CA1 cell loss (see Fig. 1). Grafts contained cells resembling CA1 pyramidal or dentate granule cells, and were innervated by cholinergic fibers from the host medial septum. There were, however, several problems with this study that required clarification. First, grafts were tested in experienced rats, so that their efficacy against the full-blown initial acquisition deficit was not examined. Second, CA1 grafts (see Fig. 1) appeared to be more uniformly sized and thriving than the DG grafts, some of which were large but others much smaller, with signs of rejection. Morphologic studies (7) have shown that DG cells develop later than pyramidal cells, so that the age of the donor may have favored survival of CA1 rather than DG grafts. If so, functional efficacy may have been related to graft viability rather than to type of cell. We therefore set up a second study comparing effects of E18 to 19 CA1 with DG grafts, dissected at postnatal day 1 to 2 to optimize their chances of survival. We also included E18 to 19 CA3 grafts to provide a more stringent test of structural specificity, by comparing effects of two pyramidal cell grafts.

Comparison of CA1 and CA3 Grafts after Global Ischemia

Cell suspension grafts, dissected from CA1 and CA3 fields at E18 to 19, and from the dentate gyrus at postnatal day 1 to 2, were implanted in the alveus above the dorsal CA1 area 3 weeks after 15 min of 4-VO, as in the first experiment (116). However, subsequent histologic examination revealed that none of the DG grafts survived, and only 50% of the CA3, as opposed to 80% of the CA1 grafts survived. Thus, only 2 days increase in maturity would appear to put DG cells at further risk for grafting. These results suggest that the environment of the host favored homotypic grafts, possibly by release of growth factors more favorable to CA1 than to other types of cell. Target regulation of grafts by growth factors has been indicated in other models (185). For statistical analysis, animals without grafts in the CA1 and CA3 groups were excluded, so that results were compared in animals with comparable and healthy grafts in the CA1 and CA3 areas. However, the "DG" group was retained as a second ischemic quasi-control group (indeed, results of these two groups were very similar). Thus, it should be borne in mind that the "ISC + DG" group shown in Figs. 2b and 3b consisted of ischemic animals with additional glial scarring and tissue loss after graft rejection. When tested in water-maze acquisition 11 to 12 weeks after grafting (65), rats with CA1 grafts showed a very substantial degree of improvement, against the marked navigational deficits shown by ischemic controls or ischemic groups with CA3 and rejected DG grafts. The CA1 group found the platform as rapidly as controls, spent a larger proportion of time in the training quadrant than the other ischemic groups, and less time searching in the vicinity of the platform without finding it. However, ischemic rats learned to locate the platform over training trials, and they spent nearly as long as controls in searching in the quadrant formerly containing the platform on the probe trial. In terms of precise recall of the platform position on the probe trial, as shown by time spent in the counter area, all ischemic groups showed less accuracy on the probe trial than nonischemic controls. Ischemic groups also were less accurate in heading angle, a measure of the direct path to the platform. Thus, the CA1 graft dramatically improved efficiency of spatial learning, but not accuracy of retention or initial orientation relative to ischemic controls or ischemic rats with CA3 grafts. The selectivity of the effects of the CA1 grafts was confirmed by testing the animals in the three-door runway (159) for 12 days, 5 months after grafting. All the groups made a similar number of errors on the first cued trial, but on the matching to position trials (2–6), nonischemic controls and ischemic rats with CA1 grafts made significantly fewer errors of nudging closed doors than the other ischemic groups. The long-lasting nature of ischemic deficits and the persistence of recovery in the CA1 grafted group was assessed by retesting acquisition in a novel water maze 6 months after grafting, with results comparable to those seen initially in these animals and in the first study (116; see Figs. 2a and 2b). Superiority of the CA1 group in the water-maze working memory test also was replicated (see Figs. 3a and 3b). This experiment, therefore, confirmed that ischemic deficits in spatial information processing are long-lasting, and that selective improvements with the CA1 grafts were maintained. Unfortunately, the brains suffered from freezing artifacts, so that the tracing studies planned for this experiment could not be carried out, although the presence and siting of grafts was determined by Nissl staining, which revealed the lack of survival in the DG group and relatively poor survival in the CA3 group. Thus, detailed anatomic studies of graft connectivity have yet to be carried out, and animals have been prepared for this purpose. Nevertheless, the behavioral data permit some preliminary conclusions. First, the failure of glutamate-releasing cells from the dentate gyrus (exp. 1) and of pyramidal cells from the CA3 field (exp. 2) to promote functional recovery suggests that a high degree of cell-type specificity is involved. If, in grafts of comparable size and viability, there is evidence for richer connections between the host and CA1 grafts than grafts from the other fields, the results would be consistent with a point-

to-point action by the CA1 grafts to repair the area of CA1 cell loss induced by ischemia, as well as with a greater capacity for their survival.

A COMPARISON MODEL OF FIELD-SELECTIVE FUNCTIONAL RECOVERY: EFFECTS OF DENTATE GRANULE GRAFTS IN RATS WITH LESIONS OF THE DENTATE GYRUS

Injections of colchicine into the dentate gyrus (6) or neonatal x-irradiation (102) have been found to produce highly selective loss of granule cells, and behavioral changes including hyperactivity, stereotypy, deficits in passive avoidance, and spatial impairment. Deficits in water-maze learning resemble effects of global ischemic damage to the CA1 field, although they are more severe in rats with extensive damage to the dentate gyrus (191). Both Barone et al. (6) and Mickley et al. (102) found transient alleviation of deficits after dentate gyrus damage, the former with NGF infusion and the latter with fetal hippocampal grafts. The lack of efficacy of grafts in the Barone et al. study may have arisen because of large lesions, or use of tissue from the whole hippocampus. Our first study (191) found that in rats with extensive dentate gyrus damage and profound impairment of spatial navigation, fetal cell suspension dentate gyrus grafts produced no significant recovery. However, in rats with smaller lesions, which produced water-maze deficits comparable to those of global ischemia, solid DG grafts, but not CA1 grafts, promoted functional recovery in animals tested 8 weeks after grafting, at a point when neural connections between graft and host would have formed (Xavier et al., in preparation). These results are precisely the reverse of those found with CA1 grafts in ischemic animals, and strengthen the possibility that recovery from damage at different points in the trisynaptic hippocampal circuit may be field dependent.

Long-term potentiation (LTP) can be elicited in hippocampal grafts placed in the lesion cavity of rats with fornix–fimbria lesions, indicating that hippocampal grafts contain mechanisms for changes in synaptic efficiency (18). Our electrophysiologic examination of connectivity between E19 to 20 graft fragments from the CA1 and DG fields, placed in the lesion sites of rats with colchicine DG lesions, has revealed important dissociations (33). In both cases, field potentials and single-unit activity in the graft were evoked by stimulation in the mid-molecular layer of the host. Delivery of tetanizing trains at this site produced short-term potentiation and LTP in the grafted CA1 and DG fields, measured at 1 min and 15 min posttetanization. In lesioned rats with DG grafts, short-term potentiation reached control amplitudes, and was greater than in rats with CA1 grafts. However, LTP was found only in rats with DG grafts, and was not detected in animals with CA1 grafts. These findings provide the first evidence for field-specific differences in electrophysiologic response, according to whether grafts matched or differed from the lesioned cells in the host. Long-term potentiation of excitatory hippocampal synapses has been identified as an important early correlate of learning, analogous to Hebb's (59) "reverberating circuits," and is associated with activity at NMDA receptors (24,107). Lesions at any point along the trisynaptic circuit, or treatment with NMDA antagonists that prevent induction of LTP, are associated with deficits in learning and memory (107). Thus, Dawe et al.'s findings (33) may provide an important clue as to why grafts from hippocampal fields differ in their functional efficacy in ischemic or colchicine-lesioned animals: Homotypic grafts that replace the damaged cells may restore synaptic plasticity more effectively than grafts from other fields. Field et al.'s (39) evidence that host projections from the dentate gyrus formed richer connections with grafted CA3 and CA1 cells is consistent with Dawe's evidence for normalized induction of LTP in DG but not CA1 cells within the lesioned dentate gyrus. It is important, therefore, to examine electrophysiologic response in slices from grafted ischemic rats with CA1 damage, to see if host-activated LTP can be initiated in CA1 but not DG or CA3 grafts.

POTENTIAL THERAPEUTIC APPLICATIONS OF NEURAL TRANSPLANTATION AFTER ISCHEMIC DAMAGE

Although there is preliminary evidence that grafts survive in quite large areas of infarction in the rodent brain, the use of grafts after focal ischemia is still at a very early stage and lacks functional investigation. Given the order of magnitude of difference between the sizes of the human and rat brains, it is important to know if grafts can be scaled up, and for this non-human primate models are an essential first step. Because stroke damage (particularly via MCAO) involves both cortical and striatal areas, it also is necessary to investigate effects of multiple grafts into both of these regions. Use of growth factors may provide a viable approach, because there is preliminary evidence that these protect against secondary retrograde degeneration (91) and nitric oxide toxicity induced by ischemia (92,93). Co-grafts of neuronal tissue and growth factors may be particularly effective. It is possible that grafts in infarcted regions may operate in a nonspecific way, for instance to provide a matrix to sustain outgrowth from host neurons, or to prevent retrograde degeneration. Current evidence points strongly to the conclusion that grafts in infarcted or lesioned areas are richly innervated by the host, but do not extend long processes, and hence do not serve to reconstruct normal pathways. Hence, alternative types of tissue (e.g., cerebellum) might prove more robust, while being as functionally effective as homotypic grafts.

An important issue that has not yet been addressed in focal models is whether grafts might actually interfere with normal recovery. After stroke, approximately 50% of surviving patients show moderate to good recovery, with the most rapid progress over the first 8 to 10 weeks, followed by a more static plateau (36). Neuroimaging techniques indicate a succession of changes in regional blood flow and oxygen and glucose use that relate initially to the development of infarction, and then to spontaneous reorganization of functional activity. Thus, 24 hr after stroke, perfusion is reduced in the territory of the affected artery, and a day later the margins of the infarct show increases in CBF, possibly with rebound circulation (luxury perfusion). From days 6 to 15, there are marked increases in contralateral flow, with large, vivid areas of reactive hyperemia, coinciding with return of stretch reflexes, followed by intentional movement in proximal muscles. Differences from normal regional changes in metabolic activity in response to movement can be detected long after resting levels have stabilized (27,87). It is not known how grafts would interact with these spontaneous processes of reorganization, which may be present to some extent even in patients with poor recovery who might be potential recipients.

Grafting in the global ischemic model has several features that make it more promising in terms of eventual therapeutic application in humans than the use of transplants in focal models of ischemia, or in models of neurodegenerative disease, particularly those of Alzheimer's disease [see Sinden et al., (this volume)]. First, many systems are disrupted in neurodegenerative disease or after stroke, and pathology is widespread, so that grafts based on delivery of particular transmitters or tissue from a limited brain region may be ineffective. In contrast, damage after global ischemia in animals is highly localized, and there is good evidence that circumscribed hippocampal damage after heart attack in humans underlies the re-

sulting cognitive deficits (157). Because damage is localized, small grafts can be used, targeted to the region of cell loss, and these grafts would not be required to extend long processes. Moreover, localized areas of damage can be detected by neuroimaging techniques, to identify patients likely to benefit from grafting, and to monitor the growth of grafts (158,197). Second, patients with neurodegenerative disease usually are elderly and fragile in health, and would be particularly at risk from transplant surgery, whereas victims of heart attack often are quite young, better able to withstand surgery, and, provided that precipitating lifestyle factors are controlled, may have many healthy years ahead of them. Third, animal models do not as yet mimic the defining pathology of Alzheimer's disease, so we do not know whether grafted neurons would integrate in brain regions containing plaques and tangles, or indeed succumb to the disease processes. Grafts in heart attack victims with localized damage would be placed within otherwise healthy brains. However, grafted neurons may be as vulnerable or even more vulnerable than normal CA1 cells to effects of ischemia and, given our recent findings for optimal recovery with CA1 grafts (64,116), we may not have the option to choose more resistant types of cell. There has been no examination as yet of the effects of ischemia on CA1 grafts. However, Tønder et al. (166) examined effects of 4-VO ischemia in rats with dentate gyrus grafts sited in the ibotenate-lesioned dentate gyrus of the host. Loss of cells was found not only in the host CA1 field and hilus, but in grafted DG and CA3 pyramidal cells, which normally are resistant to ischemia. Thus, grafted neurons may indeed be more susceptible than the host to effects of a second heart attack. This is disappointing from the viewpoint of clinical applications, but repeated ischemia may be a useful method to achieve experimental graft "rejection" (166) to see how far behavioral recovery depends on the continuing presence of CA1 grafts.

CURRENT OBJECTIVES AND FUTURE PROSPECTS FOR ANIMAL MODELS OF ISCHEMIA

Before transplants can be envisaged as treatment for effects of heart attack or stroke in humans, there are several ways in which animal models can be developed to provide more information about the cognitive effects of ischemia, graft efficacy, and mechanisms of action. The primary requirement is for the demonstration of graft efficacy in the primate models of ischemia that have been developed for global and focal ischemia (8,198; see section on primate models of ischemia with hippocampal damage).

Second, there is a need for more refined and reliable behavioral tests of the effects of ischemia, particularly in focal models. Even neurologic assessment is relatively undeveloped, so that we do not know how persistent impairment in grasping and fine motor control is, although the gross rotation and locomotor deficits appear to be transient. The possibility that MCAO produces cognitive deficits (118), perhaps through loss of cortical cholinergic function, requires further investigation. Deficits in discrimination learning, found in animals with cortical lesions, have not been investigated in animals with cortical infarcts. In models of global ischemia, where cognitive effects have been linked to hippocampal function and more thoroughly investigated, there still is a need for more sensitive and reliable tests, because effects of discrete CA1 subfield damage may be smaller and more subtle than those of large hippocampal lesions (70). Because both cortical and hippocampal damage is found with longer durations of 4-VO (107), there also is a need for tests to discriminate between effects of cell loss at the two sites (e.g., win-shift/lose-stay conditional discrimination; 151). Steady-state measures of behavioral deficit are required to examine the time course and stability of behavioral recovery after transplantation. Acquisition in the water maze is extremely sensitive to effects of global ischemia, but animals show marked improvement with repeated testing (116; see section on comparison of CA1 and DG grafts), so that this task is not optimal for long-term studies.

Third, there is a need for more detailed analysis of the connectivity between transplant and host. Elegant histologic analyses have been undertaken to trace connections between hippocampal field grafts and host (39,165,197; see section on grafts from hippocampal fields: connectivity studies), but not extensively in ischemic rats, and still more rarely after behavioral testing. Electrophysiologic studies also will contribute substantially to our understanding of the functional links between graft and host. For instance, the demonstration that LTP can be evoked in DG but not CA1 grafts in animals with colchicine lesions of the dentate gyrus (33) calls for extension of LTP studies to rats with ischemic loss of CA1 cells. Restoration of LTP in ischemic rats with CA1 grafts would provide powerful support for the behavioral evidence of selective, field-dependent functional recovery, and would indicate that synaptic plasticity provided by the grafts may be related to the recovery of spatial learning ability. Electrophysiologic studies also will provide a method of assessing possible deleterious effects of grafts, particularly if sited in the hippocampus. Buzsaki et al. (17,19) have shown, both in intact rats and in those with subcortical hippocampal denervation, that grafts of fetal hippocampal tissue in the hippocampus can act as a focus for epileptic activity, or reduce the threshold for picrotoxin-induced seizures. It also is possible that paroxysmal activity could be triggered by cortical or striatal grafts in MCAO-induced infarcted regions. Although we have not observed seizures in ischemic rats over 6 to 8-month periods after grafting, the possibility that hippocampal grafts may trigger epileptic attacks and create further brain damage warrants investigation.

Finally, alternatives to neuronal fetal homografts and methods to increase graft out-growth require investigation, because clinical development of transplantation will require nonfetal sources of donor tissue. Xenografts are the simplest alternative, but without immunosuppression (and often with it) these grafts are rejected, with deleterious pathologic consequences to the host, including edema, macrophage invasion, demyelination, and cell death (153). Consequently, much recent effort has gone into the development of cells for grafting that are more immunologically inert, including glial cells to deliver growth factors; neuroblastoma cells chemically treated to promote differentiation; potentially autologous cells from myenteric plexus, or autologous fibroblasts, which may be genetically transfected so as to express desired characteristics (e.g., transmitters, growth factors); and cells encapsulated in polymer to allow diffusion of low–molecular-weight substances, but otherwise minimize contact between graft and host (152). Response to growth factors in both cortical infarcted tissue (187) and ischemic hippocampal cell cultures (92) provides encouraging evidence that neurons damaged by ischemia are receptive to trophic influences. Recent findings that NT-3 (23), in cultures of developing hippocampal cells, stimulates the number of neurons expressing calbindin suggest that this factor supports the differentiation and survival of discrete populations of hippocampal neurons, in particular those (e.g., DG cells) that are resistant to glutamate toxicity. A similar strategy may be applicable to CA1 cells. A still more interesting possibility is that application of growth factors may stimulate *de novo* growth of cells of neuronal morphology *in situ*. Richards et al. (138) identified neuronal cells arising from dividing precursors in dissociated cell populations of adult mouse brain that grew optimally when stimulated with bFGF and exposed to a medium conditioned by an astrocytic cell line, Ast-1. If the signals for proliferation and differentiation of these precursor cells can be

identified, the possibility exists for replacement of damaged cells within the area of cell loss. A major new approach has been the development of neuroepithelial stem cell lines from primordial hippocampus that differentiate on transplantation into identifiable neurons and glia with phenotypes and connectivity appropriate to the host site (137,155). This may provide transplant tissue that is immunologically safe, and fosters normal, homotypic-like cell development *in situ*. Immortal stem cells also may be transfected, for instance with a temperature-sensitive oncogene (152), to permit them to differentiate when placed in host. These cells, therefore, offer the possibility of donor tissue, with a low potential to evoke immune responses, with neuronal phenotype potential, and into which it is possible to include additional desired genes, so that it may be applicable to both focal and global models of ischemic brain damage.

CONCLUSIONS

Although effects of neural transplantation only recently have been investigated in models of ischemic brain damage, several important findings have emerged. First, successful survival of fetal homografts has been shown within large areas of infarction after MCAO, and the capacity of these grafts to improve cognitive deficits has been demonstrated. Second, there is evidence for reduction in ischemic brain damage after delivery of growth factors. Third, grafts of fetal hippocampal tissue in animals subjected to global ischemia, which preferentially damages cells in the hippocampal CA1 field, have been shown to form appropriate connections within the host and to ameliorate deficits in spatial navigation. Fine-grained analysis, permitted by use of grafts dissected from discrete fetal hippocampal fields, has indicated a surprising degree of functional specificity, in that grafts dissected from the fetal CA1 field were

CEREBRAL TRANSPLANTATION IN ISCHEMIA *379*

found to be significantly superior to grafts of DG or CA3 cells in improving deficits in spatial learning and working memory in rats with selective CA1 cell loss after global ischemia. The detailed comparison of connectivity of CA1 grafts with those from other hippocampal fields in ischemic rats has not yet been undertaken. However, in rats with colchicine lesions of the dentate gyrus, which also showed field-specific improvement of spatial navigation with DG but not CA1 grafts, LTP was elicited in rats with DG but not CA1 grafts, suggesting that homotypic cell replacement reestablishes neuronal plasticity. Subfield graft-induced recovery from the effects of ischemic CA1 lesions, therefore, provides an opportunity to investigate "point-to-point" mechanisms of functional recovery. In terms of future therapeutic efficacy, use of grafts to promote recovery from widespread effects of stroke will require extensive further investigation in animal models, and possibly combined use of cortical, striatal, and growth factor grafts. In contrast, loss of CA1 hippocampal cells after heart attack may be identified by neuroimaging techniques, and provides a relatively limited target for specific grafts.

ACKNOWLEDGMENTS

Our research was supported by the British Heart Foundation, the Wellcome Trust, the Medical Research Council, the Bethlem Maudsley Trust, and CNPq, Brasil.

REFERENCES

1. Andiné P, Jacobson I, Hagberg H. Enhanced calcium uptake by CA1 pyramidal cell dendrites in the postischemic phase despite subnormal evoked field potentials: excitatory amino acid receptor dependency and relationship to neuronal damage. *J Cereb Blood Flow Metab* 1992;12:733–783.
2. Arendt T, Allen Y, Marchbanks R, et al. Cholinergic system and memory in the rat: effects of chronic ethanol, embryonic basal forebrain transplants and excitotoxic lesions of the forebrain cholinergic projection system. *Neuroscience* 1989;33:435–462.
3. Arvin B, Moncada C, Le Peillet E, Chapman A, Meldrum BS. GYKI 52466 blocks the increase in extracellular glutamate induced by ischemia. *NeuroReport* 1992;3:235–238.
4. Auer RN, Jensen ML, Whishaw IQ. Neurobehavioral deficit due to ischemic brain damage limited to half of the CA1 sector of the hippocampus. *J Neurosci* 1989;9:1641–1647.
5. Baddeley A. Amnesia: a minimal model and interpretations. In: Cermak L, ed. *Human memory and amnesia.* Hillsdale, NJ: Erlebaum; 1984:305–336.
6. Barone S, Tandon P, McGinty J, Tilson HA. Effects of NGF and fetal cell transplantation on spatial learning after intradentate administration of colchicine. *Exp Neurol* 1991;114:351–363.
7. Bayer SA. Development in the hippocampal region in the rat: 1. neurogenesis examined with 3H-thymidine autoradiography. *J Comp Neurol* 1980;190:87–114.
8. Bechevalier J, Mishkin M. Mnemonic and neuropathological effects of occluding the posterior cerebral artery in *Macacca mulatta*. *Neuropsychologia* 1989;27:83–105.
9. Björklund A, Stenevi U. Intracerebral neural transplants: neuronal replacement and reconstruction of damaged circuitries. *Annu Rev Neurosci* 1984;7:279–308.
10. Bode-Greuel KM. 5-H$_{1A}$ receptor agonists as neuroprotective agents in cerebral ischemia. In: Kriegelstein J, ed. *Pharmacology of cerebral ischemia.* Stuttgart: Wissenschaftliche Verlagsgesellschaft mbH;1990.
11. Boissard CG, Lindner MD, Gribkoff VK. Hypoxia produces cell death in the rat hippocampus in the presence of A$_1$ adenosine receptor antagonist: an anatomical and behavioral study. *Neuroscience* 1992;48:807–812.
12. Bradbury E, Kershaw T, Marchbanks R, Sinden J. Foetal basal forebrain cell type transplants and behavioural recovery. *Rest Neurol Neurosci* 1992;4:145.
13. Brierley JB, Graham DI. Hypoxia and vascular disorders of the central nervous system. In: Hulme Adams J, Corsellis JAN, Duchen LW, eds. *Greenfield's neuropathology.* London: Edward Arnold; 1984:125–207.
14. Buchan AM. The N-methyl-D-aspartate antagonist MK-801 fails to protect against neuronal damage caused by transient severe forebrain ischemia in adult rats. *J Neurosci* 1991;11:1049–1056.
15. Buchan AM, Yue D, Slivka A. A new model of temporary focal neocortical ischemia in the rat. *Stroke* 1992;23:273–279.
16. Busto R. Hank SI, Yoshida S, Scheinberg P, Ginsberg MD. Cerebral norepinephrine depletion enhances recovery after brain ischemia. *Ann Neurol* 1985;18:329–336.
17. Buzsaki G, Ponomareff G, Bayardo F, Shaw T, Gage FH. Suppression and induction of epilep-

tic activity by neuronal grafts. *Proc Natl Acad Sci USA* 1988;85:9327–9330.

18. Buzsaki G, Wiesner J, Henriksen SJ, Gage FH. Long-term potentiation of evoked and spontaneous neuronal activity in the grafted hippocampus. *Exp Brain Res* 1989;76:410–408.

19. Buzsaki G, Maslieh E, Chen LS, Horvath Z, Terry R, Gage FH. Hippocampal grafts into the intact brain induce epileptic patterns. *Brain Res* 1991;554:30–37.

20. Castro AJ, Hogan TP, Shaw PL, Schulz MK. Connectivity of neocortical transplants placed into the N-methyl-D-aspartate (NMDA) ablated cortex of adult rats. *Rest Neurol Neurosci* 1992;4:216.

21. Cenci MA, Kalen P, Mandel RJ, Wictorin K, Björklund A. Dopaminergic transplants normalise amphetamine- and apomorphine-induced fos expression in the 6-hydroxydopamine-lesioned striatum. *Neuroscience* 1992;46:943–957.

22. Churn SB, Yaghmai A, Povlishock J, Rafiq A, De Lorenzo R. Global forebrain ischemia results in decreased immunoreactivity of calcium/calmodulin dependent protein kinase II. *J Cereb Blood Flow Metab* 1992;12:784–793.

23. Collazo D, Takahashi H, McKay RDG. Cellular targets and trophic functions of neurotropin-3 in the developing rat hippocampus. *Neuron* 1992;9:643–656.

24. Collingridge GL. Long-term potentiation in the hippocampus: mechanisms of initiation and modulation by neurotransmitters. *Trends Neurosci* 1985;6:407–411.

25. Combs DJ, D'Alecy LG. Motor performance in rats exposed to severe forebrain ischemia: effects of fasting and 1,3-butanediol. *Stroke* 1987;18:503–511.

26. Comelli MC, Guidolin D, Seren MS, et al. Time course, localization and pharmacological modulation of immediate early inducible genes, brain-derived neurotrophic factor and trkB messenger RNAs in the rat brain following photochemical stroke. *Neuroscience* 1993;55:473–490.

27. Costa DC, Ell PJ. *Brain blood flow in neurology and psychiatry.* Edinburgh: Churchill-Livingstone; 1991.

28. Cummins JL, Tomiyasu U, Read S, Benson DF. Amnesia with hippocampal lesions after cardiopulmonary arrest. *Neurology* 1984;34:679–681.

29. Damsma G, Boisvert DP, Mudrick LA, Wenkstem D, Fibiger HC. Effects of transient forebrain ischemia and pargyline on extracellular concentrations of dopamine, serotonin, and their metabolites in the rat striatum as determined by in vivo microdialysis. *J Neurochem* 1990;54:801–808.

30. Davis HP, Tribuna J, Pulsinelli WA, Volpe BT. Reference and working memory of rats following ischemic hippocampal damage. *Physiol Behav* 1986;37:387–392.

31. Davis HP, Baranowski JR, Pulsinelli WA, Volpe BT. Retention of reference memory following ischemic hippocampal damage. *Physiol Behav* 1987;39:783–786.

32. Davis HP, Volpe BT. Memory performance after ischemic or neurotoxin damage of the hippocampus. In: Squire LR, Lindenlaub E, eds. *The biology of memory.* Stuttgart, New York: Symposia Medica Hoechst 23, FK Schattauer Verlag; 1990:477–507.

33. Dawe GS, Gray JA, Sinden JD, Stephenson JD, Segal M. Extracellular recordings in the colchicine-lesioned rat dentate gyrus following transplants of fetal dentate gyrus and CA1 hippocampal subfield tissue. *Brain Res* 1993;625:63–74.

34. Dawson GR, Heyes CM, Iversen SD. Pharmacological mechanisms and animal models of cognition. *Behav Pharmacol* 1992;3:285–297.

35. Dewar D, Chalmers DT, Graham DI, McCullogh T. Glutamate metabotropic and AMPA sites are reduced in Alzheimer's disease: an autoradiographic study of the hippocampus. *Brain Res* 1991;553:58–64.

36. Dombovy ML, Bach-y-Rita P. Clinical observations on recovery from stroke. *Adv Neurol* 1988;47:265–276.

37. Dunnett SB, Björklund A, Stenevi U, Iversen SD. Behavioural recovery following transplantation of substantia nigra into rats subjected to 6-OHDA lesions of the nigrostriatal pathway: 1. unilateral lesions. *Brain Res* 1981;215:147–161.

38. Eichenbaum H, Stewart C, Morris RGM. Hippocampal representation in place learning. *J Neurosci* 1991;10:3531–3542.

39. Field PM, Seeley PJ, Frotscher M, Raisman G. Selective innervation of embryonic hippocampal transplants by adult host dentate granule cell axons. *Neuroscience* 1991;41:713–727.

40. Fine A, Meldrum BS, Patel S. Modulation of experimentally induced epilepsy by intracerebral grafts of fetal GABAergic neurons. *Neuropsychologia* 1990;28:627–634.

41. Fischer W, Wictorin K, Björklund A, Williams LR, Varon S, Gage FH. Amelioration of cholinergic neuron atrophy and spatial memory impairment in aged rats by nerve growth factor. *Nature* 1987;329:65–68.

42. Frim DM, Uhler TA, Short MP, et al. Effects of biologically delivered NGF, BDNF and bFGF on striatal excitotoxic lesions. *NeuroReport* 1993;4:367–370.

43. Gage FH, Björklund A, Stenevi U, Dunnett SB, Kelly PAT. Intrahippocampal septal grafts ameliorate learning impairments in aged rats. *Science* 1984;225:533–536.

44. Gage FH, Kawaja MD, Fisher LJ. Genetically modified cells: applications for intracerebral grafting. *Trends Neurosci* 1991;14:328–333.

45. Garthwaite J, Meldrum BS. Excitatory amino acid neurotoxicity and neurodegenerative disease. *Trends Pharm Sci* 1990;11:379–387.

46. Gibbs RB, Yu J, Cotman CW. Entorhinal transplants and spatial memory abilities in rats. *Behav Brain Res* 1987;26:29–35.

47. Globus MYT, Busto R, Dietrich WD, Martinez E, Valdes I, Ginsberg MD. Effects of ischemia

on the in vivo release of striatal dopamine, glutamate and γ-amino butyric acid studied by intracerebral microdialysis. *J Neurochem* 1988; 51:1455–1464.

48. Globus MYT, Busto R, Dietrich WD, Martinez E, Valdes I, Ginsberg MD. Direct evidence for acute and massive norepinephrine release in hippocampus during transient ischemia. *J Cereb Blood Flow Metab* 1989;9:892–896.

49. Goedert M, Fine A, Hunt SP, Ullrich A. Nerve growth factor mRNA in peripheral and central rat tissues and in the human central nervous system: lesion effects in the rat brain and levels in Alzheimer's disease. *Mol Brain Res* 1986; 1:85–92.

50. Grabowski M, Nordberg C, Johansson BB. Sensorimotor performance and rotation correlates to lesion size in right but not left hemisphere brain infarcts in the spontaneously hypertensive rat. *Brain Res* 1991;547:249–257.

51. Grabowski M, Brundin P, Johansson BB. Fetal neocortical grafts implanted in adult hypertensive rats with cortical infarcts following a middle cerebral artery occlusion: ingrowth of afferent fibres from the host brain. *Exp Neurol* 1992;116:105–121.

52. Grabowski M, Christofferson RH, Brundin P, Johansson BB. Vascularization of fetal neocortical grafts implanted in brain infarcts in spontaneously hypertensive rats. *Neuroscience* 1992; 51:673–82.

53. Grabowski M, Brundin P, Johansson BB. Paw-reaching, sensorimotor, and rotational behavior after brain infarction in rats. *Stroke* 1993; 24:889–895.

54. Graham DI. Hypoxia and vascular disorders. In: Hulme Adams J, Duchen LW, eds. *Greenfield's neuropathology*. London: Edward Arnold; 1992:153–268.

55. Greenamyre JT, Young AB. Excitatory amino acids and Alzheimer's disease. *Neurobiol Aging* 1989;10:593–602.

56. Guan J, Williams C, Gunning M, Mallard C, Gluckman P. The effects of IGF-1 treatment after hypoxic–ischemic brain injury in adult rats. *J Cereb Blood Flow Metab* 1993;13:609–616.

57. Gustafson I, Westerberg EJ, Wieloch T. Extracellular brain cortical levels of noradrenaline in ischemia: effects of desipramine and postischemic administration of idazoxan. *Exp Brain Res* 1991;86:555–561.

58. Hagan BJ, Beaughard M. The effects of forebrain ischemia on spatial learning. *Behav Brain Res* 1990;41:151–160.

59. Hebb DO. *The organisation of behavior*. New York: Wiley;1949.

60. Herranz AS, Cannon-Spoor HE, Freed WJ. Attempted reconstruction of the corticostriatal pathway using fetal cortical tissue transplants. *Rest Neurol Neurosci* 1992;4:216.

61. Heyes MP, Brew BJ, Martin A, et al. Quinolinic acid in cerebrospinal fluid and serum in HIV-1 infection: relationship to clinical and neurological status. *Ann Neurol* 1991;29:202–209.

62. Hillered L, Hallstrom A, Segersvard S, Persson L, Ungerstedt U. Dynamics of extracellular metabolites in the striatum after middle cerebral artery occlusion in the rat monitored by intracerebral microdialysis. *J Cereb Blood Flow Metab* 1989;9:607–616.

63. Hodges H, Allen Y, Kershaw T, Lantos PL, Gray JA, Sinden JD. Effects of cholinergic-rich neural grafts on radial maze performance of rats after excitotoxic lesions of the forebrain cholinergic projection system: 1. amelioration of cognitive deficits by transplants into cortex and hippocampus but not into basal forebrain. *Neuroscience* 1991;45:587–607.

64. Hodges H, Sinden JD, Netto CA, et al. Graft-induced recovery of cognitive function after focal or diffuse brain damage. *Rest Neurol Neurosci* 1992;4:133.

65. Hodges H, Sowinski P, Fleming P, et al. Foetal CA1 grafts selectively alleviate ischaemic deficits in spatial learning and working memory. *J Cereb Blood Flow Metab* 1993;13(Suppl 1):S51.

66. Hoffman MC, Nitsch S, Scotti AZ, Reinhard E, Monarch D. The prolonged presence of glia-derived nexin, an endogenous protease inhibitor, in the hippocampus after ischemia-induced delayed neuronal death. *Neuroscience* 49;1992: 397–408.

67. Horel JA. The neuroanatomy of amnesia. *Brain* 1978;101:403–445.

68. Iizuka H, Sakatani K, Young W. Neural damage in the rat thalamus after cortical infarcts. *Stroke* 1990;21:790–794.

69. Irle E, Wowra B, Kunert HJ, Hampl J, Kunze S. Memory disturbances following anterior communicating artery rupture. *Ann Neurol* 1992;31:473–480.

70. Jarrard LE. Selective hippocampal lesions and behavior: implications for current research and theorizing. *The Hippocampus* 1986;4:93–126.

71. Jaspers RMA, Block F, Heim C, Sontag K-H. Spatial learning is affected by transient occlusion of common carotid arteries (2-VO): comparison of behavioral and histopathological changes after "2-VO" and "four vessel occlusion" in rats. *Neurosci Lett* 1990;117:149–153.

72. Johansen FF, Jørgenson MB, Diemer NH. Ischemic CA1 pyramidal cell loss is prevented by pre-ischemic colchicine destruction of dentate gyrus cells. *Brain Res* 1986;377:344–347.

73. Jørgenson MB, Johanson FF, Diemer NH. Removal of the entorhinal cortex protects hippocampal CA1 neurons from ischemic damage. *Acta Neuropathol* 1987;73:189–194.

74. Kar S, Baccichet A, Quirion R, Poirier J. Entorhinal cortex lesion induces differential responses in [^{125}I]insulin-like growth factor I, [^{125}I]insulin-like growth factor II and [^{125}I]insulin receptor binding sites in the rat hippocampal formation. *Neuroscience* 1993;55:69–80.

75. Kataoka K, Hayakawa T, Ryotaro K, Yuguchi T, Yamada K. Cholinergic deafferentation after focal cerebral infarct in rats. *Stroke* 1991;22: 1291–1296.

76. Kataoka K, Yamada K, Tokuno T, et al. Single unit changes in VPL neurons after cortical ablation in rats and effect of b-FGF treatment. *J Cereb Blood Flow Metab* 1993;13(Suppl 1):S58.

77. Katayama Y, Tsubokawa T, Koshinaga M, Miyazaki S. Temporal pattern of survival and dendritic growth of fetal hippocampal cells transplanted into ischemic lesions of the adult rat hippocampus. *Brain Res* 1991;562:352–355.

78. Kawaja MD, Gage FH. Reactive astrocytes are substitutes for the growth of adult central nervous system axons in the presence of elevated levels of nerve growth factor. *Neuron* 1991; 7:1019–1030.

79. Kesslack JP, Nieto-Sampedro M, Globus J, Cotman CW. Transplants of purified astrocytes promote behavioral recovery after frontal cortex ablation. *Exp Neurol* 1986;92:377–390.

80. Kesslack JP, Walencewicz A, Calin L, Nieto-Sampedro M, Cotman CW. Hippocampal, but not astrocyte transplants enhance recovery on a forced choice alternation task after kainate lesions. *Brain Res* 1988;454:347–354.

81. Kiessling M, Mies G, Paschen W, Thilman R, Detmar M, Hossman K-A. Blood flow and metabolism in heterotypic cerebellar grafts during hypoglycaemia. *Acta Neuropathol* 1988;77: 142–151.

82. Kimble DP, Bremiller R, Stickrod G. Fetal brain implants improve maze performance in hippocampal-lesioned rats. *Brain Res* 1986; 363:358–363.

83. Kitigawa K, Matsumoto M, Niinobe M, et al. Microtubule-associated protein 2 as a sensitive marker for cerebral ischemic damage: immunohistochemical investigation of dendritic damage. *Neuroscience* 1989;31:410–411.

84. Kiyota Y, Miyamoto M, Nagaoka A. Relationship between brain damage and memory impairment in rats exposed to transient forebrain ischemia. *Brain Res* 1991;538:295–302.

85. Kohmura E, Tsuruzono K, Tamada K, Yuguci, T, Hayakawa T. Neurotoxicity caused by hypoxia and excitatory amino acids: modulation by basic fibroblast growth factor (bFGF). *J Cereb Blood Flow Metab* 1993;13(Suppl 1):S62.

86. Lanier WL, Perkins WJ, Karlsson BR, et al. The effects of dizocilpine maleate (MK-801), an antagonist of the N-methyl-D-aspartate receptor on neurologic recovery and histopathology following complete cerebral ischemia in primates. *J Cereb Blood Flow Metab* 1990;10:252–261.

87. Lenzi GL, Frackowiak RSJ, Jones T. Cerebral oxygen metabolism and blood flow in human cerebral ischaemic infarction. *J Cereb Blood Flow Metab* 1982;2:321–335.

88. Le Peillet E, Arvin B, Moncada C, Meldrum BS. The non-NMDA antagonists NBQX and GYKI 52466 protect against cortical and striatal cell loss following transient global ischaemia in the rat. *Brain Res* 1992;571:115–120.

89. Leranth C, Ribak CE. Calcium binding proteins are concentrated in the CA2 field of the mon-key hippocampus: possible key to this region's resistance to epileptic damage. *Exp Brain Res* 1991;85:129–136.

90. Lescaudron L, Stein DG. Functional recovery following transplants of embryonic brain tissue in rats with lesions of visual, frontal and motor cortex: problems and prospects for future research. *Neuropsychologia* 1990;28:585–599.

91. Liberini P, Pioro EP, Maysinger D, Ervin FD, Cuello AC. Cortical devascularizing lesion model in primates: long term effect of human recombinant nerve growth factor and mono-sialganglioside treatment. *Soc Neurosci Abstr* 1992;18:774.

92. Maiese K, Boniece I, Wagner JA. Peptide growth factors are neuroprotective during ischemic-induced nitric oxide toxicity in primary hippocampal cell cultures. *Soc Neurosci Abstr* 1992;18:1453.

93. Maiese K, Boniece D, DeMeto D, Wagner JA. Neuroprotection by peptide growth factors during anoxia and nitric oxide toxicity. *J Cereb Blood Flow Metab* 1993;13(Suppl 1):S43.

94. Mampalam TJ, Gonzalez MF, Weinstein P, Sharp FR. Neuronal changes in fetal cortex transplanted to ischemic adult rat cortex. *J Neurosurg* 1988;69:904–912.

95. Mattson MP, Chang B, Davis D, Bryant K, Lieberburg L, Rydel RE. B amyloid peptides destabilize calcium homeostasis and render human cortical neurons vulnerable to excitotoxicity. *J Neurosci* 1992;12:376–389.

96. Meldrum BS. Excitatory amino acids in epilepsy and in acute and chronic neuronal degenerative disorders. In: Huether G, ed. *Amino acid availability and brain function in health and disease*. Berlin and Heidelberg: Springer Verlag; 1988:325–332.

97. Meldrum B. Protection against ischaemic neuronal damage by drugs acting on excitatory neurotransmission. *Cerebrovasc Brain Metab Rev* 1990;2:27–57.

98. Meldrum BS, Arvin B, Chapman AG, Durmuller N, Lees GT. Modulation of excitotoxicity by monoamines. In: Krigelstein J, Oberpichler H, eds. *Pharmacology of cerebral ischemia*. Stuttgart: Wissenschaftliche Verlagsgesellschaft mbH; 1990:459–467.

99. Meldrum BS. Protection against ischemic brain damage by excitatory amino acid antagonists. In: Bazan NG, Braquet P, Ginsberg MD, eds. *Advances in neurochemistry*. New York: Plenum Press; 1992:245–263.

100. Meldrum BS. Excitatory amino acid receptors and disease. *Current Opp Neurol Neurosurg* 1992;5:508–513.

101. Memezawa H, Minamisawa H, Smith M-L, Siesjo BK. Ischemic penumbra in a model of reversible cerebral artery occlusion in the rat. *Exp Brain Res* 1992;89:67–78.

102. Mickley GA, Ferguson JL, Mulvihill MA, Nemeth TJ. Early neural grafts transiently reduce the behavioral effects of radiation-induced fascia dentata granule cell hypoplasia. *Brain Res* 1991;550:24–34.

103. Mishkin M. Memory in monkeys is severely impaired by combined but not by separate removal of amygdala and hippocampus. *Nature* 1978;273:297–298.

104. Mitani A, Kataoka K. Cortical levels of extracellular glutamate mediating gerbil hippocampal delayed neuronal death during hypothermia: brain microdialysis study. *Neuroscience* 1991;42:661–670.

105. Moncada C, Lekieffre D, Arvin B, Meldrum BS. Effect of NO synthase inhibition on NMDA- and ischemia-induced hippocampal lesions. *NeuroReport* 1992;3:530–532.

106. Morris RGM, Garrud P, Rawlins JNP, O'Keefe J. Place navigation is impaired in rats with hippocampal lesions. *Nature* 1982;297:681–683.

107. Morris RGM, Anderson E, Lynch GS, Baudry M. Selective impairment of learning and blockade of long-term potentiation by an N-methyl-D-aspartate receptor antagonist AP5. *Nature* 1986;319:774–776.

108. Mudrick LA, Baimbridge KG, Peet MJ. Hippocampal neurons transplanted into ischemically lesioned hippocampus: electroresponsiveness and re-establishment of circuitries. *Exp Brain Res* 1989;76:333–342.

109. Mudrick LA, Baimbridge KG. Hippocampal neurons transplanted into ischemically lesioned hippocampus: anatomical assessment of survival, maturation and integration. *Exp Brain Res* 1991;86:233–247.

110. Mufson EJ, Labbe R, Stein DG. Morphological features of embryonic neocortex grafts in adult rats following frontal cortical ablation. *Brain Res* 1987;86:233–247.

111. Murase K, Kato H, Liu X-H, Katoh-Semba R, Kato K, Kogure K. Alterations of nerve growth factor (NGF) content and glial reactions following lethal and non-lethal ischemia in gerbil brain. *J Cereb Blood Flow Metab* 1993;13 (Suppl 1):S47.

112. Myers R, Margil LG, Cullen BM, Price GW, Frackowiak SJ, Cremer JE. Macrophage and astrocyte populations in relation to [³H] PK 11195 binding in rat cerebral cortex following local ischemic lesion. *J Cereb Blood Flow Metab* 1991;11:314–322.

113. Nakuma M, Araki M, Oguro K, Masuzawa T. Differential distribution of 68 Kd and 200 Kd neurofilament proteins in the gerbil hippocampus and their early distributional changes following transient forebrain ischemia. *Exp Brain Res* 1992;89:31–39.

114. Nemeth G, Cintra A, Herb J-M, et al. Changes in striatal dopamine neurohistochemistry and biochemistry after incomplete transient cerebral ischemia in the rat. *Exp Brain Res* 1991;86:545–554.

115. Nemoto EM, Bleyaert AL, Stezoski SW, et al. Global brain ischemia: a reproducible monkey model. *Stroke* 1977;8:558–564.

116. Netto CA, Hodges H, Sinden JD, et al. Effects of foetal hippocampal field grafts on ischaemic-induced deficits in spatial navigation in the water maze. *Neuroscience* 1993;54:69–92.

117. Nilsson OG, Björklund A. Behaviour dependent changes in acetylcholine release in normal and graft-reinnervated hippocampus: evidence for host regulation of grafted cholinergic neurons. *Neuroscience* 1992;49:33–44.

118. Nishino H, Koide K, Aihara N, Mitzukawa K, Nagai H. Striatal grafts in infarct striatum after occlusion of the middle cerebral artery improve passive avoidance/water maze learning, GABA release and GABA_A receptor deficits in the rat. *Rest Neurol Neurosci* 1992;4:178.

119. Nozaki K, Finklestein S, Beal MF, Uemura Y, Kikuchi H. Basic fibroblast growth factor protects against hypoxia–ischemia and NMDA toxicity in neonatal rats. *J Cereb Blood Flow Metab* 1993;13(Suppl 1):S54.

120. Nunn JA, Le Peillet E, Netto CA, et al. CA1 cell loss produces deficits in learning and memory in the water maze regardless of additional intra- and extra-hippocampal damage. *J Cereb Blood Flow Metab* 1991;11(Suppl 2):S338.

121. Nunn JA, Le Peillet E, Netto CA, et al. CA1 cell loss produces deficits in the water maze but not in the radial maze. *Soc Neurosci Abstr* 1991;17:108.

122a.Nunn JA, Cerebral ischaemia: hippocampal pathology and spatial deficits in the rat. PhD Thesis, Faculty of Science, London University, 1993.

122b.Nunn JA, Le Peillet E, Netto CA, Hodges H, Gray JA, Meldrum BS. Global ischaemia, hippocampal pathology, and special deficits in the water maze. *Behav Brain Res (in press)*.

123. O'Keefe J, Nadel L. *The hippocampus as a cognitive map.* Oxford: Clarendon Press; 1978.

124. Olney JW. Neurotoxicity of excitatory amino acids. In: McGeer E, Olney JW, McGeer P, eds. *Kainic acid as a tool in neurobiology.* New York: Raven Press; 1978:201–217.

125. Olton DS, Becker JT, Handelman GE. Hippocampus, space and memory. *Behav Brain Sci* 1979;2:313–365.

126. Onadera H, Sato G, Kogure K. Lesions to Schaffer collaterals prevent ischemic death of CA1 pyramidal cells. *Neurosci Lett* 1986;68:169–174.

127. Onadera H, Sato G, Kogure K. Autoradiographic analysis of muscarinic cholinergic and adenosine A1 binding sites after transient forebrain ischemia in the gerbil. *Brain Res* 1987;415:309–322.

128. Onifer SM, Low WC. Spatial memory deficit resulting from ischemia-induced damage to hippocampus is ameliorated by intra-hippocampal transplants of foetal hippocampal neurons. *Prog Brain Res* 1990;82:359–366.

129. Ott BR, Saver JL. Unilateral amnesic stroke. *Stroke* 1993;24:1033–1042.

130. Perlow MF, Freed WF, Hoffer B, Seiger A, Olson L, Wyet RJ. Brain grafts reduce motor abnormalities produced by destruction of the nigrostriatal dopamine system. *Science* 1979;204:643–647.

131. Perry EK, Tomlinson BE, Blessed G, Bergman K, Gibson PH, Perry RH. Correlation of cho-

linergic abnormalities with senile plaques and mental test scores in senile dementia. *Br Med J* 1978;2:1457–1459.

132. Petito CK, Feldman E, Pulsinelli WA, Plum F. Delayed neuronal hippocampal damage in humans following cardiorespiratory arrest. *Neurology* 1987;37:1281–1286.

133. Phillips S, Sangalang V, Sterns G. Basal forebrain infarction: a clinicopathologic correlation. *Arch Neurol* 1987;44:1134–1138.

134. Pulsinelli WA, Brierley MD, Plum F, Temporal profile of neuronal damage in a model of transient forebrain ischemia. *Ann Neurol* 1982; 11:491–498.

135. Rawlins JNP. Associations across time: the hippocampus as a temporary memory store. *Behav Brain Sci* 1985;8:479–496.

136. Regli L, Anderson RE, Meyer FB. Basic fibroblast growth factor increases cerebral blood flow in vivo. *J Cereb Blood Flow Metab* 1993;13(Suppl 1):S66.

137. Renfranz PJ, Cunningham MC, McKay RDG. Region-specific differentiation of the hippocampal stem cell line Hi BS upon implantation into the developing mammalian brain. *Cell* 1991;66:713–729.

138. Richards LJ, Kilpatrick TJ, Bartlett PF. De novo generation of cells from the adult mouse brain. *Proc Natl Acad Sci USA* 1992;89:8591–8595.

139. Ridley RM, Baker HF. A critical evaluation of monkey models of amnesia and dementia. *Brain Res Rev* 1991;16:15–37.

140. Rod MR, Whishaw IQ, Auer RN. The relationship of structural ischemic brain damage to neurobehavioural deficit: the effect of postischemic MK-801. *Can J Psychol* 1990;44:196–209.

141. Rod MR, Auer RN. Combination therapy with nimodipine and dizocilpine in a rat model of transient forebrain ischemia. *Stroke* 1992;23:196–209.

142. Sakaguchi T, Yamada K, Yuguchi E, et al. Focal cerebral ischaemia induces mRNA expression of fibroblast growth factor receptor. *J Cereb Blood Flow Metab* 1993;13(Suppl 1):S49.

143. Sakai N, Ryu JH, Yanai K, Nagasawa H, Watanabe T, Kogure K. Behavioral studies on transient cerebral ischemia induced by middle artery occlusion in rats. *J Cereb Blood Flow Metab* 1993;13(Suppl 1):S76.

144. Scheller MS, Grafe MR, Zornow MH, Fleischer JH. Effects of ischemia duration on neurological outcome, CA1 histopathology and nonmatching to sample learning in monkeys. *Stroke* 1992;23:1471–1478.

145. Schmidt-Kastner R, Freund TF. Selective vulnerability of the hippocampus in brain ischaemia. *Neuroscience* 1991;40:599–636.

146. Scoville WB, Milner B. Loss of recent memory after bilateral hippocampal lesions. *J Neurol Neurosurg Psychiatry* 1957;20:11–21.

147. Seubert P, Lee K, Lynch G. Ischemia triggers NMDA receptor-linked cytoskeletal proteolysis in hippocampus. *Brain Res* 1991;492:366–370.

148. Shimohama S, Tamura Y, Akaike A, et al. Protection by recombinant human nerve growth factor against glutamate cytotoxity in the cultured cortical neurons. *J Cereb Blood Flow Metab* 1993;13(Suppl 1):S65.

149. Simon RP, Griffiths T, Evans MC, Swan JH, Meldrum BS. Calcuim overload in selectively vulnerable neurons of the hippocampus during and after ischemia: an electron microscopy study in the rat. *J Cereb Blood Flow Metab* 1984;4:350–361.

150. Simon RP, Swan JH, Griffith T, Meldrum BS. Blockade of N-methyl-D-aspartate receptors may protect against ischemic damage in the brain. *Science* 1984;226:850–852.

151. Sinden JD, Allen YS, Rawlins JNP, Gray JA. The effects of ibotenic acid lesions of the nucleus basalis and cholinergic-rich neural transplantation on win-stay/lose-shift and win-shift/lose-stay performance in the rat. *Behav Brain Res* 1990;36:229–249.

152. Sinden JD, Patel SN, Hodges H. Neural transplantation: problems and prospects for therapeutic application. *Current Opp Neuropathol* 1992;5:902–908.

153. Sloan DJ, Wood MJ, Charlton HM. The immune response to intracerebral neural grafts. *Trends Neurosci* 1991;14:341–346.

154. Smith SE, Meldrum BS. Cerebroprotective effect on a non-N-methyl-D-aspartate antagonist, GYKI 52466, after focal ischemia in the rat. *Stroke* 1992;23:861–864.

155. Snyder EY, Deitcher DL, Walsh C, Arnold-Alden S, Hartwieg EA, Cepko CL. Multipotent neural cell lines can engraft and participate in development of mouse cerebellum. *Cell* 1992; 68:33–51.

156. Sprick U. Transient and long-lasting beneficial behavioral effects of grafts in the damaged hippocampus of the rat. *Behav Brain Res* 1991; 42:187–199.

157. Squire LR. Mechanisms of memory. *Science* 1986;232:1612–1619.

158. Squire LR, Amaral DG, Press GA. Magnetic resonance imaging of the hippocampal formation and mamillary nuclei distinguish medial temporal lobe and diencephalic amnesia. *J Neurosci* 1990:3110–3117.

159. Sugimachi K, Izawa K, Nakamura K, et al. Impairment of working memory by neuronal degeneration with NMDA in rat hippocampal CA1. *Behav Pharmacol* 1992;3:379–385.

160. Sutherland RJ, McDonald RJ. Hippocampus, amygdala, and memory deficits in rats. *Behav Brain Res* 1990;37:57–79.

161. Takeda A, Onadera H, Sugimoto A, Kogure K, Obinata M, Shibahara S. Coordinated expression of messenger RNAs for nerve growth factor, brain-derived neurotrophic factor and neurotrophin-3 in the rat hippocampus following transient forebrain ischaemia. *Neuroscience* 1993;55:23–31.

162. Tamura A, Nagashima H, Tsujita Y, Nakayama H, Kirino T, Sano K. Behavioral changes after cerebral infarction in rats. *J Cereb Blood Flow Metab* 1993;13(Suppl 1):S53.

163. Tandon P, McLamb RL, Novicki D, Shuey D, Tilson HA. Fetal hippocampal cell suspensions ameliorate behavioral effects of intradentate colchicine in the rat. *Brain Res* 1988;473:241–248.

164. Tønder N, Sørenson T, Zimmer J, Jørgenson MB, Johanson FF, Diemer NH. Neural grafting to ischemic lesions of the adult rat hippocampus. *Exp Brain Res* 1989;74:512–526.

165. Tønder N, Sorenson T, Zimmer J. Grafting of CA3 neurons to excitotoxic axon-sparing lesions of the hippocampal CA3 area in adult rats. *Prog Brain Res* 1990;83:391–409.

166. Tønder N, Aznar S, Johansen FF, Diemer NH, Zimmer J. Fascia dentata transplants in axon-sparing lesions of the adult rat hippocampus are susceptible to cerebral ischemia. *Rest Neurol Neurosci* 1992;4:216.

167. Tsuchiya M, Sako K, Yura S, Yonemasu Y. Cerebral blood flow and histopathological changes following permanent bilateral carotid ligation in Wistar rats. *Exp Brain Res* 1992;89:87–92.

168. Tsukahara T, Yonekawa Y, Yanaka K, Kimura T, Taniguchi T. Brain-derived neurotrophic factor after transient forebrain ischemia in the rat hippocampus. *J Cereb Blood Flow Metab* 1993;13(Suppl 1):S57.

169. Tsuda T, Kogure K, Nishioka K, Watanabe T. Mg^{2+} administered up to twenty four hours following reperfusion prevents ischemic damage of the CA1 neurons in the rat hippocampus. *Neuroscience* 1991;44:335–341.

170. Turner JJ, Hodges H, Sinden JD, Gray JA. Comparison of radial maze performance of rats after ibotenate and quisqualate lesions of the forebrain cholinergic projection system: effects of pharmacological challenge and changes in training regime. *Behav Pharmacol* 1992;3:359–373.

171. Ulas J, Brunner LC, Jades JW, Shoe W, Cotman CW. N-methyl-D-aspartate receptor complex in the hippocampus of elderly normal individuals, and those with Alzheimer's disease. *Neuroscience* 1992;49:45–61.

172. Varon S, Agate, Manthorpe M. Neuronal growth factors. In: Seil FJ, ed. *Neural regeneration and transplantation*. New York: Alan R. Liss; 1989:101–121.

173. Van Horne CG, Stromberg I, Young D, Olson L, Hoffer B. Functional enhancement of intrastriatal dopamine-containing grafts by the cotransplantation of sciatic nerve tissue in 6-hydroxydopamine lesioned rats. *Exp Neurol* 1991;113:143–154.

174. Vass K, Welch WJ, Nowack TS. Localization of 70-KDa stress protein induction in gerbil brain after ischemia. *Acta Neuropathol* 1988;77:128–135.

175. Voll CL, Whishaw IQ, Auer RN. Postischemic insulin reduces spatial learning deficit following transient forebrain ischemia in rats. *Stroke* 1989;20:646–651.

176. Volpe BT, Pulsinelli WA, Tribuna J, Davis HP. Behavioral performance of rats following transient forebrain ischemia. *Stroke* 1984;15:558–562.

177. Volpe BT, Petito CK. Dementia with bilateral medial temporal lobe ischemia. *Neurology* 1985;35:1793–1797.

178. Volpe BT, Colombo P, Davis HP. Preoperative training modifies radial maze performance in rats with ischemic hippocampal injury. *Stroke* 1989;20:1700–1706.

179. Volpe BT, Davis HP, Towle A, Dunlap WP. Loss of hippocampal CA1 neurons correlates with memory impairment in rats with ischemic or neurotoxin lesions. *Behav Neurosci* 1992;106:457–464.

180. Wahl F, Allix M, Plotkine M, Bouhi RG. Neurological and behavioral outcomes of focal cerebral ischemia in rats. *Stroke* 1992;23:267–272.

181. Weinrauch V, Safar P, Fisherman S, Kuboyama K, Radovsky A. Beneficial effect of mild hypothermia and detrimental effect of deep hypothermia after cardiac arrest in dogs. *Stroke* 1992;23:1454–1462.

182. Wenk GL, Walker LC, Price DL, Cork LC. Loss of NMDA but not $GABA_A$ binding in the brain of aged rats and monkeys. *Neurobiol Aging* 1991;12:93–98.

183. Wets KM, Sinden J, Hodges H, Allen Y, Marchbanks R. Specific brain protein changes correlated with behaviourally effective brain transplants. *J Neurochem* 1991;57:1661–1670.

184. Widmer HR, Knussel B, Hefti F. BDNF protection of basal forebrain cholinergic neurons after axotomy: complete protection of p75NGFR-positive cells. *NeuroReport* 1993;4:363–366.

185. Whittemore SR, White LA. Target regulation of neuronal differentiation in a temperature-sensitive cell line derived from medullary raphe. *Brain Res* 1993;615:27–40.

186. Wieloch T, Koide T, Westerberg E. Inhibitory transmitters and neuromodulators as protective agents against ischemic brain damage. In: Krigelstein J, ed. *Pharmacology of ischemia brain damage*. Amsterdam: Elsevier; 1986:191–197.

187. Williams CE, Guan J, Dragunow M, Glickman P. Effects of insulin-like growth factor-1 (IGF-1) treatment two hours after hypoxic–ischemic injury. *Soc Neurosci Abstr* 1992;18:1260.

188. Winn SR, Fresco PA, Zeilinski B, Greene LA, Jaeger CB, Aebischer P. Behavioral recovery following intrastriatal implantation of microencapsulated PC 12 cells. *Exp Neurol* 1991;113:322–329.

189. Woodhams PL, Kawano H, Raisman G. The OM series of terminal field-specific monoclonal antibodies demonstrate reinnervation of the adult rat dentate gyrus by embryonic entorhinal transplants. *Neuroscience* 1992;46:71–82.

190. Woodruff MI, Baisden RH, Nonneman AJ. Effects of transplantation of fetal hippocampal or hindbrain tissue into brains of adult rats with hippocampal lesions on water maze acquisition. *Behav Neurosci* 1992;118:39–50.

191. Xavier GF, Kershaw TR, Gray JA, Sinden JD. Foetal dentate and CA1 subfield transplants and spatial orientation following colchicine le-

sions of the dentate gyrus. *Eur J Neurosci* 1991;(Suppl 4):103.

192. Yamada K, Otsuki H, Kohmura E, et al. Neurotrophic activity detected in the peri-infarcted brain tissue is partly mediated by basic FGF. *J Cereb Blood Flow Metab* 1993;13(Suppl 1):S55.

193. Yamaguchi T, Takahashi K, Yamamoto M. YM796, a novel M1-selective agonist, improves the impairments of learning behavior in a rat model of chronic focal cerebral ischemia. *J Cereb Blood Flow Metab* 1993;13(Suppl 1):S71.

194. Yuguchi T, Yamada K, Kohmura K, Otsuki H, Kishiguchi T, Hayakawa T. Expression of basic FGF receptor in CNS injury: gene expression and protein dynamics. *J Cereb Blood Flow Metab* 1993;13(Suppl 1):S45.

195. Zheng J, Onadera H, Kogure K. Mapping signal transduction systems in the kainate-lesioned hippocampus after transplantation of fe-

tal hippocampal neurons. *J Cereb Blood Flow Metab* 1993;13(Suppl 1):S50.

196. Zhou FC, Li Y, Raisman G. Embryonic entorhinal transplants project selectively to the deafferented entorhinal zone of the adult mouse hippocampi as demonstrated by the use of Thy-1 allelic immunohistochemistry: effect of timing of transplantation in relation to deafferentation. *Neuroscience* 1989;32:349–362.

197. Zola-Morgan S, Squire LR, Amaral DG. Human amnesia and the medial temporal region: enduring memory impairment following a bilateral lesion limited to field CA1 of the hippocampus. *J Neurosci* 1986;6:2950–2967.

198. Zola-Morgan S, Squire LR, Rempel NL, Clower RP, Amaral DG. Enduring memory impairment in monkeys after ischemic damage to the hippocampus. *J Neurosci* 1992;12:2582–2596.

Functional Neural Transplantation,
edited by S. B. Dunnett and A. Björklund.
Raven Press, Ltd., New York © 1994.

15

Grafts in Models of Epilepsy

Olle Lindvall, Johan Bengzon, Eskil Elmér, Merab Kokaia, and Zaal Kokaia

*Restorative Neurology Unit, Department of Neurology, University Hospital,
S-221 85 Lund, Sweden*

Compared to studies in models of neurodegenerative diseases, considerably less work has been performed with cell transplantation to the CNS in experimental epilepsy. One major explanation is that, unlike the situation in, for example, Parkinson's disease, the deficit that should be corrected for by grafts in epilepsy is not known. Epileptic seizures are characterized by hyperexcitability and synchronization of activity among populations of central neurons. Impairment of inhibitory γ-aminobutyric acid (GABA)ergic transmission and abnormal increase of excitatory (e.g., glutamatergic) mechanisms have been suggested to play a major role (73). Long-loop neuronal circuitries, such as the inhibitory noradrenergic locus coeruleus system (20), also might be able to influence the development and generalization of epileptiform activity.

Cell transplantation to the brain has several attractive features, both as a research tool to elucidate pathophysiologic mechanisms underlying seizure activity and, in a longer perspective, as a possible therapeutic strategy to dampen human epilepsy. For example, fetal CNS tissue rich in neurons producing a certain transmitter can be implanted at different sites in the normal or lesioned brain to clarify the role both of these neurons, and of the target region innervated by the graft, for seizure development and generalization. Cell transplantation also offers a possibility for long term delivery of an inhibitory transmitter locally in the epileptic focus or in a region critical for seizure spread. Finally, neural grafting may be carried out with epileptic tissue into a nonepileptic host, which allows for detailed studies of the anatomic, biochemical, and physiologic basis of epileptogenesis.

The initial transplantation studies have been carried out to explore the possibility that intracerebral neural grafts are able to influence seizure activity in the CNS, and to obtain basic information on how grafts can operate in epilepsy. There are several reasons why implantation of fetal noradrenaline (NA)-rich tissue from the locus coeruleus region has become particularly useful as a model system: First, considerable evidence has accumulated indicating that intrinsic locus coeruleus neurons act to dampen epileptic activity in the CNS (see, e.g., ref. 20); second, the anatomy of this system is well known, and the locus coeruleus neurons can easily be demonstrated microscopically and also are susceptible to relatively specific destruction using 6-hydroxydopamine (6-OHDA; see, e.g., ref. 12); third, there is extensive knowledge of the biochemical, pharmacologic, and physiologic characteristics of presynaptic and postsynaptic noradrenergic mechanisms (see, e.g., ref. 29); and fourth, grafted locus coeruleus neurons have been shown to grow into the host brain and modify the function and behavior of the host (see, e.g., ref. 54).

The objectives of the present chapter are twofold: first, to describe how neural graft-

TABLE 1. *Summary of studies using transplantation to the central nervous system in animal models of epilepsy*[a]

Authors	Epilepsy model	Lesion	Type/location of implant	Control implant	Functional effects	Graft survival/ingrowth/correlation to effects
Barry et al. (1987)	Hippocampal kindling	6-OHDA i. vent.	Fetal NA-rich locus coeruleus/hippocampus	Saline	Suppression of kindling rate	>100 NA neurons per side/NA reinnervation of dorsal hippocampus/yes
Cassel et al. (1987)	Subcortically denervated hippocampus	Fimbria–fornix	Fetal ACh-rich basal forebrain/hippocampus	Saline	Increased reactivity to PTZ and decreased reactivity to sound	AChE-positive grafts in most rats/poor AChE-positive reinnervation/no
Holmes et al. (1987)	Amygdala kindling	No	Fetal neocortex/hippocampus	Ringer	No effects on kindling rate	Good survival/not shown/no
Buzsáki et al. (1988)	Subcortically denervated hippocampus	Fimbria–fornix	Fetal NA-rich locus coeruleus or hippocampus/hippocampus	Fetal hippocampus or locus coeruleus	Increased latency to picrotoxin-evoked behavioral seizures and reduced frequency of interictal spikes (locus coeruleus grafts); increased incidence of interictal spikes and behavioral seizures (hippocampus grafts)	Survival of NA or GABA neurons/NA ingrowth/not shown
Stevens et al. (1988)	Amygdala kindling	No	Fetal GABA-rich cerebellum or cerebral cortex/deep prepiriform area	No	Transient changes of seizure threshold in a minority of rats	Survival of grafts but no GABA neurons/not shown/not shown
	Genetically epilepsy-prone rats	Removal of occipital poles	Fetal GABA-rich cerebellum or cerebral cortex/inferior colliculi	No	No changes in seizure characteristics in grafted rats	Poor graft survival/not shown/not shown
	Genetically epilepsy-prone rats	No	Catecholamine-rich adrenal medulla/lateral ventricle	No	Minor change of seizure intensity in one of six rats	Scattered catecholamine cells/not shown/not shown
Barry et al. (1989)	Hippocampal kindling	6-OHDA i. vent.	Fetal NA-rich locus coeruleus/amygdala–piriform cortex	Saline	Suppression of kindling rate	NA neurons in all rats/NA ingrowth/not shown
Buzsáki et al. (1989)	Subcortically denervated hippocampus	Fimbria–fornix	Fetal hippocampus/solid pieces in lesion cavity, suspension in hippocampus	No	Interictal spikes and epileptic activity in graft, behavioral seizures in host	Survival of all solid grafts and most suspension grafts/reciprocal connections with solid grafts/not shown
Bengzon et al. (1990)	Hippocampal kindling	6-OHDA i. vent.	Fetal NA-rich locus coeruleus/hippocampus	No	Suppression of kindling rate in grafted rats blocked by idazoxan (α_2 adrenoreceptor antagonist)	>200 NA neurons per side/NA reinnervation of dorsal hippocampus/not shown

388

continued

Reference	Model	Pretreatment/lesion	Graft tissue/location	Control	Results	Survival/integration
Camu et al. (1990)	Olfactory bulb kindling	5,7-DHT in olfactory bulb	Fetal 5-HT-rich raphe/ olfactory bulb	Fetal cortex or vehicle	Suppression of kindling rate and reduction of AD duration	5-HT neurons in most rats/5-HT ingrowth/not shown
Fine et al. (1990)	Systemic pilocarpine	Bilateral intrastriatal ibotenic acid	Fetal GABA-rich striatum/substantia nigra pars reticulata	Sciatic nerve	Reduced seizure severity score also in controls	Survival of GABA neurons not shown/not shown/not shown
Bengzon et al. (1991)	Hippocampal kindling	6-OHDA i. vent.	Fetal NA-rich locus coeruleus/ hippocampus	No	Suppression of kindling rate; restoration of basal and seizure-evoked NA release in hippocampus	114–374 NA neurons per side/NA reinnervation of dorsal hippocampus/yes
Buzsáki et al. (1991)	Intact brain	No	Fetal hippocampus/ hippocampus	Fetal cerebellum	Interictal spikes in host hippocampus, stimulus-evoked behavioral seizures	Survival in 6 or 10 rats/not shown/ effects only with surviving grafts
Cassel et al. (1991)	Subcortically denervated hippocampus	Fimbria–fornix	Fetal ACh-rich septum or hippocampus/ hippocampus	No	Decreased reactivity to PTZ by both grafts at 3 but not at 7 and 12 months; increased reactivity to sound at 3 and 7 (only hippocampal grafts) but not at 12 months	Survival in all animals, AChE-positive grafts/septal grafts reinnervate hippocampus/no
Clough et al. (1991)	Genetically epilepsy-prone rats	No	Fetal NA-rich locus coeruleus/dorsal hippocampus or third ventricle	Fetal neocortex	No group effects; decreased severity of audiogenic seizures in some animals with i. vent. grafts	NA neurons in most rats/NA ingrowth not shown/not shown
Holmes et al. (1991)	Kainic acid	No	Fetal locus coeruleus, cerebellum, neocortex or hippocampus/lateral ventricle	Saline	Slight reduction of frequency of spontaneous seizures in hippocampus and locus coeruleus grafted groups; no change in percentage of rats with spontaneous recurrent seizures or in kindling rate	Survival of graft tissue but NA or GABA cells not shown/not shown/ not shown
Teillet et al. (1991)	Genetic epilepsy in F. epi (intermittent light stimulation)	No	Defined areas of neuroepithelium in F. epi/substitution of same areas in normal chicken at E2	Neuroepithelium of normal chicken	Transplantation of both prosencephalon and mesencephalon for full epileptic phenotype	Good survival of graft/integration with host brain/yes
Guy et al. (1992)	Genetic epilepsy in F. epi	No	Prosencephalon alone or + mesencephalon/ substitution of same areas in normal chicken at E2	No	Less severe motor seizures with prosencephalon alone; lower threshold to PTZ seizures in chimeras than in normal controls	Good survival of graft/integration with host brain/yes

TABLE 1. *Continued.*

Holmes et al. (1992)	Genetically epilepsy-prone rats	No	Fetal NA-rich locus coeruleus, neocortex or cerebellum/inferior colliculi or lateral ventricle	Ringer	Longer latency to tonic phase and shorter duration of clonic phase after audiogenic stimulation in all grafted groups, seizure severity unchanged; no influence on kindling rate	Survival of graft tissue but NA or GABA cells not shown, no change of NA in CSF/not shown/not shown
Bengzon et al. (1993)	Hippocampal kindling	6-OHDA i. vent.	Fetal NA-rich locus coeruleus/hippocampus	Saline	No change of seizure characteristics in kindled rats	200–300 NA neurons per side/NA reinnervation of dorsal hippocampus/not shown
	Hippocampal kindling	No	Fetal NA-rich locus coeruleus/hippocampus	Saline	No effects on kindling rate	300 NA neurons per side/NA innervation in the vicinity of the grafts/not shown
	Hippocampal kindling	No	Fetal NA-rich locus coeruleus/hippocampus	Fetal cerebellum	Restoration of kindling-induced decrease of basal NA release; no effect on seizure characteristics	350 NA neurons/NA innervation in the vicinity of the grafts/not shown
Kokaia et al. (1994)	Amygdala kindling	No	GABA-releasing polymer matrix/substantia nigra	Polymer matrix without GABA	Prevention of generalized seizures in kindled rats after 2 days but not 7 and 14 days	Good/no/GABA release high during first 3 days
	Hippocampal kindling	6-OHDA i. vent.	NA-releasing polymer matrix/hippocampus	Polymer matrix without NA	No effects on kindling rate	Good/no/NA release high during first 2 weeks

[a]All studies except those by Teillet et al. (76) and Guy et al. (39), which were carried out in chicken, have been performed on rat epilepsy models. ACh, acetylcholine; AChE, acetylcholinesterase; AD, after discharge; 5,7-DHT, 5,7-dihydroxytryptamine; F. epi, Fayoumi chicken; GABA, γ-aminobutyric acid; 5-HT, 5-hydroxytryptamine; i. vent., intraventricular; NA, noradrenaline; 6-OHDA, 6-hydroxydopamine; PTZ pentylenetetrazol.

ing has been used as a tool either to reduce or to increase neuronal excitability in a variety of seizure models (summarized in Table 1), and how it has provided interesting data on pathophysiologic mechanisms in experimentally induced seizures; and secondly, to discuss some current research strategies—in particular, those aiming at the development of transplantation approaches to dampen epileptic activity in the brain.

CHOICE OF EPILEPSY MODEL FOR GRAFTING STUDIES

Not all animal seizure models are suitable for neural grafting, although they still may be useful for other types of implants, such as neurotransmitter-releasing polymer matrices or genetically engineered, nonneuronal cells. The epileptic syndromes are either too variable, or transient and resolve before the graft-derived innervation is complete, or the seizure-inducing agent is toxic to the transplanted fetal neurons. The time course of axonal outgrowth from the fetal CNS graft and synapse formation with neuronal elements in the host brain must be taken into account when the experimental model is chosen. For example, reinnervation of the denervated hippocampus by noradrenergic axons from an intrahippocampal locus coeruleus graft occurs over a period of 2 to 3 months. Obviously, no meaningful information will be obtained if locus coeruleus neurons are implanted into animals with experimental epilepsy that will resolve spontaneously within 1 or 2 months. An alternative approach is then to induce the epileptic syndrome in grafted animals after reinnervation has been completed, and to compare the results with those obtained in appropriate controls.

Even under optimal conditions in rat-to-rat grafting experiments, there is a variability in the degree of graft survival within a group of recipients. To allow for correlation analysis between, for example, cell number or density of reinnervation from the graft,

and various parameters of the epileptic syndrome (e.g., seizure threshold), it is of great importance that the model used has a high reproducibility. Furthermore, the epileptogenic agent must not have any toxic effects on the grafted neurons. This could cause either poor cell survival or inhibited outgrowth, or degeneration if the induction of epilepsy is carried out after the graft has grown into the host brain. The repeated electrical stimulations performed in kindling seem to have no such adverse effects on grafted locus coeruleus neurons (3,4, 7,8). In contrast, the application of cobalt leads to few surviving noradrenergic neurons and restricted axonal ramifications from locus coeruleus implants (Trottier et al., unpublished).

GRAFTS IN KINDLING

The Kindling Model

Kindling is one of the most extensively studied animal models of epilepsy (38). It refers to a process whereby repeated administration of an initially subconvulsive electrical stimulus results in progressive intensification of stimulus-induced seizure activity, culminating in a generalized seizure (see, e.g., ref. 70). The initial stimulus evokes focal seizure activity (so-called afterdischarge) recorded on EEG without overt clinical signs of convulsions. The following stimulations lead to the development of kindled seizures, which generally proceed through five distinguishable grades (69): grade 0, normal behavior, arrest, wet-dog shakes; grade 1, facial twitches; grade 2, chewing, head nodding; grade 3, forelimb clonus; grade 4, rearing; grade 5, rearing and falling on the back. When the animal has exhibited grade 5 seizures, it is said to be kindled. This effect is permanent, and even if the animal is left unstimulated for as long as 12 months, it will respond to one of the first electrical stimuli with a grade 5 seizure (79). Kindling triggered by electrical stimulation of the limbic system has been proposed to be analogous to complex partial epilepsy (60), which is the most frequent type of epilepsy in adult humans (36).

Noradrenaline-Releasing Implants

Rats with extensive lesions of NA neurons in the forebrain (induced by intraventricular injection of 6-OHDA) exhibit a marked acceleration in the rate of kindling evoked by electrical stimulation in the amygdala or hippocampus (Fig. 1). This is caused by removal of the powerful inhibitory influence on the development of kindled seizures normally exerted by the locus coeruleus system (1,22,56–58). A series of grafting experiments has been carried out in such animals with the following main ob-

jectives: first, to explore the possibility that locus coeruleus grafts can reverse the functional deficit induced by the 6-OHDA lesion, that is, retard the kindling rate in NA-depleted, hyperexcitable rats; second, to clarify how these grafts exert their functional effects in kindled seizures; and, third, to obtain more information on the role and mode of action of the intrinsic locus coeruleus system in kindling. Fetal locus coeruleus grafts implanted bilaterally into the hippocampus retarded the development of hippocampal kindling in NA-depleted rats (Fig. 1) (3). The NA neurons in the grafts reinnervated the dorsal two thirds of the hippocampal formation, whereas only a few graft-derived NA axons were observed outside the hippocampus (Figs. 2, 3). The retardation of kindling was observed in ani-

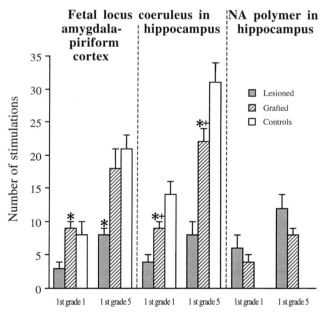

FIG. 1. Number of hippocampal kindling stimulations to reach the first grade 1 and grade 5 seizure in 6-OHDA-treated, NA-depleted rats (lesioned); 6-OHDA-treated animals with bilateral fetal locus coeruleus grafts in either the amygdala or the hippocampus or with bilateral NA-releasing polymer matrices in the hippocampus (grafted); and intact rats. Rats with fetal locus coeruleus grafts in hippocampus or amygdala developed seizures more slowly than NA-depleted rats without transplants. In contrast, implantation of NA-releasing polymer matrices in 6-OHDA-treated rats, which increased hippocampal NA levels to normal or supranormal levels (data not shown), had no significant effect on the development of kindling. *Significantly different from lesioned rats without grafts ($p < 0.05$). +Different from intact controls at $p < 0.05$. Modified from Barry et al. (4) and Kokaia et al. (49).

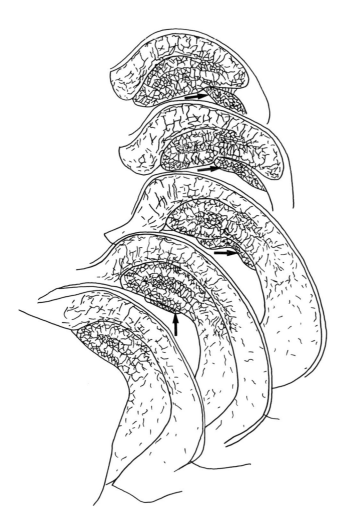

FIG. 2. Semischematic illustration of the distribution and density of the graft-derived noradrenergic reinnervation produced by implantation of fetal locus coeruleus tissue into the previously 6-OHDA-denervated hippocampus. *Arrows* indicate the location of the graft tissue containing noradrenergic neurons. Modified from Barry et al. (3).

mals with more than 100 surviving grafted NA neurons on each side and was significantly correlated to the degree of noradrenergic axonal ingrowth from the graft into the host hippocampus, supporting that the seizure-suppressant action of the grafts was mediated via NA mechanisms. In a subsequent study, this effect was obtained only with bilateral grafts, and could not be demonstrated after implantation of locus coeruleus tissue unilaterally into the hippocampus ipsilateral to the stimulating electrode (3). Interestingly, because the grafts reinnervated only a minor part of the NA-denervated forebrain, the results of Barry et al. (3) suggest that reinstatement

of NA transmission locally in the hippocampus is sufficient to suppress the development of seizures.

The functional capacity of locus coeruleus grafts also has been tested after implantation into a region distant to the stimulating electrode (4). The amygdala–piriform cortex was chosen as implantation site because this region has been proposed to be of central importance for the development and expression of kindled seizures (59,70). The locus coeruleus grafts, placed bilaterally into the amygdala–piriform cortex, retarded the kindling rate evoked by hippocampal stimulation to the same degree as if they had been implanted into the

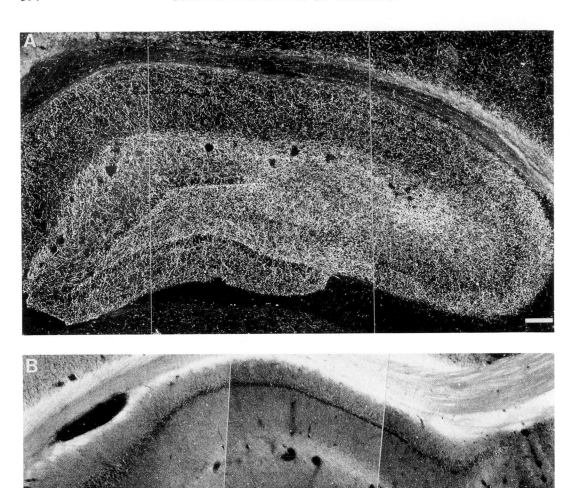

FIG. 3. A: Dark-field photomicrograph of a coronal section through the dorsal hippocampus showing a dense terminal network of dopamine-β-hydroxylase-positive, presumed noradrenergic fibers derived from a locus coeruleus graft implanted in the previously denervated host hippocampal formation. Bar = 0.30 mm. **B**: Dark-field photomicrograph of a dopamine-β-hydroxylase-immunostained coronal section through the dorsal hippocampus in a 6-OHDA-treated, nongrafted rat showing the complete lack of noradrenergic fibers. Bar = 0.30 mm. Modified from Bengzon et al. (9).

hippocampus (Fig. 1). In this experiment, it was not possible to determine the degree of noradrenergic reinnervation by the grafts, and their mechanisms of action therefore remain to be elucidated. However, Barry et al. (4) proposed that the grafted locus coeruleus neurons influenced kindling rate through NA release at denervated postsynaptic sites in the amygdala–piriform cortex. Restoration of NA neurotransmission in this area, remote from the stimulation site, thus seems to be sufficient to normalize the susceptibility of the NA-depleted animals to kindled seizures, elicited by stimulation in the hippocampus. These findings point to the interesting possibility that implants in a restricted region of critical importance for the spread and generalization of seizures could influence seizure susceptibility in widespread areas of the CNS, including the epileptic focus.

A major objective for subsequent studies has been to explore further how locus coeruleus grafts exert their seizure-suppressant effect. Bengzon et al. (7) administered the α_2 adrenergic receptor blocker idazoxan systemically before each hippocampal kindling stimulation in normal rats and in a group of 6-OHDA-denervated rats with bi-

lateral intrahippocampal locus coeruleus transplants. Another group of grafted rats received vehicle injections. The development of seizures (Fig. 4) was significantly faster in the grafted and normal rats that had been given idazoxan than in the grafted rats that had not been subjected to α_2 receptor blockade. The results of Bengzon et al. (7) provided further evidence that the seizure-suppressant action of locus coeruleus grafts in hippocampal kindling is mediated via noradrenergic mechanisms. Similar to what has been shown for the intrinsic locus coeruleus system (37), the grafted neurons seem to exert this effect through activation of postsynaptic α_2 adrenergic receptors.

Much information has been obtained using intracerebral microdialysis to monitor NA release during and between seizures. The steady-state output of NA in the hippocampus of grafted, previously 6-OHDA-denervated animals was found to be similar to the baseline level in normal rats (8). A generalized seizure (lasting about 2 min) gave rise to a threefold increase of hippocampal NA levels in both normal and grafted animals (Fig. 5). The maximal increase of NA output occurred within 2 to 4 min after the onset of seizure activity, and

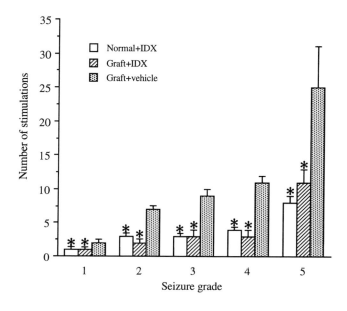

FIG. 4. Effects of α_2-adrenoceptor blockade on the number of hippocampal kindling stimulations to reach different seizure grades in normal rats and in 6-OHDA-treated, NA-depleted rats with bilateral locus coeruleus grafts in the hippocampus. The α_2 adrenoceptor antagonist idazoxan (IDX) was administered systemically before every stimulation in the normal group and in one of the grafted groups. The kindling rate in the groups given IDX was much faster than that in rats not subjected to α_2 receptor blockade. *Significantly different from non IDX treated rats. Modified from Bengzon et al. (7).

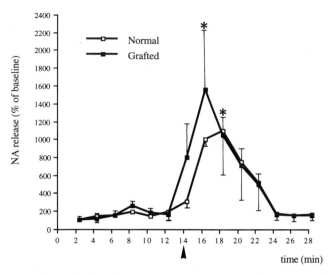

FIG. 5. Noradrenaline release in the hippocampus in response to a generalized kindled seizure (lasting about 2 min) in animals with an intact noradrenergic system (normal) and in 6-OHDA-treated, NA-depleted rats with locus coeruleus grafts in the hippocampus (grafted). The NA uptake blocker desipramine was continuously present in the perfusion fluid. The *arrowhead* indicates the time point for hippocampal stimulation. Maximal increase of NA output is observed 2 to 4 min after the onset of seizure activity, and the extracellular level then tapers off, reaching baseline after another 6 to 8 min. The data have been corrected for the delay in the probe outlet tubing. *Significantly different from the preceding baseline level. Modified from Bengzon et al. (8).

the extracellular levels then tapered off, reaching baseline after another 6 to 8 min. From the microdialysis experiments it can be concluded that epileptic seizures lead to a temporally defined, well regulated increase of NA output both from intrinsic and grafted locus coeruleus neurons occurring concurrently with their seizure-suppressant action. Despite the ectopic location in the hippocampus, the grafted locus coeruleus neurons seem to be functionally integrated with the host brain, at least in terms of increased release of NA during generalized kindled seizures.

The intrahippocampal locus coeruleus grafts form a noradrenergic terminal plexus very similar to the normal one in the denervated hippocampal formation. They establish synaptic contacts with host hippocampal neurons and also seem to be innervated by the host (63). This afferent input, the origin of which is not known, may mediate the regulatory influence of the recipient's

brain on NA release from the graft in response to seizures. Experiments performed on the intrinsic locus coeruleus system have provided further information regarding the regulation of transmitter release from locus coeruleus neurons in response to seizure activity. Transection of the ascending projection from the locus coeruleus caused a marked attenuation of hippocampal NA release induced by focal and generalized seizures after hippocampal kindling stimulation (8,9). These findings indicate that a major part of the NA release in the hippocampus depends on nerve impulse flow in the noradrenergic locus coeruleus neurons. Increased firing rate in these neurons has, in fact, been recorded during generalized kindled seizures (45). However, both focal and generalized seizures caused a significant increase in NA levels in the hippocampus after the transection as well. This observation suggests that part of the release of NA in kindling-evoked seizures is regulated locally at the level of the terminals. Evidence for such local regulatory mechanisms of NA release not requiring nerve impulse flow has been provided in kainic acid-induced seizures (65). It remains to be elucidated to what extent NA release from grafted locus coeruleus neurons, located in the hippocampus, is regulated via afferent inputs on the cell bodies or through local mechanisms at the terminal level.

In the experiments of Barry et al. (3,4), the locus coeruleus grafts had an antiepileptogenic effect, that is, they counteracted the development of hyperexcitability in response to stimulations in previously nonkindled rats. To explore the possibility that the grafts also could be anticonvulsant, locus coeruleus neurons were implanted bilaterally into the hippocampus in 6-OHDA-denervated animals after kindling had been established. The number of surviving grafted NA neurons and the extent and density of their axonal outgrowth in the hippocampus of these animals would most likely have retarded the kindling rate (3). However, no effect on the duration and severity of seizures in fully kindled rats was observed (Table 2) (10). These findings argue against an anticonvulsant action of grafted locus coeruleus neurons in kindling epilepsy. Such an effect cannot yet be totally excluded, however, because it may require graft-derived

innervations in widespread areas outside the hippocampus or in regions critical for seizure generalization.

Not least from the clinical point of view, it seems highly warranted to address the question whether NA-rich grafts can reduce neuronal excitability after implantation into a region without prior lesion-induced denervation of the intrinsic noradrenergic input. However, grafting of locus coeruleus neurons into the nondenervated hippocampus, which gave rise to a noradrenergic hyperinnervation, did not influence seizure development in kindling; that is, the "extra" NA input had no antiepileptogenic effect (10). When implanted into intact, kindled animals, the grafts increased both basal and seizure-evoked NA release in the stimulated hippocampus (10), but whether this increase led to any change in neuronal excitability within the area of hippocampus innervated by the graft is unknown.

To test the hypothesis that inhibition of seizure development in kindling requires a synaptic, well regulated release of NA, polymer matrices containing NA were implanted bilaterally into the hippocampus of NA-denervated, 6-OHDA-treated rats (49). A polymer matrix can release transmitters over several weeks and is a useful tool for establishing which functional properties of the implants (e.g., synaptic or diffuse, reg-

TABLE 2. *Effects of bilateral intrahippocampal locus coeruleus grafts or saline injections on seizure characteristics in previously 6-OHDA-treated, fully kindled rats[a]*

	Pre-LC graft	Post-LC graft	Presaline	Postsaline
Seizure grade	4.0 ± 0.3	3.6 ± 0.4	3.6 ± 0.2	4.4 ± 0.4
Threshold (μA)	44 ± 8	114 ± 55	87 ± 27	195 ± 89
AD duration (sec)	83 ± 5	102 ± 8	92 ± 7	83 ± 10
Duration of convulsion (sec)	48 ± 2	63 ± 7	50 ± 3	54 ± 4

Modified from Bengzon et al., ref. 10.

[a]Means ± SEM in response to ten daily hippocampal stimulations before and eight stimulations at 10 weeks after locus coeruleus implantation or saline injection. The locus coeruleus grafts had no effect on any seizure parameter despite giving rise to a noradrenergic reinnervation of normal or supranormal density in major parts of the hippocampal formation.

AD, afterdischarge; LC, locus coeruleus.

ulated or nonregulated release) are necessary to exert a certain effect. No influence on the number of stimulations needed to reach the different seizure grades in hippocampal kindling was observed (Fig. 1). The extracellular NA levels, as measured by intracerebral microdialysis about 1 mm from the polymer matrix, were 473 and 104 fmol/30 μl at 7 and 14 days, respectively, after implantation. Interestingly, these levels exceeded those measured in the hippocampus of locus coeruleus-grafted (58 fmol/30 μl) and intact rats (40 fmol/30 μl), respectively. Furthermore, NA release from the matrices was in the same order of magnitude as the seizure-induced release in locus coeruleus-grafted (240 fmol/30 μl) and intact rats (190 fmol/30μl).

The lack of effect of the polymer matrix implants may have several different explanations. First, these data might indicate that a well regulated release of NA at synaptic sites is necessary for the retardation of kindling development. Second, there was a dramatic fall of extracellular NA levels between 1 and 2 mm from the matrix, probably caused by limited diffusion of NA in the denervated hippocampus as well. The NA release from the matrix may therefore reach an insufficient volume of the hippocampus. Third, NA release from the polymers gradually tapered off with time and had reached control levels at 3 weeks after implantation. However, it seems unlikely that this decline of NA release facilitated the kindling process, because the transmitter level was high during the early phases of kindling, when NA has been shown to exert its major inhibitory effect (23). Fourth, a downregulation of hippocampal adrenergic receptors in response to the abnormally high NA levels after implantation of matrices also may influence NA transmission during seizure development.

GABA-Releasing Implants

Enhancement of GABA neurotransmission in the substantia nigra pars reticulata has a powerful anticonvulsant effect in a variety of animal models of epilepsy (31). Muscimol (a $GABA_A$ receptor agonist) and γ-vinyl-GABA (a GABA transaminase inhibitor) injected into the substantia nigra efficiently suppress generalized, nonconvulsive seizures (24), as well as seizures induced by flurothyl (84), pentylenetetrazol (43), bicuculline (35), electroshock (43), ethanol withdrawal (30), pilocarpine (77), and kindling (51,61). These findings have raised the possibility that GABA-secreting grafts placed in the substantia nigra region might exert an anticonvulsant action. To test this hypothesis, Kokaia et al. (49) implanted GABA-releasing polymer matrices bilaterally immediately dorsal to the substantia nigra in rats previously kindled in the amygdala. Two days after implantation, rats with GABA-releasing matrices showed only focal limbic seizures in response to electrical stimulation, whereas animals with control matrices, not containing GABA, exhibited generalized convulsions (Fig. 6A). GABA release from the polymer matrices was high during the first days after implantation, as demonstrated both *in vitro* and *in vivo* using microdialysis (Fig. 6B, C). The anticonvulsant effect was no longer observed at 7 and 14 days, when GABA release was found to be low (Fig. 6A–C). The marked inhibition of motor seizures observed after 2 days correlates well with the elevated GABA levels in the region of substantia nigra at this time point. Similarly, the lack of any seizure-suppressant effect at 7 and 14 days after matrix implantation probably can be ascribed to a decline in GABA release. However, it cannot be excluded that the disappearance of the effect also could result from downregulation of postsynaptic nigral GABA receptors in response to the high levels of GABA release by the matrices.

The results of Kokaia et al. (49) indicate that grafts not only can inhibit epileptogenesis, as shown previously for locus coeruleus neurons, but dampen seizure generalization in already established kindling epilepsy. Furthermore, implantation in the

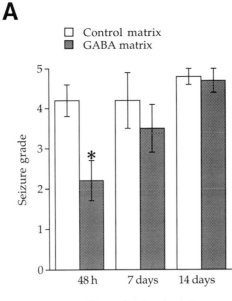

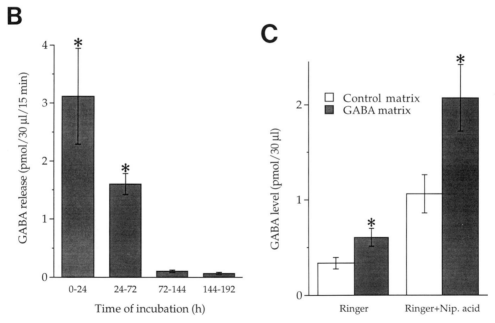

FIG. 6. A: Severity of seizures in response to amygdala stimulation after bilateral implantation of GABA-releasing or control (without GABA) polymer matrices dorsal to the substantia nigra in previously fully kindled rats. Generalized convulsions were inhibited at 48 hr after GABA polymer implantation, but this effect had disappeared at 7 and 14 days. *Significantly different from control at $p <$ 0.05. **B**: *In vitro* GABA release from the GABA-containing polymer matrices during different time intervals after the start of incubation in Ringer solution. During the first 3 days, GABA release from the matrices was high but at later time points had decreased to the control level. *Significantly different from control matrix without GABA at $p <$ 0.0001. **C**: *In vivo* GABA release at 48 hr after matrix implantation as monitored by intracerebral microdialysis probes located about 1 mm from the GABA-releasing or control polymer matrices in the substantia nigra. Rats with GABA polymers showed markedly higher levels of GABA both under basal conditions and during GABA reuptake blockade (produced by nipecotic acid in the dialysis perfusion fluid) than animals implanted with control matrices without GABA. *Significantly different at $p <$ 0.05. Modified from Kokaia et al. (49).

vicinity of the substantia nigra seems to be a useful model to test both *in vivo* GABA release from various types of GABA-containing implants, and the duration and efficacy of their seizure-suppressant action. Although the seizure suppression exerted by the GABA polymers was transient in the experiment of Kokaia et al. (49), a sustained effect might be achieved by the use of coated polymer matrices with long-term transmitter release or, alternatively, by implantation of GABA-producing, genetically engineered cells. It seems likely, on the basis of these observations, that the anticonvulsant effect on already generalized seizures can be exerted by grafts acting as biologic minipumps in the region of the substantia nigra, and does not require a synaptic, well regulated release of GABA.

Stevens et al. (75) reported that grafts of fetal cerebellar or cortical tissue placed in the deep prepiriform area of amygdala-kindled rats (intended to provide the host brain with additional GABA neurons at a site important for seizure generalization) transiently raised seizure thresholds in a minority of animals. However, no glutamic acid decarboxylase (GAD)-immunopositive, presumed GABAergic neurons could be demonstrated in the grafts.

5-Hydroxytryptamine-Releasing Implants

Kindling epilepsy also can be induced by electrical stimulations in the olfactory bulb. Although the role of the serotonergic system in kindling evoked from other structures (e.g., amygdala and hippocampus) is unclear, serotonergic afferents seem to inhibit kindling in the olfactory bulb (52). Specific neurotoxin-induced lesions of the serotonergic innervation of the olfactory bulb lead to facilitation of seizure development in kindling. In analogy with the experiments in which NA-rich tissue from the locus coeruleus region was implanted in the NA-depleted hippocampus (see earlier), fetal 5-hydroxytryptamine (5-HT)-rich tissue from the raphe region was grafted into the

5-HT-depleted (using 5,7-dihydroxytryptamine injections) olfactory bulb of adult rats. The grafted serotonergic neurons exhibited extensive axonal outgrowth, predominantly to the glomerular layer, and the raphe implants reversed the facilitation of olfactory bulb kindling caused by the neurotoxin lesion (17).

Cortical Implants

With the idea of providing a source of neurotransmitters and neurotrophic factors, Holmes et al. (40) implanted fetal neocortical tissue unilaterally into the hippocampus of rats. Two experiments were carried out. In the first experiment, 16-day-old rats were kindled in the right amygdala and grafted in the contralateral hippocampus 3 days later. No influence on kindling rate evoked by stimulation in the left amygdala (transfer kindling) at 84 days was observed in the group with neocortical implants. In the second experiment, previously unkindled 19-day-old animals were grafted similarly and subjected to kindling in the ipsilateral amygdala at 84 days of age. No difference in kindling rate was observed between grafted and control rats. Good graft survival was reported in all rats. The results suggest that implantation into the hippocampus of any fetal CNS tissue is not sufficent to change seizure susceptibility in kindling.

GRAFTS IN THE PILOCARPINE-INDUCED SEIZURE MODEL

Systemic administration of the muscarinic cholinergic agonist pilocarpine to rats gives rise to seizures that are considered to resemble complex partial epilepsy in humans (for references, see ref. 27). Susceptibility to such pilocarpine-induced seizures is increased by lesions of the striatonigral GABAergic projection produced by neurotoxin injections in the caudate–putamen (27). Transplantation of GABA-rich tissue from the fetal striatum into the substantia nigra attenuated the lesion-induced increase of seizure susceptibility (27). However, in this study no attempt was made to assess the degree of survival of GABAergic neurons in the graft. Furthermore, the control grafts consisting of sciatic nerve had the same effects on seizure susceptibility as the implants of striatal tissue. Thus, the functional effects observed after transplantation could not be attributed to increased GABAergic inhibition provided by the grafts.

GRAFTS IN THE INTACT OR SUBCORTICALLY DENERVATED HIPPOCAMPUS

Another epilepsy model, suitable for transplantation experiments, is created by transection of the fimbria–fornix (FF), thus removing major parts of the subcortical inhibitory input to the hippocampus (13). More specifically, the lesion involves aspiration of the medial portion of the parietal cortex and cingulate cortex, and transects the cingulate bundle, the supracallosal stria, the corpus callosum, the dorsal fornix, the fimbria, and the ventral hippocampal commissure. According to Buzsáki et al. (13), this lesion leads to the removal of cholinergic and GABAergic afferents from the septal area, noradrenergic afferents from the locus coeruleus, serotonergic afferents from the mesencephalic raphe, several minor pathways from other subcortical nuclei, and the commissural pathways and subcortical efferent projection of the hippocampal formation. Animals with subcortically denervated hippocampus show increased susceptibility to behavioral seizures induced by picrotoxin (a GABA receptor antagonist), and a higher frequency of interictal spikes in the hippocampus both before and after repeated hippocampal seizures evoked by electrical stimulation of the perforant path (13). Grafts of fetal locus coeruleus tissue implanted bilaterally into the hippocampus of lesioned animals reduced the incidence of interictal spikes in the host hippocampus (Fig. 7), and protected against picrotoxin-induced behavioral seizures. Control grafts consisting of fetal hippocampal tissue had the opposite effect. The locus coeruleus grafts contained noradrenergic neurons from which axonal processes extended into the host hippocam-

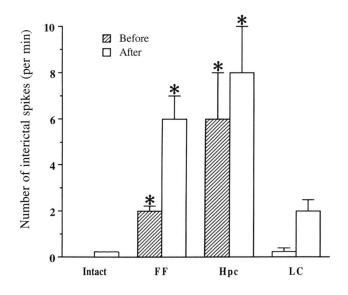

FIG. 7. Interictal spike frequency in the hippocampus 1 day before (hatched bars) and 1 day after (open bars) six seizures induced by perforant path stimulation in intact rats, animals with lesions of the fimbria–fornix (FF), and in FF-lesioned rats with intrahippocampal grafts of either fetal hippocampus (Hpc) or locus coeruleus (LC). The locus coeruleus grafts reduced the incidence of interictal spikes, whereas the hippocampal implants had the opposite effect. *Significantly different from intact rats ($p < 0.01$). Modified from Buzsáki et al. (13)

pus. Buzsáki et al. (13) proposed that the grafted locus coeruleus neurons may have influenced seizure susceptibility in this model either through a direct action of NA on hippocampal pyramidal cells or by competing for vacant (after the lesion) postsynaptic sites with sprouting axons of host neurons, thereby limiting excessive collateral excitation.

Buzsáki et al. (14) have described in more detail the electrical patterns of solid and dissociated hippocampal grafts placed in or close to the subcortically denervated hippocampus, and the physiologic and anatomic interactions between the grafted tissue and the host brain. Both interictal spikes and seizure activity, frequently invading the host hippocampus, were recorded from the hippocampal grafts. Spontaneous behavioral seizures were observed in about half of the grafted rats. There were reciprocal anatomic connections between the graft and the host brain. Buzsáki et al. (14) proposed that the increased excitability of the hippocampal graft, observed despite the presence of large numbers of GABAergic neurons, was caused by the high incidence of recurrent excitatory collaterals terminating on or close to the somata of pyramidal neurons. The grafted hippocampus seems to serve as an epileptic focus, which kindles the host brain by repeated seizures, leading to the spontaneous behavioral convulsions.

Neural grafting into the subcortically denervated hippocampus also was used by Cassel et al. (18), who implanted dissociated fetal basal forebrain, rich in cholinergic neurons, into the hippocampus of 6-week-old rats with FF lesions. Twelve months after grafting, the rats were tested for reactivity to intraperitoneal injection of pentylenetetrazol and to audiogenic stimulation. The grafted animals showed more and stronger convulsive reactions than nongrafted controls in response to pentylenetetrazol, but were less reactive to sound. It is unclear to what extent specific effects exerted by the grafts (e.g., mediated via cholinergic transmission) could explain the observed changes of seizure susceptibility. Reactivity to pentylenetetrazol was correlated with body weight and degree of graft-induced hippocampal damage, but not with graft size. Although acetylcholinesterase-positive staining was observed in all surviving grafts, indicating survival of grafted cholinergic neurons, the grafts did not reinnervate, or reinnervated only poorly, the deafferented hippocampus.

In a subsequent study, Cassel et al (19) reported the time course of the effects of intrahippocampal fetal septum or hippocampus grafts on susceptibility to pentylenetetrazol and audiogenic seizures in FF-lesioned rats. At variance with their previous data (18), septal grafts in this study were found to *reduce* the reactivity to pentylenetetrazol and to *increase* the reactivity to sound at 3 months but not at 7 and 12 months posttransplantation. The fetal hippocampal implants had similar effects. As described earlier, opposite changes of reactivity had been reported previously for septal grafts at the 12-month time point. Acetylcholinesterase-positive staining was observed in the grafts as well as "a significant acetylcholinesterase-positive reinnervation" of the host hippocampus. No clear explanation of the discrepancy between the two studies of Cassel et al. (18,19) was given.

Fetal hippocampal tissue implanted into the intact rat hippocampus also induced epileptic patterns (15). The host hippocampus exhibited putative interictal spikes (Fig. 8), and electrical stimulation of the perforant path induced behavioral seizures in 50% of the animals with hippocampal grafts. This was not observed in the control rats. Thus, the implanted hippocampal tissue can both increase excitability and give rise to seizure activity in the host brain. Grafting hippocampal tissue to the intact brain seems to be a useful model to study various anatomic, biochemical, and physi-

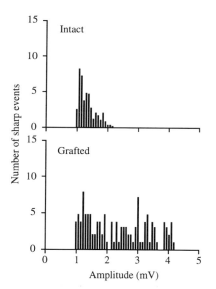

FIG. 8. Amplitude histograms showing the frequency of sharp events (< 100 msec) recorded from the dentate gyrus hilus during a 30-min period of immobility in normal rats (*top*) and in animals with fetal hippocampal grafts implanted bilaterally in the intact hippocampal formation (*bottom*). Large-amplitude (> 3 mV) events occurred more frequently in grafted rats, illustrating the increased excitability and induction of seizure activity in the host hippocampus. Modified from Buszáki et al. (15).

ologic changes in the normal hippocampus associated with the development of an epileptic syndrome.

GRAFTS IN THE KAINIC ACID MODEL

Systemic, intraventricular, or intracerebral administration of the excitotoxin kainic acid leads to a chronic model of epilepsy resembling complex partial seizures in humans (5,6,64). The hippocampus seems to be the primary brain region involved in kainic acid-induced seizures, and is particularly vulnerable to neuronal necrosis after kainic acid. Rats given intraperitoneal injections of kainic acid exhibit recurrent, spontaneous seizures, which can be quantified and scored. The behavioral and electroencephalographic features of the kainic

acid-induced seizures are similar to those observed in hippocampal kindling.

Holmes et al. (41) injected immature rats (1 month old) with a convulsant dosage of kainic acid intraperitoneally. Ten days later, the rats exhibited severe seizures and were grafted bilaterally in the lateral ventricle with fetal locus coeruleus, cerebellar, neocortical, or hippocampal tissue. Control rats received saline alone. The frequency of spontaneous seizures was monitored for 230 days. No differences in the percentage of rats developing spontaneous seizures were observed between the transplant groups and control rats. There was a slight reduction of the frequency of spontaneous seizures in the hippocampus- and locus coeruleus-transplanted groups, but not in animals with cerebellar or neocortical grafts. At the age of 270 days, the rats were subjected to angular bundle kindling. However, both afterdischarge thresholds and kindling rates were similar in the four transplanted groups and in the control group.

Although Holmes et al. (41) concluded that "the anticonvulsant effects of neural transplants, using this animal model are mild," their interpretation may be questioned for the following reasons: First, the size, location, and survival of the transplants varied considerably. No attempts to correlate graft size with seizure parameters were made. Second, the survival of specific neuronal populations, such as the NA-producing neurons in the locus coeruleus grafts, and their growth into the host brain, were not assessed.

GRAFTS IN GENETIC EPILEPSY MODELS

In certain human epilepsies, localized or diffuse alterations of the brain are found, whereas in others the origin is unknown. Some forms of cryptogenic epilepsy in humans have a genetic origin. Several animal models of genetic epilepsy exist, and two of them have been used for grafting experiments. Genetically epilepsy-prone rats (GEPRs) are susceptible to seizure induction by sound and exhibit a lack of seizure-suppressant mechanisms, including deficits in both NA and GABA transmission (46). In the first grafting experiments using this genetic epilepsy model, Stevens et al. (75) implanted fetal cerebellar, GABA-rich tissue into the inferior colliculi of GEPRs. Surviving graft tissue (but no GAD-positive cells) was observed in one of nine animals. Another group of GEPRs received catecholamine-containing adrenal medulla grafts bilaterally into the lateral ventricle. Graft survival (but only few scattered TH-positive cells) was found in five of six animals. Consistent with very poor survival of grafted, presumably inhibitory GABAergic neurons and NA-releasing cells, no reduction of the intensity of the seizures evoked by audiogenic stimulation was observed.

Fetal NA-rich locus coeruleus tissue was, in a preliminary study (21), implanted into GEPRs to elucidate if restoration of NA transmission by grafts may have a suppressant effect on the severity of audiogenic seizures. The locus coeruleus grafts were implanted either in the hippocampus or in the third ventricle of GEPRs. No effect was observed in any of the animals with hippocampal implants, whereas some of the rats with grafts in the third ventricle displayed decreased seizure severity. However, there were no significant group effects and no correlation between seizure suppression and number of surviving noradrenergic neurons. Furthermore, no attempts were made to clarify the distribution and density of the graft-derived noradrenergic reinnervation.

In the same genetic epilepsy model, Holmes et al. (42) explored the effects of implantation of fetal locus coeruleus, neocortical, and cerebellar tissue either bilaterally into the inferior colliculi or into the lateral ventricle. After audiogenic stimulation, the grafted rats had a longer latency to the tonic phase and a shorter duration of the clonic phase than sham-operated controls. However, seizure severity score was not altered by grafting. No differences in the effects were observed between animals receiving cerebellar, locus coeruleus, or neocortical transplants. When the animals were subjected to electrical stimulation of the angular bundle, the kindling rate was the same in grafted and sham-operated animals. Holmes et al. (42) hypothesized that the locus coeruleus grafts would release NA and the implanted cerebellar tissue release a variety of neurotransmitters, including GABA, which may have a seizure-suppressant action. Although Holmes et al. (42) reported survival of grafted tissue using routine histologic techniques, no evidence for survival and axonal outgrowth from grafted noradrenergic and GABAergic neurons in the implants was presented. In fact, NA concentration in cerebrospinal fluid was unchanged in the grafted animals. Therefore, no conclusions can be drawn from the results of Holmes et al. (42) about the possible anticonvulsant effects of grafted GABA- or NA-producing cells in GEPRs.

In contrast to the studies using kindling and the subcortically denervated hippocampus (see earlier), these experiments with the GEPR model were not based on prior lesioning in the brain but on a naturally occurring deficit. In that way, transplantation in GEPRs more closely resembled the situation of testing grafts in a human epileptic disorder. Whether NA- or GABA-rich grafts can change seizure susceptibility in GEPRs must, however, be analyzed further.

Another transplantation approach to elucidate pathophysiologic mechanisms in genetic epilepsy was introduced by Teillet et al. (76). Fayomui chickens, with a spontaneous recessive autosomal mutation responsible for increased seizure susceptibility in response to intermittent light stimulation, were used. On embryonic day 2, different regions of the brain anlage from the genetically epileptic chickens were transplanted to normal chickens, substituting the equivalent areas of the encephalic neuroepithelium. Transplantation of all four primitive encephalic vesicles (i.e., the whole brain or both the prosencephalon and mesencephalon) led to the transfer of the full disease as observed in adulthood. In contrast, chickens only with prosencephalic grafts showed interictal paroxysms on EEG, but not complete epileptic seizures. The susceptibility to pentylenetetrazol-evoked seizures was higher in the chimeras than in control chickens (39). Grafts of mesencephalon, rhombencephalon, or both did not give rise to the epileptic phenotype. The results indicate that the cooperation of forebrain and midbrain is necessary to generate the full epileptic syndrome in this genetic model.

CURRENT RESEARCH STRATEGIES

Experimental evidence obtained over the past 7 years has clearly demonstrated that intracerebral transplants can both suppress and induce epileptic phenomena in the brain. It seems possible to draw three major conclusions: (1) *Fetal neural grafts can dampen epileptogenesis in the lesioned, hyperexcitable brain.* This effect has been clearly demonstrated in hippocampal kindling using NA-rich locus coeruleus grafts placed in the hippocampus or amygdala–piriform cortex of NA-depleted rats, and seems to occur also in olfactory bulb kindling after implantation of 5-HT-rich raphe grafts in the 5-HT-depleted olfactory bulb. Furthermore, the suppression of epileptic activity by locus coeruleus grafts in the subcortically denervated hippocampus probably is an antiepileptogenic effect. (2) *Fetal neural grafts can serve as an epileptic focus.* Fetal hippocampal tissue implanted both in the intact and subcortically denervated hippocampus exhibits epileptic activity that spreads to the host hippocampus and may lead to behavioral seizures. (3) *Embryonic grafts of selected regions of brain anlage may transfer the epileptic phe-*

notype. Transplantation of the prosencephalic and mesencephalic neuroepithelium from genetically epileptic chickens generates the full epileptic syndrome in normal chickens.

Studies performed so far have not been able convincingly to show if neural grafts can exert anticonvulsant effects in the epileptic brain. Intrahippocampal locus coeruleus grafts do not lead to seizure suppression in fully kindled rats despite good survival of implanted NA neurons and extensive reinnervation of the host hippocampus. Other attempts to explore the possibility of an anticonvulsant effect by grafting NA- or GABA-rich tissue in the kindling, kainic acid, pilocarpine, and genetic epilepsy models have documented only minor changes. Unfortunately, these data are largely inconclusive because survival of NA and GABA neurons in the grafts, intended to lead to seizure suppression, has either been poor or has not been investigated. The report by Kokaia et al. (49) that intranigral implants of GABA-releasing polymer matrices can suppress generalized kindled seizures provides the first direct evidence suggesting that cell transplants may have a major anticonvulsant effect.

The cell transplantation strategy is already an important research tool for studies on the pathophysiologic role in epilepsy of defined transmitter systems and brain regions. However, the major challenge for transplantation research in epilepsy, not least from the clinical point of view, is to explore further if and how grafts could be used to suppress the generation, spread, severity, and duration of convulsive activity in the brain with an established epileptic syndrome. The principal strategy underlying the transplantation approach seems very simple: to reduce neuronal hyperexcitability in an epileptic brain region by implanting cells leading to increased inhibition. The further progress of this research is, however, complicated by two major problems. First, there is the lack of any identified deficit in a particular transmitter system underlying most forms of experimental as well as clinical epilepsy. This is in contrast to the situation for transplantation in Parkinson's disease, in which the implantation of neural tissue aims at restoring dopamine synthesis, storage, and release at synaptic sites through a reinnervation of the striatum by grafted mesencephalic dopaminergic neurons. Second, it is largely unknown whether the addition of inhibitory neurons to an epileptic brain region without a deficit in that particular neuron system leads to increased inhibition. For example, if GABA-producing cells are implanted, it remains to be established to what extent they are anatomically and functionally integrated with the host brain. If so, one must consider the possibility not only of a seizure-suppressant effect but also that the resultant functional action exerted by these cells, particularly if they are placed at an ectopic site, could be an increased excitation (e.g., through inhibition of inhibitory interneurons).

In the following, some of the scientific problems that should be addressed with transplantation in experimental epilepsy models are discussed. The main emphasis is put on GABA- and NA-releasing implants, which seem to be the most suitable ones to reduce neuronal excitability. A new approach is intracerebral transplants of cells producing neurotrophic factors to elucidate their role in the sprouting and synaptic reorganization underlying hyperexcitability in epilepsy. Furthermore, the use of transplants as a model system for epileptogenesis in the host brain is mentioned.

Noradrenaline-Releasing Implants

In previous kindling experiments (3,4, 7,8), grafting was performed before the start of stimulations. Similarly, in subcortically denervated animals (13), cell implantation took place about 1 week after the FF lesion. In both models the influence of the locus coeruleus grafts was primarily anti-epileptogenic, that is, they counteracted the development of hyperexcitability. If locus coeruleus neurons were implanted after kindling had been established, no effects on the duration and severity of seizures were observed (10). These findings argue against an anticonvulsant action of grafted locus coeruleus neurons in kindling epilepsy, which is in good agreement with the lack of effects on seizure characteristics if NA depletion is performed in the fully kindled animal (82). However, an anticonvulsant effect cannot yet be totally excluded in kindling because it may require graft-derived innervations in widespread areas outside the hippocampus or in regions critical for seizure generalization (e.g., amygdala–piriform cortex).

Two major scientific questions should now be addressed: First, can NA-releasing implants inhibit convulsive activity when transplanted to animals with a fully developed epileptic syndrome? Second, how do the NA grafts exert their seizure-suppressant effect (e.g., is it dependent on release at synaptic sites and functional integration with the host brain)? Although an anticonvulsant action of NA grafts seems unlikely in kindling, such an effect may occur in other models of epilepsy, in which the intrinsic locus coeruleus system seems to play this role. Stimulation in the area of the locus coeruleus, which causes increased turnover of NA in the forebrain, leads to suppression of epileptiform activity produced by focal application of cobalt (28) or penicillin (66), or by systemic administration of pentylenetetrazol (53). Conversely, lesions of the locus coeruleus projection to the forebrain potentiate electroshock- and pentylenetetrazol-induced convulsions (55). Furthermore, indices of NA transmission are reduced in GEPRs (46). It seems highly warranted to analyze in detail (1) if NA-releasing implants can have an anticonvulsant effect in these epilepsy models; (2) which target regions for implantation are critical (e.g., hippocampus or piriform cortex) to obtain a graft effect; and (3) how large the areas need to be that are reached by NA released from the transplant. Of special interest will be transplantation of locus coeruleus neurons and other NA-releasing implants into GEPRs. In these animals, the intrinsic NA system is present, although there are functional impairments. Both the kainic acid and genetic models, which have been used in initial, largely inconclusive grafting studies, seem to be highly suitable for testing the anticonvulsant action of NA-releasing grafts.

Implantation of NA-releasing grafts in the kindling model constitutes a highly useful model system to elucidate which properties of grafts are necessary to dampen epileptic phenomena in the brain. Seizure properties of regions provided with a regulated NA release and a synapse-forming noradrenergic innervation can be compared to regions with a diffuse, nonsynaptic transmitter release by grafting locus coeruleus neurons and genetically modified, NA-producing nonneuronal cells, respectively. Furthermore, this model system can provide basic information on the functional importance of anatomic connections between the graft and the host brain, and on a regulatory influence by the host on the activity of the graft.

GABA-Releasing Implants

A major problem for the strategy of increasing GABA transmission within a brain region using neural grafts has been the difficulty of finding a suitable source of fetal GABA-rich tissue. Although GABA neurons from the striatum can survive both in the normal and in the kainic acid-treated, epileptic hippocampus, the grafts often are small and poorly integrated with the host brain (72). This is in contrast to when the grafts are placed in the lesioned striatum, where they form extensive afferent and efferent connections with the host brain and release GABA [see Björklund et al. *(this volume)*]. Other possible sources of GABA

neurons, such as fetal cerebellum, have been tested, but grafts from these regions are unfavorable when implanted at ectopic sites. A new, attractive possibility may be the implantation of genetically engineered, GABA-producing cells made by insertion of the gene encoding GAD.

In the experiments carried out so far (Lindvall et al., *unpublished observations*), cell lines made to express the GAD gene have been shown to secrete high amounts of GABA *in vitro*. However, after implantation in the rat hippocampus, no clear-cut GABA release from the graft could be detected by microdialysis, and there were no changes of seizure characteristics in hippocampal kindling. The downregulation of GABA production in the transduced cells was probably caused by a decline in the expression of the GAD gene. Of major importance now is first to find nontumorigenic cells that can be efficiently transduced *in vitro,* and that exhibit sustained and long-lasting expression of the transgene after transplantation to the brain. As a second step, both neuronal and nonneuronal GAD-expressing cells should be tested for their possible seizure-suppressant action in different models of epilepsy. It is not known if such an effect requires a synaptic release of GABA, regulated by the host brain. The observations in the kindling model of seizure suppression by intranigral GABA-releasing polymer matrices indicate that it may be sufficient with a graft acting as a biologic minipump.

As mentioned earlier, the hypothesis that GABA implants would effect increased inhibition in an epileptic brain region remains to be confirmed. In fact, hippocampal implants containing GABA neurons have been shown to serve as an epileptic focus (13–15). On the other hand, the effects of intranigral polymer implants (49) suggest that, in this location at least, short-term seizure suppression can be obtained with GABA-releasing grafts. Achievement of long-term effects depends both on the duration of the GABA-secreting capacity of the implants as well as on possible changes (e.g., downregulation) in postsynaptic receptors due to continuous GABA release.

Available experimental evidence suggest that GABA-producing cells might influence epileptic phenomena after implantation into at least two, principally different sites: first, in the epileptic focus, where some reports have described a deficit of GABAergic transmission, for example, after hippocampal kindling (47,48) and application of cobalt (25) or alumina cream (71). However, even without deficits in intrinsic GABAergic transmission, grafting of GABA cells to the epileptic focus might possibly counteract the hyperexcitability caused by perturbations in other neuronal systems. The second sites are the regions of importance for the spread and generalization of epileptic seizures. As discussed in detail earlier, one such site is the substantia nigra pars reticulata. In particular, it seems highly warranted to test whether an anticonvulsant effect, similar to that obtained by GABA-releasing polymer matrices, could also be exerted by GABA-producing cells implanted into the substantia nigra. Another region that might be suitable for transplantation of GABA neurons is the area tempestas within the deep prepiriform cortex (68). GABA-mediated inhibition is believed to control the seizure-triggering output from this region (32), and enhancement of GABA transmission in the area tempestas can block both chemical- and kindling-induced seizures (32,74).

Other Implants

Implants Releasing Other Neurotransmitters

In addition to NA and GABA neurons, several other transmitter systems have been proposed to be involved in the development and expression of epileptic syndromes. Transplantation of a more-or-less pure population of cells releasing a particular transmitter to the intact or lesioned brain could add valuable data on the pathophysiologic role of these systems. Some of the reported findings are of particular interest in relation to grafting studies. Recently, Pasini et al. (67) reported that bilateral intranigral injection of the 5-HT uptake inhibitor fluoxetine produced a dose-dependent anticonvulsant effect on seizures evoked by bicuculline administration into the area tempestas of rats. Blockade of GABA receptors in the substantia nigra did not influence, whereas depletion of serotonin prevented the anticonvulsant action of fluoxetine. Pasini et al. (67) concluded that endogenous 5-HT in the substantia nigra has a seizure-suppressant role independent of GABA transmission. This raises the possibility that 5-HT-releasing implants placed bilaterally in the substantia nigra could dampen seizure susceptibility, which could be tested both in intact and 5-HT-depleted animals.

Interestingly, serotonergic deficits have been shown in several brain areas in GEPRs (46). These deficits may contribute to the increased seizure susceptibility in this genetic model. Implantation of 5-HT-releasing implants at various sites should be a valuable approach to test this hypothesis.

Dopamine (DA) neurons have been considered to play only a minor role in seizures. However, Turski et al. (78) reported that bilateral injections of the DA agonist apomorphine directly into the striatum protect against seizures in the pilocarpine epilepsy model. Conversely, intrastriatal or systemic application of the DA receptor antagonist haloperidol lowered the threshold for pilocarpine-induced seizures. Furthermore, Wahnschaffe and Löscher (80) showed anticonvulsant effects on kindled seizures by a DA D_2 agonist injected into the ipsilateral nucleus accumbens. These results indicate that enhanced dopaminergic transmission in the striatum can lead to elevated seizure threshold. Grafts of fetal mesencephalic tissue, rich in DA neurons, survive transplantation and innervate both the DA-denervated and intact striatum [see Brundin *(this volume)*], and the results of Turski et al. (78) and Wahnschaffe and Löscher (80) suggest that such grafts may change seizure susceptibility.

The involvement of cholinergic neurons in epileptic seizures has been suggested by several studies using the kindling model. For example, infusion of cholinomimetics into various brain regions results in kindling (16,81), and systemic administration of the muscarinic receptor antagonist scopolamine retards amygdala kindling (83). To explore further the pathophysiologic role of cholinergic mechanisms in epilepsy, fetal basal forebrain, rich in cholinergic neurons, should be implanted in various regions of the intact brain or after specific lesions.

Implants Releasing Neurotrophic Factors

As shown in a variety of epilepsy models, seizure activity induces elevated mRNA levels for the neurotrophins, brain-derived neurotrophic factor (BDNF) and nerve growth factor (NGF), in cortical and hippocampal neurons (2,11,26,33,34,44). During kindling epileptogenesis, each brief, stimulus-evoked seizure gives rise to transient increases of mRNA expression for BDNF and NGF. These changes are confined to the dentate gyrus after the first stimuli, but generalized seizures cause increases in hippocampal CA1–CA3 regions, amygdala, piriform cortex, and neocortex as well (11). In contrast, kindled seizures lead to reduced mRNA expression for neurotrophin-3 (NT-3) in dentate granule cells (11). Furthermore, there is an increased expression of the high-affinity receptor for BDNF, called trkB, in dentate granule cells after kindling (62). Brain-derived neurotrophic factor and trkB are coexpressed in cortical and hippocampal neurons, suggesting an autocrine or paracrine mode of action (50).

The seizure-evoked cascade of changes in neurotrophin levels may be involved in the regulation of plastic changes, synaptic reorganization, and development of hyperexcitability characteristic of kindling. If this was the case, the neurotrophins also could play an important role in the development of human epilepsy. Grafting of genetically engineered cells made to produce the neurotrophins through the insertion of the BDNF, NGF, or NT-3 genes should be a valuable tool to test this hypothesis. These grafts will provide a continuous local supply of one or more of the neurotrophins. The effect on development of seizure susceptibility as well as on the plastic changes can be determined after implantation into various regions critically involved in epileptogenesis, such as the hippocampal formation and amygdala–piriform cortex.

Epileptic Implants

The possibility of using neural grafts to induce epileptic patterns in the host brain has been clearly documented by Buzsáki et al. (13–15) and Teillet et al. (76). Implantation of solid fetal hippocampal grafts in the subcortically denervated or intact hippocampus seems particularly suitable for studies of the interaction between the primary epileptic focus and the rest of the brain, both during epileptogenesis and in the generalization of convulsive activity. In this chronic epilepsy model, both afferent and efferent connections between the graft and host brain can be mapped, and their relative importance for various parts of the epileptic syndrome can be determined after selective surgical lesions. Complete removal of the graft allows for studies on permanent anatomic, biochemical, and electrophysiologic changes induced in the host brain, and the significance and nature of secondary epileptic foci. This model also can be used to investigate the influence of different behavioral states on the interictal transitions. For example, Buzsáki et al. (14) found that eruption of seizure activity often occurred when grafted rats spontaneously arose from sleep or drowsiness. Factors other than synaptic connections seemed to be able to trigger seizures, because they also were observed in animals with poor integration of the grafts with the host, and for interictal spikes and epileptiform activity that propagated poorly from the graft to the host.

CONCLUDING REMARKS

The use of cell transplantation as an investigative tool in epilepsy research is still in its infancy. The potential value of this approach is, however, strongly supported by experimental evidence showing that neural grafts can (1) suppress epileptic phenomena in the CNS, (2) serve as an epileptic focus and induce hyperexcitability and behavioral seizures in the host, and (3) transfer the epileptic phenotype. Further studies should characterize in detail to what extent different parts of the epileptic syndrome can be influenced by cell implants releasing transmitters or neurotrophic factors. For example, can grafts have both antiepileptogenic and anticonvulsant effects? Where should the grafts be placed—in the epileptic focus, in regions of critical importance for seizure generalization, or as multiple implants to innervate large volumes of the epileptic brain? For further progress, it is mandatory that in each study, survival of, and, if possible, transmitter release from the cells of interest are assessed after transplantation. The mechanisms of action of grafts in epilepsy should be explored further. Do the grafts have to act via a controlled synaptic release of transmitter, or is a biologic minipump, delivering the compound in a more diffuse, hormonal manner, sufficient to influence seizure activity? Which level of anatomic and functional integration into the host neuronal circuitry is necessary for grafts to modulate neuronal excitability and convulsive phenomena? Are the changes in the levels of certain neurotrophic factors, induced by brief periods of seizure activity, directly involved in epileptogenesis? Obviously, more general advancements in the field of cell transplantation also will have a direct impact on its application in epilepsy research. These include the production of genetically engineered cells, making possible implantation of a "pure" population of transmitter-characterized (e.g., GABA-producing) cells. It is conceivable that this research will give more insights into the pathophysiology of seizures and, it is hoped, also will provide the necessary experimental basis for future attempts at reducing neuronal hyperexcitability in human epilepsy using cell transplantation.

ACKNOWLEDGMENTS

We are most grateful to Marie Lundin for valuable secretarial help. Our own research reviewed here was supported by grants from the Swedish Medical Research Council (14X-8666), the Thorsten and Elsa Segerfalk Foundation, the Kock Foundation, the Wiberg Foundation, the Bergvall Foundation, and the Medical Faculty, University of Lund.

REFERENCES

1. Araki H, Aihara H, Watanabe S, Ohta H, Yamamoto T, Ueki S. The role of noradrenergic and serotonergic systems in the hippocampal kindling effect. *Jpn J Pharmacol* 1983;33:57–64.
2. Ballarin M, Ernfors P, Lindefors N, Persson H. Rapid induction of mRNA for brain derived neurotrophic factor after intrahippocampal injection of kainic acid. *Exp Neurol* 1991;114:35–43.
3. Barry DI, Kikvadze I, Brundin P, Bolwig TG, Björklund A, Lindvall O. Grafted noradrenergic neurons suppress seizure development in kindling-induced epilepsy. *Proc Natl Acad Sci USA* 1987;84:8712–8715.
4. Barry DI, Wanscher B, Kragh J, et al. Grafts of fetal locus coeruleus neurons in rat amygdala–piriform cortex suppress seizure development in hippocampal kindling. *Exp Neurol* 1989;106:125–132.
5. Ben-Ari Y, Tremblay E, Ghilini G, Nacquet R. Electrographic, clinical and pathological alterations following systemic administration of kainic acid, bicuculline or pentrazole: metabolic mapping using the deoxyglucose method with special

reference to the pathology of epilepsy. *Neuroscience* 1981;6:1361–1391.

6. Ben-Ari Y. Limbic seizure and brain damage produced by kainic acid: mechanisms and relevance to human temporal lobe epilepsy. *Neuroscience* 1985;14:375–403.

7. Bengzon J, Kokaia M, Brundin P, Lindvall O. Seizure suppression in kindling epilepsy by intrahippocampal locus coeruleus grafts: evidence for alpha-2-adreno-receptor-mediated mechanism. *Exp Brain Res* 1990;81:433–437.

8. Bengzon J, Brundin P, Kalén P, Kokaia M, Lindvall O. Host regulation of noradrenaline release from grafts of seizure-suppressant locus coeruleus neurons. *Exp Neurol* 1991;111:49–54.

9. Bengzon J, Kikvadze I, Kokaia M, Lindvall O. Regional forebrain noradrenaline release in response to focal and generalized seizures induced by hippocampal kindling stimulation. *Eur J Neurosci* 1991;4:278–288.

10. Bengzon J, Kokaia Z, Lindvall O. Specific functions of grafted locus coeruleus neurons in the kindling model of epilepsy. *Exp Neurol* 1993; 122:143–154.

11. Bengzon J, Kokaia Z, Ernfors P, et al. Regulation of neurotrophin and trkA, trkB and trkC tyrosine kinase receptor mRNA expression in kindling. *Neuroscience* 1993;53:433–446.

12. Björklund A, Lindvall O. Catecholaminergic brain stem regulatory systems. In: Bloom FE, ed. *Handbook of physiology: the nervous system IV, intrinsic regulatory systems in the brain.* Bethesda, MD: American Physiological Society; 1986:155–235.

13. Buszáki G, Ponomareff G, Bayardo F, Shaw T, Gage FG. Suppression and induction of epileptic activity by neuronal grafts. *Proc Natl Acad Sci USA* 1988;85:9327–9330.

14. Buzsáki G, Bayardo F, Miles R, Wong RKS, Gage FH. The grafted hippocampus: an epileptic focus. *Exp Neurol* 1989;105:10–22.

15. Buzsáki G, Masliah E, Chen LS, Horvath Z, Terry R, Gage FH. Hippocampal grafts into the intact brain induce epileptic patterns. *Brain Res* 1991;554:30–37.

16. Cain DP. Bidirectional transfer of electrical and carbachol kindling. *Brain Res* 1983;260:135–138.

17. Camu W, Marlier L, Lerner-Natoli M, Rondouin G, Privat A. Transplantation of serotonergic neurons into the 5,7-DHT-lesioned rat olfactory bulb restores the parameters of kindling. *Brain Res* 1990;518:23–30.

18. Cassel JC, Kelche C, Will BE. Susceptibility to pentylenetetrazol-induced and audiogenic seizures in rats with selective fimbria–fornix lesions and intrahippocampal septal grafts. *Exp Neurol* 1987;97:564–576.

19. Cassel JC, Kelche C, Will BE. Susceptibility to pentylenetetrazol-induced and audiogenic seizures in rats given aspirative lesions of the fimbria–fornix pathways followed by intrahippocampal grafts: a time-course approach. *Rest Neurol Neurosci* 1991;3:55–64.

20. Chauvel P, Trottier S. Role of noradrenergic ascending system in extinction of epileptic phenomena. *Adv Neurol* 1986;44:475–487.

21. Clough RW, Browning RA, Maring ML, Jobe PC. Intracerebral grafting of fetal dorsal pons in genetically epilepsy-prone rats: effects on audiogenic-induced seizures. *Exp Neurol* 1991; 112:195–199.

22. Corcoran ME, Mason ST. Role of forebrain catecholamines in amygdaloid kindling. *Brain Res* 1980;190:473–484.

23. Corcoran ME. Characteristics of accelerated kindling after depletion of noradrenaline in adult rats. *Neuropharmacology* 1988;27:1081–1084.

24. Depaulis A, Snead OI, Marescaux C, Vergnes M. Suppressive effects of intranigral injection of muscimol in three models of generalized nonconvulsive epilepsy induced by chemical agents. *Brain Res* 1989;498:64–72.

25. Emson P, Joseph M. Neurochemical and morphological changes during the development of cobalt-induced epilepsy in the rat. *Brain Res* 1975;93:91–110.

26. Ernfors P, Bengzon J, Kokaia Z, Persson H, Lindvall O. Increased levels of messenger RNAs for neurotrophic factors in the brain during kindling epileptogenesis. *Neuron* 1991;7:165–176.

27. Fine A, Meldrum BS, Patel S. Modulation of experimentally induced epilepsy by intracerebral grafts of fetal GABAergic neurons. *Neuropsychology* 1990;28:627–634.

28. Fisher W, Kästner I, Lanck R, Müller M. Wirkung der Reizung des Locus coeruleus auf Kobalt-induzierte epileptiforme Aktivität bei der Ratte. *Biomed Biochim Acta* 1983;1179–1187.

29. Foote SL, Bloom FE, Aston-Jones G. Nucleus locus coeruleus: new evidence of anatomical and physiological specificity. *Physiol Rev* 1983; 63:844–914.

30. Frye GD, McCown TJ, Breese GR. Characterization of susceptibility to audiogenic seizures in ethanol-dependent rats after microinjection of gamma-aminobutyric acid (GABA) agonists into the inferior colliculus, substantia nigra or medial septum. *J Pharmacol Exp Ther* 1983;227:663–670.

31. Gale K. GABA and epilepsy: basic concepts from preclinical research. *Epilepsia* 1992;33 (Suppl 5):3–12.

32. Gale K. Focal trigger zones and pathways of propagation in seizure generation. In: Schwartzkroin PA, ed. *Epilepsy: models, mechanisms, and concepts.* Cambridge: Cambridge University Press; 1993:48–93.

33. Gall CM, Isackson PJ. Limbic seizures increase neuronal production of messenger RNA for nerve growth factor. *Science* 1989;245:758–761.

34. Gall C, Murray K, Isackson PJ. Kainic acid-induced seizures stimulate increased expression of nerve growth factor mRNA in rat hippocampus. *Brain Res* 1991;9:113–123.

35. Garant DS, Gale K. Intranigral muscimol attenuates electrographic signs of seizure activity induced by intravenous bicuculline in rats. *Eur J Pharmacol* 1986;124:365–369.

36. Gastaut H, Gastaut JL, Goncalves e Silva GE, Fernandez Sanchez GR. Relative frequency of different types of epilepsy: a study employing the classification of the International League Against Epilepsy. *Epilepsia* 1975;16:457–461.

37. Gellman RL, Kalianos JA, McNamara JO. Alpha-2 receptors mediate an endogenous noradrenergic suppression of kindling development. *J Pharmacol Exp Ther* 1987;241:891–898.

38. Goddard GV, McIntyre DC, Leech CK. A permanent change in brain function resulting from daily electrical stimulation. *Exp Neurol* 1969; 25:295–330.

39. Guy N, Teillet M, Schuler B, et al. Pattern of electroencephalographic activity during light induced seizures in genetic epileptic chicken and brain chimeras. *Neurosci Lett* 1992;145: 55–58.

40. Holmes GL, Thompson JL, Smeyne RJ, Wallace RB. Failure of neocortical transplants to alter seizure susceptibility in previously kindled rats. *Epilepsia* 1987;28:242–250.

41. Holmes GL, Thompson JL, Huh K, Stuart JD, Carl GF. Effect of neural transplants on seizure frequency and kindling in immature rats following kainic acid. *Dev Brain Res* 1991;64:47–56.

42. Holmes GL, Thompson JL, Huh K, Stuart JD, Carl GF. Effects of neural transplantation on seizures in the immature genetically epilepsy-prone rat. *Exp Neurol* 1992;116:52–63.

43. Iadarola MJ, Gale K. Substantia nigra: site of anticonvulsant activity mediated by γ-aminobutyric acid. *Science* 1982;218:1237–1240.

44. Isackson PJ, Huntsman MM, Murray KD, Gall CM. BDNF mRNA expression is increased in adult rat forebrain after limbic seizures: temporal patterns of induction distinct from NGF. *Neuron* 1991;6:937–948.

45. Jimenez-Rivera CA, Weiss GK. The effect of amygdala kindled seizures on locus coeruleus activity. *Brain Res Bull* 1989;22:751–758.

46. Jobe PC, Mishra PK, Ludvig N, Dailey JW. Genetic models of the epilepsies. In: Schwartzkroin PA, ed. *Epilepsy: models, mechanisms, and concepts.* Cambridge: Cambridge University Press; 1993:94–140.

47. Kamphuis W, Wadman WJ, Buijs R, Lopes da Silva FH. Decrease in number of hippocampal gamma-aminobutyric acid (GABA) immunoreactive cells in the rat kindling model of epilepsy. *Exp Brain Res* 1986;64:491–495.

48. Kamphuis W, Huisman E, Wadman WJ, Lopes da Silva FH. Decrease in GABA immunoreactivity and alteration of GABA metabolism after kindling in the rat hippocampus. *Exp Brain Res* 1989;74:375–386.

49. Kokaia M, Aebischer P, Elmér E, et al. Seizure suppression in kindling epilepsy by intracerebral implants of GABA- but not by noradrenaline-releasing polymer matrices. *Exp Brain Res* 1994 (*in press*).

50. Kokaia Z, Bengzon J, Metsis M, Kokaia M, Persson H, Lindvall O. Coexpression of neurotrophins and their receptors in neurons of the central nervous system. *Proc Natl Acad Sci USA.* 1993;90:6711–6715.

51. LeGal LaSalle G, Kaijima M, Feldblum S. Abortive amygdaloid kindled seizures following microinjection of gamma-vinyl-GABA in the vicinity of substantia nigra in rats. *Neurosci Lett* 1983;36:69–74.

52. Lerner-Natoli M, Rondouin G, Malafosse A, Sandillon F, Privat A, Baldy-Moulinier M. Facilitation of olfactory bulb kindling after specific destruction of serotonergic terminals in the olfactory bulb of the rat. *Neurosci Lett* 1986; 66:299–304.

53. Libet B, Gleason CA, Wright EW Jr, Feinstein B. Suppression of an epileptiform type of electrocortical activity in the rat by stimulation in the vicinity of locus coeruleus. *Epilepsia* 1977; 18:451–462.

54. Lindvall O, Bengzon J, Brundin P, Kalén P, Kokaia M. Locus coeruleus grafts in hippocampal kindling epilepsy: noradrenalin release, receptor specificity and influence on seizure development. *Prog Brain Res* 1990;82:339–346.

55. Mason ST, Corcoran ME. Catecholamines and convulsions. *Brain Res* 1979;170:497–507.

56. McIntyre DC, Saari M, Pappas BA. Potentiation of amygdala kindling in adult or infant rats by injections of 6-hydroxydopamine. *Exp Neurol* 1979;63:527–544.

57. McIntyre DC, Edson N. Facilitation of amygdala kindling after norepinephrine depletion with 6-hydroxydopamine in rats. *Exp Neurol* 1981;74:748–757.

58. McIntyre DC, Edson N. Effect of norepinephrine depletion on dorsal hippocampus kindling in rats. *Exp Neurol* 1982;77:700–704.

59. McIntyre DC, Racine RJ. Kindling mechanisms: current progress of an experimental epilepsy model. *Prog Neurobiol* 1986;27:1–12.

60. McNamara JO. Kindling: an animal model of complex partial epilepsy. *Ann Neurol* 1984; 16(Suppl):72–76.

61. McNamara JO, Galloway MT, Rigsbee LC, Shin C. Evidence implicating substantia nigra in regulation of kindled seizure threshold. *J Neurosci* 1984;4:2410–2417.

62. Merlio J-P, Ernfors P, Kokaia Z, et al. Increased production of the trkB protein tyrosine kinase receptor after brain insults. *Neuron* 1993;10: 151–164.

63. Murata Y, Chiba T, Brundin P, Björklund A, Lindvall O. Formation of synaptic graft–host connections by noradrenergic locus coeruleus neurons transplanted into the adult rat hippocampus. *Exp Neurol* 1990;110:258–267.

64. Nadler JV. Kainic acid as a tool for the study of temporal lobe epilepsy. *Life Sci* 1981;29:2031–2042.

65. Nelson MF, Zaczek R, Coyle JT. Effects of sustained seizures produced by intrahippocampal injection of kainic acid on noradrenergic neurons: evidence for local control of norepinephrine release. *J Pharmacol Exp Ther* 1980; 214:694–702.

66. Neuman RS. Suppression of penicillin-induced focal epileptiform activity by locus coeruleus stimulation: mediation by an alpha1-adrenoceptor. *Epilepsia* 1986;27:359–366.

67. Pasini A, Tortorella A, Gale K. Anticonvulsant effect of intranigral fluoxetine. *Brain Res* 1992; 593:287–290.
68. Piredda S, Gale K. A crucial epileptogenic site in deep prepyriform cortex. *Nature* 1985;317: 623–625.
69. Racine RJ. Modification of seizure activity by electrical stimulation: II. motor seizure. *Electroencephalogr Clin Neurophysiol* 1972;32:281–294.
70. Racine RJ, Burnham WM. The kindling model. In: Schwartzkroin PA, Wheal HV, eds. *Electrophysiology of epilepsy*. London: Academic Press; 1984:153–171.
71. Ribak CE, Harris A, Vaughn J, Roberts E. Inhibitory, GABAergic nerve terminals decrease at sites of focal epilepsy. *Science* 1979;205:211–214.
72. Schwartzkroin PA, Kunkel D. Viability of GABAergic striatal neurons grafted into normal hippocampus. *Soc Neurosci Abstr* 1988;233:8.
73. Schwartzkroin PA. *Epilepsy: models, mechanisms, and concepts*. Cambridge: Cambridge University Press; 1993.
74. Stevens JR, Phillips I, deBeurepaire R. Gammavinyl GABA in endopiriform area suppresses kindled amygdala seizures. *Epilepsia* 1988;29: 404–411.
75. Stevens JR, Phillips I, Freed WJ, Poltorak M. Cerebral transplants for seizures: preliminary results. *Epilepsia* 1988;29:731–737.
76. Teillet MA, Naquet R, LeGal LaSalle G, Merat P, Schuler B, LeDouarin NM. Transfer of genetic epilepsy by embryonic brain grafts in the chicken. *Proc Natl Acad Sci USA* 1991;88:6966–6970.
77. Turski L, Cavalheiro EA, Schwarz M, et al. Susceptibility to seizures produced by pilocarpine in rats after microinjection of isoniazid or gamma-vinyl-GABA into the substantia nigra. *Brain Res* 1986;370:294–309.
78. Turski L, Cavalheiro EA, Bortolotti ZA, Ikonomidou-Turski C, Kleinrok Z, Turski WA. Dopamine-sensitive anticonvulsant site in the rat striatum. *J Neurosci* 1988;8:4027–4037.
79. Wada JA, Sato M, Corcoran ME. Persistent seizure susceptibility and recurrent spontaneous seizures in kindled cats. *Epilepsia* 1974;15:465–478.
80. Wahnschaffe U, Löscher W. Anticonvulsant effects of ipsilateral but not contralateral microinjections of the dopamine D2 agonist LY 171555 into the nucleus accumbens of amygdala-kindled rats. *Brain Res* 1991;553:181–187.
81. Wasterlain CG, Jonec V. Chemical kindling by muscarinic amygdaloid stimulation in the rat. *Brain Res* 1983;271:311–323.
82. Westerberg V, Lewis J, Corcoran ME. Depletion of noradrenaline fails to affect kindled seizures. *Exp Neurol* 1984;84:237–240.
83. Westerberg V, Corcoran ME. Antagonism of central but not peripheral cholinergic receptors retards amygdala kindling in rats. *Exp Neurol* 1987;95:194–206.
84. Xu SG, Garant DS, Sperber EF, Moshe SL. Effects of substantia nigra gamma-vinyl-GABA infusions on flurothyl seizures in adult rats. *Brain Res* 1991;566:1–2.

Functional Neural Transplantation
edited by S. B. Dunnett and A. Björklund.
Raven Press, Ltd., New York © 1994.

16

Cortical Graft Function in Adult and Neonatal Rats

Bryan Kolb and *Bryan Fantie

*Psychology Department, University of Lethbridge, Lethbridge, Alberta, Canada T1K 3M4; *Human Neuropsychology Laboratory, The American University, Washington, DC 20001*

There is now little doubt that cortical grafts grow when transplanted into neocortex. Over a century has passed since Thompson (96) published a brief description of the first attempt to graft central nervous system (CNS) tissue into the brain. Almost 30 years later, Dunn (10) demonstrated that grafts taken from neonatal donors would survive for extended periods in adult rat hosts. Until relatively recently, however, most of the work that used CNS transplants exercised this technique as a means to understand the structure of the nervous system, particularly in relation to development and recovery from injury.

There is little doubt that the grafts possess at least some of the cytologic and neurochemical characteristics of the cortex that they replace and that they acquire at least some of the connections of normal cortex (see 12 for review). The fundamental, and clinically significant, question that remains unanswered, however, is whether the transplanted tissue actually assumes the function of the original tissue. Stated differently, one can ask whether functions lost as a result of cortical injury can actually be restored by replacing the lost cortical tissue. This question forms the basis of the current chapter. We begin by considering theoretical issues surrounding the proposition of graft-induced functional restitution. We then

consider the practical problems in assessing recovery. Finally, we review the existing evidence for behavioral recovery and attempt to draw conclusions that might guide future research.

THEORETICAL ISSUES

The rodent neocortex offers an excellent model system for graft-induced recovery of function in humans; yet, not without formidable difficulties. It is excellent insofar as (a) it is easily accessible for surgical procedures; (b) its cytoarchitecture and connectivity are well described; and (c) there is considerable knowledge about its functional organization. Thus, in principle, it ought to be relatively straightforward to determine the cytoarchitecture and connectivity of host and graft. Furthermore, it would seem a forthright proposition to assess function after the introduction of a graft. Unfortunately, it is here that the researcher finds at least two substantial problems. First, we must ask what we might expect a graft to do considering how the neocortex is normally organized and how important that organization is to function. Second, we must consider the general principle of science that requires different researchers to agree about what constitutes the phenomenon that they are studying. In the current context, this means that there must be consensus about what will be taken as evidence of graft-induced recovery of function. We consider these problems in turn.

How Is the Neocortex Normally Organized?

To determine how a cortical transplant might be affecting brain function, one must make assumptions about how the cortex customarily operates. The classic notions of mass action and equipotentiality presumed that the brain worked as an integrated whole (in contrast with the varied and assorted independent organs of phrenology) and that any piece of cerebral cortex had the potential to assume the duties of any other piece. Although Lashley (62) clearly showed that the size of lesions was positively correlated with the magnitude of the resulting deficits in maze learning, it does not follow that simply replacing cortical tissue will allow restitution of function. Even though the precise localization of complex faculties proposed by Gall and Spurzheim is no longer given serious consideration (59), it is now generally recognized that even the relatively simple rodent cortex is highly differentiated both cytoarchitectonically and functionally. Furthermore, the cortex clearly has intrinsic structural and connectivity characteristics that are crucial to its normal role in behavior. An understanding of the functional properties of grafts, therefore, must consider briefly the basic intrinsic properties of cortical organization (for a detailed discussion see 18,40,95).

The intrinsic organization of the cortex is characterized by at least three fundamental attributes. First, the cortex has a laminar organization (40). Hence, cells of like somata tend to be aggregated together in layers. Furthermore, it appears that like somata within a layer have similar patterns of efferent, and perhaps afferent, connectivity. Therefore, the second basic feature of cortical organization is connectivity. The output cells of the cortex are the pyramidal cells, the output targets varying with the laminar location of the somata. Third, the cortex has a modular structure. This is perhaps best illustrated by Szentágothai's beautiful diagrammatic representations of the internal neuronal connectivity. Thus, Szentágothai (94), as well as others (18), have emphasized that the neocortex is subdivided into a mosaic of modules that form the basic functional units of the neocortex. The loss of specific modules, therefore, compromises cortical processing. The addition of modules in evolution enhances cortical processing and behavioral flexibility.

All regions of neocortex share these three primary characteristics. Therefore, modular and laminar organization, as well as the pyramidal outputs, are fundamental features of neocortical structure. Since this is so, it is reasonable to ask if they are necessary for "normal" neocortical function. This is a difficult question to answer definitively because the neocortex rarely fails to bear these attributes. Indeed, even major surgical or chemical intervention in perinatal animals results in only minor deviations from the normal modular and laminar organization in the remaining tissue. Interestingly, neocortical grafts often do not possess this normal laminar or modular structure, even when they completely fill the lesion cavity (Fig. 1). Surprisingly, this

---

FIG. 1. Photomicrographs showing an example of the growth of a frontal cortical transplant. **A**: Nissl-stained section showing the transplant filling the entire lesion cavity. Note that the cells do not respect cortical laminae within the graft. **B**: Adjacent myelin-stained section from the same brain. **C**: Higher magnification of the section illustrated in B. Note the relatively heavy myelinization and lack of laminar organization.

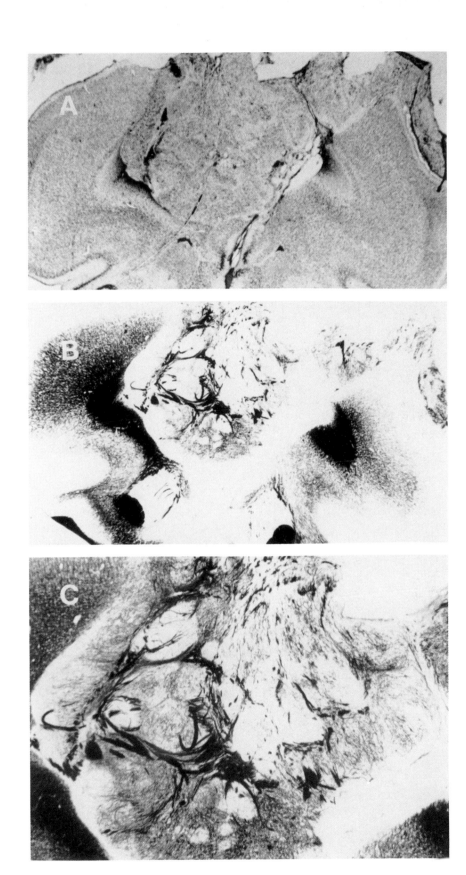

aberrant cortical cytoarchitecture is sometimes still associated with amazing functional properties. For instance, Girman and
Golovina (32) replaced portions of the occipital cortex in adult rats with embryonic
cortical grafts and later made electrophysiologic recordings from the implants. Remarkably, they not only found visually
evoked responses from cells in the transplanted tissue, but they also found that
there was an orderly visual field representation in at least some of the transplants.
Unfortunately, it is unknown whether the
visual input had any behavioral significance
and provided information that could be
used by the animal in some meaningful way.
Nonetheless, their results raise the possibility that, at least in some limited circumstances, neocortex may be able to function
relatively normally in the absence of the
usual modular–laminar structure. It is possible that, when the gross appearance of the
cortex lacks the usual laminar structure,
there may still be a highly ordered intrinsic
organization such as the patch–matrix of
the striatum.

There is an additional related question.
Is the mere presence of laminar–modular
structure sufficient to produce normal cortical function? Under the appropriate surgical conditions it is sometimes possible to
obtain remarkably normal-appearing laminar and modular organization in transplants
that have been introduced into neonatal
brains (2,74), but it has not yet been shown
whether or not these transplants function
like normal tissue. Although it is tempting
to assume that apparently normal structure
implies normal function, it is not necessarily so. In fact, the primary determinant of
normal functioning is likely to be relevant
and effective connectivity. Similarly, although early cortical injuries may allow the
relatively normal development of laminar
and modular organization, function may be
significantly more compromised than that
observed following a seemingly comparable
cortical injury later in development (49).
Viewed in this light, it is clear that the mere
presence of laminar and modular structure

in a cortical transplant provides little information about its functional viability.

What Happens When the Nervous System Is Compromised?

Cortical injuries may alter behavior directly and indirectly. The purest form of a
direct, primary deficit would arise when the
essential circuit for a given behavioral function was wholly or partially lost. Secondary
deficits may result when the missing neural
circuit was responsible for inhibiting another circuit. In one case, its absence might
lead to the release of some function that
either interferes with the operation of one
or more other circuits or disrupts the performance of the behavior itself (e.g., by
producing an incompatible, competing motor pattern). For instance, loss of the dopaminergic input to the basal ganglia can
produce tremors that seriously disturb
handwriting.

Another indirect source of behavioral
disruption can occur when circuits become
disorganized by the loss of either specific or
nonspecific afferents. For example, if an
animal sustains damage to the somatosensory cortex, it is difficult to conclude
whether the behavioral loss represents a direct loss of somatosensory function, or an
indirect change brought about by lost afferents to the motor cortex. Further compli-
cating the interpretation, how the organism
attempts to redress the loss also colors the
net behavioral change. This can include
compensation at the anatomic (e.g., sprouting), the physiologic (e.g., redundant circuitry), and the behavioral (e.g., alternative
strategies) levels. Brain damage rarely, if
ever, results in a purely subtractive behavioral deficit. It is only when other sources
of data, such as electrophysiologic measurements from the intact brain, complement the evidence of behavioral change
that we are able to approach making valid
inferences concerning the functional organization of the cortex. The interpretation of
behavioral change in an animal with a cor-

tical lesion is further complicated by the addition of a specific treatment, such as the implantation of fetal tissue. The graft can have direct effects that will likely be coupled with the host organism's reactions to its presence. It is difficult, therefore, to delineate clearly the precise nature of the origin of each facet of damage-produced deficits. This leads us to another basic question: "What constitutes recovery of function?"

What Constitutes Recovery of Function?

There is no conventional definition of what constitutes recovery of function. Hence, behavioral recovery can refer to different things to different investigators. Restitution of function could be complete, or it could be partial. It might be absolute, or relative. Just as the amount of improvement can vary, so can the quality, and this is much more difficult to quantify. Deficits themselves can vary greatly in both configuration and magnitude. This interaction complicates the picture. Even if we assume that a cortical injury alters behavior consistently in some meaningful way, we still have a variety of different possible forms of functional restitution, each of which has a different implication for studies of recovery.

First, one type of injury may normally be expected to cause a given behavior to disappear permanently. In this case, recovery might constitute (a) a complete return of the behavior, or (b) a partial return of the behavior. These two forms of recovery are fundamentally different. A complete return implies a total reversal of the process that caused the behavioral loss in the first place. A less than complete restoration of function could occur for many reasons, including a partial reversal of the original loss, which could mean that a graft partially replaced the original tissue. In contrast with total recovery, however, partial recovery could occur indirectly because a graft facilitated plastic changes somewhere else in the host

brain. It is unlikely that a similar mechanism could be invoked to create a total remedy.

Second, a given behavior might disappear after an injury, but then, in normal circumstances, return slowly, either partially or completely, over the ensuing weeks, months, or years. Here, enhanced recovery might constitute (a) a faster return of the behavior to its expected level of competence, or (b) a more complete return of the behavior. These two outcomes are by no means equivalent.

Third, when considering complex behaviors, a cortical injury might lead either to the total inability to solve a problem (such as a maze), or to the retarded solution of the problem. Here, graft-induced recovery could mean that the animal could (a) solve the problem as efficiently as intact animals, (b) perform the problem better than similarly injured animals without the treatment in question, or (c) solve the problem more quickly than expected after the injury. Again, these outcomes are not equivalent.

Finally, we must make a distinction between the expected outcomes of injury at different ages, particularly during the period of development before adulthood. If the cortex is injured before a behavior completely appears, or if that behavior has reached final maturity, one might expect that (a) because of the injury, the behavior(s) will fail to emerge at all; (b) behaviors will emerge later in development than expected; (c) behavior that would have been lost or impaired after an adult injury of the same structures either will emerge normally in development (a condition usually referred to as sparing of function) or, at least, will be more normal than expected had the injury occurred later in the life span; or (d) a form of the behavior will emerge on schedule and be abnormal, but will later improve so that it appears normal or, at least, more normal than for an injury in adulthood. Treatments, such as cortical grafts, may affect each of these possibilities differently.

Clearly, there are multiple definitions of

recovery. Few investigators studying recovery of function appear to consider precisely what has occurred, and there is a tendency to accept any quantitative improvement in performance after a treatment as evidence of "functional recovery." Albeit this optimism is obviously well-meaning, nevertheless, it may be misguided and unintentionally misleading. The difficulty is that dramatically different mechanisms likely mediate different forms of recovery. Furthermore, when multiple measures of function are used to assess behavioral restitution, it is often observed that "recovery" is not equivalent across the different measures. Again, this has important implications for the issue of what the graft is actually doing.

For the present review, we will assume that *recovery* means simply that behavior is different in cortically injured animals with and without cortical grafts. Our intent is to search for evidence that the grafts influence the operation of the host brain. We will return to the issue of why at the end of the chapter.

PRACTICAL ISSUES

Before one can seriously examine the evidence for graft-induced recovery of function, one needs some idea of what the usual "rules" concerning the untreated recovery from cortical injury might be. This is a complex issue that has been reviewed in detail elsewhere (52), so here we will focus only on issues that are likely to influence studies of the functional consequences of cortical implantation.

Factors Influencing Recovery From Cortical Injury and Cortical Grafting

Lesion Size

The work of Lashley (62) demonstrated that there is a positive correlation between lesion size and behavioral loss. The relation is somewhat more complicated than Lashley envisioned, however. Although often true, the larger the lesion, the greater the deficit is likely to be, this principle is not inviolable. For example, the extent of recovery can be strikingly greater following unilateral cortical injuries, compared with quantitatively equivalent bilateral insults. Furthermore, it appears that even small bilateral lesions may allow less recovery than large unilateral injuries. What is particularly surprising about this is that it seems that the bilateral injury need not necessarily include homologous tissue in the two hemispheres to produce significantly greater behavioral deficits (97).

Thus, this effect is not merely because unilateral lesions spare destruction of specific corresponding contralateral circuitry that may have had the potential to maintain some degree of residual function. A more likely scenario, considering the experimental data, would suggest that damage anywhere within a hemisphere compromises many functions, including its capability to respond to new demands. In a unilateral lesion, the unaffected hemisphere remains at its full capacity and is able to offer some degree of compensation. In contrast, a bilateral injury not only destroys the tissue at the site of the insult, but it removes the possibility that an intact hemisphere can contribute fully to offsetting the loss.

That bilateral lesions can allow less recovery than unilateral ones is important for studies of the efficacy of grafts to restore function. Not only do differential ceiling or floor effects of the respective recovery potential confound the detection of improvement, but the mechanisms through which the grafts mediate recovery from unilateral and bilateral injury may be entirely different. We are not aware of any experiments that have systematically considered this issue after cortical grafts, but it is our impression from our own work that one is far more likely to observe some functional restitution after unilateral, rather than after bilateral, lesions. This difference may represent the indirect effect of the grafts on the undamaged hemisphere in the unilateral cases, or it may simply reflect that unilateral injury allows more plasticity, essentially providing a more permissive environment for transplanted tissue to affect function.

Lesion Location

As a rule of thumb, it appears that damage to primary sensory or motor areas are less amenable to complete restoration of function than is damage to "association" regions. From a practical standpoint, this is sensible because the maintenance of an internal representation of the external sensory world can be accomplished only by an exquisite pattern of specific neural connectivity. These connections are wholly dependent on finite populations of sensory receptors and are functionally subordinate to an accurate topographic organization. There is limited redundancy in the circuits between receptors and the level of the first synapse in primary sensory cortices. Similarly, the operation of primary motor cortex may require precise corticofugal connectivity, which is unlikely to be regained after its loss. The portions of neural circuits closest to the periphery, whether the first stages of the inwardly expanding branches of afferents or the later stages of efferent pathways converging on spinal motor nerves, have a decreasing number of possible alternate transmission routes. In contrast, higher-level behaviors, such as spatial maze learning, presumably can be accomplished in numerous ways through multiple analogous circuits. Indeed, it is rare for cortical lesions to eliminate completely the ability to accomplish cognitive tasks in laboratory animals. Instead, one generally sees an inferior performance, rather than a complete abolition. Relative to graft efficacy, one might predict that cortical grafts would be more likely to enhance recovery after damage to association cortex than after primary sensory or motor cortical injury, especially

in adult animals. We expect that grafted neurons would be more likely to form potentially meaningful connections in the local circuitry associated with higher-level associations than they would relink the correct specific inputs or outputs of primary motor and sensory pathways.

Age at Injury

Damage to a given area of the brain at different times in life may lead to markedly disparate behavioral symptoms. The degree of resilience of the embryonic mammalian CNS during the course of development varies enormously, depending on the particular stage that is in progress (tempered, of course, by the size of the lesion). For example, if a lesion is made early, during cellular proliferation, before developmental events determine the morphology, location, and function of the newborn neurons, the damaged cells are replaced and no apparent deficit follows. In contrast, an injury that hampers mitosis or confounds neuronal migration, disrupts subsequent development and typically produces severe behavioral loss. Injury during the period of cortical differentiation and maturation, on the other hand, can allow remarkable sparing of function, presumably because, at this time, there are sufficient redundant neurons, which in normal circumstances would disappear during programmed cell death, that can replace the circuitry and take over the functions of the lost cells. Injury in aged animals may produce greater or lesser effects than in younger animals, depending on the region injured and the behavioral measure used (22,56). The important point here is that there may be times when the brain is especially able to compensate for injury, and other periods when it is not so capable. Perinatal cortical lesions in prefrontal, motor, and parietal cortex of rats are more debilitating than similar lesions made at 7 to 10 days of age (58). What transplantation at 7 to 10 days might do, however, is not yet known, since studies showing functional improvement in animals with neonatal cortical injuries have consistently involved perinatal injuries. What would one expect from grafts into brains with lesions at 7 to 10 days?

The timing of cortical tissue transplantation needs to be considered in the light of this evidence of the brain's changing capacity to respond to injury. Indeed, several of our own studies lead us to suspect that grafts may be most effective at times when the brain is not normally able to compensate. A corollary of this prediction is that grafts might be ineffective, or even a hindrance, when transplantation occurs at times when the brain normally shows good compensation (24,51). Perhaps the main restorative effect of transplantation is not direct, that is, originating from the graft itself, but rather the graft works indirectly by altering the host brain's ability to recuperate.

A further complication of age-related differences in recovery relates to the question of bilateral versus unilateral injury at different times in life. This issue has not been studied systematically in animals without cortical grafts, let alone in conjunction with implantation. Nonetheless, we are struck by the fact that studies showing enhanced recovery of forelimb movements after neonatal cortical transplantation have all used animals with unilateral injuries. Would similar recovery be observed after bilateral injury? If it was not, what would that imply about the mechanism(s) of graft-induced recovery?

Injury-to-Transplant Interval

The most common procedure is to wait 7 to 14 days after making the lesions before implanting donor tissue into adult animals because the grafts are more likely to survive after such a delay (68). The general assumption is that factors such as the increased vascularity in the lesion cavity, a reduction or absence of posttraumatic blood clots, the peak production of trophic factors or glia, and so forth, enhance graft survival. Curiously, there does not seem to be any systematic study of the optimal time to implant tissue after perinatal damage. In fact, virtually all studies implant the tissue immediately after the injury. Although this convention reduces the trauma to the young animal by eliminating the necessity for a second surgery, and this may indeed be the optimal time for graft survival in perinatal animals, this has not been established empirically. The timing of transplantation is not only relevant to graft survival, but it determines the stage of recovery to the insult in which the host brain is engaged. Therefore, the efficacy of the graft to interact with the various mechanisms that may be at work naturally in the recovery process will vary differentially depending on the time of implantation. If maximum recovery calls for a specific interaction between the implant and one of these processes, timing may be crucial. This issue clearly needs more study.

Lesion Method

Cortical lesions may be produced by a variety of methods, including ablation by suction or electrolysis, neurotoxins, vascular occlusion, or head trauma. Few studies have attempted to directly compare the behavioral sequelae of comparable lesions produced by different techniques, although it is our impression that head trauma produces greater effects than ablations which, in turn, produce larger effects than toxins. This remains to be investigated directly. In view of the dearth of data concerning the comparative effects of different lesion techniques, it is not surprising that there are as yet no studies that compare graft efficacy after different forms of lesions. Since most investigators prefer to implant cortical chunks, it is convenient to have a cavity for implantation, but this may not be the optimal experimental paradigm for those interested in clinical applications after cerebral vascular accidents or trauma. Of course, how one hopes and expects that the graft will function in promoting recovery will determine what type of dysfunction will be improved most by implants. At the present state of the art, it is more likely that grafts will be better able to ameliorate the deficits that result from degenerated neurotransmitter sources in disorders such as Parkinson's disease, or even Huntington's chorea, than they will reverse the widespread neuronal damage caused by cerebral vascular accidents or traumatic head injury. In a similar vein, neuronal transplants will likely be better suited to result in improvement when traumatic damage is focal as opposed to diffuse.

Sex of Host and Donor

There is now little doubt that there is sexual dimorphism in the structure of the cerebral cortex (42). For example, Kolb and Stewart (53) found that pyramidal cells in the prefrontal cortex of rats were sexually dimorphic: cells in the medial prefrontal regions had more extensive dendritic arbor in males, whereas cells in the orbital regions had more arbor in females. These anatomic results run parallel to behavioral studies finding sex-related differences in frontal lesion effects in both humans (46) and rats (50). Hence, it appears that gonadal steroids affect both cortical structure and function. What might then be the role of gonadal steroids in graft growth and function? In a preliminary study of this issue we implanted frontal cortical tissue from male or female newborn rats into adult male or female rats with medial prefrontal lesions. Our principal finding was that the grafts from either sex of donors grew pyramidal cells, with more extensive aborization in male hosts than female hosts (Fig. 2). This result suggests that gonadal steroids might influence graft growth, and possibly function. It is unknown, however, whether such effects might be true in other cortical regions.

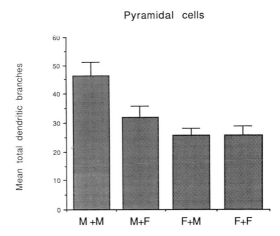

FIG. 2. Summary of quantified dendritic branching in the transplants of adult male or female rats given E21 grafts from either male or female donors. Note that the type of host differentially influenced the extent of dendritic growth, as the male hosts had greater arborization than the female hosts, regardless of the sex of the donor. *M + M,* male host + male donor; *M + F,* male host + female donor; *F + M,* female host + male donor; *F + F,* female host + female donor.

Behavioral Measure

Cortical injuries normally produce a constellation of behavioral effects that are not equally likely to show recovery. For example, Kolb and Whishaw (55,57) showed that, although rats or hamsters with frontal lesions at about 7 days of age showed impressive sparing of performance on tests of maze learning relative to rats with similar lesions in adulthood, the same animals showed absolutely no recovery on tests of species-typical behavior, such as food hoarding or defensive burying. Nonneman and Kolb (72) found parallel results in their study of rats with serial frontal lesions in adulthood. Thus, a single behavioral measure is simply inadequate for making valid generalizations about the degree, or even mere presence, of recovery after cortical injury. This has important implications for studies of graft-induced recovery, since it is common for studies to use a single measure of behavior. A recent study of ours illustrates the problem. Rats received medial prefrontal lesions in adulthood, followed by cortical transplants from donors aged E17, E19, E21, or E23 days. Two months later the animals were trained on a spatial alternation task, and those animals with E21 implants showed no functional deficit relative to control animals, whereas all other groups were impaired. However, when the same animals were subsequently trained on another spatial navigation task (Morris water task) the animals with E21 grafts were as impaired as the other groups, but the animals with E19 transplants now showed a partial restitution of function. Thus, although both behavioral tasks are commonly used to assess the integrity of prefrontal function in rats, the measures were not equally sensitive to the effects of prefrontal grafts. Indeed, we have no reason to believe that other measures might not have shown beneficial effects of either the E17 or E23 grafts. The important lesson here is that behavioral analysis is not easy and that a thorough behavioral analysis is needed before generalizations concerning the extent of graft-induced recovery, or the mechanisms underlying the recovery, may be made. We are not aware of a single behavioral study of the functional effects of cortical grafts that has done a truly thorough behavioral analysis, although several have used at least multiple measures (14,23).

Postoperative Recovery Time

Different behaviors show different rates of recovery after neocortical lesions, the rate of change varying with factors such as lesion size and location. Furthermore, there is accumulating evidence that cortical grafts may influence behavior in different ways at different times during recovery. For example, both we (51) and Dunnett and coworkers (14) showed that frontal transplants reduced the behavioral deficits when animals with prefrontal lesions were studied soon after implantation, but that the be-

havioral gain was actually reversed when behavior was retested weeks later. The reasons for the behavioral changes have not been established, but it is clear that behavioral assessment at only one time or the other would have been misleading.

What Might We Expect Cortical Grafts to Do?

When the cortex is damaged, there are two intimately related, but essentially dissociable, mechanisms that attempt to mediate recovery. On the neurobiologic level, some or all of a variety of processes (that include collateral sprouting, the disinhibition of previously silent redundant circuits, and so forth) act to compensate the remaining brain tissue, at least partially, for its loss. On the behavioral level, new strategies develop, where possible, to accomplish tasks that relied on specific lost skills. These changes are not static, but continue to evolve for months, and in humans, even years. Any treatment, such as a cortical graft, that is introduced after cortical injury could have a variety of effects. First, the lost tissue could be wholly replaced by the graft, much as if one replaced a broken component in a radio. This appears to be very unlikely in an adult animal. An adult brain has a lifetime of experiences that have altered the details of the intrinsic circuitry (4). There would simply be no easy way for a newly grown neural region to integrate into the existing neural circuits in the same manner as the original tissue. Indeed, it seems likely that reintegration with existing circuits could prove disruptive (14,20,51). In contrast, however, it appears that transplants into a perinatal brain could integrate into circuits as they develop and, thus, could form relatively normal connections (8,75). Accordingly, O'Leary and Stanfield (75) showed that when they transplanted late fetal neocortex into heterotopic positions in newborn rodents, the grafted tissue established connectivity characteristic of the new location. Furthermore, the grafted tissue had the cytoarchitectonic characteristics of the new area. For example, when occipital cortex was grafted into the presumptive barrel-field region, the transplanted tissue developed morphologic features resembling barrels (73). The mere fact that transplantation occurs in infancy is no guarantee of "normal" development, however. Indeed, it is our impression that most studies of early transplants do not find very normal-appearing tissue. Studies of neonatal animals with occipital (39), motor (77), or prefrontal (52) grafts, all failed to observe normal cytoarchitectonic characteristics in the transplants.

Second, the lost tissue could be partially replaced. This might imply that only some of the original characteristics were returned or that most of the original characteristics were replaced, but not to the original levels. There is evidence that this does indeed happen. Thus, transplanted cortical tissue shows many types of somata (39) that resemble normal cortical neurons. Furthermore, there is histochemical evidence of a variety of normal neurochemical characteristics of neocortical neurons. These include immunocytochemical identification of glutamic acid decarboxylase, choline acetyltransferase, vasoactive intestinal polypeptide, and somatostatin reactive neurons (17,27,33,84,90). In addition, binding sites for particular transmitters have also been described (29).

Third, the graft might affect function because it either prevented the death of traumatized neurons, or it reduced the transneuronal changes in regions not directly affected by the injury. For example, Haun et al. (37) reported that occipital cortex grafts reduced the transneuronal degeneration normally observed in the frontal eye fields after visual cortex lesions. Similarly, several studies have shown that grafts into neonatal animals reduce the thalamic atrophy normally observed after neonatal injury (35,36,83,88). Curiously, these rescue effects may be specific to certain types of

targets. Thus, Kolb and Muirhead (52) found that, although frontal grafts reduced thalamic atrophy after perinatal prefrontal lesions, they had no effect on cortical thinning in the undamaged cortical regions. Although they did not comment on it in the paper, a similar result can be seen in the illustration of the findings of Sørensen et al. (88): motor cortex implants reduced thalamic, but not cortical, atrophy.

Fourth, cortical transplants might have some type of trophic action on the remaining brain, leading to changes in the host that subsequently support recovery. This trophic action could result from the implantation of glial elements, such as astrocytes (44,45), the stimulation of nerve growth factor or similar substances (60), or effects on protein synthesis in the host brain (41). Astrocytes produce neurotrophic and neurite-promoting factors, and these factors may promote reactive synaptogenesis (71). Although there is no direct evidence that graft-induced trophic actions function to affect reactive synaptogenesis after cortical injury, there have been clear demonstrations of synaptic remodeling (49,92,101).

EVIDENCE OF CORTICAL GRAFT FUNCTION

There are three general types of functional studies. Those in which embryonic grafts are placed into (a) adult animals with cortical lesions, (b) infant animals with cortical lesions, and (c) intact, aged animals or animals with lesions of nonspecific cortical afferents. We consider each of these separately.

Functional Outcome After Cortical Grafts in Adulthood

Prefrontal Cortex

Labbe et al. (61) were the first to show that implantation of cortical tissue might have the capacity to restore lost cognitive function. They made medial prefrontal lesions in rats and found that rats given transplants of embryonic frontal tissue had an improvement in performance of spatial delayed alternation in a T-maze. This finding was novel and suggested that cortical transplants had the capacity to restore complex circuits in the cortex. Subsequent investigators replicated the Labbe et al. finding (Table 1) but it has become evident that we are far from understanding under what conditions frontal transplantation will restore lost functions. Kesslak et al. (45) first showed that, although frontal transplants were effective, they were not necessary because implanted purified astrocytes were as effective as neural tissue in restoring function. Next, Dunnett et al. (14) found beneficial effects of grafts only when they studied the animals shortly after the transplantation. In fact, we found that, when animals were tested immediately after transplantation, they performed better than nongrafted control operates. Whereas, if the rats were tested a month or later after transplantation, the grafted animals performed more poorly than the nongrafted frontal operates (51). Finally, it is now clear that the beneficial effects of frontal grafts may be restricted to specific behavioral measures (14). In sum, although the prefrontal cortex appears to provide a good model system for studying the functional effects of fetal transplants, there is now no evidence that the beneficial effects result from the reconstruction of damaged prefrontal circuitries. The majority of evidence to date is consistent with a hypothesis of graft action that is nonspecific.

Occipital Cortex

The first evidence that cortical grafts might improve sensory function after cortical injury came from a report by Stein et al. (89) that implantation of frontal, but not occipital, tissue reduced deficits in a brightness discrimination after visual cortex removal in rats. Because it was frontal, rather than occipital, tissue that promoted recovery the authors concluded that the recovery was due to some trophic action of the grafts on the remaining brain, rather than a replacement of visually responsive neurons. More direct evidence of visual function in cortical transplants has come from electrophysiologic experiments by Girman and Golovina (32). These authors implanted "caudal telencephalic" tissue into the cav-

TABLE 1. *Behavioral effects of adult cortical lesions and fetal grafts*

Region[a]	Task	Outcome	Refs.
Pfc (B)	Place alternation	Improved performance[b]	14,23,44,45,61,91
	Water task	Worse or no effect	14,21,23,51
		Improved performance[b]	23
	Activity	No effect	14
Occ (B)	Brightness disk	Occ graft had no effect	89
		Pfc graft improved	89
Occ (B)	Pattern disk	No effect	66
Gus (B)	Conditioned taste aversion	Partial or total recovery	3,19,26,67,102
Motor (U)	Reaching	No effect	50,87
Motor (B)	Walking	Gait improved	98
		No gait improvement	38,86
Parietal (U)	Activity	Partial decrease	43
Ent (B)	Radial arm maze	Improved performance	31

[a]B, bilateral lesion; Ent, entorhinal cortex; Occ, occipital cortex; Pfc, prefrontal cortex; U, unilateral lesion.
[b]Improved performance true only under certain conditions.

ity made from an aspiration lesion centered in Zilles' area Oc_1. Following a recovery period of 2 to 10 months, the animals were again anesthetized and both extracellular field potentials and neuronal activity were recorded in response to visual stimulation. Although many of the transplants had abnormal electrical activity, many others showed clear responses to visual stimulation that were generally similar to those observed in normal visual cortex in rats. The visual input apparently reached the cortex by the visual thalamus, since stimulation of lateral geniculate nucleus also stimulated grafted neurons. One explanation for the positive physiologic results of Girman and Golovina and the negative behavioral results of Stein is that, although the grafted neurons in the Girman and Golovina study were visually responsive, they were not connected with the normal efferent systems in the brain. A study by Nakamura and Mishkin (69) is instructive here. With monkeys as experimental subjects, these authors found that disconnection of visual cortex from normal output targets produced behavioral blindness in the presence of normal electrophysiologic activity in the visual cortex. The Nakamura and Mishkin results provide two important lessons for graft studies. First, they confirm that the presence of what appears to be typical electrophysiologic activity at one point in a circuit does not necessarily mean that one can expect normal, behaviorally relevant function. Second, they imply that the absence of behavior need not indicate a lack of activity in a particular area. What is needed in the current context is to replicate the Stein et al. behavioral study before measuring electrophysiologic activity as Girman and Golovina did.

Gustatory Cortex

The most compelling evidence for graft-induced functional recovery in adult rats comes from studies of the implantation of gustatory cortex. In a remarkable series of experiments, Bermudez-Rattoni and his colleagues have shown that (a) deficits in conditioned taste aversion can be reduced or eliminated by cortical implants in rats with bilateral gustatory cortex lesions, and (b) the recovery correlates with the morphologic maturity and connectivity of the grafts (see Table 1). These findings are novel in that, whereas most studies of graft growth in adult rats report only limited connectivity between the host and implant, Bermudez-Rattoni and his coworkers have demonstrated truly massive regrowth of connections between gustatory cortex and the gustatory regions of the ventromedial thalamus (26). Although the Bermudez-Rattoni studies represent the best evidence of graft-induced recovery from a cortical injury in adulthood, the data must still be interpreted with caution. There is no evidence that the graft itself is responsible for the recovery and no physiologic evidence that the cells in the transplant are actually responsive to gustatory stimuli.

Motor Cortex

Damage to the motor cortex produces clear long-term deficits in the use of forepaws to reach (100) as well as in the normal walking gait (28). Because these movements are easily quantified, the motor cortex ought to provide a good site for functional studies of cortical grafts. However, there is as yet little evidence that cortical grafts ameliorate behavioral loss after motor cortex lesions (see Table 1). Held et al. (38) make an important point here. They found that, although the walking gait of rats with transplants of motor cortex were grossly abnormal, the grafted animals ran more quickly than rats without grafts. The authors conclude that behavioral measures based upon achievement (obtaining food, traversing a runway, and such) may not be sufficient to describe and assess the complex nature of recovery of motor function after cortical transplantation.

Parietal Cortex

In general, damage to the parietal cortex in rodents produces a loss or reduction of their ability to make certain sensory discriminations (9). Unfortunately, recovery of this behavior has not yet been studied in animals with transplants. Such focal lesions of the right parietal cortex, on the other hand, typically generate a transient period of hyperactivity (80). Treating these lesions with cortical grafts yielded equivocal results, depending on the particular criterion used to assess activity and when the measurement was made (43). Indeed, on some measures the lesion effect was actually exacerbated.

The vibrissal barrel field of the rat provides a nice potential model for studying graft efficacy, since it is topographically organized, it has a unique anatomic organization, and it is easily accessible for neuronal recording. Studies in several laboratories (Table 2), therefore, have tried to evaluate the extent to which specific morphologic and electrophysiologic characteristics might be reproduced by transplants. As with implants into other cortical regions, there is little evidence of normal modular or laminar structure in the barrels. Nevertheless, cells in the grafts respond to vibrissae stimulation. The receptive fields tend to be much wider in these fields, and the receptive areas of grafted neurons are not limited to a single vibrissa, as in the normal barrel field neurons. In fact, many of the grafted cells are responsive to tactile stimulation beyond the vibrissae, extending as far as the limbs and body surface (5). Cortical grafts located in somatosensory cortex also have an increased 2-deoxyglucose uptake in response to vibrissae stimulation, which also suggests functional connectivity with the periphery (65).

In one elegant experiment, Bragin et al. (7) bilaterally ablated the barrel field and then transplanted fetal tissue into the cavities. Immediately after surgery the vibrissae were trimmed unilaterally and kept trimmed for the subsequent 4 months. The grafts in the two hemispheres were then compared anatomically and electrophysiologically. The grafts contralateral to the trimmed vibrissal field grew less well and were less responsive both to thalamic and somatic stimulation, indicating poorer functional integration with the host brain in the "deprived" hemisphere. These results are provocative for a couple of reasons. First, the data suggest that, as in normal development, sensory stimulation is important for the functional development of neurons in sensory cortical regions. It is not clear, however, how much sensory input might be required. It could be argued that visual stimulation in standard laboratory cages is insufficient to influence graft integration. Second, one wonders whether the failure to find better outcomes from grafts in the motor or prefrontal cortex might, at least partly, be due to a failure of standard laboratory housing to provide an environment that effectively stimulates these regions. This possibility is not without precedent, since it has been claimed that amphetamine is able to accelerate recovery following motor cortex lesions only if the animals are given specific motor training under the influence of the drug (25). Since the beneficial effect of amphetamine is abolished in

TABLE 2. *Summary of electrophysiologic measures in fetal cortical grafts*

Region[a]	Measure and outcome	Refs.
Parietal (A)	Barrel field response to vibrissae stimulation	5–7,16,47,63
Parietal (N)	Response to thalamic or somatic electrical stimulation	70
Occ (A)	Retinotopic map	32

[a]A, adult lesions and grafts; N, neonatal lesions and grafts.

animals that remain in laboratory cages after drug administration, it is conceivable that animals restricted to cages after motor cortex grafts might be disadvantaged for graft growth.

Functional Outcome After Cortical Grafts in Infancy

One might expect that fetal tissue transplanted into a developing brain might be better able to integrate more normally with the host and provide better functional outcome than it would in an adult animal. Somewhat surprisingly, there have not been many functional studies after grafts in infancy, and those that are available have not been encouraging (Table 3). One exception, however, is a series of studies on forepaw-reaching after motor cortex transplants. Thus, in contrast with the negative results in adult operates, several groups have found that transplants into the damaged forepaw motor representation area resulted in at least partial restitution of reaching (34,77,81). Furthermore, anatomic analyses in these animals indicate more extensive connectivity with the host brain than typically found in adults. For example, Plumet et al. (77) found that the transplants sent fibers to the spinal cord, striatum, thalamus, and homotopic contralateral cortex, whereas they received connections from the thalamus and contralateral cortex. However, the recovery from neonatal motor cortex lesions may not extend to movements other than skilled reaching, as Swenson et al. (93) failed to find recovery of hind limb

deficits in the traversing of a narrow beam after neonatal motor cortex transplants. This discrepancy may reflect a specificity in the anatomic connectivity, although this is not proved.

There are surprisingly few other functional transplant studies in neonatal animals with cortical lesions. In one study of rats with visual cortex lesions, there was a partial restitution of pattern discrimination performance (37). This finding is difficult to interpret, however, since the animals had unilateral lesions. The authors suggested that the beneficial effect might have been on visual attention, rather than visual discrimination per se, but this was not studied directly. The one remaining behavioral study of neonatal grafts was in animals with prefrontal lesions (52). These animals showed no beneficial effects on forelimb-reaching or the learning of a spatial navigation problem in the Morris water task. The failure to find an improvement in forelimb-reaching appears to conflict with the results of the studies of motor cortex injury. One significant difference between these studies is that our prefrontal experiment used bilateral lesions, whereas the motor cortex studies were all done with unilateral injuries. This difference needs to be explored systematically.

There is but a single electrophysiologic study of fetal transplants into neonatal rats. Neafsey et al. (70) found that transplanted sensorimotor neurons responded to electrical stimulation of both the thalamus and contralateral forepaw. Additionally, the spontaneous neuronal activity was comparable with that in normal cortex. This result con-

TABLE 3. *Behavioral effects of neonatal cortical lesions and fetal grafts*

Region[a]	Task	Outcome	Refs.
Motor (U)	Reaching	Parietal restitution	34,76,77,81
Motor (U)	Walking	No hindlimb gait recovery	93
Occ (U)	Pattern discrimination	Partial restitution	37
Pfc (B)	Reaching	No effect	52
	Water task	No effect	52

[a]D, bilateral lesion; Occ, occipital cortex; Pfc, prefrontal cortex; U, unilateral lesion.

trasts with that reported in Bragin et al.'s (5,6) studies of adult rat hosts in which the spontaneous activity in the transplanted neurons was not normal. The difference between the neonatal and adult hosts may reflect a better integration of the transplants in the neonatal hosts, although there were methodologic differences in the studies that might also be responsible for the differences.

Effects of Nonspecific Cortical Implants in Adulthood

To this point we have considered only the attempts to repair damage to specific cortical regions. Certain conditions, such as dementia, do not represent the sequelae of focal lesions, but are hypothesized to reflect more generalized losses (82). In disorders such as Alzheimer's disease and Huntington's chorea, this loss may include one or more transmitter systems. In addition, many forms of dementia (e.g., Alzheimer's disease) are also characterized by other neuropathologic signs, such as cell death in relatively isolated regions (e.g., nucleus basalis of Meynert or entorhinal cortex), or changes in cortical morphologic structure (e.g., plaques and tangles). The possibility that the replacement of specific cell populations, such as basal forebrain cholinergic cells, might ameliorate some of the symptoms of dementia has led to considerable interest in neural transplantation as a possible treatment (see 11 for review). Studies of this sort have been of two general types. In the first, young adult animals are given lesions of regions such as the basal forebrain, to simulate the typical effects of pathologic deterioration, and then cholinergic grafts are placed into the cortex. Subsequently, the animals negotiate various mazes as an assessment of their learning or memory. In the second type of study, aged animals are simply given the grafts. In some of these studies the animals are first screened to pick out those who show age-associated deficits in particular tasks, and the transplantations are restricted to this subpopulation.

These experiments are difficult to conduct and to interpret for various reasons. First, it remains to be resolved whether cholinergic deafferentation of the cortex produced by basal forebrain lesions or aging is the critical factor common to the observed behavioral impairments associated with dementia.

Second, since there is no known selective cholinergic neurotoxin, various lesion methods have been used. These methods produce differing behavioral effects, including many that are not easily ascribed to cortical cholinergic systems (1,99). For example, three excitotoxins, ibotenic acid, kainic acid, and quisqualic acid, all destroy cholinergic neurons, but their behavioral effects are not equivalent. It is particularly noteworthy that quisqualic acid is as effective in killing cholinergic cells as the other two neurotoxins, but the treated animals have relatively smaller behavioral impairments (15,78,79). Nonetheless, Dunnett (11) concludes that rats with quisqualate lesions do manifest a sufficiently severe range of impairments to provide a viable model for study.

The third difficulty arises from an enigmatic conventional procedure. Although it is well documented that behavioral deficits can be localized to reasonably small regions of the neocortex in rats (see 54 for review), many studies of cholinergic implants have placed the grafts in curious cortical regions, such as sensorimotor cortex, that are unlikely to be involved in learning or memory.

Fourth, cholinergic grafts placed into the cortex invaginate only a small region of the depleted cortex. This leads one to question what role the grafts are playing in enhancing recovery. There is an additional related problem. Basal forebrain lesions do not cause complete cholinergic depletion of the cortex, and the intrinsic cholinergic cortical cells remain intact. One wonders why the remaining cholinergic innervation is insufficient to mediate recovery.

Finally, the recovery reported in animals that receive acetylcholine-producing grafts is often restricted to a particular behavior (85). Whether this task-specific recovery is attributable to additional noncholinergic damage is not resolved. In view of the methodologic difficulties, we are inclined to agree with Dunnett's (11) conclusion that the cognitive deficits that result from basal forebrain lesions may often be due to noncholinergic damage in this area. In addition, age-related deficits in memory may reflect the involvement of prefrontal, posterior cingulate, or hippocampal regions. If this proves correct, then it follows that cholinergic grafts into the prefrontal or cingulate regions might be the most efficacious cortical locations in reversing the effects of either aging or basal forebrain lesions. There is tentative evidence favoring this interpretation (13).

CONCLUSIONS

One of the most perplexing and significant questions facing modern neuroscience is the issue of how to repair the injured cerebral cortex. In principle, neural transplantation represents a promising avenue for both basic and clinical investigation. At present, however, the extent of our ignorance about the efficacy of neural implantation as a treatment far exceeds our rudimentary knowledge. We shall now attempt to take stock of what we do know and reach some conclusions about where we go from here.

What Do We Know?

There is little doubt that cortical implants grow and connect with the host brain, although the integration with the host is by no means normal and probably varies with the cortical region of implantation. Grafts grow better and there is more integration between implant and host in the immature brain. One obvious reason for this is that the grafted cells receive the advantage of the normally occurring optimal growth conditions of the developing brain. This includes appropriate cell and surface adhesion molecules, extracellular matrix, and various trophic factors, including transiently expressed transmitters and proteins with specific signals. There are now several clear examples of improvement in behavioral outcome in brain-injured animals given grafts either in infancy or adulthood. It has not yet been proved, however, that the grafts are directly responsible for the "recovery." In the definitive experimental paradigm, the grafts must be removed, either directly through surgery or by inducing rejection by the host, and the behavioral recovery must reverse as a consequence. There are also many examples of failed functional improvement from cortical transplants. Indeed, in view of the lower likelihood of authors publishing negative results, the published negative results may underestimate the failure rate. Electrophysiologic studies in both occipital and parietal transplants have found cells to be physiologically responsive both to appropriate peripheral sensory stimulation as well as to thalamic stimulation. The physiologic responses are less specific than in normal brain and may be more normal when grafts are made in developing brains than in adulthood. There is, however, no evidence that the physiologically responsive cells function to affect behavior. Few studies have done a thorough behavioral analysis of the response capabilities of grafted animals. This is important because there is consistent evidence that different measures may find different functional outcomes. There is suggestive evidence that the functional integration of the graft with the host is activity-dependent. This is reminiscent of the importance of activity in normal brain development. Finally, there is more optimism in the literature concerning the potential benefits from nonspecific grafts, such as cholinergic implants, than for the regrowth of intrinsic circuits of specific cortical regions. In sum, we believe that there is sufficient evidence that supports the claim that cortical transplants may be functional under appropriate circumstances to warrant continued research.

What Questions Remain?

One of the goals of scientific inquiry into a new problem is to identify what the significant questions are. When studies of cortical transplantation began, the question was simple: Do neural grafts grow and might they assume any function? As we have seen, the answer was a simple, "yes." The next level of question to be addressed will be far more difficult to answer and promises to lead to more questions. We list some of the questions that strike us as the most interesting.

First, what is the difference between those studies that result in functional recovery and those that do not? Studies of animals with prefrontal grafts in adulthood have shown that the recovery time after implantation negatively influences the functional outcome, but this is not the only explanation for discrepancies in outcome in different studies. Other explanations may include the specific behavioral measure used, the definition of recovery, the age or sex of the host or donor, and so on. One would hope that there is some systematic relation between cortical implantation and the conditions under which one finds or fails to find recovery. In view of the evidence that recovery from both infant lesions and serial lesions in adulthood is better with cognitive tests than with tests of species-typical behavior, a direct comparison of these types of measures might be a promising route to follow.

Second, what is the relation between the physiologic, metabolic, and behavioral measures of the function of transplanted tissue? Different processes may mediate recovery through different mechanisms, depending on the behavior in question, the site of the lesion, and the residual plasticity of the host brain. Studies that use multiple measures are needed.

Third, when grafts alter behavior, why do they do so? There is currently no evidence that behavioral recovery is directly related to the graft. Improved function may result from a positive trophic action of the graft, or from effects on structures functionally related to the injured cortex. This could involve other heterotopic or homotopic cortical regions. A related question asks whether the lesion size is important and why. It is our impression that grafts grow better if the lesion is small, but there are no direct studies of this. Furthermore, there are no systematic studies of whether or not bilateral grafts are more, or are less, likely to alter function than unilateral grafts.

Fourth, when is the optimal time for grafting? Grafts have been made in very young (usually day of birth or the day after), adult, or geriatric rats. There are now no experiments that directly compare animals with similar lesions and grafting procedures at different ages. It appears that there is an assumption that grafts will function more effectively in the developing animal, but this is not proved. A related question comes from the observation that implantations have been made in animals at ages at which the brain normally shows rather little recovery of specific cortical functions. Specifically, what happens if grafts are made in rats at about days 7 to 15, which is a time that the brain is more plastic and recovery is usually far better?

Fifth, how important is a laminar or modular organization to function? Laminar–modular function is a consistent characteristic of cortical organization that can be manipulated with appropriate experimental procedures in perinatal animals. Does the anatomic organization correlate with behavioral or electrophysiologic recovery? This question is not only of interest relative to grafting procedures, but is of more general interest relative to the question of how the cortex functions.

Sixth, what is the role of experience? Since vibrissae stimulation is apparently necessary for the growth of barrel field transplants, one wonders if housing animals in laboratory cages to recover after motor, visual, or prefrontal grafts might not be equivalent to cutting off the vibrissae?

Finally, in the transplantation of nonspecific tissue, such as cholinergic cells, there are the questions of where the optimal locations for transplantation might be, how many implants are optimal, and what the grafts actually do to alter behavior?

To conclude, it is now an established fact that cortical transplantation is possible and that implants both survive and have behavioral consequences. Future studies must address the large gaps in our knowledge to exploit the vast possibilities offered by this technique that loom, tantalizingly, just beyond our grasp.

REFERENCES

1. Abrogast RE, Kozlowski MR. Quantitative morphometric analysis of the neurotoxic effects of the excitotoxin, ibotenic acid, on the basal forebrain. *Neurotoxicology* 1988;9:39–46.
2. Andres FL, Van der Loos H. Removal and reimplantation of the parietal cortex of the neonatal mouse: consequences for the barrelfield. *Dev Brain Res* 1985;20:115–121.
3. Bermudez-Rattoni F, Fernandez J, Sanchez MA, Aguilar-Roblero R, Drucker-Colin R. Fetal brain transplants induce regeneration of taste aversion learning. *Brain Res* 1987;416: 147–152.
4. Black JE, Greenough WT. Developmental approaches to the memory process. In: Martinez JL Jr, Kesner RP, eds. *Learning and memory, a biological view.* New York: Academic Press; 1991:61–91.
5. Bragin AG, Bohne A, Vinogradova OS. Transplants of the embryonal rat somatosensory neocortex in the barrel field of the adult rat: responses of the grafted neurons to sensory stimulation. *Neuroscience* 1988;25:751–758.
6. Bragin AG, Bohne A, Kitchigina VF, Vinogradova OS. Functional integration of neurones in

7. Bragin AG, Vinogradova OS, Stafekhina VS. Sensory deprivation prevents integration of neocortical grafts with the host brain. *Restor Neurol Neurosci* 1992;4:279–283.
8. Chang FL, Steedman JG, Lund RD. The lamination and connectivity of embryonic cerebral cortex transplanted into newborn rat cortex. *J Comp Neurol* 1986;244:401–411.
9. Chapin JK, Lin C-S. The somatic sensory cortex of the rat. In: Kolb B, Tees R, eds. *Cerebral cortex of the rat.* Cambridge, MA: MIT Press; 1990:341–380.
10. Dunn E. Primary and secondary findings in a series of attempts to transplant cerebral cortex in the albino rat. *J Comp Neurol* 1917;27:565–582.
11. Dunnett SB. Neural transplantation in animal models of dementia. *Eur J Neurosci* 1990;2: 567–587.
12. Dunnett SB. Neural transplantation in the cerebral cortex. In: Kolb B, Tees R, eds. *Cerebral cortex of the rat.* Cambridge, MA: MIT Press; 1990:589–612.
13. Dunnett SB, Badman F, Rogers DC, Evenden JL, Iversen SD. Cholinergic grafts in the neocortex or hippocampus of aged rats: reduction of delay-dependent deficits in the delayed nonmatching to position task. *Exp Neurol* 1988; 102:57–64.
14. Dunnett SB, Ryan CN, Levin PD, Reynolds M, Bunch ST. Functional consequences of embryonic neocortex transplanted to rats with prefrontal cortex lesions. *Behav Neurosci* 1987; 101:489–503.
15. Dunnett SB, Whishaw IQ, Jones GH, Bunch ST. Behavioural, biochemical and histological effects of different neurotoxic amino acids injected into the nucleus basalis magnocellularis of rats. *Neuroscience* 1987;20:653–669.
16. Ebner FF, Erzurumlu RS, Lee SM. Peripheral nerve damage facilitates innervation of brain grafts in adult sensory cortex. *Proc Natl Acad Sci USA* 1989;86:730–734.
17. Ebner FF, Olschowska JA, Jacobowitz DM. The development of peptide-containing neurons within neocortical transplants in adult mice. *Peptides* 1984;5:103–113.
18. Eccles JC. The cerebral neocortex: a theory of its operation. In: Jones EG, Peters A, eds. *Cerebral cortex, vol 2.* New York: Plenum Press; 1984:1–36.
19. Escobar M, Fernandez J, Guevara-Aguilar R, Bermudez-Rattoni F. Fetal brain grafts induce recovery of learning deficits and connectivity in rats with gustatory neocortex lesions. *Brain Res* 1989;478:368–374.
20. Fantie BD, Kolb B. Cortical grafts impair spatial learning in adult rats with medial frontal cortex lesions. *Soc Neurosci Abstr* 1985;11: 616.
21. Fantie BD, Kolb B. An examination of prefrontal lesion size and the effects of cortical grafts

on performance of the Morris water task by rats. *Psychobiology* 1990;18:74–80.

22. Fantie BD, Kolb B. The problems of prognosis. In: Dywan J, Kaplan KD, Pirozzolo FJ, eds. *Neuropsychology and the law.* New York: Springer-Verlag; 1991:186–238.

23. Fantie BD, Kolb B. Functional consequences of transplantation of frontal neocortex vary with age of donor tissue and behavioral task. *Restor Neurol Neurosci* 1993;5:141–149.

24. Fantie BD, Reynolds B, Di Lullo D, Anchan R, Kolb B. Some factors affecting the influence of cortical grafts on the behavioural recovery of rats with medial frontal cortex lesions. *Soc Neurosci Abstr* 1987;13:163.

25. Feeney DM, Gonzalez A, Law WA. Amphetamine, haloperidol, experience interact to affect rate of recovery after motor cortex injury. *Science* 1982;217:855–857.

26. Fernandez-Ruiz J, Escobar ML, Pina AL, Diaz-Cintra S, Cintra-McGlone FL, Bermudez-Rattoni F. Time-dependent recovery of taste aversion learning by fetal brain transplants in gustatory neocortex-lesioned rats. *Behav Neural Biol* 1991;55:179–193.

27. Floeter MK, Jones EG. Transplantation of fetal postmitotic neurons to rat cortex survival, early pathway choices and long-term projections of outgrowing axons. *Dev Brain Res* 1985;22:19–38.

28. Gentile AM, Green S, Nieburgs A, Schmelzer W, Stein DG. Disruption and recovery of locomotor and manipulatory behavior following cortical lesions in rats. *Behav Biol* 1978; 22:417–455.

29. Getz RL, Moody TW, Rosenstein JM. Neuropeptide receptors are present in fetal neocortical transplants. *Neurosci Lett* 1987;79:97–102.

30. Gibbs RB, Cotman CW. Factors affecting survival and outgrowth from transplants of entorhinal cortex. *Neuroscience* 1987;21:699–706.

31. Gibbs RB, Harris EW, Cotman CW. Replacement of damaged cortical projections by homotypic transplants of entorhinal cortex. *J Comp Neurol* 1985;237:47–65.

32. Girman SV, Golovina IL. Electrophysiological properties of embryonic neocortex transplants replacing the primary visual cortex of adult rats. *Brain Res* 1990;523:78–86.

33. Gonzalez MF, Sharp FR. Fetal frontal cortex transplanted to injured motor/sensory cortex of adult rats. I. NADPH-diaphorase neurons. *J Neurosci* 1987;7:2991–3001.

34. Gonzalez MF, Sharp FR. Fetal cortical transplants surviving in injured sensorimotor cortex of rats: cellular composition and function. *Prog Brain Res* 1990;82:309–312.

35. Haun F, Cunningham TJ. Cortical transplants reveal CNS trophic interactions in situ. *Dev Brain Res* 1984;15:290–294.

36. Haun F, Cunningham TJ. Specific neurotrophic interactions between cortical and subcortical visual structures in the developing rat: in vivo studies. *J Comp Neurol* 1987;256:561–569.

37. Haun F, Cunningham TJ, Rothblat LA. Neurotrophic and behavioral effects of occipital cortex transplants in newborn rats. *Vis Neurosci* 1989;2:189–198.

38. Held JM, Basso DM, Gentile AM, Stein DG. Homotopic or heterotopic fetal transplants and recovery of locomotion *(in preparation).*

39. Jaeger CB, Lund RD. Transplantation of embryonic occipital cortex to the tectal region of newborn rats: a Golgi study of mature and developing transplants. *J Comp Neurol* 1981; 194:571–597.

40. Jones EG. Anatomy of cerebral cortex: columnar input–output organization. In: Schmidt FO, Worden FG, Edelman G, Dennis SG, eds. *The organization of the cerebral cortex.* Cambridge, MA: MIT Press; 1981:199–235.

41. Jorgensen OS, Stein DG. Transplant and ganglioside GM_1 mediated neuronal recovery in rats with brain lesions. *Restor Neurol Neurosci* 1992;3:311–320.

42. Juraska JM. The structure of the rat cerebral cortex: effects of gender and the environment. In: Kolb B, Tees R, eds. *Cerebral cortex of the rat.* Cambridge, MA: MIT Press; 1990:483–505.

43. Justice A, Moran TH, Deckel AW, Robinson RG. The use of fetal neocortical transplants to treat the hyperactivity resulting from cortical suction lesions in adult rats. *Behav Brain Res* 1989;33:97–104.

44. Kesslak JP, Brown L, Steichen C, Cotman CW. Adult and embryonic frontal cortex transplants after frontal cortex ablation enhance recovery on a reinforced alternation task. *Exp Neurol* 1986;94:615–626.

45. Kesslak JP, Nieto-Sampedro M, Globus J, Cotman CW. Transplants of purified astrocytes promote behavioral recovery after frontal cortex ablation. *Exp Neurol* 1986;92:377–390.

46. Kimura D. Sex differences in the brain. *Sci Am* 1992;267(3):118–125.

47. Kitchigina VF, Vinogradova OS, Bragin AG. Neuronal activity of the septum transplanted into the neocortical barrel field of the rat. *Restor Neurol Neurosci* 1991;2:109–122.

48. Kolb B. Sex-related differences in the effects of prefrontal lesions in rats. 1994 *(submitted).*

49. Kolb B, Gibb R. Anatomical correlates of behavioral change after neonatal prefrontal lesions in rats. *Prog Brain Res* 1990;85:241–256.

50. Kolb B, Griffith C, Muirhead D, de Brabander H. A comparison of the effects of unilateral and bilateral embryonic grafts on the recovery of motor skills in rats. 1994 *(in preparation).*

51. Kolb B, Reynolds B, Fantie B. Frontal cortex grafts have different effects at different postoperative recovery times. *Behav Neural Biol* 1988;50:193–206.

52. Kolb B, Muirhead D, Cloe J. Neonatal frontal cortex grafts fail to attenuate behavioral deficits or abnormal cortical morphogenesis. *Brain Res* 1994 *(in press).*

53. Kolb B, Stewart J. Sex-related differences in dendritic branching of cells in the prefrontal cortex of rats. *J Neuroendocrinol* 1991;3:95–99.

54. Kolb B, Tees R, eds. *The cerebral cortex of the rat.* Cambridge, MA: MIT Press; 1990.

55. Kolb B, Whishaw IQ. Neonatal frontal lesions in the rat: sparing of learned but not species typical behavior in the presence of reduced brain weight and cortical thickness. *J Comp Physiol Psychol* 1981;95:863–879.

56. Kolb B, Whishaw IQ. Earlier is not always better: behavioral dysfunction and abnormal cerebral morphogenesis following neonatal cortical lesions in the rat. *Behav Brain Res* 1985; 17:25–43.

57. Kolb B, Whishaw IQ. Neonatal frontal lesions in hamsters impair species-typical behaviors and reduce brain weight and cortical thickness. *Behav Neurosci* 1985;99:691–704.

58. Kolb B, Whishaw IQ. Brain and behavioral development after neonatal cortical lesions in rats: a review. *Prog Neurobiol* 1989;32:235–276.

59. Kolb B, Whishaw IQ. *Fundamentals of human neuropsychology,* 3rd ed. San Francisco: WH Freeman; 1989.

60. Kromer LF. Nerve growth factor treatment after brain injury prevents neuronal death. *Science* 1987;235:214–216.

61. Labbe R, Firl A Jr, Mufson EJ, Stein DG. Fetal brain transplants: reduction of cognitive deficits in rats with frontal cortex lesions. *Science* 1983;221:470–472.

62. Lashley KH. *Brain mechanisms and intelligence.* Chicago: University of Chicago Press; 1929.

63. Lee SM, Ebner FF. Response characteristics of neocortical graft neurons to host somatosensory input. *Prog Brain Res* 1990;82:301–308.

64. Lescaudron L, Stein DG. Function recovery following transplants of embryonic brain tissue in rats with lesions of visual, frontal and motor cortex: problems and prospects for future research. *Neuropsychologia* 1990;28:585–599.

65. Levin BE, Dunn-Meynell A, Sced AF. Functional integration of fetal cortical grafts into the afferent pathway of the rat somatosensory cortex (Sml). *Brain Res Bull* 1987;19:723–734.

66. Lindsay JF, McDaniel WF. Neural tissue transplants in rats with lateral peristriate lesions. II. Behavior. *Med Sci Res* 1987;15:655–656.

67. Lopez-Garcia JC, Fernandez-Ruiz J, Bermudez-Rattoni F, Tapia R. Correlation between acetylcholine release and recovery of conditioned taste aversion induced by fetal neocortex grafts. *Brain Res* 1990;523:105–110.

68. Manthorpe M, Nieto-Sampedro M, Skaper SD, Lewis ER, Bardin G, Longo FM, Cotman CW, Varon S. Neuronotrophic activity in brain wounds of the developing rat. Correlation with implant survival in the wound cavity. *Brain Res* 1983;267:47–56.

69. Nakamura RK, Mishkin M. Blindness in monkeys following non-visual cortical lesions. *Brain Res* 1980;188:572–577.

70. Neafsey EJ, Sørenson JC, Tønder N, Castro AJ. Fetal cortical transplants into neonatal rats respond to thalamic and peripheral stimulation in the adult. An electrophysiological study of single unit activity. *Brain Res* 1989;493:33–40.

71. Nieto-Sampedro M, Cotman CW. Growth factor induction and temporal order in central nervous system repair. In: Cotman CW, ed. *Synaptic plasticity.* New York: Guilford Press; 1985:407–456.

72. Nonneman AJ, Kolb B. Functional recovery after serial ablation of prefrontal cortex in the rat. *Physiol Behav* 1979;22:895–901.

73. O'Leary DDM. Do cortical areas emerge from a proto-cortex? *Trends Neurosci* 1989;12.400–406.

74. O'Leary DDM, Schaggar BL, Stanfield BB. The specification of sensory cortex: lessons from cortical transplantation. *Exp Neurol* 1992; 115:121–126.

75. O'Leary DDM, Stanfield BB. Selective elimination of axons extended by developing cortical neurons is dependent on regional locale: experiments utilizing fetal cortical transplants. *J Neurosci* 1989;9:2230–2246.

76. Plumet J, Cadusseau J, Roger M. Fetal cortical transplants reduce motor deficits resulting from neonatal damage to the rat's frontal cortex. *Neurosci Lett* 1990;109:102–106.

77. Plumet J, Cadusseau J, Roger M. Skilled forelimb use in the rat: amelioration of functional deficits resulting from neonatal damage to the frontal cortex by neonatal transplantation of fetal cortical tissue. *Restor Neurol Neurosci* 1991;3:135–147.

78. Robbins TW, Everitt BJ, Marston HM, Wilkinson J, Jones GH, Page KJ. Comparative effects of ibotenic acid- and quisqualic acid-induced lesions of the substantia innominata on attentional function in the rat: further implications for the role of the cholinergic neurons of the nucleus basalis in cognitive processes. *Behav Brain Res* 1989;35:221–241.

79. Robbins TW, Everitt BJ, Ryan CN, Marston HM, Jones GH, Page KJ. Comparative effects of quisqualic and ibotenic acid-induced lesions of the substantia innominata and globus pallidus on the acquisition of a conditional visual discrimination: differential effects on cholinergic mechanisms. *Neuroscience* 1989;28:337–352.

80. Robinson RG, Shoemaker WJ, Schlumpf M, Valk T, Bloom FE. Effect of experimental cerebral infarction in rat brain on catecholamines and behavior. *Nature* 1975;225:332–333.

81. Sandor R, Gonzalez MF, Mosebey M, Sharp FR. Motor deficits are produced by removing some cortical transplants grafted into injured somatosensory cortex of neonatal rats. *J Neural Transpl Plast* 1991;2:221–233.

82. Selkoe DJ. Aging brain, aging mind. *Sci Am* 1992;267(3):135–142.

83. Sharp FR, Gonzalez MF. Fetal cortical transplants ameliorate thalamic atrophy ipsilateral to neonatal frontal cortex lesions. *Neurosci Lett* 1986;71:247–251.

84. Sharp FR, Gonzalez MF, Sagar SM. Fetal frontal cortex transplanted to injured motor/sensory cortex of adult rats. II. VIP-, somatostatin-, NPY-immunoreactive neurons. *J Neurosci* 1987;7:3002–3015.

85. Sinden JD, Allen YS, Rawlins JNP, Gray JA.

The effects of ibotenic acid lesions of the nucleus basalis and cholinergic-rich neural transplants on win–stay/lose–shift and win–shift/lose–stay performance in the rat. *Behav Brain Res* 1990;36:229–249.

86. Slavin MD, Held JM, Basso DM, Lesensky S, Curran E, Gentile AM, Stein DG. Fetal brain tissue transplants and recovery of locomotion following damage to sensorimotor cortex in rats. *Prog Brain Res* 1988;78:33–38.

87. Sofroniew MV, Dunnett SB, Isacson O. Remodelling of intrinsic and afferent systems in neocortex with cortical transplants. *Prog Brain Res* 1990;82:313–320.

88. Sørensen JC, Zimmer J, Castro AJ. Fetal cortical transplants reduce the thalamic atrophy induced by frontal cortical lesions in newborn rats. *Neurosci Lett* 1989;98:33–38.

89. Stein DG, Labbe R, Attella MJ, Rakowsky HA. Fetal brain tissue transplants reduce visual deficits in adult rats with bilateral lesions of the occipital cortex. *Behav Neural Biol* 1985;44:266–277.

90. Stein DG, Mufson EJ. Morphological and behavioral characteristics of embryonic brain tissue transplants in adult, brain damaged subjects. *Ann NY Acad Sci* 1987;495:444–463.

91. Stein DG, Palatucci C, Kahn D, Labbe R. Temporal factors influence recovery of function after embryonic brain tissue transplants in adult rats with frontal cortex lesions. *Behav Neurosci* 1988;102:260–267.

92. Stewart O, Vinsant SV. The process of reinnervation of the dentate gyrus of the adult rat: a quantitative electron microscopic analysis of terminal proliferation and reactive synaptogenesis. *J Comp Neurol* 1983;214:370–386.

93. Swenson RS, Danielsen EH, Klausen BS, Erlich E, Zimmer J, Castro AJ. Deficits in beamwalking after neonatal motor cortical lesions are not spared by fetal cortical transplants in rats. *J Neural Transpl Plast* 1989;1:129–133.

94. Szentágothai J. The "module concept" in cerebral cortex architecture. *Brain Res* 1975; 95:475–496.

95. Szentágothia J. Local neuron circuits of the neocortex. In: Schmitt FO, Worden FG, eds. *Neurosciences fourth study program.* Cambridge, MA: MIT Press; 1979:399–415.

96. Thompson WG. Successful brain grafting. *NY Med J* 1890;51:701–702.

97. Vargha-Khadem F, Watters G, O'Gorman AM. Development of speech and language following bilateral frontal lesions. *Brain Lang* 1985;37:167–183.

98. Vereschak NK, Lenkov DN. The recovery of locomotion following partial extirpation of the motor cortex and transplantation of cortical tissue in the white rat. *Neurosci Behav Physiol* 1990;20:371–377.

99. Whishaw IQ, O'Connor WT, Dunnett SB. Disruption of central cholinergic systems in the rat by basal forebrain lesions or atropine: effects on feeding, sensorimotor behaviour, locomotor activity, spatial navigation. *Behav Brain Res* 1985;17:103–115.

100. Whishaw IQ, O'Connor WT, Dunnett SB. The contributions of motor cortex, nigrostriatal dopamine and caudate putamen to skilled forelimb use in the rat. *Brain* 1986;109:805–843.

101. Williams R, Lynch G. Terminal proliferation and synaptogenesis following partial deafferentiation: the reinnervation of the inner molecular layer of the dentate gyrus following removal of its commissural afferents. *J Comp Neurol* 1978;180:581–616.

102. Yirmiya R, Zhou FC, Holder MD, Deems DA, Garcia J. Partial recovery of gustatory function after neural tissue transplantation to the lesioned gustatory neocortex. *Brain Res Bull* 1988;20:619–625.

Functional Neural Transplantation,
edited by S. B. Dunnett and A. Björklund.
Raven Press, Ltd., New York © 1994.

17

Anatomic and Functional Correlates of the Regeneration of Retinotectal Projections in Adult Mammals

Michael Rasminsky, Garth M. Bray, and Albert J. Aguayo

*Center for Research in Neuroscience,
McGill University and Montreal General Hospital, Montreal, Quebec H3G 1A4 Canada*

The survival of damaged neurons, the extension of axons toward appropriate targets, and the restoration of afferent and efferent connections are essential requirements for the recovery of neural function after injury. In adult mammals, recovery from central nervous system (CNS) injury is hindered by the loss of many damaged nerve cells and the failure of most axons to regrow when they are severed in the brain or spinal cord.

Components of the nonneuronal environment that surrounds the nerve cell somata and their appendages appear to exert powerful influences on neuronal viability, axonal elongation, terminal differentiation, and synapse formation. Such components include growth-inhibiting molecules in glial cells (53), changes in the extracellular matrix (48), and modifications in the expression of trophic molecules and their receptors (16,43). In spite of remarkable advances in the identification of molecules involved in these interactions, much work will be required to define their relative importance in the complex setting of the injured mammalian nervous system.

To investigate *in vivo* the role of the nonneuronal environment in the success or failure of axonal regeneration from injured CNS neurons, the CNS glial substrate present in the adult mammalian brain or spinal cord was replaced by nonneuronal components of the peripheral nervous system (PNS) (2,4). The experimental strategy applied in these studies consisted of bypassing portions of the CNS of laboratory animals with transplanted, axon-free, peripheral nerve segments the distal end of which was either left unconnected or used as a bridge to reach CNS targets. This approach has provided insight into the intrinsic capacities of different mature CNS neurons to overcome injury and form new synapses under conditions that permit, promote, and guide the extension of their interrupted axons to a selected target.

In this review we focus on experiments in the retinotectal system of rodents, in which we have carried out studies that center on the responses of axotomized retinal ganglion cells (RGCs), a population of CNS neurons that normally project from the eye to the superior colliculus by way of the optic nerve and tract. In adult Sprague–Dawley rats or Syrian hamsters, an autologous segment of peripheral nerve was attached to the ocular stump of the optic nerve transected near the eye (Fig. 1). In some of these animals, the remainder of the periph-

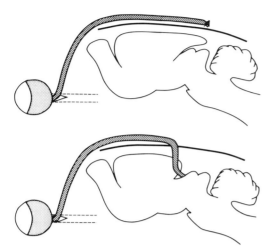

FIG. 1. Peripheral nerve grafts are sutured to the eye; the distal end can either be left unconnected (**above**) or is directed into the superior colliculus (**below**), the normal major target of retinal projections in the rodent. (Adapted from ref. 5 with permission.)

eral nerve graft was left blind-ended beneath the scalp. In other animals, the distal end of the graft was inserted into the superior colliculus, the region of the mesencephalon that normally receives most retinal afferents in rodents.

The purpose of the initial experiments was to study the survival of RGCs (61,62) and the regrowth of axons in the absence of terminal connectivity with a CNS target (60). In later experiments, the regeneration of cut RGC axons along the peripheral nerve graft and the formation of RGC terminals and synapses in the superior colliculus were documented by anterogradely labeling the axonal projections with neuroanatomic tracers (horseradish peroxidase, tritiated amino acids, or fluorescent dyes) (14,59,60). The peripheral nerve graft and the superior colliculus were then examined by light and electron microscopy to identify axons or axon terminals containing these markers. In complementary electrophysiologic experiments, responses to visual stimulation of the retina were sought in both the RGC axons and in the superior colliculus, to characterize functional correlates of the

formation of RGC synapses in the superior colliculus (25).

AXOTOMY AND NEURONAL SURVIVAL

Loss of Axotomized Retinal Ganglion Cells

As with other injured neuronal populations (34), the interruption of RGC axons is followed by the death of many of the axotomized nerve cells. The survival of RGCs was studied in adult rats with optic nerves transected near (0.5 mm) or far (8–10 mm) from the posterior pole of the eye (61,62); each of these lesions permanently disconnected the RGCs from all synaptic targets in the brain. When RGC populations were determined between 15 days and 15 months after optic nerve transection, the axotomy not only caused an early, abrupt loss of RGCs, but also led to a gradual, but sustained decrease in the number of RGCs.

The severity of the early, sudden, postaxotomy loss of RGCs related closely to the proximity of the site of injury to the neuronal soma (62). These findings suggest that the survival of RGCs injured near their neuronal somata may be strictly dependent on an increased supply of trophic molecules, a dependency that is a known feature of neuronal development, but may decline in the adult (36). Furthermore, the loss of cells may be greater when potential sources of trophic support residing in the optic nerve itself are removed by the loss of most of the optic nerve stump after transection near the eye. The greater survival of the RGCs, the axons of which are interrupted in the optic nerve far from the eye (62), and the effects of peripheral nerve grafts on RGC survival (59,61) suggest that nonneuronal elements surrounding axonal projections in both the CNS and PNS may play a role in the protection of neurons from the effects of axonal injury.

The documentation of a gradual and prolonged phase of neuronal loss after axotomy raises the possibility that this pattern of cell death is common to other conditions in which terminal contacts with fields of innervation are lost and cells become dependent on vicarious, non–target-related sources of trophic support.

Enhancement of Neuronal Survival in the Retina

The extent of RGC loss that follows optic nerve transection close to the eye can be reduced in adult rats by the apposition of a segment of peripheral nerve to the ocular stump of the transected optic nerve (8,61). These effects may be explained by the presence in the peripheral nervous system of factors that can promote the survival of injured neurons. Brain-derived neurotrophic factor (BDNF), one of several proteins related to nerve growth factor (NGF) (33), enhances RGC survival *in vitro* (24,58) and is found in peripheral nerves (1). Peripheral nerves also contain other trophic molecules that can enhance neuronal survival: fibroblast growth factor (FGF; 6,55), and ciliary neurotrophic factor (CNTF; 39,54). Because Schwann cells, fibroblasts, and macrophages participate in the synthesis and regulation of several trophic molecules (35), the peripheral nerve grafts used in these studies may meet the specific requirements of a wide spectrum of neurons. However, the ability of peripheral nerve grafts to enhance the survival of RGCs may be only temporary (61), perhaps because there is a decreased synthesis of trophic molecules, such as NGF, when the regenerating axons grow along the peripheral nerve segment (23).

Additional *in vivo* evidence for the role that specific molecules may play in rescuing the axotomized RGCs is the finding of an increase in the number of surviving RGCs in retinas of adult rats treated by single or repeated injections of BDNF into the vitreous chamber following optic nerve transection within the orbit (38).

Other experiments have provided further evidence that synaptic interactions are, in the long-term, essential for the maintenance of the anatomic integrity of axotomized neurons. In rats in which peripheral nerve grafts bridged the eye and the superior colliculus, there was no apparent reduction in the extent of superior colliculus reinnervation by the RGCs between 2 and 18 months after grafting (59), a finding that suggests that the population of RGCs that re-forms synapses with neurons in the superior colliculus persists for the entire life of the animal.

REGENERATION AND SYNAPSE FORMATION

Elongation of Cut Central Nervous System Axons Along Nerve Grafts

Although densities of surviving RGCs fell to nearly 20% by 1 month and to 5% at 3 months after an intraorbital axotomy (62), up to 12% of the normal RGC population (60) and an average of 20% of the surviving RGCs regenerated lengthy axons along peripheral nerve grafts apposed to the optic nerve stump (61). Within peripheral nerve grafts, the RGC axons regrow at rates of 1 to 2 mm/day (17) for 3 or 4 cm, distances that are approximately twice the length of the normal retinocollicular projection of intact adult rats (60). In the peripheral nerve grafts, growth cones extended in close apposition to Schwann cells and their basal laminae (12), an anatomic relation that suggests such contacts mediate neuronal interactions with these substrates through soluble and surface molecules (7,48).

Studies of the expression of certain cytoskeletal proteins illustrate the wide spectrum of neuronal responses that are possible in the injured CNS of adult mammals in response to changes in the growth cone substrate. In the ocular stumps of intracranially transected optic nerves not exposed to peripheral nerve grafts, there was a tenfold decrease in the transport of tubulin and neurofilaments (42). This decrease in rats of slow transport was not accompanied by comparable changes in fast axonal transport. In contrast, when the optic nerve was replaced by a peripheral nerve graft, the rates of tubulin and neurofilament transport doubled (41), a pattern that resembles the transport in axons of the developing optic nerve (65).

Changes in gene expression were also investigated in axotomized RGCs by determining levels of mRNAs encoding β-tubulin under conditions that inhibit or permit the regrowth of damaged axons. After axotomy, in the optic nerve β-tubulin mRNAs decreased and remained at nearly one-half the normal level for the 1-month period studied. In the peripheral nerve-grafted retinas, in which approximately 20% of the surviving RGCs regenerate their axons, there were β-tubulin mRNA "hotspots" that corresponded to RGCs that had regenerated an axon into the peripheral nerve graft. In these RGCs, the β-tubulin signal increased to an average of 286% over that detected in the intact RGCs. Thus, these injured CNS neurons appear capable of

marked changes in gene expression, presumably triggered by molecular interactions between RGC growth cones and components of the microenvironment that promote or inhibit growth (40).

Formation of New Synapses in the Injured Central Nervous System

In adult rats and hamsters, autologous peripheral nerve grafts attached to the ocular stump of transected optic nerves (see Fig. 1) were used as bridges to guide RGC axons to the superior colliculus (14,60) to determine if axonal regeneration could restore synaptic connections in the CNS. After different time intervals, RGCs were labeled intravitreally with tracer substances, and the region of the superior colliculus near the end of the peripheral nerve graft was surveyed by light or electron microscopy. In the animals with bridging grafts connecting the retina and the midbrain, the

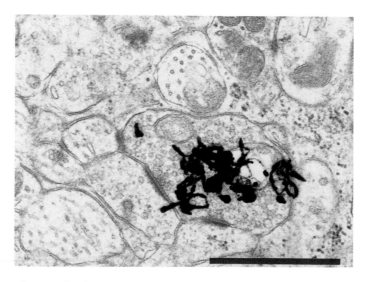

FIG. 2. Electron micrograph of a regenerated retinocollicular axon terminal observed 16 months after the eye and the superior colliculus were linked by a peripheral nerve graft. The RGC terminal, labeled after [³H]amino acids were injected intravitreally, contains pale mitochondria, clear vesicles, and asymmetric synapses. (Calibration bar, 1 μm.) (From ref. 59, with permission.)

RGC axons grew into the superficial layers of the superior colliculus for up to 500 μm at 2 months (14) and 1000 μm at 8 to 10 months (15). Although such limited extension into the superior colliculus contrasts sharply with the sustained growth of the RGC axons along the peripheral nerve grafts, such penetrations into the CNS are long enough to reach most of the neurons in the retinorecipient layers of the targeted tectum. However, likely as a result of the massive loss of axotomized RGCs, the maximal density of reinnervation observed in the superior colliculus of these animals was 11% of normal (15).

On penetration into the tectum, the regenerating RGC axons extended toward the superficial laminae of the superior colliculus that normally receive most retinal projections and formed normal-appearing terminals and synapses (Fig. 2) (14,59,60). Moreover, the proportion of contacts made by the RGC terminals on the dendritic shafts and on the spines of superior colliculus neurons closely resembled the normal pattern of postsynaptic neuronal domains (14).

The continued regrowth of RGC axons into the superior colliculus was accompanied by a 30-fold increase in the number of terminals formed by these axons between 2 and 6 months after the insertion of the caudal end of the graft into the dorsal mesencephalon. In addition, the newly formed terminals and synapses underwent a gradual remodeling toward normal (15).

Although the striking predilection of the regenerating RGC axons for certain superior colliculus laminae and neuronal domains could be dictated by the extensive tectal denervation caused by optic nerve interruption, or by molecular affinities between pre- and postsynaptic elements, studies of the synaptic distribution of RGC axons guided to abnormal targets (66) suggest that conditions other than denervation may play a role in determining these synaptic preferences.

FUNCTION OF AXOTOMIZED NEURONS THAT REGENERATE AXONS

Electrophysiologic Recording From Regenerated Retinal Ganglion Cell Axons

Retinal ganglion cells of vertebrates have a variety of morphologies and respond to visual stimulation in a variety of ways. Cells may have either transient or sustained responses to the onset or offset of light within a restricted visual field, and these responses may be altered by visual stimulation within the surrounding field. This large repertoire of responses reflects various patterns of dendritic organization and the functional innervation of RGCs from the other nervous elements in the retina (19). Preservation of normal patterns of response to visual stimulation in axotomized RGCs with regenerated axons would imply preservation of much of the normal afferent innervation of these cells.

The function of rodent RGCs with axons regenerated into peripheral nerve grafts was examined by recording responses to light from regenerated axons teased from peripheral nerve grafts apposed to the retina (27; Fig. 3). The responses to light of RGCs with regenerated axons were similar to those of normal rat RGCs (13,47). Their visual receptive fields were comparable in both size and suppressive surround organization to those of RGCs in intact animals. Examples of the various types of responses to light that are characteristic of normal RGCs were observed. These included both phasic and tonic, on, off, and on–off responses. The number of functional RCGs with regenerated axons in the peripheral nerve grafts that were not connected with the mesencephalon dropped precipitously with time. Fewer units responsive to light were found in grafts examined 25 to 28 weeks after graft insertion, and almost no visually responsive units could be found in animals with grafts implanted for 44 to 48 weeks (26,27).

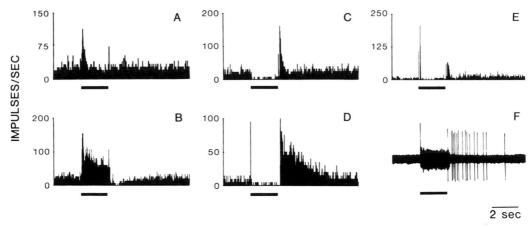

FIG. 3. Responses to light of axotomized rat retinal ganglion cells with regenerated axons. **A–E:** Peristimulus time histograms (bin width 10 msec) of unitary responses to diffuse light presented during periods indicated by the *bars.* In some histograms, artifacts related to shutter opening and closing (as seen in F) are represented by accumulations in single bins at 2 and 4 sec. **A:** A transient on unit in which a short, high-frequency burst in response to the beginning of illumination is followed by a rapid return to baseline. **B:** A sustained on unit in which an initial transient increase in firing is followed by maintained increased activity for the duration of the stimulus. **C:** A transient off unit in which a short, high-frequency burst occurred at the cessation of the light stimulus. **D:** A sustained off unit in which a more protracted increase in firing was observed at the cessation of the light stimulus. **E:** An on–off unit. **F:** The responses of an on and off unit simultaneously recorded from the same small filament to presentation of a circle of light 2° in diameter during the period indicated by the *black bar.* The centers of the receptive fields for the two units were identical. (From ref. 27, with permission.)

Similar physiologic experiments have recently been carried out in cats, in which there has been a more thorough classification of RGCs on both a morphologic (11) and physiologic (56) basis. Feline RGCs with axons regenerated into peripheral nerve grafts also respond to visual stimulation with discharge patterns characteristic of all of the main physiologically classified types of feline RGCs, including various types of Y, X, and W cells (64). This finding is in keeping with the anatomic demonstration that cells with somatic and dendritic morphologies characteristic of alpha, beta, and gamma cells, all regenerate axons into peripheral nerve grafts apposed to the cat eye (63). Although there may be differences in survival and regrowth of axons among different populations of axotomized RGCs (63), it appears that no group of retinal neu-rons is singled out for failure of functional regeneration.

The major conclusion to be drawn from these studies of RGCs and from similar experiments on injured brain stem neurons that had regenerated axons into peripheral nerve grafts (22,32,45), is that at least some of the CNS neurons that have successfully regenerated their axons into peripheral nerve grafts can retain or regain function. This implies preservation of afferent innervation of at least some injured cells with sufficient complexity to subserve the variety of responses found in intact animals. The protracted decrease of functionally responsive neurons with regenerated axons observed several months after peripheral nerve grafting into the retina (26,27) or the brain stem (22) may reflect anatomic loss of axotomized neurons that are prevented from making connections in the brain.

Functional Synapses Made by Regenerated Retinal Ganglion Cell Axons

The experimental preparation initially used to demonstrate synaptic transmission between axons regenerated from RGCs and superior colliculus neurons is illustrated in Fig. 4. Peripheral nerve grafts were first at-tached to the ocular stump of the transected optic nerve. After allowing a period of 7 to 8 weeks to permit regeneration of RGCs axons into the graft, the distal end of the graft was inserted into the lateral aspect of the superficial layer of the ipsilateral superior colliculus. Two to three weeks later, the contralateral optic nerve was transected to vacate synaptic sites on neurons in the tar-geted superior colliculus at the time that the regenerating RGC axons reached the supe-rior colliculus. Bilateral optic nerve tran-

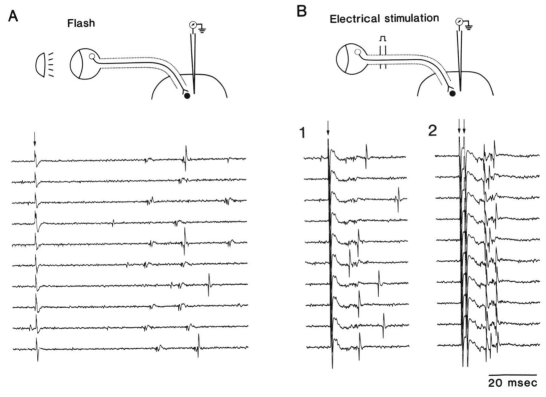

FIG. 4. Excitatory postsynaptic responses in a reinnervated SC neuron of a hamster with a periph-eral nerve graft directed from the eye to the SC. **A**: A single unit 250 μm below the surface responds to light flashes to the eye (*arrow*) with a single spike on four of ten trials. This response could represent a recording from either a presynaptic RGC axon or a postsynaptic SC neuron. **B**: Electrical stimulation of the graft distinguishes between these possibilities. The same unit responds erratically with inconstant latency to (**traces 1**) single electrical stimuli (*arrow*) delivered to the graft, but at a more constant latency, often with multiple spikes, to (**traces 2**) paired electrical stimuli (*arrows*) of the same intensity. The latter response would not be expected if the recording were made from a presynaptic RGC axon, but reflects postsynaptic summation to threshold of successive subthreshold EPSPs elicited by the afferent input. (From ref. 25, with permission.)

section also ensured that all visual input to the superior colliculus would be by RGC axons that had regenerated through the peripheral nerve graft.

Microelectrode recordings were made from the vicinity of graft insertion 15 to 18 weeks later (27). Both excitatory and inhibitory unitary responses to light were found in the region of graft insertion. The excitatory responses were proved to be postsynaptic by demonstrating an enhanced response to paired subthreshold electrical stimulation of the graft (see Fig. 4). In more recent experiments, we have been able to demonstrate more directly synaptic interactions between regenerated RGC axons and superior colliculus neurons by selectively abolishing postsynaptic, but not presynaptic, responses to visual stimulation with iontophoretic application of γ-aminobutyric acid (GABA), an inhibitory synaptic transmitter (51). Sawai et al. (52) have also reported visual responses from the superior colliculus in hamsters in which a peripheral nerve was used to bridge the brachium of the superior colliculus and the superior colliculus following transection of the brachium.

Functional Consequences of Reconnectivity

Pupillary Light Reflex

Because the pupillary light reflex can be quantitated and has a well-defined circuitry, it offers a particularly attractive assay system for the study of functional reinnervation of pretectal neurons by retinofugal fibers. In this reflex pathway, excitation of RGCs by light elicits activity in neurons in the olivary pretectal (OPT) nucleus. The OPT neurons project to neurons in the nucleus of Edinger–Westphal in the midbrain which, in turn, project to ciliary ganglion neurons, the activity of which results in pupilloconstriction.

When grafts of fetal rat retina are placed on the tectum and pretectum of neonatal rats, RGCs within the graft grow axons into the underlying tectum and pretectum (37). Light shown on such grafts elicits a pupillary light reflex (29–31) in the normally innervated eye of the grafted animal. The innervation of the host pretectum by axons growing from the transplant can thus functionally replace the retinopretectal limb of the pathway that normally mediates the pupillary light reflex.

Thanos (57) has recently shown that a functional retinopretectal pathway can also be reconstructed with a peripheral nerve graft. From 6 to 7 weeks after placement of a one-stage peripheral nerve graft between the eye and the ipsilateral pretectum of adult rats, pupillary constriction was seen in response to light shown in the grafted eye (Fig. 5). Abolition of the pupillary response by transection of the graft established that this response was mediated by the graft. Pupillary responses to light were found in 9 of 22 animals with histologically verified placement of the grafts in either the pretectum or the pretectum and the superior colliculus. Responses were not found in animals in which the graft tips were directed exclusively to the superior colliculus.

Light-Directed Behavior Mediated by Nerve Grafts

Preliminary behavioral studies have suggested that retinotectal grafts may convey sufficient information to permit rodents to respond appropriately to light in a conditioned–avoidance behavioral paradigm.

Sasaki et al. (49) studied hamsters with peripheral nerve grafts directed from the retina to the superior colliculus. Grafts were prepared as a two-stage procedure. The insertion of the distal end of the graft into the ipsilateral superior colliculus was performed 8 weeks after optic nerve replacement, at which time the contralateral optic nerve was also cut to ensure that the graft provided the only route of visual input to the brain. Behavioral experiments were done 2 to 3 months after graft insertion into the superior colliculus.

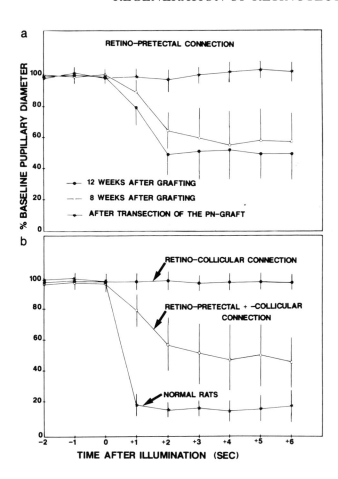

FIG. 5. Pupillary constriction following illumination of eyes that have peripheral nerve grafts directed from the retina to the midbrain. **A**: Responses of six animals with retinopretectal grafts 8 and 12 weeks after grafting and after transection of the graft. The response to light is abolished after graft transection. **B**: Pupillary responses to light in animals with retinocollicular grafts, with combined retinopretectal and retinocollicular grafts, and in normal animals. The data represent mean pupillary diameters, the *bars* the range of diameters. (From ref. 57, with permission.)

Animals placed in a shuttle box were exposed to a conditioned stimulus of light from a fluorescent tube, paired with an unconditioned stimulus of scrambled electric shock. Subjected to 30 or 50 daily trials, normal animals increased the probability of an avoidance response to light from 9.3% to 42.7% between the first and tenth days of the trial (Fig. 6). There was no increase in the light-avoidance response of blind hamsters. The mean light-avoidance responses for five hamsters with retinotectal grafts increased from less than 5% on the first day to 19.5% by the tenth day of the trial, a significant difference from the performance of blind hamsters. This difference was more striking when the behavior of individual animals was considered. Three of the five hamsters with retinotectal grafts increased their avoidance responses to 23%, 28%, and 30% by the tenth day of the trial, whereas the remaining two hamsters had no significant increase in avoidance behavior. Placement of at least part of the graft within the superior colliculus was verified histologically for four of the five animals, including two of the three with significant increases in light-avoidance behavior. Histologic analysis was not performed on one of the three animals with a behavioral response. The main target of the graft was the inferior colliculus for one animal with a demonstrable behavioral response and one animal with no response. The authors do not report the depth of the tip of their grafts, and it is thus unclear which population(s) of superior colliculus neurons are contacted by the regenerated RGC axons.

Similar experiments on rats have been reported in preliminary form by Kittlerová

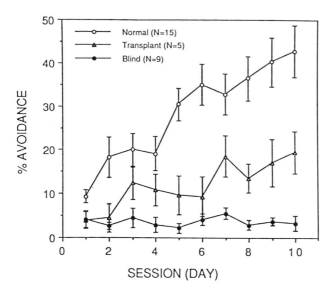

FIG. 6. Mean avoidance scores for hamsters subjected to 30 or 50 daily trials in which the conditioned light stimulus preceded an unconditioned electric shock by 10 sec. Mean avoidance scores did not increase for blinded animals, but did increase significantly for animals with retinocollicular grafts. This increase was less than that observed for intact animals. (From ref. 49, with permission.)

(28). Ipsilateral retinotectal grafts were prepared as a one-stage procedure, combined with section of the contralateral optic nerve. Persistence of retinal function was verified in the grafted animals by demonstration of preservation of the electroretinogram over many months. Behavioral experiments on these animals were performed 8 to 17 months after transplantation. Grafted animals performed significantly better than blinded animals in a light–shock–escape task.

Additional Considerations Concerning Effective Re-Formation of Functional Circuitry

The electrophysiologic and behavioral experiments, described in the foregoing, suggest that peripheral nerve grafts can mediate not only transsynaptic activation in the visual system, but also certain simple visually elicited behaviors. The functional effectiveness of graft-mediated reconnections in the visual and other systems will depend on the nature of the behavior in question. The extent to which normal circuitry needs to be replaced and the necessity for precision in rewiring of connections may vary substantially for different types of visually mediated behaviors. Certain visual behaviors appear to demand only a relatively limited amount of visual input. For example, pattern discrimination in cats appears to be retained until more than 95% of optic nerve fibers are damaged (21,46), and brightness perception can be restored in rats that have lost more than 90% of their optic nerve fibers (50). These studies, done on animals with damaged, but not regenerated, optic nerves, could not address the question of the role of topologic specificity of the remaining optic nerve fibers. Even though it has been shown anatomically that the regenerating RGC axons grow only into the superficial layers of the superior colliculus that normally receive retinal inputs, and that the RGC synapses are distributed in appropriate proportions on dendrites and dendritic spines (14), it is not known whether any retinotopy is preserved during reinnervation of the mammalian superior colliculus by regenerating RGC axons.

Among the considerations determining the effectiveness of nerve grafts in restoring function will be the properties of the reinnervated cells. Within certain well-defined pathways in the nervous system, the biophysical properties of the postsynaptic cell may permit a 1:1 input–output relation. For example, relay neurons of the cat lateral geniculate nucleus may discharge in response to an impulse in a single afferent RGC axon (18). In such cells, excitatory postsynaptic potentials (EPSPs) generated in dendrites by afferent activity in RGCs are thought to be only modestly attenuated toward the cell body, such that an impulse in a single afferent can theoretically give rise to a somatic EPSP of several millivolts (10). In a pathway such as this, re-formation of a relatively small number of synapses could be expected to have a significant functional influence. At the other extreme, there are pathways, such as that mediating the monosynaptic spinal reflex arc, in which multiple Ia afferents synapse on individual homonymous motor neurons, but inputs from individual Ia afferent fibers generate somatic EPSPs of no more than a few hundred microvolts (44). Because neurons in this type of circuit may require simultaneous inputs from a great many afferents to elicit firing, they are poor candidates as targets for *functional* reinnervation with a high degree of precision by regenerating axons.

The use of nerve grafts as conduits for functional reinnervation may be particularly useful in systems that are less dependent on the precision of synaptic input, but can be restored to more normal activity by the delivery of depleted neurotransmitters. In the striatonigral system, transplants of embryonic dopaminergic neurons reinnervate the striatum and can functionally replace dopaminergic neurons depleted from the host by administration of 6-hydroxydopamine (6-OHDA) (9). Although transplants are usually placed close to the target in such experiments, axons from fetal mesencephalic neurons placed 2 cm or more from the striatum can be directed through a peripheral nerve graft to the denervated host striatum (3). Reinnervation of the unilaterally denervated striatum by mono-

aminergic fibers is sufficient to suppress amphetamine-induced rotational asymmetry in these animals, this functional effect disappearing after transection of the graft (20).

SUMMARY AND CONCLUSIONS

The visual system has offered a useful paradigm for the demonstration of the capacity of injured mammalian CNS neurons to re-form connections. The anatomic studies described in the initial part of this review suggest that certain injured RGC neurons are capable of recapitulating essential steps required for their interrupted axons to regrow and make synaptic connections when their extension is both facilitated and guided to the immediate vicinity of their natural targets. The functional consequences of these re-formed connections have now been studied in several ways. At the simplest level, re-formed synapses have mediated transsynaptic excitation and inhibition. Furthermore, the experiments demonstrating pupillary reactivity to light in animals with retinopretectal grafts suggest that neurons influenced by newly formed synapses in the adult can transmit information forward within the nervous system. Finally, at a more complex level of integration, preliminary experiments suggest that some animals with nerve grafts from the eye to the brain can acquire light-avoidance behavior. Strategies aimed at further enhancing the survival and regrowth of axotomized CNS neurons should provide new opportunities to determine if regeneration in the CNS of adult mammals can lead to a useful recovery of function.

ACKNOWLEDGMENTS

Work in the authors' laboratories is supported by the Medical Research Council of Canada and the Multiple Sclerosis Society of Canada. The authors are members of the Canadian Network for the Study of Neural Regeneration and Recovery of Function.

REFERENCES

1. Acheson A, Barker PA, Alderson RF, Miller FD, Murphy RA. Detection of brain-derived neurotrophic factor-like activity in fibroblasts and Schwann cells: inhibition by antibodies to NGF. *Neuron* 1991;7:265–275.
2. Aguayo AJ. Axonal regeneration from injured neurons in the adult mammalian central nervous system. In: Cotman C, ed. *Synaptic plasticity.* New York: Guilford Press; 1985:457–484.
3. Aguayo AJ, Björklund A, Stenevi U, Carlstedt T. Fetal mesencephalic neurons survive and extend long axons across peripheral nervous system grafts inserted into the adult rat striatum. *Neurosci Lett* 1984;45:53–58.
4. Aguayo AJ, Rasminsky M, Bray GM, Carbonetto S, McKerracher MP, Villegas-Pérez M, Vidal-Sanz M, Carter DA. Degenerative and regenerative responses of injured neurons in the central nervous system of adult mammals. *Philos Trans R Soc Lond B* 1991;331:337–343.
5. Aguayo AJ, Vidal-Sanz M, Villegas M-P, Bray GM. Growth and connectivity of axotomized retinal neurons in adult rats with optic nerves substituted by PNS grafts linking the eye and the midbrain. *Ann NY Acad Sci* 1987;495:1–7.
6. Bähr M, Vanselow J, Thanos S. Ability of adult rat ganglion cells to regrow axons in vitro can be influenced by fibroblast growth factor and gangliosides. *Neurosci Lett* 1989;96:197–201.
7. Barde Y-A. Trophic factors and neuronal survival. *Neuron* 1989;2:1525–1534.
8. Berry M, Rees L, Sievers J. Regeneration of axons in the mammalian visual system. *Exp Brain Res* 1986;13(suppl):18–33.
9. Björklund A, Lindvall O, Isacson O, Brundin P, Wictorin K, Strecker RE, Clarke DJ, Dunnet SB. Mechanisms of action of intracerebral neural implants: studies on nigral and striatal grafts to the lesioned striatum. *Trends Neurosci* 1987;10:509–516.
10. Bloomfield SA, Sherman SM. Dendritic current flow in relay cells and interneurons of the cat's lateral geniculate nucleus. *Proc Natl Acad Sci USA* 1989;86:3911–3914.
11. Boycott BB, Wässle H. The morphological types of ganglion cells of the domestic cat's retina. *J Physiol* 1974;240:397–419.
12. Bray GM, Vidal-Sanz M, Villegas-Perez M-P, Carter DA, Zwimpfer T, Aguayo AJ. Growth and differentiation of regenerating CNS axons in adult mammals. In: Letourneau PC, Kater SB, Macagno ER, eds. *The nerve growth cone.* New York: Raven Press; 1991:489–504.
13. Brown JE, Rojas JA. Rat retinal ganglion cells: receptive field organization and maintained activity. *J Neurophysiol* 1985;28:1073–1090.
14. Carter DA, Bray GM, Aguayo AJ. Regenerated retinal ganglion cell axons can form well-differentiated synapses in the superior colliculus of adult hamsters. *J Neurosci* 1989;9:4042–4050.
15. Carter DA, Bray GM, Aguayo AJ. Long-term growth and remodelling of regenerated retinocollicular connections in adult hamsters. *J Neurosci* 1994;14:590–598.
16. Chao MV. Growth factor signaling: where is the specificity? *Cell* 1991;68:995–997.
17. Cho EYP, So K-F. Rate of regrowth of damaged retinal ganglion cell axons regenerating in a peripheral nerve graft in adult hamsters. *Brain Res* 1987;419:369–374.
18. Cleland BG, Dubin MW, Levick WR. Sustained and transient neurons in the cat's retina and lateral geniculate nucleus. *J Physiol* 1971;217:473–496.
19. Dowling JE. *The retina.* Cambridge, MA: Belknap Press of Harvard University Press; 1987.
20. Gage FH, Stenevi U, Carlstedt T, Foster G, Björklund A, Aguayo AJ. Anatomical and functional consequences of grafting mesencephalic neurons into a peripheral nerve "bridge" connected to the denervated striatum. *Exp Brain Res* 1985;60:584–589.
21. Galambos R, Norton TT, Frommer GP. Optic tract lesions sparing pattern vision in cats. *Exp Neurol* 1967;18:8–25.
22. Gauthier P, Rasminsky M. Activity of medullary respiratory neurons regenerating axons into peripheral nerve grafts in the adult rat. *Brain Res* 1988;438:225–236.
23. Heumann R, Lindholm D, Bandtlow C, Mayer M, Radeke MJ, Misko TP, Shooter E, Thoenen H. Differential regulation of nerve growth factor (NGF) and NGF-receptor mRNA in the rat sciatic nerve during development, degeneration, and regeneration; role played by macrophages. *Proc Natl Acad Sci USA* 1987;84:8735–8739.
24. Johnson JE, Barde Y-A, Schwab M, Thoenen H. Brain-derived neurotrophic factor supports the survival of cultured rat retinal ganglion cells. *J Neurosci* 1986;6:3031–3038.
25. Keirstead SA, Rasminsky M, Fukuda Y, Carter DA, Aguayo AJ, Vidal-Sanz M. Electrophysiological responses in hamster superior colliculus evoked by regenerating retinal axons. *Science* 1989;246:255–258.
26. Keirstead SA, Rasminsky M, Vidal-Sanz M, Aguayo AJ. Functional studies of central nervous system neurons regenerating axons into peripheral nerve grafts. In: Gordon T, Stein RB, Smith PA, eds. *The current status of peripheral nerve regeneration.* New York: Alan R Liss; 1988:143–155.
27. Keirstead SA, Vidal-Sanz M, Rasminsky M, Aguayo AJ, Levesque M, So K-F. Responses to light of retinal neurons regenerating axons into peripheral nerve grafts in the rat. *Brain Res* 1985;359:402–406.
28. Kittlerová P. [MSc dissertation], Charles University, Prague, 1992.
29. Klassen H, Lund RD. Retinal transplants can drive a pupillary reflex in host rat brains. *Proc Natl Acad Sci USA* 1987;84:6958–6960.
30. Klassen H, Lund RD. Anatomical and behavioural correlates of a xenograft-mediated pupillary reflex. *Exp Neurol* 1988;102:102–108.
31. Klassen H, Lund RD. Retinal graft-mediated pupillary responses in rats: restoration of a reflex function in the mature mammalian brain. *J Neurosci* 1990;10:578–587.
32. Lammari-Barreault N, Rega P, Gauthier P. Axonal regeneration from central respiratory neu-

types of cat retinal ganglion cells following axotomy and axonal regeneration. *Neurosci Res* 1992;17(suppl):S241.

Willard MB, Simon C. Modulations of neurofilament axonal transport during the development of rabbit retinal ganglion cells. *Cell* 1983;35:551–559.

66. Zwimpfer TJ, Aguayo AJ, Bray GM. Synapse formation and preferential distribution in the granule cell layer by regenerating retinal ganglion cell axons guided to the cerebellum of adult hamsters. *J Neurosci* 1992;12:1144–1159.

rons of the adult rat into peripheral nerve autografts: effects of graft location within the medulla. *Neurosci Lett* 1991;125:121–124.

33. Leibrock J, Lottspeich F, Hohn A, Hofer M, Herenger B, Masiakowski P, Thoenen H, Barde Y-A. Molecular cloning and expression of brain-derived neurotrophic factor. *Nature* 1989;341: 149–152.

34. Lieberman AR. Some factors affecting retrograde neuronal responses to axonal lesions. In: Bellairs R, Gray EG, eds. *Essays on the nervous system.* Oxford: Clarendon; 1974:71–105.

35. Lindholm D, Heumann R, Meyer M, Thoenen H. Interleukin-1 regulates synthesis of nerve growth factor in non neuronal cells of rat sciatic nerve. *Nature* 1987;330:658–659.

36. Lindsay RM. Nerve growth factors (NGF, BDNF) enhance axonal regeneration but are not required for survival of adult sensory neurons. *J Neurosci* 1988;8:2394–2405.

37. Lund RD, Radel JD, Hankin MH, Yee KT, Banerjee R, Coffey PJ, Horsburgh GM. Intracerebral retinal transplants. In: Lam DM-K, Bray GM, eds. *Regeneration and plasticity in the mammalian visual system.* Cambridge, MA: MIT Press; 1992:125–145.

38. Mansour-Robaey S, Bray GM, Aguayo AJ. In vivo effects of brain-derived neurotrophic factor (BDNF) and injury on the survival of axotomized retinal ganglion cells (RGCs) in adult rats. *Mol Biol Cell* 1992;3:333.

39. Manthorpe M, Skaper SD, Williams LR, Varon S. Purification of adult rat sciatic nerve ciliary neuronotrophic factor. *Brain Res* 1986;367:282–286.

40. McKerracher L, Essagian C, Aguayo AJ. Marked increase in β-tubulin mRNA expression during regeneration of axotomized retinal ganglion cells in adult mammals. *J Neurosci* 1993;13:5294–5300.

41. McKerracher L, Vidal-Sanz M, Aguayo AJ. Slow transport rates of cytoskeletal proteins change during regeneration of axotomized retinal neurons in adult rats. *J Neurosci* 1990; 10:641–648.

42. McKerracher L, Vidal-Sanz M, Essagian C, Aguayo AJ. Selective impairment of slow axonal transport after optic nerve injury in adult rats. *J Neurosci* 1990;10:2834–2841.

43. Meakin SO, Shooter EM. The nerve growth factor family of receptors. *Trends Neurosci* 1992; 15:323–331.

44. Mendell LM, Henneman E. Terminals of single Ia fibers: location, density and distribution within a pool of 300 homonymous motor neurons. *J Neurophysiol* 1971;34:171–187.

45. Munz M, Rašminsky M, Aguayo AJ, Vidal-Sanz M, Devor M. Functional activity of rat brainstem neurons regenerating axons along peripheral nerve grafts. *Brain Res* 1985;340:115–126.

46. Norton TT, Galambos R, Frommer GP. Optic tract lesions destroying pattern vision in cats. *Exp Neurol* 1967;18:26–37.

47. Partridge LD, Brown JE. Receptive fields of rat retinal ganglion cells. *Vision Res* 1970;10:455–460.

48. Reichardt LF, Tomaselli KJ. Extracellular ma-

trix molecules and their rec
neural development. *Annu*
14:531–570.

49. Sasaki H, Inoue T, Iso H, Fu
Light–dark discrimination
transplantation to the sectic
adult hamsters. *Vision Res* 1

50. Sautter J, Duvdevani R, Sch
Recovery of brightness disc
mance after graded crush of
Eur J Neurosci 1990;3(suppl)

51. Sauvé Y, Rasminsky M, Carte
and characterization of resj
reinnervated hamster superi
Neurosci Abstr 1991;17:568.

52. Sawai H, Fukuda Y, Watana
of retinocollicular pathway a
transplantation into the secti
adult hamsters. *Soc Neuros*
1322.

53. Schwab ME. Myelin-associa
neurite growth. *Exp Neurol* 19

54. Sendtner M, Kreutzberg GW,
ary neurotrophic factor preve
tion of motor neurons after
1990;345:440–441.

55. Sievers J, Hausmann B, Unsic
Fibroblast growth factors pron
of adult rat retinal ganglion cell
tion of the optic nerves. *Neu*
76:157–162.

56. Stone J, Fukuda Y. Properties c
glion cells: a comparison of W-c
Y-cells. *J Neurophysiol* 1974;37

57. Thanos S. Adult retinofugal ax
through peripheral nerve grafts
light-induced pupilloconstrictio
Neurosci 1992;4:691–699.

58. Thanos S, Bähr M, Barde Y-A, V
vival and axonal elongation of a
ganglion cells. *Eur J Neurosci* 1

59. Vidal-Sanz M, Bray GM, Aguay
ated synapses persist in the sup
after the regrowth of retinal gang
J Neurocytol 1991;20:940–952.

60. Vidal-Sanz M, Bray GM, Villeg
Aguayo AJ. Axonal regeneratio
formation in the superior collicu
ganglion cells in the adult rat
1987;7:2894–2907.

61. Villegas-Pérez MP, Vidal-Sanz 1
Aguayo, AJ. Influences of per
grafts on the survival and regrow
ized retinal ganglion cells in adul
rosci 1988;8:265–280.

62. Villegas-Pérez M-P, Vidal-Sanz N
M, Bray GM, Aguayo AJ. Rapid a
phases of retinal ganglion cell los
tomy in the optic nerve of adult rats
1993;24:23–36.

63. Watanabe M, Sawai H, Fukuda Y.
tribution and morphology of reti
cells with axons regenerated into
nerve graft in adult cats. *J Net*
13:2105–2117.

64. Watanabe M, Sawai H, Rasminsky
M, Fukuda Y. Preservation of physi

Functional Neural Transplantation,
edited by S. B. Dunnett and A. Björklund.
Raven Press, Ltd., New York © 1994.

18

Hypothalamic Grafts and Neuroendocrine Function

Matthew J. A. Wood and Harry M. Charlton

Department of Human Anatomy, University of Oxford, Oxford OX1 3QX, United Kingdom

The hypothalamus is a neural integration center that is now known to be of critical importance in the control of the endocrine, autonomic, and behavioral responses essential for the survival of the individual animal and the species. It is central to the regulation of water homeostasis, thermoregulation, food intake, aggression, reproductive processes, and sleep–wake cyclic activity (76).

In the years between 1935 and 1965, much effort was devoted to the study of the anatomic pathway by which the central nervous system (CNS) influenced the function of the anterior pituitary gland. The scientific evidence that established the central importance of the hypothalamus in the regulation of neuroendocrine mechanisms and that culminated in the formulation of the neurohumeral hypothesis of anterior pituitary function was described in the Dale lecture delivered in 1972 by Geoffrey Harris (31). The experimental approach of tissue transplantation was of fundamental importance for much of this work. Studies in which pituitary tissue was grafted to different sites within the brain thus proved to be of value in defining the the neurovascular relations between the hypothalamus and the anterior pituitary gland. Only those transplants that were vascularized directly from the median eminence of the hypothalamus were fully functional and could abolish the physiologic effects of hypophysec-

tomy. Thus, a model system of a surgically lesioned host animal into which tissue transplants were placed became productive for understanding neuroendocrine mechanisms.

More than 20 neuropeptides have now been localized in the endocrine hypothalamus (9). Besides the hypothalamic peptides with neurohormonal effects, such as those that control the release of growth hormones—the gonadotropic hormones, thyroid-stimulating hormone, and adrenocorticotropic hormone, which all have been isolated and their respective genes cloned—there are those that may have neurotransmitter (neuromodulator) activity. The latter, which include opioid peptides, brain-borne gastrointestinal peptides, and vasoactive peptides, may influence hypothalamohypophysial regulatory mechanisms, or they may constitute a neuronal link between the endocrine hypothalamus and extrahypothalamic brain regions, especially the limbic system and autonomic regulatory centers in the lower brain stem. With the advent of immunoassays, immunocytochemistry, and messenger RNA (mRNA) hybridization, our knowledge of the sites of production of these peptides and the factors controlling their synthesis and release has advanced greatly in recent years.

Of the early methods that were developed to investigate the specific areas of the hypothalamus involved in pituitary control, some involved electrolytic lesioning or deafferentation techniques using knife cuts, others used electrical stimulation, but several authors favored the intraparenchymal transplantation of anterior pituitary tissue as a model system. In this way, the hypophysiotropic region of the hypothalamus was defined. More recently the transplantation of hypothalamic tissue in various model systems has become a rewarding strategy for investigating not only the functional integration of hypothalamic neurons with the pituitary gland, but also for analyzing the complex interactions between the hypothalamus and extrahypothalamic brain regions.

THE HYPOPHYSIOTROPIC AREA

In the early 1960s, several reports were published describing the functional consequences of pituitary tissue grafted directly into the brain. Knigge demonstrated that reproductive function could be restored in hypophysectomized rats by grafting such tissue into the tuberoinfundibular recess of the third ventricle (38). This work was subsequently extended by Halasz et al. (28–30) to show that gonadotropic hormone secretion could be restored to the normal range following pituitary transplantation into the medial basal hypothalamus of hypophysectomized rats. The histologic evidence from these studies suggested that direct vascularization from capillaries of the pituitary portal vessels was not required for the recovery of full reproductive function. However, the maintenance of normal thyroid and adrenal activity did apparently require contact with the median eminence. From these studies, the concept of a hypophysiotropic region within the medial basal hypothalamus developed, within which pituitary grafts had the capacity to elicit normal physiologic responses.

In the studies of Halasz et al. (30) the suggestion was put forward that a local diffusion of releasing factors in the graft vicinity was the likely explanation for pituitary gonadotropin stimulation. However in subsequent studies in which the median eminence was also ablated, the evidence has pointed to the integrity of the median eminence and the fenestrated vessels within the medial basal hypothalamus as both being essential for the stimulatory effects of pituitary grafts (67).

In contrast, the work of Shechter et al. (68) has indicated that pituitary grafts placed in the cerebral cortex may possess active gonadotrophs. They have postulated that hypophysectomy could result in the excessive hypothalamic secretion of gonadotropin-releasing hormone (GnRH), sufficient to activate cells of the cortical grafts. However, in this work, no mention was made of the reproductive status of the recipient animals. Nevertheless, it would seem that this unresolved area of brain transplantation probably deserves reexamination with the more modern techniques now at our disposal. In addition, the grafting of pituitary tissue to extracerebral sites in hypophysectomized rats is beginning to yield information concerning intrinsic mechanisms of the anterior pituitary gland that might modulate hormone release (18). Although it is premature to assess the effects of such work, it is likely that this will become an important area of study.

In the foregoing examples, direct perturbation of normal function was an integral part of the experimental procedures. Such lesioning, whether by chemical or surgical means, is again frequently becoming essential to generate animal model systems amenable to the study of hypothalamic function. The use of transgenic approaches is becoming more widespread, but occasionally mutant animals have arisen spontaneously, in which the gene mutation has affected physiologic function, resulting in precisely lesioned animal models. Two such neuroendocrine models are the antidiuretic hormone (ADH)-deficient Brattleboro rat and the GnRH-deficient hypogonadal (hpg) mouse.

THE BRATTLEBORO RAT

The roles of the posterior pituitary gland hormones in the control of milk ejection and water balance are well documented (76). The Brattleboro rat, derived from the Long–Evans strain, was discovered and characterized by Valtin (77,78), and it is an animal model for vasopressin-deficient diabetes insipidus. In this animal, the deletion of a single nucleotide in the second exon of the gene for the peptide hormone vasopressin has resulted in a frame-shift mutation, with the subsequent production of an aberrant vasopressin mRNA that cannot be translated into the mature hypothalamic hormone (63). Since both alleles of the gene are transcribed, the trait is recessive. The genetics of the Brattleboro rat are not yet fully understood, since several anomalies require explanation. Namely, that normal amounts of vasopressin are found in both the adrenal glands (53) and the ovaries (42) and, second, that revertant magnocellular neurons exhibiting apparently heterozygotic phenotypes are found with low frequency and in an age-dependent manner in the hypothalami of homozygous animals. The most provocative explanation for these observations would be to invoke a DNA repair mechanism occurring postmitotically in somatic cells, but there are other possibilities that require experimental exclusion (36). Nevertheless, there can be no doubt that a failure of production of hypothalamic vasopressin results in the severe diabetes insipidus observed in this animal. Little or no immunoreactive ADH is observed within the posterior pituitary gland, and the mutants excrete large volumes of hypotonic urine.

At first glance, this mutant might seem to be an excellent model in which to monitor the survival, by immunocytochemical methods and the function, with measurements of water intake and urine output, of transplanted vasopressin neurons. The potential of such neural transplants to alleviate the physiologic disorder of this mutant was examined by Gash et al. (22). In these studies the survival of vasopressinergic fibers within the grafts was readily detected with immunohistochemical techniques, and these axons densely innervated the median eminence, a finding confirmed in other reports (75). In subsequent studies, axonal projections toward other specific target areas were noted (7). The functional effects of such grafts, however, were equivocal, with the reversal of diabetes insipidus in only a small proportion of mutant animals in the study reported by Gash et al. (22), and a failure to confirm even these findings in subsequent studies (6,65).

The failure of neural transplants to ameliorate the diabetes insipidus of the Brattleboro rat in almost all trials has reduced the usefulness of this model system. Nevertheless, several important neurobiologic points have emerged from these studies. The outgrowth of vasopressinergic fibers to the median eminence suggests an active influence of this region in attracting such axons, even in the adult animal. Second, as the Brattleboro rat strain is not specifically inbred, it is conceivable that immunologic factors may play a role in the failure of many grafts to provide functional compensation. Thus, to test the hypothesis of whether vasopressin cells are the specific osmoreceptors of the hypothalamus, it may be of use to include some form of immunosuppression in the experimental procedures to guarantee maximal long-term graft survival.

More recently, an alternative paradigm has been used to address the slightly different question of whether neural implants can stimulate recovery from the diabetes insipidus resulting from an impairment of the hypothalamic neurosecretory system (45). In this model system, neurohypophysectomized Long–Evans rats were used. Neurohypophysectomy in rodents results in the degeneration of about 75% of magnocellular neurons; however, the remaining 25% may regenerate and establish new neurohemal connections with the reorganized vasculature of the median eminence (32). Such animals received anterior hypothalamic grafts transplanted into the third ventricle, and complete functional recovery occurred in over 50% of animals. The mechanisms by which such functional recovery occurs have been investigated. The experimental evidence now suggests that such hypothalamic transplants can promote the functional regeneration of axotomized supraoptic vasopressinergic neurons, and that it is this, rather than the formation of specific synaptic contacts, that is thought to be the dominant mechanism of physiologic recovery in this system (45).

THE HYPOGONADAL MOUSE

The hypogonadal (hpg) mouse arose in a breeding colony at the MRC Radiobiology Unit at Harwell, United Kingdom, and was originally characterized by Cattanach et al. (11). This mutant mouse has a congenital deficiency of the hypothalamic-releasing factor GnRH, which regulates the synthesis and release of the pituitary gonadotropins luteinizing hormone (LH) and follicle-stimulating hormone (FSH). As a result, pituitary LH and FSH content is drastically reduced, and there is a failure of postnatal gonadal development in both sexes. The structure of the mammalian GnRH gene was determined by Adelman et al. (1), and there is probably a single copy consisting of four exons encoding the decapeptide sequence of GnRH and a 56-amino acid sequence gonadotropin-associated peptide, or GAP. The genetic cause of the hypogonadism of the hpg mouse was shown by Mason et al. (46) to be a deletion of at least 33.5 kilobases in the distal half of the gene for the common biosynthetic precursor of GnRH and GAP. This results in a failure of GnRH gene transcription and translation. Although there is some evidence that the partially deleted GnRH gene is transcriptionally active, as revealed by in situ hybridization (46), there is an absolute failure

to detect GnRH-positive cell bodies or fibers using immunohistochemical methods.

The hpg pituitary gland contains immunohistochemically identifiable gonadotroph cells, but these are smaller, fewer, and contain fewer granules than those of normal mice (44). They also possess fewer GnRH receptors than those of normal control littermates (84). The cells contain biologically active LH (20), and they respond to injections of GnRH by releasing LH (35). Such synthetic GnRH injections increase the number of GnRH receptors into the normal range, result in increased LH and FSH synthesis and secretion, and stimulate of ovarian and testicular activity with concomitant increases in the mass of these organs (84). Furthermore, the atrophic nature of the seminal vesicles and uteri in male and female hpg mice, respectively, provides a natural bioassay for any gonadal steroid production elicited by experimental manipulation of the animals.

Transplantation in the hpg Mouse

Thus, the hpg mouse is an animal model that lends itself to a study of the effects of transplanting hypothalamic tissue containing normal GnRH neurons into the brain. The functional effects of such transplants may be usefully monitored at several different levels. The surviving GnRH neurons may be readily detected by immunostaining; the effects of such grafts on the pituitary can be detected by radioimmunoassay of hormone content, by the analysis of hormone-specific mRNA levels, and by changes in the gland ultrastructure; the action of these pituitary hormones on the gonads may also be followed in terms of organ weight, structure, steroid production, and gene expression.

The first study in which normal fetal hypothalamic preoptic area (POA) tissue was transplanted into the third ventricles of hpg mice was that of Krieger et al. (39), and the functional consequences of such grafts were remarkable. Complete reversal of the hypogonadism of mutant male hpg mice was observed, with increased pituitary LH and FSH synthesis and secretion and the stimulation of all stages of spermatogenesis in the seminiferous epithelium within 2 months of grafting. Dramatic increases in testicular weight occurred, although normal adult levels were not achieved. Pituitary GnRH receptor and testicular LH receptor levels have also been restored to the normal range after transplantation (85). Not every male in which the testicular weight had increased displayed evidence of seminal vesicle growth, which indicated that, in some animals, the testes had been stimulated to produce sufficient steroid only for local intragonadal activity, but not necessarily enough for export (85). Where positive physiologic results were obtained, there was always evidence of a graft within the third ventricle, and GnRH-immunopositive cell bodies were detected with fibers specifically directed toward the median eminence to abut on pituitary portal vessels. This suggests that, even in the adult mutant, the median eminence seems to maintain mechanisms that can attract GnRH axons in a specific manner. Fiber outgrowth appeared to follow the normal pattern, with a greater concentration noted in the lateral sulci of the median eminence (23).

In female hpg mice, POA transplants restored pituitary and ovarian function, and evidence of uterine stimulation was noted (23,85). However, such grafted female mice failed to demonstrate normal estrus cyclic activity and did not ovulate. Histologic analysis of the ovaries revealed numerous ripe follicles, and vaginal smears indicated prolonged periods of estrus. The production of gonadal steroids in the grafted females stimulated female sexual behavior, and many of them mated with normal male mice. (Grafted male hpg mice fail to demonstrate sexual behavior because of the absolute requirement for early neonatal androgen stimulation of the gonads.) A most remarkable result in this study was that a significant proportion of the grafted female hpg mice became pregnant (23). The reflex release of pituitary LH has been subsequently demonstrated in such mated female hpg mice bearing POA grafts (24).

Regulation of Preoptic Area Graft Function

The failure to initiate spontaneous estrus cycles in grafted female hpg mice and, therefore, the absence of spontaneous GnRH surges every 4 to 5 days indicates that the grafts have not become completely integrated with the host structures. Nevertheless, Gibson et al. (26) have demonstrated that frequently pituitary LH is released in a pulsatile fashion. The precise location of such a putative pulse generator remains unknown, but several possibilities suggest themselves. It could be that such pulsatility is an inherent property of the grafted neurons themselves, and there is now some evidence in support of this idea from the analysis of immortalized GnRH neurons in culture, which exhibit release of GnRH in a pulsatile manner (48). Alternatively, pulsatility may be transduced from a host pulse generator at the level of the median eminence. In a recent report, pulsatile LH secretion in the rat was impaired following posteroanterior hypothalamic deafferentation (54). Subsequent transplantation of fetal mediobasal hypothalamus, lacking GnRH neurons, restored some pulsatile secretory activity, which suggests that pulsatile GnRH secretion can be modulated by this region. Finally, it may be that pulsatility is due to the innervation of donor GnRH cells by host axons. This last suggestion would appear to be the least probable, since little interchange of axons between host and graft across the third ventricular wall has been demonstrated (33). These physiologic results suggest that, although hypothalamic POA grafts can survive and release GnRH, usually neurons within the graft are not capable of transducing much of the information that would normally impinge on GnRH neurons within the preoptic area of normal mice. The failure of the peripheral administration of the excitatory amino acid *N*-methyl-D-aspartic acid (NMDA) to stimulate LH secretion in POA-grafted male hpg mice, in contrast with normal mice, supports this idea (61). Indeed, subsequent studies using the expression of Fos protein as an index of NMDA stimulation suggest that NMDA does not activate GnRH neurons directly (62).

In an extension of the above physiologic studies, the hpg mouse has been of value in analyzing the possible sites of negative-feedback of gonadal steroids on LH and FSH synthesis and secretion. In normal male mice, subcutaneous implants of testosterone cause a massive reduction in pituitary LH and FSH content. If the site of steroid feedback were primarily at the level of the pituitary gland, then testosterone implants in hpg mice would prevent the synthesis of gonadotropic hormones stimulated by GnRH injections. In fact, such injections increase pituitary gonadotropic hormone content in both untreated and testosterone-treated hpg male mice, which indicates that a major site of negative-feedback is above the level of the gonadotroph (12). In male hpg POA-grafted mice, a drastic reduction in LH and FSH synthesis would be expected following testosterone treatment, should such feedback act directly on GnRH neurons within the grafted. However, subcutaneous testosterone pellets had no effect on the graft-induced increase in gonadotropic hormone synthesis, suggesting that the site of negative-feedback may reside in other neurons that normally interact with GnRH cells in the preoptic area. It would thus appear that dissection of the graft tissue and its subsequent transplantation disrupts the innervation essential for normal negative-feedback (13,14). The situation in female mice appears to be more equivocal. Some investigators have failed to find evidence of negative-feedback in estrogen-treated mice with POA grafts (25), whereas others have dem-

onstrated a consistent negative-feedback effect on pituitary LH content and LHβ mRNA levels (66). In the latter report, the authors have argued that the negative-feedback effect might be exerted on cografted estrogen-sensitive neurons or on steroid-sensitive neurons normally projecting to the median eminence.

Mechanisms of Action of Gonadotropin-Releasing Hormone Grafts

The mechanism by which such third ventricular POA grafts exert their functional effects in hpg mice has been the subject of considerable study. It might be considered that the grafts simply act as minipumps within the third ventricle, releasing GnRH into the ventricular compartment and into the brain. However, when POA tissue has been transplanted into the lateral ventricle, the survival of GnRH neurons has been noted, but axonal outgrowth toward the median eminence was not observed, and there was no restoration of pituitary and gonadal function. When third ventricular POA grafts have stimulated reproductive activity, axon terminals have always innervated the median eminence. Indeed, greater than 95% of GnRH-immunopositive fibers exiting from the graft have terminated close to pituitary portal vessels (69). Although such fibers are often observed to course through the arcuate nucleus en route to the median eminence, the guidance of GnRH axons has been found not to depend on the presence of neurons within the arcuate nucleus. Thus, in hpg mice in which neurons of the arcuate nucleus have been destroyed by neonatal injections of the excitatory neurotoxin monosodium glutamate, GnRH axons are still found to specifically innervate the median eminence (72).

Thus, the question arises as to what factors may determine the specificity of outgrowth of GnRH fibers to the basal hypothalamus. In studies using the fluorescent retrograde tracer fluorogold, very few non-

GnRH graft cells capture the tracer. Thus, axons that project to the median eminence and, therefore, are outside the blood–brain barrier, would seem to be GnRH-specific (71). Indeed, studies using the carbocyanine dye DiI suggest that non-GnRH total efferent outgrowth is very restricted (74). The gliosis that occurs following POA transplantation and the possible permissive nature of this glial environment on the outgrowth of GnRH axons has been studied (73). The GnRH axons at the graft–host interface appeared to be confined to glial channels and, thus, glia may indeed have growth-promoting effects on GnRH neurons. Nevertheless, reactive glia were not restricted to the area of GnRH outgrowth, which suggested that other cues must be present to guide the orientation of GnRH growth cones.

The GnRH axons terminate precisely where the portal vessels leading from the hypothalamus to the pituitary gland are found and, in intimate association with these vessels, is the pars tuberalis of the pituitary gland. Also, the GnRH axons from the preoptic area grow toward anterior pituitary tissue when slice preparations of GnRH neurons are cocultured with pituitary tissue (81). However, arguing against such in vitro observations are the findings of Daikoku et al. (17), suggesting that when pituitary and POA are cografted to the third ventricle, the GnRH axons tend to enclose the pituitary grafts, rather than infiltrate between cells. Furthermore, our own observations of anterior pituitary and POA cografts placed in the lateral ventricle of hpg mice have indicated that, even after 9 months, there is no evidence of a robust innervation of the anterior pituitary tissue (H. M. Charlton and M. J. Wood, unpublished, 1991). For the stimulation of pituitary function by GnRH neurons to occur, only the innervation of fenestrated capillaries reaching the glandular tissue would necessarily be required. Daikoku et al. (17) have claimed that when POA tissue was grafted with medial basal hypothalamic tissue, median eminence-like structures could be visualized within the grafts, and GnRH axons terminated on these structures. However, their analysis did not extend to electron microscopy to determine whether the blood vessels associated with these structures were indeed fenestrated. A.-J. Silverman and M. J. Gibson (personal communication) have found that exuberant outgrowth of GnRH axons toward the median eminence occurs, even in hypophysectomized hpg mice, which further argues against a major role for the pituitary gland in guidance mechanisms. In the study of Daikoku et al. and that of Silverman and Gibson, the pars tuberalis of the pituitary gland is likely to have been adherent to the median eminence. Nevertheless, GnRH axons also innervate the organum vasculosum of the lamina terminalis and the subfornical organ, and at both of these sites, there is no adjacent pituitary tissue. The regrowth of damaged neurosecretory axons toward fenestrated vessels of implanted peripheral tissues has recently been described (37). Three different types of tissue containing fenestrated capillaries—pineal, adrenal medulla, and pituitary neural lobe—were grafted to the retrochiasmatic region of the hypothalamus, and the degree of innervation of these tissues by regenerating neurosecretory nerve terminals was determined. However, no obvious specificity of innervation of the neural lobe compared with pineal gland and adrenal medulla was noted. It may thus be that fenestrated vessels themselves possess neurotrophic properties.

During neural development, GnRH neurons are generated in the olfactory placode and, from there, migrate to the anterior hypothalamus before the extension of axons to the median eminence (64). This cell migration is highly specific and is defective in patients with Kallmann's syndrome, such patients being characterized by hypogonadism and anosmia as a consequence. It has recently been determined that a gene deleted in the X-linked form of Kallmann's syndrome shares homology with neural cell adhesion molecules (21), suggesting that such molecules are essential to the process of GnRH neuron migration during development. The in situ hybridization studies of Mason et al. (46) suggest that GnRH cell bodies are found within preoptic area in hpg mice, indicating that this migration is not dependent on successful expression of the GnRH gene. Whatever the guidance cues are for the journey from the olfactory placode to the final neuroanatomic site during embryogenesis, would such cells from normal fetal olfactory placode be capable of migrating into the hpg POA? It might be expected that there exists some temporal program for fetal GnRH cell bodies that first dictates the migration pattern of cells to the POA and, later, controls axonal guidance to the median eminence. In recent experiments, grafts derived from embryonic nasal septum have been transplanted to sites within the hpg brain (43). Despite the few animals examined, the neurons did show the capacity to differentiate, migrate, and innervate appropriate host structures in the adult hpg brain, and in few animals testicular stimulation was evident.

Functional Preoptic Area Xenografts in hpg Mice

An interesting extension of the transplant work in the field of guidance mechanisms has come from experiments in which monoclonal antibody (MAb) blockade of T-lymphocyte activation has allowed us to graft rat POA into the hpg mouse, with the result that indefinite graft survival is obtained. It has long been recognized that allograft rejection is especially dependent on thymus-derived T lymphocytes (4). More recently, two major subsets of T lymphocytes have been defined, according to function and surface antigen characteristics, namely, helper or $CD4^+$ T cells and cytotoxic T cells, which bear the CD8 antigen. By making use of monoclonal antibodies against the CD4 and CD8 antigens we have been able to obtain specific subset depletion and, thereby, to investigate the respective roles of these particular T-lymphocyte subsets in the rejection of neural xenografts.

It has emerged that the $CD4^+$ T-cell subset is critically important for the immune response to neural xenoantigens to proceed successfully, and profound depletion of these cells, using the anti-CD4 monoclonal antibody YTA 3.1, has allowed us to obtain the indefinite survival of rat xenografts implanted into the mouse striatum (80). Early results in male hpg mice, using a different anti-CD4 monoclonal antibody (YTS 191.1) from that used in the previous study (YTA 3.1), suggested that $CD4^+$ T-cell depletion could prolong the survival of rat POA xenografts for up to 30 days, with accompanying evidence of detectable GnRH-immunopositive fibers and an increase in paired testicular weight (34). However, by 60 days, GnRH immunoreactivity had decreased, and the paired testicular weight had declined to approach hpg values. In preliminary experiments, we have now shown that a decline in detectable pituitary mRNA levels for the common α-subunit, LHβ, and FSHβ genes is a sensitive, early index of graft failure in such cases. Subsequent work involving manipulations of the monoclonal antibody dosage and administration regimens and using combinations of anti-CD4 (YTA 3.1) and anti-CD8 antibodies has allowed rat POA xenografts to survive and function in the hpg mouse third ventricle, with steadily increasing testicular weight (Table 1), for in excess of 110 days (M. J. A. Wood et al., in preparation). Of particular interest in these studies is, first, the small number of GnRH-immunopositive neurons that are consistently required to provide functional compensation in the mutant, often only between 5 and 15 being detectable. Second, the rat GnRH axons, as with mouse fibers, have been found, to specifically innervate the median eminence, with the greatest concentration of fibers once again detectable at the lateral sul-

TABLE 1. *Preoptic area xenograft function in male hypogonadal mice*

Experiment[a]	Day[b]	Testis weight[c] (mg ± SEM)
Mouse POA allograft	30	53.7 ± 11.7
Untreated	110	112.1 ± 12.1
Rat POA xenograft	30	6.1 ± 0.3
Untreated	110	5.9 ± 0.8
Rat POA xenograft	30	49.6 ± 4.9
Anti-CD4 MAb treatment (YTA 3.1), low-dose	110	12.1 ± 3.2
Rat POA xenograft	30	53.4 ± 8.4
Anti-CD4 MAb treatment (YTA 3.1), high-dose	110	77.4 ± 9.2

[a]Male hpg mice received rat or control mouse preoptic area (POA) grafts on day 1. Animals were untreated or treated with low- or high-dose YTA 3.1 anti-CD4 monoclonal antibody (MAb) therapy.

[b]Animals were analyzed on day 30 or day 110 after transplantation.

[c]The mean paired testis weight (± standard error of the mean; SEM) was measured as an index of graft function.

cus. Thus, whatever the guidance cues are for GnRH axon extension to the median eminence, they are sufficiently homologous between the two species to allow precise outgrowth of fibers from rat xenografts.

Transplantation of Gonadotropin-Releasing Hormone Cell Lines

A particularly promising recent development, with much potential for transplantation studies in the GnRH-deficient hpg mouse, has been the production of immortalized GnRH neuronal cell lines (48,57). In the studies reported by Mellon et al. (48), the potent SV-40 T-antigen oncogene was specifically targeted to hypothalamic GnRH neurons in transgenic mice, using the rat GnRH promoter. This resulted in the production of specific tumors of GnRH-secreting neurons and, from one of these, which was located in the anterior hypothalamus, was derived the immortalized cell line GT1. A similar approach was used by Radovick et al. (57), who used the human GnRH pro-

moter. These studies are of importance not only because they constitute an experimental model for the study of neuroendocrine regulation, but also because the derivation of these cell lines has demonstrated the feasibility of immortalizing differentiated neurons by targeting tumorigenesis in transgenic mice to specific neurons of the CNS.

The properties of immortalized GnRH neurons have now been extensively characterized in vitro. These cells have many neuronal properties; they extend neurites in culture that end in growth cones or contact distant cells; they have fast Na^+ channels that can be regulated in neurons; and they express neuronal, but not glial, cell markers. In addition, many properties characteristic of differentiated GnRH cells are displayed by the immortalized cells. The endogenous mouse GnRH mRNA is expressed, and the cells immunostain for GnRH and GnRH-associated peptide and, furthermore, they release GnRH in response to depolarization (48). At the ultrastructural level, the GT1 cells have the distinct characteristics of neurosecretory neurons, with prominent Golgi apparatus, rough endoplasmic reticulum, and evidence of mature neurosecretory granules. Subsequent studies have found that GnRH release by these immortalized cells in culture is pulsatile and, thus, as alluded to previously, it seems that inherent pulsatility may exist within GnRH neurons (79). Interestingly, this pattern of secretion by the immortalized cells in culture may have a morphologic basis, in that it appears that the GT1 cells establish numerous synapse-like connections among themselves as well as showing biochemical evidence of coupling.

The hpg mouse represents a highly sensitive assay system for the presence of GnRH and, thus, constitutes an ideal model system in which to test the capacity of immortalized GnRH cell lines to provide functional compensation in vivo. This question has recently been examined by Silverman et al. (70), who used the GT1 cell line and, in this work, intraparenchymal implants of varying numbers of cells were made at the border of the anterior hypothalamus and the ventromedial nucleus. The results of these experiments have indicated that implanted immortalized GnRH cells are capable of sufficient differentiation in the hpg brain to stimulate testicular growth; however, neither the proportion of animals exhibiting growth nor the degree of spermatogenesis observed was high. There was no evidence that the migration of GnRH cells or their axonal outgrowth was specifically directed toward normal sites and targets; nevertheless, the greatest gonadal growth was noted in those mutants in which axons were found in the median eminence region. A particular, but not unexpected, problem encountered in these experiments was the observation of tumor formation. In the original transgenic lines (48), the gonads and accessory sex organs were underdeveloped, and all mice were infertile. This suggested the possibility that the expression of the transgene interfered with sexual maturation and, even in those mice bearing anterior hypothalamic tumors, the specific extension of axons to the median eminence was not observed. Therefore, it would seem that for these cell lines to fulfill their obvious potential for in vivo studies, the problem of tumor formation will need to be addressed and successfully circumvented.

THE SUPRACHIASMATIC NUCLEUS

The suprachiasmatic nucleus (SCN) receives afferent inputs conveying environmental information that allows the animal to synchronize a variety of diurnal events, including neuroendocrine control mechanisms, with the dark–light cycle. The SCN is thus thought to be central to the organization of endogenous rhythms in mammals (47). Destruction of the SCN abolishes circadian rhythms in locomotor activity, drinking, sleeping, photoperiodic response, and endocrine function (9). Recently, several reports have addressed the potential of neural transplantation to compensate for defects in endogenous rhythms (59). Although this subject is reviewed in detail in Chapter 19, the model systems used and the challenging questions in this area are briefly reviewed here, in particular, as they relate to hypothalamic transplantation and neuroendocrine mechanisms in general.

The question of whether the SCN is the master oscillator that drives endogenous rhythms and what cellular components of this nucleus possess such properties is obviously of great importance. In a model system in which the SCN has been electrolytically lesioned, the subsequent effects of transplantation of fetal SCN on circadian activity may be difficult to discern from the possible trophic effects of the transplant, as has been noted in the earlier discussion concerning animal models of diabetes insipidus. An alternative model system in which to specifically address this question is the *tau* mutant hamster. Although the precise genetic defect of this mutant is unknown, the physiologic effect of the mutation is to set the endogenous circadian clock of the homozygote to about 20 hours. The SCN tissue from the mutant strain was grafted into normal hamsters in which the SCN had been ablated and that were, therefore, arrhythmic (58). These animals were placed on running wheels after the operation, and in 80% of the arrhythmic hosts a circadian running pattern was generated, typical of the donor tissue. This use of mutant and normal strains has demonstrated conclusively that the endogenous rhythm of the SCN is maintained in the transplants, and that the host is driven by the donor tissue.

In several reports the transplantation of fetal SCN into lesioned animals has resulted in the restoration of circadian patterns of running activity (59). However, in these grafted animals the restored locomotor rhythms did not become synchronized with light–dark cycles, suggesting that the

SCN tissue had not become fully integrated with the hosts normal afferent inputs. Thus, the questions of how such grafts produce their functional effects and to what extent specific connections with host centers are essential to this process remain to be answered. There is evidence that such transplants demonstrate limited graft–host connectivity (9). In these studies, SCN transplants developed the morphologic and functional (in terms of electrical activity and glucose utilization) features characteristic of normal SCN (2). Thus, transplants with no recognizable neural connections with the host may still elicit a circadian response, which argues for some communication mechanism based on a humoral route. This stands in contrast to much of the evidence discussed for the hpg mouse. The use of dissociated and cultured SCN cells for transplantation, which has now been established (59), with the associated possibilities of cellular enrichment, depletion, or genetic manipulation, will undoubtedly offer approaches for defining the mechanisms of SCN graft function and host interaction more precisely.

THE PINEAL GLAND

The mammalian pineal gland has evolved in function during phylogenetic development from that of a photoendocrine to that of a neuroendocrine organ (55), with its basic biochemical function being the synthesis of melatonin from serotonin with a diurnal rhythm (60). The gland receives a rich innervation of sympathetic catecholaminergic nerve fibers from the superior cervical ganglion (51). The use of transplantation techniques has enabled questions concerning pineal differentiation and the development of glandular innervation to be addressed. In addition, the analysis of pineal physiology in functional transplantation models is becoming productive and of interest.

In recent years, studies have reported the transplantation of pineal tissue to many different sites, including the anterior chamber of the eye, beneath the renal capsule, into the cerebral ventricular spaces, and into the cerebral cortex (40). Nonaka et al. (52) have transplanted pineal tissue to the cerebral cortex or cerebral interhemispheric fissure and have addressed the question of pinealocyte differentiation in a foreign environment in vivo. Pineal gland differentiation was judged to have proceeded normally in such grafts by the expression of high levels of serotonin for up to 6 months after transplantation. However, the extension of neurites by these cells, often noted previously in culture (3), was not observed. This has suggested that neurite extension may be a pinealocyte property that is actively suppressed in the intact organ. Tyrosine hydroxylase-immunopositive fibers innervated only the periphery of the pineal tissue at the cortical site, but dense innervation of interhemispheric grafts was noted, and these fibers often accompanied blood vessels, suggesting that they were derived from sympathetic ganglia. However, the possible effects of this apparently specific innervation on diurnal rhythms of melatonin synthesis were not determined.

Early work by Moore in 1975 (49), in which pineal glands were transplanted into the anterior chamber of the eye, demonstrated a dense innervation of such grafts by sympathetic fibers of the iris. In addition, day–night rhythms in N-acetyltransferase activity and, therefore, presumably in melatonin synthesis, were restored to the transplanted tissue. In more recent studies, questions concerning the postnatal development and specificity of pineal innervation have been addressed. The pineal glands of hamsters are innervated by a dense mesh of tyrosine hydroxylase (TH)- and neuropeptide Y (NPY)-immunopositive fibers by the seventh postnatal day of development (40). However, in the same study, neonatal pineal grafts placed at various locations within the hamster third ventricle survived and integrated well into their new locations, but TH or NPY fibers seldom entered the graft parenchyma, despite their observed abundance adjacent to the transplants. Such grafts exhibited levels of S-antigen (a protein characteristic of retinal photoreceptors) and glial fibrillary acidic protein expression, comparable with normal pineal tissue, suggesting that normal development had occurred (41). These results suggested the possibility that pineal tissue may have attractive properties only for fibers originating in peripheral sympathetic ganglia. In attempts to refine this hypothesis, an investigation of the innervation of pineal tissue transplanted beneath the renal capsule was undertaken; however, this produced equivocal results. Thus, although it seems that pineal catecholaminergic innervation must derive from the sympathetic ganglia, whether such fibers need to be of superior cervical ganglion origin remains unresolved (40).

For an assessment of pineal graft function, an animal model in which rats have been pinealectomized before grafting into the third ventricle has been employed (82). Physiologic function was monitored with measurements of serum melatonin levels, which were noted to have decreased in pinealectomized animals. In almost 50% of grafted rats, melatonin levels had significantly increased within 6 weeks of transplantation, and this was accompanied by evidence of graft vascularization, with fenestrated vessels and ultrastructural observations of pinealocyte secretory activity. Furthermore, this functional recovery in pinealectomized animals was correlated with innervation by TH-positive fibers that appeared to originate from the median eminence. However, whether these fibers innervated the graft core was unclear. Subsequent work, however, has failed to demonstrate circadian day–night rhythms of melatonin secretion by such transplants (83), suggesting that functional integration

with the appropriate hypothalamic centers has not been achieved.

MISCELLANEOUS HYPOTHALAMIC TRANSPLANTATION

Very few neural transplantation studies have yet addressed the growth hormone axis, which is surprising, because of the number of animals exhibiting genetic lesions of this system. However, few of these mutants would appear to be amenable to functional repair with neural grafts. Growth hormone-releasing factor (GRF) immunoreactive neurons are located in the arcuate nucleus of the hypothalamus and are central to the regulation of growth hormone (GH) secretion by the pituitary gland (15). An alternative approach to create an adequate animal model of growth hormone deficiency has thus been to use the excitatory neurotoxin monosodium glutamate to ablate the arcuate nucleus. Despite the lack of specificity of such lesions, animals treated in this way demonstrate a marked reduction in GRF immunoreactivity in the arcuate nucleus and median eminence, reduced pituitary GH secretion, and growth retardation (5). A recent study (8), has used such a model in which to evaluate the structure of GRF-positive neuronal transplants. In these experiments, grafts located in close proximity to the host median eminence survived and demonstrated numerous GRF-immunopositive terminals at the median eminence. This suggests that such transplants may indeed provide functional compensation, although this remains to be demonstrated.

A second area of developing interest is that concerning the transplantation of hypothalamic histaminergic neurons. There is evidence to suggest that histamine is synthesized in the posterior hypothalamus and that axons originating in this center project widely to different areas of the brain (27). Such observations suggest that histamine may function as a neurotransmitter and influence diverse functions in the nervous system. Thus, recent work has sought to use the intraocular transplantation technique, used successfully to study the properties of monoaminergic neurons, to evaluate the developmental characteristics of hypothalamic histaminergic neurons (27). In this study, such grafts survived the transplantation procedure well, but innervation of the iris was notably less dense than commonly found with other monoaminergic neurons. Of particular interest, however, was the dense histaminergic innervation of cografted hippocampal tissue. Thus, such a transplantation strategy would appear to offer an in vivo approach for studying the interactions between hypothalamic neurons and their extrahypothalamic target regions.

A final area of potential importance concerns the role of the hypothalamus in the pathogenesis of genetic hypertension. Although the precise genetic lesion in the spontaneously hypertensive rat (SHR) is uncharacterized, it is thought that the defect manifests itself primarily in the hypothalamus (50). In such animals, the levels of vasoactive intestinal polypeptide (VIP) mRNA in the SCN have been noted to be increased, whereas hypothalamic vasopressin levels are commonly reduced. In an interesting report Eilam et al. (19) have demonstrated the induction and maintenance of hypertension in normal normotensive rats grafted with fetal hypothalamic tissue from SHR. These results thus support the hypothesis that the hypothalamus is the primary site involved in generating spontaneous hypertension in mammals, and offer an interesting model to further dissect the cellular mechanisms underlying the pathophysiology of this condition.

CONCLUSIONS AND FUTURE PERSPECTIVES

Natural mutations, rather than drug or experimentally induced lesions, provide precise animal model systems in many fields of study. The hpg mouse is an example of such a precise genetic defect and, as a consequence, this model has become a useful tool for the neurobiologist. The capacity to generate specific transgenic animals to study functional aspects of neuroendocrine systems will undoubtedly be of importance in the future. Provided the gene of interest is a single copy, then the approach of homologous recombination will allow the insertion of defined mutant DNA into the original site (10). Furthermore, with such a strategy, investigation of the temporal and spatial regulation of gene expression is possible with the site-directed mutagenesis of the associated regulatory elements.

The generation of immortalized GnRH neurons now offers the prospect that many other differentiated neuronal cell lines will be created by similar approaches. This will obviously have important implications for the transplantation neurobiologist, in addition to which the possibility of genetically manipulating any established cell line exists. For such cell lines to be of maximum benefit for in vivo studies, their potential for tumor formation will need to be reduced. There are a number of strategies by which this may be achieved. The use of antimitotic agents, although likely to be effective, may have benefits of only short duration. Alternatively, the use of antisense oligonucleotides to hybridize with, and block the function of, the oncogenic mRNA may be more rewarding. However, recently the catalytic potential of RNA itself has begun to be explored (16). Such RNA molecules, or ribozymes, can be modified to target certain RNA species, catalyze their cleavage and, thereby, regulate the expression of specific genes. Moreover, the introduction of genes for such ribozymes into cells, to precisely target their activity, may be a feasible prospect.

By using these approaches, more precise animal models should be generated, and genetically defined neuronal cell populations will become available for transplantation studies. This, in turn, should enable more specific questions concerning neural graft function to be asked.

ACKNOWLEDGMENTS

We would like to acknowledge the collaboration of all those colleagues cited in joint publications and the financial assistance from The Wellcome Trust, The Medical Research Council, The International Spinal Research Trust, and The Beit Trust.

REFERENCES

1. Adelman JP, Mason AJ, Hayflick JS, Seeburg PS. Isolation of the gene and hypothalamic cDNA for the common precursor of GnRH and prolactin release inhibiting factor in human and rat. *Proc Natl Acad Sci USA* 1986;83:179–183.
2. Aguilar-Roblero R, Shibata S, Speh JC, Drucker-Colin R, Moore RY. Morphological and functional development of the suprachiasmatic nucleus in transplanted foetal hypothalamus. *Brain Res* 1992;580:288–296.
3. Araki M, Watanabe K, Tokunaga F, Nonaka T. Phenotypic expression of photoreceptor and endocrine cell properties by cultured pineal cells of the newborn rat. *Cell Differ Dev* 1988;25:155–164.
4. Billingham RE, Brent L, Medawar PB. Quantitative studies on tissue transplantation. *Proc R Soc Lond* 1954;143:58–80.
5. Bloch B, Ling N, Benoit R, Guillemin R. Specific depletion of immunoreactive growth hormone releasing factor by monosodium glutamate in rat median eminence. *Nature* 1984;307:272–273.
6. Boer GJ, Schluter N, Gash DM. A procedure for small volume brain grafting vasopressin cells in neonatal and adult Brattleboro rats. *J Neurosci Methods* 1984;11:39–46.
7. Boer GJ, Gash DM, Dick L, Schluter N. Vasopressin neuron survival in neonatal Brattleboro rats. *Neuroscience* 1985;15:1087–1109.
8. Bruhn TO, Tresco PA, Jackson IMD. Transplantation of fetal growth hormone-releasing factor-immunoreactive neurons into the ventricular system of adult MSG-treated rats. *Peptides* 1991;12:957–961.
9. Canbeyli RS, Lehman M, Silver R. Tracing SCN afferents with DiI. *Brain Res* 1991;554:15–21.
10. Cappechi MR. The new mouse genetics: altering the genome by gene targeting. *Trends Genet* 1989;5:70–76.
11. Cattanach BM, Iddon CA, Charlton HM, Chiappa SA, Fink G. Gonadotropin-releasing hormone deficiency in a mutant mouse with hypogonadism. *Nature* 1977;269:338–340.
12. Charlton HM, Halpin DMG, Iddon C, et al. The effects of daily administration of single and multiple injections of gonadotrophin-releasing hormone on pituitary and gonadal function in the hypogonadal (hpg) mouse. *Endocrinology* 1983; 113:535–544.
13. Charlton HM, Jones AJ, Ward BJ, Detta A, Clayton RN. The effects of castration or testosterone upon pituitary function in hypogonadal (hpg) mice bearing normal foetal preoptic area (POA) grafts. *Neuroendocrinology* 1987;45:376–380.
14. Charlton HM, Porter Goff AE, Cox BS, et al. The hypogonadal mouse: a model for brain–pituitary–gonadal interactions. In: Imura H, Shizume K, Yoshida S, eds. *Progress in endocrinology.* Amsterdam: Excerpta Medica; 1988: 525–530.
15. Clark RG, Robinson ICAF. Growth induced by pulsatile infusion of an amidated fragment of human growth hormone releasing factor in normal and GHRF–deficient rats. *Nature* 1985;314:281–283.
16. Cotten M. The in vivo application of ribozymes. *Trends Biotechnol* 1990;8:174–178.
17. Daikoku Ishido H, Okamura Y, Yanaihara N, Daikoku S. Development of the hypothalamic luteinising hormone-releasing hormone containing neurone system in the rat. In vivo and in transplantation studies. *Dev Biol* 1990;140;374–387.
18. DePaulo LV, Bald LN, Fendly BM. Passive immunoneutralisation with a monoclonal antibody reveals a role for endogenous activin-B in mediating FSH hypersecretion. *Endocrinology* 1992; 130:1741–1743.
19. Eilam R, Malach R, Bergman F, Segal M. Hypertension induced by hypothalamic transplantation from genetically hypertensive to normotensive rats. *J Neurosci* 1991;11:401–411.
20. Fink G, Sheward WJ, Plant TM. The hypogonadal mouse pituitary contains bioactive LH. *J Reprod Fertil* 1984;70:277–280.
21. Franco B, Guioli S, Ballabio A, et al. A gene deleted in Kallmann's syndrome shares homology with neural cell adhesion and axonal pathfinding molecules. *Nature* 1991;353:529–536.
22. Gash DM, Sladek JR Jr, Sladek CD. Functional development of grafted vasopressin neurons. *Science* 1980;210:1367–1369.
23. Gibson MJ, Krieger DT, Charlton HM, Zimmerman EA, Silverman AJ, Perlow MJ. Mating and pregnancy can occur in genetically hypogonadal mice with preoptic area brain grafts. *Science* 1984;225:949–951.
24. Gibson MJ, Moscovitz HC, Kokoris GJ, Silverman AJ. Plasma LH rises rapidly following mating in hypogonadal female mice with preoptic area (POA) brain grafts. *Brain Res* 1987;424:133–137.
25. Gibson MJ, Silverman A-J. Effects of gonadectomy and treatment with gonadal steroids of lu-

teinising hormone secretion in hypogonadal mice. *Endocrinology* 1989;125:1525–1532.

26. Gibson MJ, Miller GM, Silverman AJ. Pulsatile luteinizing hormone secretion in normal female mice and in hypogonadal female mice with preoptic area implants. *Endocrinology* 1991; 128:965–971.

27. Granholm A-C, Bergman H, Blomqvist A. Intra-ocular hypothalamic transplants containing his-taminergic neurons. *Exp Neurol* 1990;108:189–197.

28. Halasz B, Pupp L, Uhlarik S. Hypophysi-otrophic area in the hypothalamus. *J Endocrinol* 1962;25:147–159.

29. Halasz B, Pupp L, Uhlarik S, Tima L. Growth of hypophysectomised rats bearing pituitary transplants in the hypothalamus. *Acta Physiol Acad Sci Hung* 1963;23:287–292.

30. Halasz B, Pupp L, Uhlarik S, Tima L. Further studies on the hormone secretion of the ante-rior pituitary transplanted into the hypophysi-otrophic area of the rat hypothalamus. *Endocri-nology* 1965;77:343–353.

31. Harris GW. Humors and hormones. *J Endocri-nol* 1972;53:2–23.

32. Herman JP, Marciano FF, Wiegand SJ, Gash DM. Selective cell death of magnocellular va-sopressin neurons in neurohypophysectomised rats following chronic administration of vaso-pressin. *J Neurosci* 1987;7:2564–2575.

33. Hodjkiss JP, Kelly JS. An intracellular study of grafted and in situ preoptic area neurones in brain slices from normal and hypogonadal mice. *J Physiol* 1990;423:111–135.

34. Honey CR, Charlton HM, Wood KJ. Rat brain xenografts reverse hypogonadism in mice im-munosuppressed with anti-CD4 monoclonal an-tibody. *Exp Brain Res* 1991;85:149–152.

35. Iddon CA, Charlton HM, Fink G. Gonadotro-phin release in hypogonadal mice. *J Endocrinol* 1980;85:105–110.

36. Ivell R, Burbach PH, Van Leeuwen FW. The molecular biology of the Brattleboro rat. *Front Neuroendocrinol* 1990;11:313–338.

37. Kadota Y, Pettigrew K, Brightman MW. Re-growth of damaged neurosecretory axons to fen-estrated vessels of implanted peripheral tissues. *Synapse* 1990;5:175–189.

38. Knigge KM. Gonadotrophic action of neonatal pituitary glands implanted in the rat brain. *Am J Physiol* 1962;202:387–391.

39. Krieger DT, Perlow MJ, Gibson MJ, et al. Brain grafts reverse hypogonadism of gonadotrophin releasing hormone deficiency. *Nature* 1982; 298:468–471.

40. Li K, Welsh MG. Tyrosine hydroxylase and neu-ropeptide Y immunoreactivity in pineal glands developing in situ and in pineal grafts. *Cell Tis-sue Res* 1991;264:515–527.

41. Li K, Welsh MG. S-antigen and glial fibrillary acidic protein immunoreactivity in the in situ pineal gland and in pineal grafts. *Am J Anat* 1991;92:510–522.

42. Lim ATW, Lolait SJ, Barlow JW, Funder JW.

Immunoreactive arginine vasopressin in Brattle-boro rat ovary. *Nature* 1984;310:61–64.

43. Livne I, Gibson MJ, Silverman A-J. Brain grafts of migratory GnRH cells induce gonadal recov-ery in hypogonadal mice. *Dev Brain Res* 1992; 69:117–123.

44. McDowell IFW, Morris JF, Charlton HM. Char-acterisation of the pituitary gonadotroph cells of hypogonadal male mice. *J Endocrinol* 1982; 95:321–330.

45. Marciano FF, Wiegand SJ, Sladek JR, Gash DM. Fetal hypothalamic transplants promote survival and functional regeneration of axotomised adult supraoptic magnocellular neurons. *Brain Res* 1989;483:135–142.

46. Mason AJ, Hayflick JS, Zoeller RT, et al. A deletion truncating the gonadotropin-releasing hormone gene is responsible for hypogonadism in the hpg mouse. *Science* 1986;234:1366–1371.

47. Meijer JH, Rietveld WJ. Neurophysiology of the suprachiasmatic circadian pacemaker in ro-dents. *Physiol Rev* 1989;69:671–707.

48. Mellon PL, Windle JL, Goldsmith PC, Padula CA, Roberts JL, Weiner RI. Immortalisation of hypothalamic GnRH neurons by genetically tar-geted tumourigenesis. *Neuron* 1990;5:1–10.

49. Moore RY. Pineal transplants to the anterior chamber of the eye: evidence for functional rein-nervation. *Exp Neurol* 1975;49:617–621.

50. Nelson DO, Boulant JA. Altered CNS neuroan-atomical organisation of spontaneously hyper-tensive rats. *Brain Res* 1981;226:119–130.

51. Nielson JT, Moller M. Innervation of the pineal gland in the Mongolian gerbil. *Cell Tissue Res* 1978;187:235–250.

52. Nonaka T, Araki M, Kimura H, Nagatsu I, Sa-toh F, Masuzawa T. Transplantation of the rat pineal organ to the brain: pinealocyte differen-tiation and innervation. *Cell Tissue Res* 1990; 260:273–278.

53. Nussey SS, Ang VTY, Jenkins JS, Bisset GW. Brattleboro rat adrenal contains vasopressin. *Nature* 1984;310:64–66.

54. Ohkura S, Tsukamura H, Meida K-I. Effects of transplants of foetal mediobasal hypothalamus on luteinising hormone pulses. *Neuroendocri-nology* 1992;55:422–426.

55. Oksche A, Hartwig HG. Pineal sense organs—components of photoendocrine systems. *Prog Brain Res* 1979;52:113–130.

56. Palkovits M. Peptidergic neurotransmitters in the endocrine hypothalamus. In: *Functional anatomy of the neuroendocrine hypothalamus.* Chichester: John Wiley & Sons; 1992:3–15.

57. Radovick S, Wray S, Lee E, Wondisford FE. Migratory arrest of gonadotropin-releasing hor-mone neurons in transgenic mice. *Proc Natl Acad Sci USA* 1991;88:3402–3406.

58. Ralph MR, Foster RG, Davis FC, Menaker M. Transplanted suprachiasmatic nucleus deter-mines circadian period. *Science* 1990;247:975–977.

59. Ralph MR, Lehman MN. Transplantation: a new tool in the analysis of the mammalian hypotha-

lamic circadian pacemaker. *Trends Neurosci* 1991;14:362–365.

60. Reiter RJ. The mammalian pineal gland: structure and function. *Am J Anat* 1981;162:287–313.

61. Saitoh Y, Silverman A-J, Gibson MJ. Effects of NMDA on luteinising hormone secretion in normal mice and in hypogonadal mice. *Endocrinology* 1991;128:2432–2440.

62. Saitoh Y, Silverman A-J, Gibson MJ. Norepinephrine neurons in mouse locus coeruleus express c-*fos* protein after NMDA treatment: relation to LH treatment *Brain Res* 1991;561:11–19.

63. Schmale H, Richter D. Single base deletion in the vasopressin gene is the cause of diabetes insipidus in Brattleboro rats. *Nature* 1984;308: 705–709.

64. Schwanzel-Fukuda M, Pfaff DW. Origin of luteinising hormone-releasing hormone neurons. *Nature* 1989;338:161–164.

65. Scott DE, Sherman DM. Neuronal and neurovascular integration following transplantation of foetal hypothalamus into the Brattleboro rat. *Brain Res* 1984;12:453–469.

66. Scott IS, Porter Goff AE, Cox BS, Charlton HM, Clayton RN. Effect of ovariectomy or oestrogen implants upon pituitary function in female hypogonadal mice bearing normal foetal preoptic area grafts. *J Neuroendocrinol* 1991; 3:303–307.

67. Setalo G, Horvath J, Schally AV, Arimura A, Flerko B. Effect of the isolated removal of the median eminence (ME) and pituitary stalk (PS) on the immunohistology and hormone release of the anterior pituitary gland grafted into the hypophysiotrophic area (HTA) and/or of the in situ pituitary gland. *Acta Biol Acad Sci Hung* 1977;28:333–349.

68. Shechter J, Gash D, Ahmad N. Rathke's pouch grafts in adult brain sites. *Am J Anat* 1987; 178:55–64.

69. Silverman AJ, Zimmerman EA, Gibson MJ, et al. Implantation of normal fetal preoptic area into hypogonadal mutant mice: temporal relationships of the growth of gonadotropin-releasing hormone neurons and the development of the pituitary/testicular axis. *Neuroscience* 1985;16: 69–84.

70. Silverman A-J, Roberts JL, Dong K-W, Miller GM, Gibson MJ. Intrahypothalamic injection of a gonadotrophin releasing hormone cell line results in cellular differentiation and reversal of hypogonadism in mutant mice. *Proc Natl Acad Sci USA* 1992;89:10668–10672.

71. Silverman RC, Silverman A-J, Gibson MJ. Identification of GnRH neurons projecting to the median eminence from third ventricular preoptic area grafts in hypogonadal mice. *Brain Res* 1989;501:260–268.

72. Silverman R, Gibson M, Charlton HM, Silverman A-J. Are neurones of the arcuate nucleus necessary for pathfinding by GnRH fibres arising from third ventricular grafts? *Exp Neurol* 1990;109:204–213.

73. Silverman RC, Gibson MJ, Silverman A-J. Relationship of glia to GnRH axonal outgrowth from third ventricular grafts in hpg hosts. *Exp Neurol* 1991;114:259–274.

74. Silverman RC, Gibson MJ, Silverman A-J. Application of a fluorescent dye to study connectivity between third ventricular preoptic area grafts and host hypothalamus. *J Neurosci Res* 1992;31:156–165.

75. Sladek JR, Scholer J, Notter MD, Gash DM. Immunohistochemical analysis of vasopressin neurons transplanted with the Brattleboro rat. *Ann NY Acad Sci* 1982;394:102–115.

76. Swanson LW. The hypothalamus. In: Bjorklund A, Hokfelt T, Swanson LW, eds. *Handbook of chemical neuroanatomy*. Amsterdam: Elsevier; 1987:1–14.

77. Valtin H. Hereditary hypothalamic diabetes insipidus. *J Pathol* 1976;83:633–636.

78. Valtin H. The discovery of the Brattleboro rat, recommended nomenclature and the question of proper controls. *Ann NY Acad Sci* 1982;394: 1–9.

79. Wetsel WC, Valenca MM, Merchenthaler I, Liposits Z, Lopez FJ, Weiner RI, Mellon PL, Negro-Villar A. Intrinsic pulsatile secretory activity of immortalised luteinising hormone-releasing hormone-secreting neurons. *Proc Natl Acad Sci USA* 1992;89:4149–4153.

80. Wood MJA, Sloan DJ, Wood KJ, Charlton HM. The critical role of CD4$^+$ T lymphocytes in the rejection of neural xenografts *(submitted)*.

81. Wray S, Gahwiler BH, Gainer H. Slice cultures of LHRH neurones in the presence and absence of brainstem and pituitary. *Peptides* 1988;9: 1151–1175.

82. Wu W, Scott DE, Miller E. Transplantation of the pineal gland in the mammalian third cerebral ventricle. *Exp Neurol* 1990;108:23–32.

83. Wu W, Scott DE, Reiter RJ. No difference in day–night serum melatonin concentration after pineal grafting into the third cerebral ventricle of pinealectomised rodents. *J Pineal Res* 1991; 11:70–74.

84. Young LS, Speight A, Charlton HM, Clayton RN. Pituitary GnRH receptor regulation in the hypogonadal mouse. *Endocrinology* 1983;113: 55–61.

85. Young LS, Detta A, Clayton RN, Jones A, Charlton HM. Pituitary and gonadal function in hypogonadotrophic hypogonadal (hpg) mice bearing hypothalamic implants. *J Reprod Fertil* 1985;74:247–255.

Functional Neural Transplantation,
edited by S. B. Dunnett and A. Björklund.
Raven Press, Ltd., New York © 1994.

19

Modulation and Restitution of Circadian Rhythms

Michael N. Lehman and *Martin R. Ralph

*Department of Cell Biology, Neurobiology, and Anatomy, University of Cincinnati College of Medicine, Cincinnati, Ohio 45267; *Department of Psychology, University of Toronto, Toronto, Ontario M5S 1A1 Canada*

Circadian clocks in living organisms have the primary function of organizing the daily patterns of physiologic, biochemical, and behavioral changes that allow the organism to function most efficiently in a cyclic environment (58,66,67). Endogenously generated cycles that are close to 24 hours in length allow these processes to "anticipate" recurrent changes in the internal or external environment and to be ready to respond when conditions are most likely to be optimal. This requires a central physiologic oscillator that will generate a stable rhythm with a period close to 24 hours, along with mechanisms of communicating this temporal information to the rest of the organism. It also requires that the oscillator be responsive to cyclic environmental stimuli, such as light and dark, so that the system may synchronize with the 24-hour day and, thus, function as a clock that measures local time (68).

In mammals, the suprachiasmatic nucleus (SCN) of the hypothalamus is the site of a circadian pacemaker (reviewed in 54,74,85). Photoreceptors that mediate the effects of light on the circadian system are located in the retina (61), and photic information is conveyed to the SCN by two pathways: a monosynaptic, retinohypothalamic tract (RHT; 52,53,57,65,81), and a second, multisynaptic pathway that includes the intergeniculate leaflet (IGL)

of the lateral geniculate nucleus (81; for review, see 50). Nonphotic information, that may also be involved in normal entrainment (20,60,76,83), may reach the SCN through this geniculohypothalamic projection (GHT; 36) or perhaps over other routes, including a major serotonergic projection from the raphe nuclei (56).

The evidence that the SCN is the site of a circadian pacemaker in mammals is substantial, and includes the fact that its anatomic location, directly dorsal to the optic chiasm, is ideal for receiving photic signals from the retina. Ablation studies attest to the importance of this nucleus in circadian organization (55,96). Lesions in this area of the brain, and in no other, result in the elimination of overt rhythmicity in the circadian range. In addition, explantation studies have demonstrated the persistence of circadian oscillations in vitro (19,26,28,62,91).

The ability of SCN transplants to restore circadian rhythms to arrhythmic, SCN-lesioned animals (74), has provided one of the strongest lines of evidence supporting the role of this nucleus as the site of an endogenous pacemaker. Perhaps the best demonstration of this comes from transplantation experiments in which a defining characteristic (phase, period) of a rhythm can be attributed unambiguously to the presence of the grafted SCN. This has been accomplished with cross-species xenografts in rodents, in which period is species-specific (87,94) and, in particular, in the golden hamster, in which a behavioral mutation, *tau* (75), permits the distinction of graft- and host-derived rhythmicity in cross-genotype grafts (72).

In this chapter, we will examine the uses of neural transplantation as a technique for investigating some of the basic issues in circadian biology. We will review the range of functions restored by SCN grafts and their anatomic characteristics, the use of circadian mutants in SCN transplant studies, and the use of dissociated and cultured SCN cells for grafting. In addition, we will consider the way in which SCN grafts are

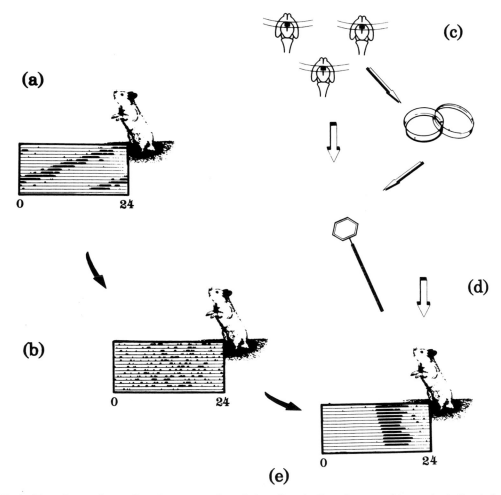

FIG. 1. Experimental paradigm for restoration of circadian rhythms by neural transplantation in hamsters. **A**: The circadian rhythmicity of the host is determined from wheel-running activity. **B**: The host SCN is ablated, and elimination of rhythmicity is confirmed from the activity record. **C**: Tissue from the embryonic SCN region (SCN and anterior hypothalamus) is removed for transplantation, cell suspension, or culture. **D**: SCN tissue (usually two donors) or cells are implanted. **E**: The success of the operation is assessed from the appearance of rhythmicity in the subsequent activity record. In this example, *tau,* a period mutation in the golden hamster is used as a behavioral marker of the transplanted SCN (see "The *tau* mutation in golden hamsters" in text). (From ref. 74, with permission.)

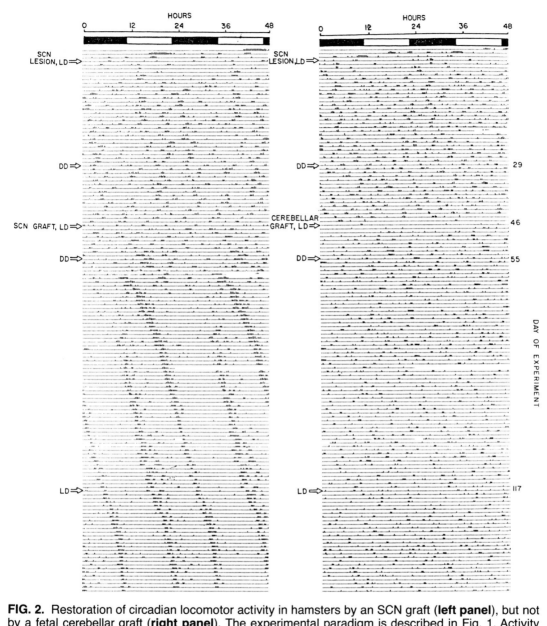

FIG. 2. Restoration of circadian locomotor activity in hamsters by an SCN graft (**left panel**), but not by a fetal cerebellar graft (**right panel**). The experimental paradigm is described in Fig. 1. Activity record is double-plotted, as is usually the convention for this type of data. *Horizontal bar* at top of record indicates the lighting schedule for periods during which the animals were exposed to a 12-hr light–12-hr dark cycle (LD). *DD* designates the onset of constant darkness.

A free-running rhythm of locomotor activity emerged 2 weeks after grafting in the animal that received a fetal SCN graft, whereas the animal given a cerebellar graft continued to be arrhythmic. Despite the recovery of locomotor rhythmicity, the SCN-grafted animal showed no entrainment to the LD cycle. (From ref. 45, with permission.)

currently being used to determine the means by which pacemakers (cells and nuclei) communicate with each other and the rest of the brain.

SUPRACHIASMATIC NUCLEUS TRANSPLANTATION: THE EXPERIMENTAL PARADIGM

The first studies of SCN transplants in rodents involved the use of whole-tissue grafts (microdissected chunks) containing the fetal or neonatal SCN, that documented recovery of locomotor and drinking rhythms after grafting of this tissue into the third ventricle of arrhythmic SCN-lesioned animals (15,16,44,88). The general paradigm that has been used for these and subsequent transplantation studies is illustrated in Fig. 1. In rodents such as hamsters, activity rhythms can be easily monitored from wheel-running activity (see Fig. 1A). The host SCN is destroyed by electrolytic lesions, and the elimination of rhythmicity is confirmed from the activity record (see Fig. 1B). Tissue from the fetal or neonatal anterior hypothalamus is harvested for transplantation (see Fig. 1C,D) and implanted into the host. Restoration of free-running activity rhythms under constant conditions is assessed from the subsequent activity record (see Fig. 1E).

Recovery of circadian function is seen only after grafting of tissue containing the SCN (Fig. 2). Grafts of fetal cortex, lateral hypothalamus (15), superior colliculus (92), or cerebellum (44) all are ineffective in restoring free-running activity rhythms (see Fig. 2B), even though some of these areas share neurochemical markers or connections in common with the SCN. A wide range of donor ages are capable of restoring circadian rhythmicity to SCN-lesioned animals; in hamsters, donor SCN tissue ranging from E13 to P5 are effective (81). The latency to recovery after SCN grafting also varies considerably: in some instances, activity rhythms reappear within several days

after grafting (see Fig. 2 in ref. 44), whereas in other animals, the latency to recovery can take up to 2 months, even though there is no obvious difference in either the anatomic characteristics or location of grafts (15,16,37,44). It may be that agents that entrain (or synchronize) grafted pacemaker cells shorten the latency to recovery after SCN grafting, since in recent studies, exogenously administered melatonin, which can entrain the fetal SCN (14), has also resulted in rapid reinstatement of locomotor rhythmicity following SCN grafting (80).

WHICH CIRCADIAN FUNCTIONS ARE RESTORED BY SUPRACHIASMATIC NUCLEUS GRAFTS?

Thus far SCN grafts have been shown to restore many, but not all circadian functions (Table 1). In addition to overt behavioral rhythms (activity, drinking and feeding, gnawing), SCN grafts reestablish endocrine rhythms, specifically that of cerebrospinal fluid (CSF) vasopressin, in the SCN-intact vasopressin-deficient Brattleboro rat (19). Preliminary results suggest that, in most recipients, rhythms in activity and sleep–wake cycles reappear simultaneously (21), suggesting that a common signal generated by the SCN controls these rhythms.

In contrast with the foregoing examples, SCN grafts have not been shown to restore reproductive rhythms, such as that underlying the timing of the preovulatory gonadotropin surge (see Table 1). The SCN grafts also fail to restore the reproductive responses of seasonally breeding mammals (e.g., hamsters) to photoperiod (44). Photoperiodic responsiveness depends on the ability of the SCN to regulate the diurnal secretion of melatonin by the pineal gland through a multisynaptic neural pathway that includes projections from the SCN to the paraventricular nucleus or subparaventricular zone (38,43,101), and subsequent

TABLE 1. *Circadian functions restored and not restored by SCN grafts*

Function	Animal	Refs.
Restored		
Locomotor/activity rhythms	Rat	88
	Hamster	15,44,72
Drinking/feeding rhythms	Rat	16,27
CSF vasopressin rhythms	Rat	19
Sleep/wake rhythms	Rat	21
Gnawing rhythms	Hamster	47
Entrainment to light	Hamster	Bittman, unpublished
Heavy water/lithium changes free-running period	Hamster	48,49
Not restored		
Photoperiodic responsiveness	Hamster	Bittman, unpublished; 44
Estrous cycles or LH surges	Hamster	Bittman, unpublished
Phase-shifts to triazolam/activity	Hamster	10

projections that eventually innervate sympathetic preganglionics in the intermediolateral spinal cord (38). The inability of SCN grafts to restore photoperiodic responses may reflect the failure of these grafts to reestablish this precise neural circuitry. It may be that SCN grafts implanted in closer proximity to sympathetic centers of the brain stem or spinal cord, or adjacent to the superior cervical ganglion, will be able to reinstate SCN control of pineal melatonin synthesis and secretion.

The question of whether the pacemaker in the grafted SCN can be entrained is an active area of investigation. Preliminary results suggest that, in a few instances, SCN-lesioned hamsters bearing SCN grafts can entrain to light, but at higher intensities than required for entrainment in SCN-intact animals (E. L. Bittman, unpublished observations). In these cases, grafts are located directly above the optic chiasm and are innervated by a few sprouting fibers from the underlying chiasm (45). The higher-light intensity required for entrainment may reflect the relatively sparse retinal input these grafts receive, as well as the fact that retinal afferents are not specifically directed toward SCN cell clusters in the graft (45). The donor pacemaker in SCN grafts, unlike the intact SCN, does not appear to be responsive to the phase-shifting effects of the benzodiazepine, triazolam (10). However, as in intact animals, both D_2O (48) and lithium (49) lengthen the free-running period of activity rhythms in SCN graft recipients. The phase responsiveness of grafted animals to other periodic environmental cues or to other pharmacologic agents remains to be investigated.

ANATOMIC CHARACTERISTICS OF GRAFTS THAT RESTORE RHYTHMICITY

One of the hallmarks of whole-tissue grafts that restore rhythmicity to SCN-lesioned rats and hamsters is the presence within the graft of clusters of peptidergic cells and fibers that are characteristic of the intact SCN (4,15,37,44). As in the intact SCN, whole-tissue SCN grafts contain clusters of cells immunoreactive for vasoactive intestinal polypeptide (VIP) and for vasopressin (VP) or its associated protein, neurophysin (Fig. 3). In the hamster, cholecystokinin (CCK)-containing neurons, which constitute a subpopulation of SCN cells (51), are also found in SCN grafts (Fig. 4). Neurons that express somatostatin or gastrin-releasing peptide (GRP) are also in-

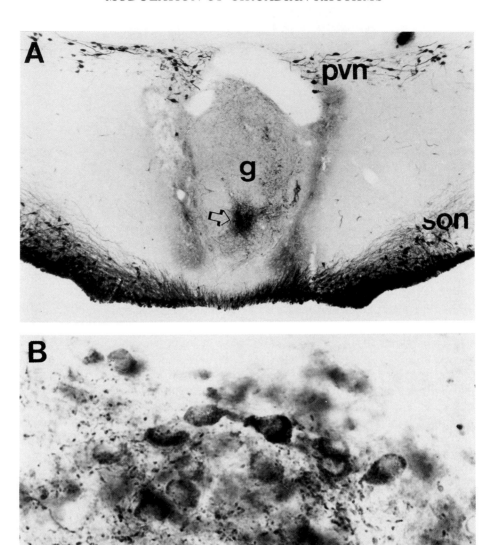

FIG. 3. A: Low-power photomicrograph of a hamster SCN graft (*g*) implanted in the third ventricle that restored rhythmicity to an SCN-lesioned host. This brain section has been immunostained with vasopressin (VP) revealing a cluster of parvicellular VP cells and fibers within the graft (*open arrow*) and magnocellular VP cells in the paraventricular (*pvn*) and supraoptic (*son*) nuclei of the host. The graft is bordered by gliotic tissue, except at its ventral edge where graft tissue appears to merge with the host brain (*double-headed arrow*). **B**: High-power photomicrograph of a cluster of immunoreactive VIP cells and fibers within a fetal SCN graft (*bar,* 10 μm). (Modified from ref. 45, with permission.)

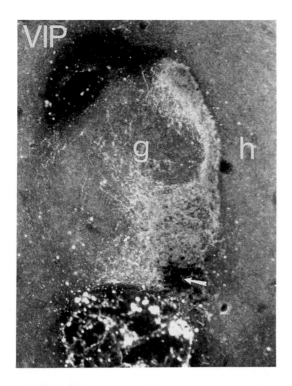

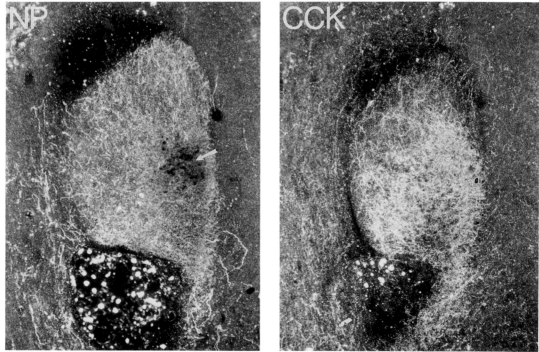

FIG. 4. Serial sections viewed under darkfield microscopy showing the component organization of *VIP*-positive cells and fibers, neurophysin (*NP*)-positive cells and fibers, and *CCK*-positive cells and fibers within an SCN graft implanted in the third ventricle that restored rhythmicity. VIP and NP cells, which appear *black* in this darkfield view, form adjacent nonoverlapping clusters (*arrows*) mimicking that organization seen in the intact SCN. The CCK cells are scattered between the VIP and NP cell clusters. Note that most VIP, NP, and CCK fibers appear to ramify within the graft (*g*): *h,* host hypothalamus. (Magnification approximately 40 ×.)

trinsic to the rodent SCN, and both soma-
tostatin- (15,27) and GRP-positive cells
(M. N. Lehman, *unpublished observations*)
have been observed in SCN grafts that restore rhythmicity.

These donor neuropeptidergic cells are
found in a component organization within
the graft almost identical with that seen in
the intact SCN (12,99). As in the intact
SCN, VIP cells are found in adjacent, but
nonoverlapping, clusters to VP cells and fibers; CCK cells and fibers partially overlap
both VIP and VP cell clusters (see Fig. 4).
This component organization also extends
to sets of neurochemically defined SCN afferents. For example, host fibers containing
neuropeptide Y (NPY) or serotonin, both of
which contact VIP cells in the intact SCN
(9,31), often innervate SCN grafts and ap-

pear to specifically target VIP cell clusters
in those grafts (Fig. 5). However, the presence of these inputs does not appear to be
critical to locomotor rhythmicity, since
some SCN grafts that restore rhythmicity
appear to lack these types of afferents (45).

Effective sites of implantation for intraventricular whole-tissue SCN grafts have
included both rostral and caudal portions of
the third ventricle (see Fig. 3A), as well as
the foramen of Monro (44,86). The question
of whether SCN grafts situated in the lateral ventricle can restore rhythmicity remains controversial. Although isolated instances have been reported of SCN grafts
in the lateral ventricle that restore rhythmicity (3,44), others have found that lateral
ventricle grafts fail to restore circadian
function, even though these grafts, similar

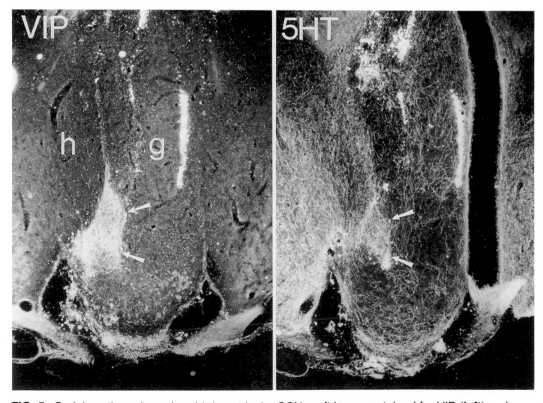

FIG. 5. Serial sections through a third ventricular SCN graft immunostained for VIP (**left**) and serotonin (5HT) (**right**). The 5HT fibers of host origin (*h*) form a dense plexus (*arrows*) that overlaps the
location of VIP cell clusters (*arrows*) in the graft (*g*). (Magnification approximately 40 ×.)

to those placed in the third ventricle, contained SCN peptidergic cells (30). The identification of effective implantation sites for the restoration of rhythmicity may be clarified by the use of dissociated cell suspension grafts (see below), which allow intraparenchymal placement of SCN cells in the host brain.

THE *tau* MUTATION IN GOLDEN HAMSTERS

Initial studies demonstrating the recovery of rhythmicity after SCN grafting, together with the demonstration of neuropeptide cell clusters within the graft, strongly suggested that these grafts were effective in restoring circadian function because they contained a functional SCN pacemaker. However, an alternative possibility was that the restorative effect was, at least partly, due to permissive or trophic influences which, in turn, allowed the expression of circadian function by another part of the brain. To distinguish between these possibilities, it was necessary to demonstrate that, following grafting, a characteristic of the donor circadian clock, such as period or phase, was transferred to the recipient.

Similar experiments had been performed previously in sparrows, in which the transplanted pineal gland was shown to determine the timing and phase of locomotor activity (102). Unfortunately, the use of embryonic tissue for SCN transplants in mammals, precludes the determination of phase before grafting; and only limited success has been achieved by retroactively inferring from the recovered locomotor rhythm, the phase of the donor clock at the time of transplantation.

As noted in the introduction, convincing demonstration of the pacemaker function of the SCN has come from transplantation studies in rodents, for which the period of the recovered rhythms reflect unambiguously the genotype of the grafted tissue. This has been done using both cross-species xenografts in rodents (87,94) and, specifically, in the golden hamster, for which a period mutation, *tau*, (75) can be used to distinguish host- and donor-derived activities in cross-genotype transplants.

The *tau* mutation was discovered in 1985 among a group of wild-type golden hamsters obtained from the Charles River breeding colony in Massachusetts. It appears to have occurred at a single, autosomal locus, and the mutant allele is semidominant (75). The allele has the behavioral effect of reducing the free-running period of the animal's circadian rhythms from about 24 hours in the wild-type, to 22 hours in heterozygotes, and about 20 hours in homozygous mutants. The three phenotypic groups are distinctive behaviorally, and frequency distributions of their periods do not overlap (70). This makes the behavioral marker ideal for transplantation experiments for which discrimination between donor and host circadian influence is critical.

Initial experiments with transplantation that used the *tau* mutation were aimed at verifying the pacemaker role of the SCN. Reciprocal transplants were performed between *tau* genotypes, and the period of the restored rhythms always reflected the genotype of the donor tissue (Fig. 6). Subsequent experiments in which circadian chimeras have been produced with two functional clocks (see later) have confirmed this result. Chimeras have been produced by transplanting SCN tissue (100) or cultured SCN cells (77) from one *tau* genotype into a host of a different genotype after its own SCN has been partially ablated. The result is an animal that exhibits two distinct rhythmic patterns in its locomotor activity, representing donor and host genotypes, with no evidence that the presence of either clock alters the function of the other. Together, these cross-genotype transplantation experiments offer proof that the SCN operates essentially independently of the rest of the brain (or organism) in producing the primary characteristics of mammalian circadian rhythms.

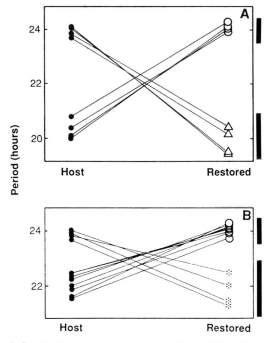

FIG. 6. Reciprocal transplantation of the SCN between wild-type and *tau* mutant hamsters. For each host, the endogenous rhythm (*left*) was eliminated by SCN lesions and restored by SCN transplants (*right*). The range of period in the intact adult population for each genotype is indicated by *vertical bars* (*right axis*). **A**: Reciprocal transplants between wild-type and homozygous mutants. **B**: Reciprocal transplants between wild-type and heterozygous mutants. Symbols represent the following: *solid circle,* host; *open circle,* SCN tissue from wild-type donor; *asterisk,* SCN tissue from heterozygous donor; *open triangle,* SCN tissue from homozygous mutant donor. (From ref. 72, with permission.)

TRANSPLANTATION OF DISSOCIATED AND CULTURED SUPRACHIASMATIC NUCLEUS CELLS

A central question in the study of circadian time-keeping is whether the pacemaker properties of the SCN arise from local interactions among groups of cells, or whether individual cells without such connections can bear those functions (35). Dissociated cell suspensions have been employed in other systems as a way of maximizing potential integration between the graft and host (7,22,90) and, in this system, have been used to determine whether isolated SCN cells, in contrast with the clusters of peptidergic neurons seen in whole-tissue grafts, can restore circadian function to arrhythmic hosts (92). The ability of cell suspension grafts of the fetal SCN to restore rhythmicity (Fig. 7) demonstrates that the intrinsic peptidergic organization of the intact SCN is not a prerequisite for functional recovery after grafting. As in whole-tissue grafts, restoration of rhythmicity is tightly correlated with the presence of VIP and other peptidergic cells characteristic of the SCN. However, unlike whole-tissue grafts, peptidergic neurons associated with cell suspension grafts are isolated and much fewer (Fig. 8).

Interestingly, the period of restored free-running rhythms in hamsters with cell suspension grafts was significantly shorter than that seen in either intact hamsters (69), or SCN-lesioned hamsters with whole-tissue grafts of the fetal SCN (44). Preliminary observations suggest that the shortened period is not due to a fewer number of cells implanted in cell suspension grafts than in whole-tissue grafts, but instead, may reflect disruption of the normal intrinsic circuitry of the SCN (M. N. Lehman, unpublished observations). Effective sites of implantation of SCN cell suspension grafts include the medial hypothalamus and midline thalamus (46,92), regions that are targets of SCN efferents in the intact brain (101). Together with the effectiveness of whole-tissue SCN grafts placed in the third ventricle and foramen of Monro, these results suggest that proximity of donor SCN cells to former postsynaptic targets of the host SCN may be required for restoration of rhythmicity.

The same dissociated fetal SCN cells used for cell suspension grafting may be grown in primary culture for several weeks, during which time they extend neurites and express SCN neuropeptides, such as VIP (Fig. 9). Primary cultures of SCN cells can be resuspended and survive subsequent grafting into adult hosts (45). Recent experiments indicate that SCN cells maintained in culture for up to 5 weeks can support locomotor rhythms following transplantation (77). This implies not only that rhythms are generated, but also that potential channels of communication with the host are present in primary culture.

The ability of cultured SCN cells to restore rhythmicity offers the possibility of genetically modifying these cells before transplantation, to perturb pacemaker function. Several approaches have been explored to achieve uptake and expression of a foreign reporter gene in primary cultures of SCN cells (42); these include lipofection of plasmid DNA, infection using a replication-defective vector based on herpes sim-plex virus (HSV), and transfection with a retroviral vector (Fig. 10A). Lipofection in these experiments resulted in transgene expression only in glial cells, whereas retroviral and HSV-based vectors resulted in expression in both neurons and glia. Infection with the HSV-based vector resulted in foreign gene expression in a larger percentage of cells than seen after retroviral transfection, but as in other studies using HSV-based vectors (24), this expression disappeared after 1 to 2 weeks *in vitro* (45). Although retroviral transfection resulted in a transgene expression in only a small subset of cultured SCN cells (presumably those still undergoing mitotic activity), transfected SCN cells continued to express the transgene for several weeks following grafting into an adult host (see Fig. 10B).

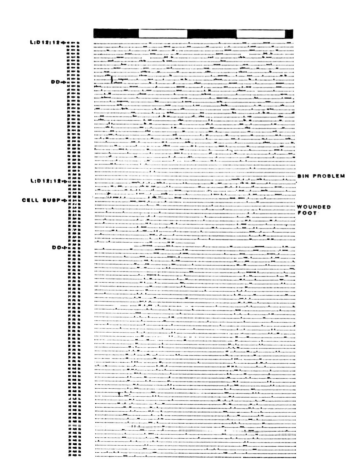

FIG. 7. Restoration of circadian locomotor activity by an SCN cell suspension graft. In contrast with the recovery seen after whole-tissue grafts (see Fig. 2), the period of the restored rhythm after cell suspension grafting was always shorter than 24 hr (abbreviations as in Fig. 2). (Modified from ref. 92, with permission.)

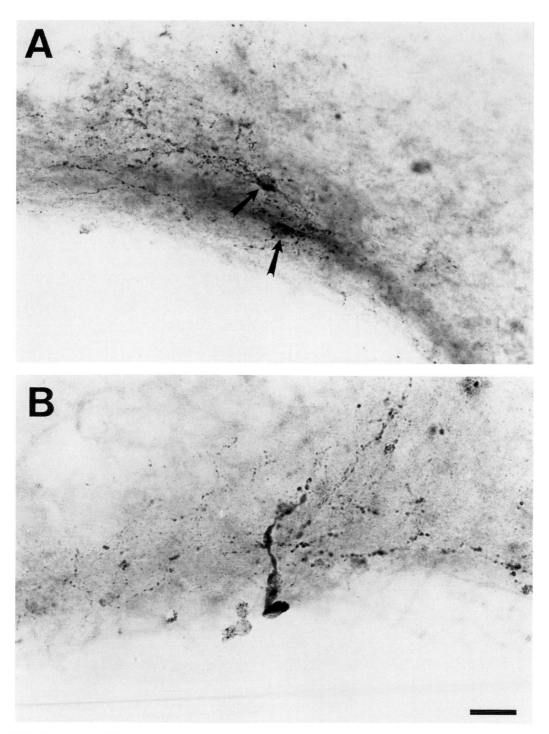

FIG. 8. Isolated VIP cells and fibers associated with a SCN cell suspension graft that restored circadian rhythmicity. **A**: Immunoreactive VIP cells (*arrows*) and fibers in close proximity to the edge of the third ventricle. **B**: Adjacent section to that in A showing another isolated VIP cell at the dorsal edge of the third ventricle (*bar,* 20 μm). (Modified from ref. 92, with permission.)

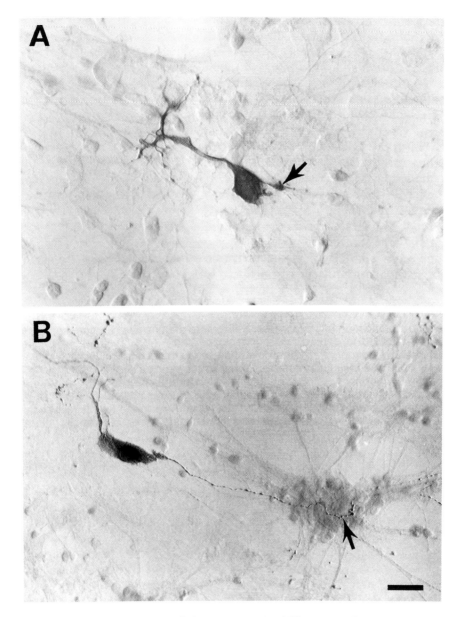

FIG. 9. SCN neurons in primary culture. **A**: Immunoreactive VIP neuron after several days in culture. Neurites, some of which have the appearance of growth cones (*arrow*), extend from the processes of this cell. **B**: Isolated VIP-positive neuron after 2 weeks in culture. A fiber with beaded varicosities extends from this cell and ramifies (*arrow*) over a cluster of nonimmunoreactive neurons (*bar, 20 μm*).

Even though further work is needed to rule out the likelihood that transfection of SCN neurons per se compromises their ability to restore circadian function, the prospect of genetically tailoring SCN neu-rons before grafting open several interesting possibilities. One application would be to use such a vector to amplify or turn off expression of genes suspected of being closely linked to either entrainment path-

One approach to determining whether the SCN communicates with the host brain by neural or humoral signals involves the use of SCN grafts encapsulated in a perm-selective polymer membrane that allows humoral communication with the host brain, but prevents neurite outgrowth (1). Both whole-tissue grafts and cell suspension grafts of the SCN remain viable when polymer-encapsulated (Fig. 11), particularly if they are mixed with extracellular matrix materials such as Matrigel before loading in the capsule, and encapsulated SCN grafts contain peptidergic cells and fibers (93). Semipermeable capsules can be prepared with different molecular weight cutoffs, and if diffusible factors are sufficient to restore rhythmicity, these capsules could be used to determine the approximate molecular weights of the critical signals. Isolation and purification of these molecules would be of particular relevance to the circadian regulation of sleep–wake cycles (21), since there has long been evidence suggesting the existence of diffusible sleep-inducing substances (8,41).

COMMUNICATION WITH OTHER PACEMAKERS

The expression of a coherent, overt rhythm requires that individual pacemaker cells within the SCN communicate with and entrain one another. The behavior of chimeric animals that have been produced by transplantation of SCN tissue or cells into hosts with partial SCN lesions, indicates that, although pacemaker coupling within the graft and host SCN are evident, the influence of one on the other is below detection. This may not be surprising from an anatomic perspective, since grafts often do not lie in close proximity to what remains of the host nucleus. It also raises the intriguing possibility that the channels of pacemaker–pacemaker communication may be quite different from those between the SCN and the rest of the organism. The appearance of rhythmicity following SCN transplantation is a highly reliable phenomenon; success rates between 80% and 100% are not uncommon in a single experiment. Yet, although the graft may strongly influence the overt behavior of an SCN-lesioned host, effects of the graft on the host rhythm itself are negligible.

In some situations, though, it may be possible to observe and study pacemaker interactions. Some limited success has been achieved when cells from two different *tau* genotypes arc thoroughly mixed before grafting. Rhythms with intermediate periods that are seen occasionally when SCN cells from wild-type and homozygous mutants are combined, attest to the ability of these cells to influence each other (71). The rarity of this finding suggests that coupling between the genotypes is weak, but this approach may provide one model with which pacemaker coupling can be observed directly.

The best demonstration of coupling between genotypes, however, has been found in chimeras when the host is particularly old. The SCN grafts are usually not expressed at all if there is no damage to the host SCN. However, Hurd et al. (33) have shown that the transplanted SCN may drive overt rhythmicity without experimental damage to the host SCN, but only if the host's rhythm of locomotor behavior has already deteriorated. Experiments are based on the notion that there is age-related degeneration within SCN that results in rhythm fragmentation and reduced amplitude. Graft–host pacemaker interactions are observed as either relative coordination between the two periodicities; as an alternation between the two; or as a complete dominance of periodicity by the grafted clock. Like mixed cell grafts, though, the most common result is the expression of two distinct rhythms; evidence for direct interaction is still difficult to obtain.

A possible explanation for the rarity of intermediate periods in these experiments may be that 20 and 24 hours are simply too far apart for synchronization to occur easily. The responsiveness of the cells to signals from other pacemakers may not be sufficient to adjust for the 4-hour difference in period. An obvious test of this is to repeat the experiment using heterozygous (22-hour) animals as one of the genotypes.

An alternative approach is to transplant tissues of the same genotype as the host, but use animals that have been raised on opposite light–dark cycles, for which the phases of donor and host clocks initially should be 180° apart. Coupling between bilateral pacemakers in the eyes of the marine snail, *Bulla gouldiana,* for which the output of the two oscillators can be monitored continuously, has been studied using this method (79). Transplantation of the clock in the mammals, however, may require 2 weeks, or more, of recovery time before the overt donor rhythm is obvious. This may allow sufficient time for donor and host to synchronize, but no evidence of interactions would be available unless the host rhythm were perturbed. To examine pacemaker synchronization, one can take advantage of the fact that metabolic activity in the SCN is itself rhythmic and 2-deoxyglucose uptake may be used as a relatively crude index of phase (89). By transplanting fetal tissue from donors raised on a 24-hour light cycle into hosts maintained on the opposite cycle, Silver and colleagues (personal communication) have shown that the rhythm in the donor SCN is rapidly synchronized to the rhythm of the host. It appears, therefore, that the ability of donor and host clocks to mutually entrain may depend on the period difference between the two pacemaker ensembles, although other factors, such as anatomic proximity or unsatisfied requirements for neural connections cannot be ruled out.

SUMMARY AND FUTURE DIRECTIONS

It is readily apparent that a consequence of having a clock, or central oscillator, is that behavioral and physiologic processes are rhythmically regulated with 24-hour periods. This means that the state or activity of this central nervous process is reflected in the phase of overt rhythms. Any phase in the cycle, hence, the physiologic state of the pacemaker, may be pinpointed; either relative to an overt reference marker, such as the onset of locomotor activity, or directly, as in continuously consulted clocks involved in orientation or migration. This window to the brain is unique among central processes that regulate behavior; not only is the assessment of state potentially continuous, but the regularity with which the clock functions allows the state of the system to be predicted, given as little as 1 day of prior activity. It is the predictability of circadian phase that allows detailed and precise evaluation of manipulations that perturb clock function.

For transplantation studies, this means that the functioning of an SCN graft and the nature of communication with the host can be evaluated with confidence. The restoration of rhythmicity to arrhythmic hosts or the expression of additional rhythmicity in intact or partially lesioned hosts, can be unambiguously attributed to activity within the graft, not simply to the presence of grafted tissue. This feature should enable the functional dissection of the SCN. Since dissociated (92) and cultured (77) cells are capable of driving overt rhythms, the potential exists to transplant subpopulations to determine what type of SCN cells do or do not retain this ability.

In addition to providing important clues to the functional organization of the circadian system, transplantation of SCN tissue provides an interesting comparison with other model systems for evaluating behavioral recovery after grafting. Unlike most transplant systems for which recovery of function is dependent on the reinnervation of specific targets, or the release of trophic factors, evidence thus far suggest that, although SCN grafts restore function by emitting a signal conveying specific time of day, the targets for that information may be relatively nonspecific, or multiple redundant signals may be used. Studies using SCN grafts are likely to reveal or to confirm both the targets and signals by which SCN pacemaker cells communicate with the rest of the brain, as well as the manner by which they communicate with each other.

For all of these studies, the use of circadian mutants, such as the *tau* hamster, will continue to possess notable advantages. By using donors and hosts that differ in the period of their endogenous circadian clock, recovery of function is unambiguous, since rhythms that reappear do so with the donor's phenotype (72). As noted earlier, temporal chimeras are sometimes produced when fetal SCN tissue (100) or cultured cells (77) from a donor of one *tau* genotype are transplanted into a host of a different genotype from which the SCN has been only partially ablated. Since these animals exhibit two distinct rhythmic patterns in their locomotor activity, representing both host and donor phenotypes, an added advantage is that these animals can also be used to assess possible trophic influences of the donor clock upon the host SCN (32,33).

An important next step in our understanding of the mammalian circadian system will be to analyze circadian pacemaker function at a cellular and molecular level. The SCN transplants may play a critical role in these efforts, particularly as a bridge between molecular and behavioral levels of analysis. For example, transplantation of genetically modified SCN cells may be useful in assessing which genes are essential to circadian pacemaker function. In addition to the use of viral-based vectors for altering SCN cells, future studies could also take advantage of the availability of transgenic animals (71) or SCN cell lines (17) as potential sources of donor tissue. The use of transgenic animals as sources of donor tissue would be one way to determine whether circadian abnormalities associated

with the transgene are due to alterations in the SCN itself (71). Even when transgenic animals do not survive until adulthood, late fetal or neonatal tissue could still be harvested for transplantation studies. By using SCN cell lines or embryonic tissue, transplant studies may also be useful for studying the potential influence of environmental factors on phenotypic differentiation in the SCN. In these ways and others, transplantation is likely to continue to play an important role in investigations of fundamental issues in circadian biology.

ACKNOWLEDGMENTS

We thank Ms. Xiao Gu for her excellent photographic assistance and Dr. Sandra J. Berriman for critical comments on the manuscript. This work is supported by NIH grant R01 NS28175 to Dr. Lehman and an AFOSR grant F49620-92-J-0517 to Drs. Ralph and Lehman. Dr. Ralph is an Alfred P. Sloan Research Fellow.

REFERENCES

1. Aebischer P, Winn SR, Galletti PM. Transplantation of neural tissue in polymer capsules. *Brain Res* 1988;448:364.
2. Aguilar-Roblero R, Garcia-Hernandez F, Aguilar R, Arankowsky-Sandoval G, Drucker-Colin R. Suprachiasmatic nucleus transplants function as an endogenous oscillator only in constant darkness. *Neurosci Lett* 1986;69:47.
3. Aguilar-Roblero RA, Morin LP, Moore RY. Is the fetal SCN sufficient to induce rhythm recovery when transplanted to SCN-lesioned hamsters? *Neurosci Abstr* 1988;14:24.2.
4. Aguilar-Roblero R, Shibata S, Speh JC, Drucker-Colin R, Moore RY. Morphological and functional development of the suprachiasmatic nucleus in transplanted fetal hypothalamus. *Brain Res* 1992;288:580.
5. Björklund A, Stenevi U. Intracerebral neural implants: neural replacement and reconstruction of damaged circuits. *Annu Rev Neurosci* 1984;1:279.
6. Björklund A, Lindvall O, Isaacson O, Brundin P, Wictorin K, Strecker RE, Clarke DE, Dunnett SB. Mechanisms of action of intracerebral neural implants: studies on nigral and striatal grafts to the lesioned striatum. *Trends Neurosci* 1987;10:509.

7. Björklund A, Stenevi U, Schmidt RH, Dunnett SB, Gage FH. Intracerebral grafting of neuronal cell suspensions. I. *Acta Physiol Scand* [*Suppl.*] 1983;522:1.
8. Borbely AA, Tobler I. The search for an endogenous "sleep substance." *Trends Pharmacol Sci* 1980;1:356.
9. Bosler O, Beaudet A. VIP neurons as prime synaptic targets for serotonin afferents in rat suprachiasmatic nucleus: a combined autoradiographic and immunocytochemical study. *J Neurocytol* 1985;14:749.
10. Canbelyi RS, Romero MT, Silver R. Neither triazolam nor activity phase advance circadian locomotor activity in SCN-lesioned hamsters bearing fetal SCN transplants. *Brain Res* 1991;566:40.
11. Canbelyi RS, Lehman MN, Silver R. Tracing SCN graft efferents with the carbocyanine dye. diI. *Brain Res* 1991;554:15.
12. Card JP, Moore RY. The suprachiasmatic nucleus of the golden hamster: immunohistochemical analysis of cell and fiber distribution. *Neuroscience* 1984;13:415.
13. Davis FC. Phase of circadian rhythms restored by suprachiasmatic nucleus (SCN) transplants. *Neurosci Abstr* 1989;15:493.
14. Davis FC, Mannion J. Entrainment of hamster pup circadian rhythms by prenatal melatonin injections to the mother. *Am Physiol Soc* 1988;255:439.
15. DeCoursey PJ, Buggy J. Circadian rhythmicity after neural transplant to hamster third ventricle: specificity of suprachiasmatic nuclei. *Brain Res* 1989;500:263.
16. Drucker-Colin R, Aguilar-Roblero R, Garcia-Hernandez F, Fernandez-Cancino F, Rattoni FB. Fetal suprachiasmatic nucleus transplants: diurnal rhythm recovery of lesioned rats. *Brain Res* 1984;311:353.
17. Earnest DJ. Establishment and characterization of a rat suprachiasmatic nucleus-derived cell line. *Abstracts EMBO workshop on molecular chronobiology.* Leicester, UK; 1992.
18. Earnest DJ, Sladek CD. Circadian rhythms of vasopressin release from individual rat suprachiasmatic explants in vitro. *Brain Res* 1986;382:129.
19. Earnest DJ, Sladek CD, Gash DM, Weigand SJ. Specificity of circadian function in transplants of the fetal suprachiasmatic nucleus. *J Neurosci* 1988;9:2671.
20. Edgar DM, Dement WC. Regularly scheduled voluntary exercise synchronizes the mouse circadian clock. *Am J Physiol* 1991;261:R928.
21. Edgar DM, Ralph MR, Seidel WF, Dement WC. Restoration of sleep–wake and body temperature circadian rhythms by fetal SCN transplants. *Abstracts third meeting Society for Research on Biological Rhythms.* Amelia Island, FL; 1992.
22. Gage FH, Dunnett SB, Brundin P, Isaacson O, Björklund A. Intracerebral grafting of embryonic neural cells into the adult host brain: an

overview of the cell suspension method and its application. *Dev Neurosci* 1983;6:137.
23. Gash DM, Sladek JR Jr. Functional and nonfunctional transplants: studies with grafted hypothalamic and preoptic neurons. *Trends Neurosci* 1984;7:391.
24. Geller AI, Breakefield XO. A defective HSV-vector expresses *Escherichia coli* β-galactosidase in cultured peripheral neurons. *Science* 1988;241:1667.
25. Gibson MJ, Charlton HM, Perlow MJ, Zimmerman EA, Davies TF, Krieger DT. Preoptic area grafts in hypogonadal (hpg) female mice abolish effects of congenital hypothalamic gonadotropin-releasing hormone (GnRH) deficiency. *Endocrinology* 1984;114:1938.
26. Green DJ, Gillette R. Circadian rhythm of firing rate recorded from single cells in the rat suprachiasmatic brain slice. *Brain Res* 1982;245:198.
27. Griffioen HA. *Suprachiasmatic nucleus transplants in rats. Growth and functional development* (Dissertation). University of Amsterdam; 1992.
28. Groos GA, Hendricks J. Circadian rhythms in electrical discharge of rat suprachiasmatic neurones recorded in vitro. *Neurosci Lett* 1982;34:283.
29. Hakim H, DeBernardo AP, Silver R. Circadian locomotor rhythms, but not photoperiodic responses, survive surgical isolation of the SCN in hamsters. *J Biol Rhythms* 1991;6:97.
30. Harrington ME, DeCoursey PJ, Bruce D, Buggy J. Circadian pacemaker (SCN) transplants into lateral ventricles fail to restore locomotor rhythmicity in arrhythmic hamsters. *Neurosci Abstr* 1987;13:213.
31. Hisano S, Chikamori-Aoyama M, Katoh S, Kagotani Y, Daikoku S, Chihara K. Suprachiasmatic nucleus neurons immunoreactive for vasoactive intestinal polypeptide have synaptic contacts with axons immunoreactive for neuropeptide Y: an immunoelectron microscopic study in the rat. *Neurosci Lett* 1988;88:145.
32. Hurd MW, Ralph MR. Patterns of circadian locomotor rhythms in aged hamsters after suprachiasmatic nucleus transplant. *Abstracts third meeting Society for Research on Biological Rhythms.* Amelia Island, FL; 1992;3:31.
33. Hurd MW, Lehman MN, Ralph MR. Circadian locomotor rhythms in aged hamsters following suprachiasmatic nucleus transplant. 1993 [submitted].
34. Inouye SE, Kawamura H. Persistence of circadian rhythmicity in a mammalian hypothalamic "island" containing the suprachiasmatic nucleus. *Proc Natl Acad Sci USA* 1979;76:5962.
35. Jacklet JW, Geronimo J. Circadian rhythm: population of interacting neurons. *Science* 1971;174:299.
36. Johnson RF, Smale L, Moore RY, Morin LP. Lateral geniculate lesions block circadian phase-shift responses to a benzodiazepine. *Proc Natl Acad Sci USA* 1988;85:5301.

37. Kawamura H, Nihonmatsu I. The suprachiasmatic nucleus as the circadian rhythm generator. Immunocytochemical identification of the suprachiasmatic nucleus within the transplanted hypothalamus. In: Hiroshige T, Honma K, eds. *Circadian clocks and zeitgebers.* Hokkaido Press; 1985.

38. Klein DC, Smoot R, Weller JL, Higa S, Markey SP, Creed GJ, Jacobowitz DM. Lesions of the paraventricular nucleus area disrupt the suprachiasmatic-spinal cord circuit in the melatonin rhythm generating system. *Brain Res Bull* 1983;10:647.

39. Krieger DT, Perlow MJ, Gibson MJ, Davies TF, Zimmerman EA, Ferin M, Charlton HM. Brain graft reverse hypogonadism of gonadotropin and releasing hormone deficiency. *Nature* 1982;298:468.

40. Kromer LF. Intracephalic embryonic transplants: new experimental preparation for developmental neurobiology. In: Sladek JR, Gash DM, eds. *Neural transplants, development and function.* New York: Plenum Press; 1984.

41. Krueger JM, Obal F, Opp M, Toth L, Johannsen L, Cady AB. Somnogenic cytokines and models concerning their effects on sleep. *Yale J Biol Med* 1990;63:157.

42. Lehman MN. Genetic modification of SCN cells prior to transplantation. *Abstracts EMBO workshop on molecular chronobiology.* Leicester, UK; 1992.

43. Lehman MN, Bittman EL, Newman SW. Role of the hypothalamic paraventricular nucleus in neuroendocrine responses to daylength in the golden hamster. *Brain Res* 1984;308:25.

44. Lehman MN, Silver R, Gladstone WR, Kahn RM, Gibson M, Bittman EL. Circadian rhythmicity restored by neural transplant: immunocytochemical characterization of the graft and its integration with the host brain. *J Neurosci* 1987;7:1626.

45. Lehman MN, Silver R, Bittman EL. Anatomy of suprachiasmatic nucleus grafts. In: Klein DC, Moore RY, Reppert SM, eds. *The suprachiasmatic nucleus: the mind's clock.* New York: Oxford University Press; 1991.

46. Lehman MN, Zimmer KA, Strother WN. Influence of the site of implantation on the restoration of circadian rhythmicity by dissociated cell grafts of the suprachiasmatic nucleus. *Neurosci Abstr* 1993;19:1055.

47. LeSauter J, Silver R. Suprachiasmatic nucleus lesions abolish and fetal grafts restore circadian gnawing rhythms in hamsters. 1993 [submitted manuscript].

48. LeSauter J, Silver R. Heavy water lengthens the period of free-running rhythms in lesioned hamsters bearing SCN grafts. *Physiol Behav* 1993 (in press).

49. LeSauter J, Silver R. Lithium lengthens period of circadian rhythms in lesioned hamsters bearing fetal SCN grafts. *Biol Psychiatry* 1993 (in press).

50. Meijer JH, Reitveld WJ. The neurophysiology of the suprachiasmatic circadian pacemaker in rodents. *Physiol Rev* 1989;69:671.

51. Miceli MO, van der Kooy D, Post CA, Della-Fera MA, Baile CA. Differential distributions of cholecystokinin in hamster and rat forebrain. *Brain Res* 1987;402:318.

52. Moore RY. Retinohypothalamic projections in mammals: a comparative study. *Brain Res* 1973;49:403.

53. Moore RY. The retinohypothalamic tract, suprachiasmatic hypothalamic nucleus and central mechanisms of circadian rhythm regulation. In: Suda M, Hyaishi O, Hakagawa H, eds. *Biological rhythms and their central mechanism.* 1979;343–354.

54. Moore RY. Organization and function of a central nervous system circadian oscillator: the suprachiasmatic nuclei. *Fed Proc* 1983;42:2783.

55. Moore RY, Eicher VB. Loss of a circadian adrenal corticosterone rhythm following suprachiasmatic lesions in the rat. *Brain Res* 1972;42:201.

56. Moore RY, Halaris AE, Jones BE. Serotonin neurones of the midbrain raphe: ascending projections. *J Comp Neurol* 1978;180:417.

57. Moore RY, Lenn N. A retinohypothalamic projection in the rat. *J Comp Neurol* 1972;146:1.

58. Moore-Ede MC, Sulzman FM, Fuller CA. *The clocks that time us.* Cambridge: Harvard University Press; 1982.

59. Morgenstern JP, Land H. Advanced mammalian gene transfer: high titre retroviral vectors with multiple drug selection markers and a complementary helper-free packaging cell line. *Nucleic Acids Res* 1990;18:3587.

60. Mrsovsky N, Reebs SG, Honrado GI, Salmon PA. Behavioral entrainment of circadian rhythms. *Experientia* 1989;45:696.

61. Nelson RJ, Zucker I. Absence of extraocular photoreception in diurnal and nocturnal rodents exposed to direct sunlight. *Comp Biochem Physiol A* 1981;69:145.

62. Newman GC, Hospod FE. Rhythm of suprachiasmatic nucleus 2-deoxyglucose uptake in vitro. *Brain Res* 1986;381:345.

63. Nishio T, Shiusaka S, Nakagawa H, Sakumoto T, Satoh K. Circadian feeding rhythm after hypothalamic knife cut isolating suprachiasmatic nucleus. *Physiol Behav* 1979;23:763.

64. Palmiter RD, Behringer RR, Quiate CJ, Maxwell IH, Brinster RL. *Cell* 1987;50:435.

65. Pickard GE. Afferent connections of the suprachiasmatic nucleus of the golden hamster with emphasis on the retinohypothalamic projection. *J Comp Neurol* 1982;211:65.

66. Pittendrigh CS. Circadian rhythms and circadian organization of living systems. *Cold Spring Harbor Symp Quant Biol* 1960;25:159.

67. Pittendrigh CS. On temporal organization in living systems. *Harvey Lect* 1961;56:93.

68. Pittendrigh CS. On the mechanism of the entrainment of circadian system by light cycles. In: Aschoff J, ed. *Circadian clocks.* Amsterdam: North-Holland; 1965:277–297.

69. Pittendrigh CS, Daan S. A functional analysis of circadian pacemakers in nocturnal rodents. V. Pacemaker structure: a clock for all seasons. *J Comp Physiol* 1976;106:333.

70. Ralph MR. SCN transplant studies using the *tau* mutation in golden hamsters. In: Klein DC, Moore RY, Reppert SM, eds. *The suprachiasmatic nucleus: the mind's clock.* New York: Oxford University Press; 1991:341–348.

71. Ralph MR. Transgenic mice for SCN transplantation studies. *Abstracts EMBO workshop on molecular chronobiology.* Leicester, UK; 1992.

72. Ralph MR, Foster RG, Davis FC, Menaker M. Transplanted suprachiasmatic nucleus determines circadian period. *Science* 1990;247:975.

73. Ralph MR, Hurd MW, Lehman MN. Culture and transplantation of a mammalian clock: circadian chimeras produced from mixed *tau* genotypes. *Abstracts third meeting Society for Research on Biological Rhythms.* Amelia Island, FL; 1992:3:68.

74. Ralph MR, Lehman MN. Transplantation: a new tool in the analysis of the mammalian circadian pacemaker. *Trends Neurosci* 1991;14:362.

75. Ralph MR, Menaker M. A mutation of the circadian system in golden hamsters. *Science* 1988;241:1225.

76. Ralph MR, Mrsovsky N. Behavioral inhibition of circadian responses to light. *J Biol Rhythms* 1992;7:353.

77. Ralph MR, Torre ER. Circadian rhythms restored by cultured suprachiasmatic cells. *Neurosci Abstr* 1990;16:769.

78. Reppert SM, Schwartz WJ. The suprachiasmatic nuclei of the fetal rat: characterization of a functional circadian clock using ^{14}C labelled deoxyglucose. *J Neurosci* 1984;4:1677.

79. Roberts MH, Block GD. Analysis of mutual circadian pacemaker coupling between the two eyes of Bulla. *J Biol Rhythms* 1986;1:55.

80. Romero M-T, Silver R. Control of phase and latency to recovery circadian locomotor rhythmicity following transplantation of fetal SCN into lesioned adult hamsters. *Neurosci Abstr* 1989;15:725.

81. Romero M-T, Lehman MN, Silver R. Age of donor influences ability of SCN grafts to restore circadian rhythmicity. *Dev Brain Res* 1993;71(1):45.

82. Rusak B, Boulos Z. Pathways for photic entrainment of mammalian circadian rhythms. *Photochem Photobiol* 1981;34:267.

83. Rusak B, Mistelberger RE, Losier B, Jones CH. Daily hoarding opportunity entrains the pacemaker for hamster activity rhythms. *J Comp Physiol A* 1988;164:165.

84. Rusak B, Morin LP. Testicular responses to photoperiod are blocked by lesions of the suprachiasmatic nuclei in golden hamsters. *Biol Reprod* 1976;15:366.

85. Rusak B, Zucker I. Neural regulation of circadian rhythms. *Physiol Rev* 1979;59:449.

86. Saitoh Y, Nihonmatsu I, Kawamura H. Location of the suprachiasmatic nucleus grafts in rats which restored circadian rhythmicity after transplantation. *Neurosci Lett* 1990;118:45.

87. Saitoh Y, Matsui Y, Nihonmatsu I, Kawamura H. Cross-species transplantation of the suprachiasmatic nuclei from rats to Siberian chipmunks (*Eutamias sibiricus*) with suprachiasmatic lesions. *Neurosci Lett* 1991;123:77.

88. Sawaki Y, Nihonmatsu I, Kawamura H. Transplantation of the neonatal suprachiasmatic nuclei into rats with complete bilateral suprachiasmatic lesions. *Neurosci Res* 1984;1:67.

89. Schwartz WJ, Gainer H. Suprachiasmatic nucleus: use of ^{14}C-labeled deoxyglucose uptake as a functional marker. *Science* 1977;197:1089.

90. Schmidt RH, Björklund A, Stenevi U. Intracerebral grafting of dissociated CNS tissue suspensions: a new approach for neuronal transplantation to deep brain sites. *Brain Res* 1981;218:347.

91. Shibata S, Oomura Y, Kita H, Hattori K. Circadian rhythmic changes of neuronal activity in the suprachiasmatic nucleus of the rat hypothalamic slice. *Brain Res* 1982;247:154.

92. Silver R, Lehman MN, Gibson M, Gladstone WR, Bittman EL. Dispersed cell suspension of fetal SCN restore circadian rhythmicity in SCN-lesioned adult hamsters. *Brain Res* 1990;525:45.

93. Silver R, LeSauter J, Romero MT, Aebischer P, Lehman MN. Encapsulated fetal SCN grafts survive transplantation to the third ventricle. *Neurosci Abstr* 1991;17:25.

94. Sollars PJ, Kimble DP. Cross-species transplantation of fetal hypothalamic tissue restores circadian locomotor rhythm to SCN-lesioned hosts. *Neurosci Abstr* 1988;14:49.

95. Stephan FK, Nunez AA. Elimination of circadian rhythms in drinking, activity, sleep, and temperature by isolation of suprachiasmatic nuclei. *Behav Biol* 1977;20:1.

96. Stephan FK, Zucker I. Circadian rhythms in behavior and locomotor activity of rats are eliminated by hypothalamic lesions. *Proc Natl Acad Sci USA* 1972;69:1583.

97. Stetson MH, Watson-Whitmyre M. Nucleus suprachiasmaticus: the biological clock of the hamster? *Science* 1976;292:197.

98. Turek FW. Circadian neural rhythms in mammals. *Annu Rev Physiol* 1985;47:49.

99. Van den Pol AN, Tsujimoto KL. Neurotransmitters of the hypothalamic suprachiasmatic nucleus: immunocytochemical analysis of 25 neuronal antigens. *Neuroscience* 1985;15:1049.

100. Vogelbaum MA, Menaker M. Temporal chimeras produced by hypothalamic transplants. *J Neurosci* 1992;12:3619.

101. Watts AG, Swanson LW, Sanchez-Watts G. Efferent projections of the suprachiasmatic nucleus: I. Studies using anterograde transport of *Phaseolus vulgaris* leucoagglutinin in the rat. *J Comp Neurol* 1987;258:204.

102. Zimmerman NH, Menaker M. The pineal gland: a pacemaker within the circadian system of the house sparrow. *Proc Natl Acad Sci USA* 1979;76:999.

Functional Neural Transplantation,
edited by S. B. Dunnett and A. Björklund.
Raven Press, Ltd., New York © 1994.

20

Recovery of Function After Spinal Cord Injury: Transplantation Strategies

Barbara S. Bregman

Department of Cell Biology, Georgetown University School of Medicine, Division of Neurobiology, Washington, DC 20007

Neural tissue transplantation techniques have been used extensively to understand mechanisms underlying central nervous system (CNS) development, anatomic plasticity, and regeneration after injury in the developing and mature nervous system and to promote recovery of function after CNS injury. Our greatest understanding of transplant-mediated CNS plasticity and recovery of function to date has derived from studies of experimental models of nigrostriatal lesions (see 2,14,18,19,25,68, and this volume, for reviews). Neural grafts may influence recovery of function within the host nervous system by a variety of mechanisms, ranging from nonspecific consequences of implantation, trophic actions on the host brain, altering the degree of anatomic sprouting of host pathways and diffuse release of hormones or neurotransmitters, to more specific mechanisms involving reinnervation of the host CNS by cells within the graft and the establishment of reciprocal connections between the host and graft (see 2,14,18,19,25,68, and other chapters in this volume for reviews). Much less is now known concerning transplant-mediated recovery of function after spinal cord injury. The requirements for anatomic and functional repair after spinal cord injury may be considerably more complex than for recovery from other types of CNS injury, in which restoration of neurotrans-

mitter levels may suffice for substantial functional improvement. Experimental studies over the past 20 years have now demonstrated that a variety of transplantation strategies alter the anatomic consequences of spinal injury, and may provide an anatomic substrate to subserve recovery of function.

Spinal cord injury in mammals is characterized by immediate and severe loss of sensory, motor, and reflex function below the level of injury, which is then succeeded by some recovery of function mediated by mechanisms intrinsic to the host nervous system. The mechanisms underlying this recovery are not entirely understood, although several possible mechanisms that might contribute to recovery have been suggested. This chapter reviews some of the mechanisms intrinsic to the host CNS that may contribute to recovery of function after spinal cord injury, reviews some of the anatomic and behavioral consequences of spinal cord injury in mammals, and examines ways in which neural tissue transplantation approaches may contribute both to enhance recovery of function and to help clarify the mechanisms underlying recovery of function. Data is reviewed that suggest that after spinal cord injury in mammals, transplantation strategies permit recovery of motor function both by specific mechanisms (i.e., permitting the regeneration of particular descending and segmental pathways, and restoring specific synaptic input to denervated targets within the spinal cord) as well as by nonspecific mechanisms (such as providing trophic support for injured neurons or by providing a terrain that permits axonal elongation). We review data to indicate that transplants of fetal spinal cord tissue mediate recovery of function after spinal cord injury in both neonatal and adult mammals and suggest that the mechanisms underlying transplant-mediated recovery differ between newborn and adult operates. In each of these studies that examine the effects of transplants on recovery of function, despite significant transplant-mediated recovery of function after spinal cord injury, permanent deficits in reflex and locomotor function persist. This suggests that combinations of interventions may be required to restore function to normal levels.

EXPERIMENTAL CONSIDERATIONS

Normal Control of Spinal Cord Function

The anatomic circuitry underlying rhythmic, alternating-stepping movements is intrinsic with the spinal cord and is known as the spinal pattern generator for locomotion (SPGL; 80,81,145; Fig. 1A). Normally, the spinal pattern generator for locomotion is under control and modulation by segmental sensory afferent influences, intersegmental (propriospinal) influences, and descending (suprasegmental) control from brain stem and cortical regions.

Research, largely from studies of normal motor control in mammals (primarily cats and, more recently, in rats) has suggested that, although the basic circuitry underlying locomotion lies within the spinal cord, particular pathways contribute particular aspects to the initiation and performance of locomotion (80,81,145). For example, most mammals are capable of goal-directed lo-

comotion, including the ability to avoid obstacles, in the absence of the cerebral cortex. Under normal conditions, the cortex appears to contribute to fine control and volitional positioning of the limbs during conditions requiring accurate foot placement during locomotion (81). Corticospinal pathways also make specific contributions to reflex motor control, mediating particular reflex responses, such as low-threshold contact-placing responses (3,31–34,57,62). Decerebrate mammals are also capable of locomotion, but lack the goal-directed initiation of locomotion and are unable to avoid obstacles. The mesencephalic locomotor region acts as a command center, capable of initiating and modulating locomotion, with the basic circuitry of the alternating-stepping movements being located at spinal cord levels. Brain stem–spinal pathways also contribute to the postural support and equilibrium required for locomotor function. Similarly, a variety of postural and segmental reflex circuits are organized at segmental (spinal cord) and brain stem–spinal levels. The extent to which similar segmental and suprasegmental circuitry underlying locomotor function exists in primates (including humans) is now unclear. Since the basic organization of locomotor control is so highly conserved during phylogeny (80,81), it is reasonable to assume that much of the basic organization may be preserved in primates.

Spinal cord lesion removes the descending suprasegmental and propriospinal control over the spinal cord circuitry either completely (transection) or partially (hemisection, contusion injury), alters the balance between excitatory and inhibitory influences, and results in a loss of function caudal to the site of injury. The loss of function after spinal cord injury is invariably followed by some subsequent recovery of function. Since those pathways that were injured (axotomized) do not regenerate, the motor behavior that recovers must be mediated by alterations in the remaining undamaged pathways. The potential intrinsic mechanisms underlying recovery of function after spinal cord injury have been the subject of several recent reviews (72,74–77). The plasticity of intrinsic host systems in response to injury is discussed briefly here, since recovery of function based on transplant–mediated interventions must be distinguished from recovery mediated by host systems (naturally occurring recovery) unrelated to the transplant and must be distinguished from the locomotor stepping movements mediated by the SPGL and independent of supraspinal and propriospinal control.

Intrinsic Mechanisms Underlying Recovery of Function

There are several potential mechanisms that may contribute to naturally occurring recovery of function after spinal cord injury. For example, in the absence of descending input to the SPGL, previously ineffective synapses (silent synapses; 174) may be recruited and may contribute to the activation of segmental reflex activity at a spinal cord level. The sensitivity of the neurons composing the SPGL may be altered as a consequence of spinal cord injury (denervation suprasensitivity, up-regulation of receptors); if so, lower levels of neurotransmitters at a segmental level may become sufficient to elicit a response. It has been suggested that such mechanisms may contribute to the early stages of recovery from spinal shock. Some of the other intrinsic mechanisms that may contribute to recovery of function after spinal cord injury include behavioral substitution, physiologic recovery (23,24), and remyelination (20,58) of injured, but intact, axonal pathways. Anatomic sprouting of undamaged pathways has also been implicated in recovery of function after spinal cord injury at birth or at maturity (69,70,72,74,75,77,119,128). These studies have demonstrated that sprout-

ing of undamaged pathways is not a random response to injury, but must be regulated in some manner, such that a hierarchy of pathways that sprout in response to a particular injury exists (69,71,72). Similarly, there appears to be a sequential and absolute hierarchy in the recovery of function that occurs. The sequence of recovery of function after spinal cord hemisection in cats is representative of the stages of recovery that occur after a variety of spinal cord injury models (32,72,74–76,85). Immediately following the lesion, there is a dramatic loss of function caudal and ipsilateral to the lesion; both reflexes and locomotion are abolished. Reflex responses (tendon reflexes, hind-limb postural reflexes, such as placing and hopping) are earliest to recover. This reflex recovery is accompanied by recovery of crude locomotion, characterized by a wide base of support and abnormal limb movement patterns. Somewhat later, accurate locomotion over difficult terrains, including more normal limb patterns returns. It has been suggested that this second stage of recovery may reflect the contribution of the contralateral descending pathways to recovery. Anatomic reorganization (sprouting) of undamaged pathways has been identified at a time that correlates with the time course of functional recovery (72,77, 85).

In most models of spinal cord injury and recovery of function that have been examined, the behavior that recovers is often not identical with that initially present. Despite recovery of function, which is often considerable, permanent deficits in motor function persist; full recovery fails to occur. Goldberger (72) has recently reviewed some of the ways in which behavioral methods can be used to predict and to understand the mechanisms underlying spinal cord plasticity. The potential mechanisms underlying plasticity and recovery of function after spinal cord injury can be used as a framework to understand and to predict neural tissue transplantation strategies that

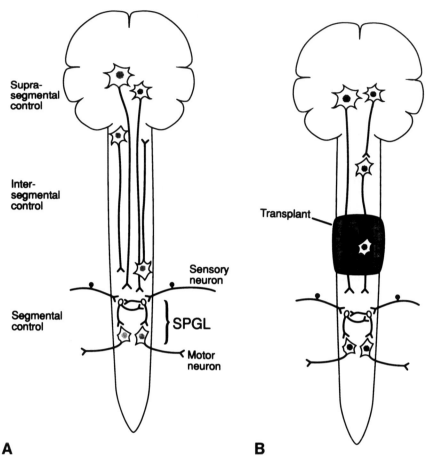

A   **B**

FIG. 1. A: Schematic representation of mechanisms contributing to normal motor control. The pair of oval neurons within the spinal cord represent the spinal pattern generator for locomotion (*SPGL*). This intrinsic circuitry is normally modulated by segmental sensory, descending (suprasegmental) and propriospinal (intersegmental) influences. Spinal cord lesions interrupt this modulation either entirely (transection) or partially (hemisection, contusion). Recovery of function after spinal cord injury occurs mediated by mechanisms intrinsic to the undamaged CNS pathways. This recovery by undamaged host pathways must be distinguished from any transplant-mediated influences. **B**: Potential mechanisms by which transplant of fetal spinal cord tissue placed into the lesion site can modify the response of the host CNS to injury and mediate recovery of function. Transplants of fetal CNS or PNS tissue may limit the initial consequences of spinal cord injury, enhance anatomic plasticity of host pathways, and subserve recovery of function. Possible mechanisms for repair: This schematic diagram illustrates several potential mechanisms by which transplants of fetal CNS tissue may repair the injured spinal cord and mediate recovery of function (see text for further discussion). Organization of the diagram is similar to A. Data exist in the literature to support each of the potential mechanisms illustrated. Transplants modify the response of immature and mature axotomized neurons to injury. Target-specific transplants rescue immature axotomized neurons from retrograde cell death and prevent the retrograde "dieback" of mature axons after injury. After lesions during development, both late-developing and regenerating axons are able to grow into and through the site of transplantation. After lesions in the adult, host axons are able to grow into both PNS and CNS transplants placed into the lesion site. At the site of injury, transplants may provide a source of trophic support for injured neurons and may provide a favorable terrain for axonal elongation. Two models of transplant function are illustrated: bridge and relay. After lesions at birth, the transplant serves as a bridge for supraspinal axons across the lesion site and to reach targets within the host spinal cord caudal to the transplant. Host axons project into the transplant and neurons within the transplant also project to the host spinal cord, setting up the potential for a relay of suprasegmental control to

will enhance functional recovery after spinal cord injury.

Potential Mechanisms Underlying Transplant-Mediated Repair

There are several possible mechanisms by which transplants of fetal CNS or peripheral nervous system (PNS) tissue can influence the response to injury and mediate recovery of function after injury. Transplants may replace particular populations of neurons, permit the reestablishment of specific connections between the host and the transplant, or replace or restore levels of neurotransmitters, hormones, or neurotrophic factors lost by the injury. There are excellent reviews of neural tissue transplantation techniques available (13, 14,18,38,42,52,59,68,118). We emphasize here the use of neural tissue transplantation approaches to mediate CNS regeneration and recovery of function after spinal cord injury in developing and mature mammals. Figure 1B illustrates some of the possible mechanisms by which transplants of fetal CNS tissue can influence the response of the developing and mature spinal cord to injury. After spinal cord injury either at birth or at maturity, the suprasegmental control over the intrinsic segmental circuitry of the spinal cord is disrupted. A transplant of fetal spinal cord tissue may serve as a bridge to permit the regrowth of axons from spinal and supraspinal levels across the site of spinal cord injury to reach targets within the cord caudal to the lesion. Transplants of fetal spinal cord tissue also provide a population of neurons at the site of injury that

may serve as a relay to convey supraspinal control to levels caudal to the lesion site. At a cellular level, the fetal transplants may provide a source of diffusible trophic support for immature and mature axotomized neurons (28,35,39,53,60,84), may inhibit the formation of a glial scar at the site of injury (91,138), may inhibit local toxic influences at the site of injury (163), may replace particular neuronal populations lost by injury (98,158), and may provide a favorable substrate (mechanical, extracellular matrix, guidance cues) to support axonal growth across the injury site (26,27,29, 30,37,136,168). In addition, transplantation of particular neuronal populations (serotonergic or noradrenergic neurons, or genetically modified cells producing particular neurotransmitters) into regions of the SPGL deprived of suprasegmental control may directly serve to restore levels of particular neurotransmitters caudal to the lesion site, reestablishing a more normal balance between excitation and inhibition of the spinal cord circuitry (44,118,120,131,132). The data supporting these potential transplant-mediated influences on anatomic repair and recovery of function are reviewed in the sections that follow. Each of these potential mechanisms of transplant influence would be expected to enhance recovery of function to levels greater than that obtained by intrinsic host mechanisms.

Behavioral Methods to Assess Recovery of Function

One of the major issues in assessing recovery of function after spinal cord or other

---

caudal spinal levels. After lesions in the adult, host axons grow into, but not through the transplant. Thus, in the adult, the transplant is in a position to serve as a relay. The transplant may modify the environment at the site of injury by limiting the glial response of the host spinal cord to injury, by providing a source of trophic support for injured host neurons, and by ameliorating some of the excitotoxic secondary effects of spinal cord injury. In addition to the mechanisms illustrated at the injury site, neural tissue transplantation of defined neuronal populations may be placed into the target area deprived of intrinsic control (by transection or by neurochemical depletion, for example) and serve to replace neurons or neurotransmitter lost by the injury and influence the activity of the spinal pattern generator for locomotion directly.

CNS injury is defining precisely what function is lost and what function recovers. Furthermore, it is essential to distinguish naturally occurring recovery of function, mediated by alterations in the host nervous system, from any recovery that is due to clinical or experimental intervention. In assessing recovery of function after spinal cord (or any other type of CNS injury), it is important to recognize that casual behavioral observation is not sufficient to determine if a particular intervention, such as transplantation, is responsible for mediating recovery of function. Some of the early studies of neural tissue transplantation on recovery of function after spinal cord injury failed to take intrinsic host mechanisms subserving functional recovery into account and erroneously attributed recovery to transplant interventions that could more properly be accounted for by plasticity of host systems. The American Paralysis Association has recently issued guidelines (73) for criteria for assessing recovery of function after spinal cord injury, similar to those established earlier to determine if regeneration of CNS pathways has occurred (82). In transplantation or other strategies designed to increase functional recovery after spinal cord or other CNS injury, it is important to address not only that recovery occurs, but also to identify the mechanisms underlying the recovery. If we can understand the mechanisms responsible for recovery of function, we will be in a better position to increase the extent of that recovery. Methods that rely on composite ratings of an animal's overall performance, although appropriate for screening groups of animals with spinal cord injury, are insufficient to demonstrate whether a particular treatment has had a specific effect on motor function, or the degree to which function is affected.

In rats, a variety of behavioral methods have been used to assess recovery of function after spinal cord injury (41,67,104,142, 166,176). Most of the methods now available, however, do not examine specific components of functional recovery and in-

dividual limb function. Specific methods to assess recovery of function are needed that not only examine the ability to move, but also examine the quality of the movement itself (73). One behavioral method commonly used to measure functional recovery is the Tarlov scale (166), which assesses open-field locomotion with a rating scale. Another method frequently used to measure behavioral recovery after spinal cord injury is the inclined plane test (142), which is a measure of an animal's ability to maintain its position on an inclined plane. More recently, both of these tests have been combined with measurements of reflexes to produce a combined behavioral score (CBS) to give an overall measure of an animal's behavioral performance (67,104,176). All of these tests assess an animal's overall performance, but are not sufficient to demonstrate whether a particular treatment has had a specific effect on functional recovery, or to demonstrate the degree to which particular sensory and motor functions are affected.

More recently, a series of sensitive quantitative methods to assess the recovery of locomotor function in rats (30,108–110) have been established. Many of these behavioral approaches have been used previously in cats to study normal locomotor function and recovery of motor function after spinal cord injury (31,32,69,70,72,74–76). The methods are designed to assess individual limb movements and to isolate the motor capacity of the involved limb(s) from compensatory movements in unaffected limbs. Both qualitative and quantitative measurements are made of reflex or triggered movements and overground and treadmill locomotion. The methods, which examine specific reflex responses and specific components of motor behavior, are sensitive to subtle differences in the pattern of locomotion and individual limb movements. Several of the tests can be used to assess the development of locomotor function as well as the mature response. Postural reflex testing and locomotor function under conditions of graded difficulty are examined, and the motor capacity of individual limbs is assessed. Animals are trained to cross runways, walk on a treadmill, and to climb onto a platform (Fig. 2). Such training is essential to ensure that any lack of movement after injury is due to an inability to move, rather than simply a reluctance to move owing to an alteration in the animal's motivation. The animal's performance is videotaped for subsequent quantitative analysis (Fig. 3). The pattern of overground and treadmill locomotion is also examined by footprint analysis (Fig. 4). Spinal cord injury alters an animal's reflex responses, and deficits are evident in locomotor function. No single test is sufficient to assess recovery of function after spinal cord injury; rather, a combination of tests, each examining particular components of normal and recovered motor function, are required. The methods used to assess recovery of locomotor function are specific, sensitive, and allow individual limb movements to be isolated. The specificity and sensitivity of these methods also enables one to begin to understand the contribution of specific anatomic pathways to the recovery of specific

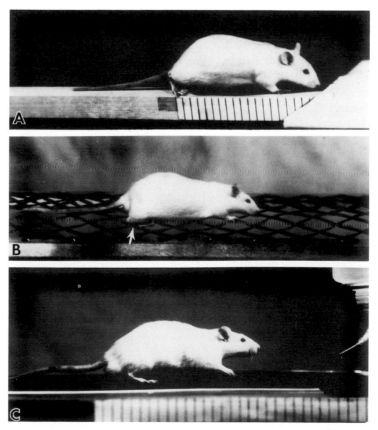

FIG. 2. A, B: Examples of some of the methods used for quantitative analysis of recovery of locomotor function. The animals cross runways of varying difficulty for a water reward. The time to cross, the number of forelimb steps, and the number of errors (footslips through the rungs of difficult runways) are determined from videotapes of the crossings. In **B,** the *arrow* indicates an error with the right hindlimb (i.e., the limb falls through the hole, rather than being placed on the rung for support). (From ref. 110, with permission.)

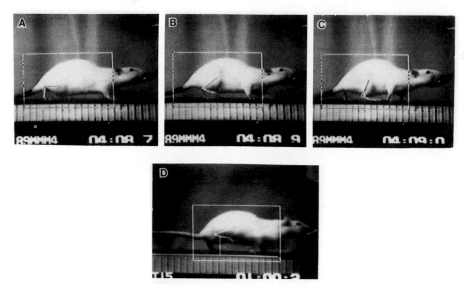

FIG. 3. Kinematic analysis. Photographs are taken from the videotapes of normal animal (**A,B,C**) and an animal that received a spinal cord hemisection at birth (**D**) on the treadmill. The images are frozen at selected phases of the step cycle. Points are digitized, and joint angles are calculated. A comparison of midswing in a normal (B) and a lesioned (D) animals indicates that the lesioned animal has a marked hypermetria during the swing phase. (From ref. 110, with permission.)

sensory and motor functions. For example, the contact-placing response has been closely associated with the corticospinal pathway. The development of contact-placing responses has been linked with the maturation of the corticospinal pathway (3,31–34,57), and the removal of the corticospinal tract results in the loss of contact-placing responses (31,32,57,109). These methods are able to differentiate between contact- and proprioceptive-placing responses and specifically examine contact-placing. This specificity in the behavioral analysis enables one to examine the contribution of a particular anatomic system to intrinsic or to transplant-mediated recovery of function. Physiologic methods also permit a more detailed analysis of the effects of spinal cord injury and subsequent recovery of function. For example, by examining the segmental spinal cord circuitry, alterations in descending control can be identified, and the influence of naturally occurring and transplant-induced interventions can be evaluated (44, 133,135,139,169). Electromyography (EMG)

can be used to determine the extent to which the sequence and duration of muscle contractions that recover after injury are similar to that in the normal pattern of locomotion.

The use of such specific methods enables one to begin to address the mechanisms underlying recovery of function following spinal cord injury. This specificity permits identification of particular behavioral deficits after spinal cord injury and allows one to determine which functional capacities recover after such injury and which fail to recover. In addition, the sensitivity of the tests enables one to evaluate the effects of potential treatments to enhance the intrinsic recovery of function (36,108,110,111, 164).

Spinal Cord Injury Models

Several different experimental models have been used in studies of spinal cord injury, repair, and recovery of function. Each

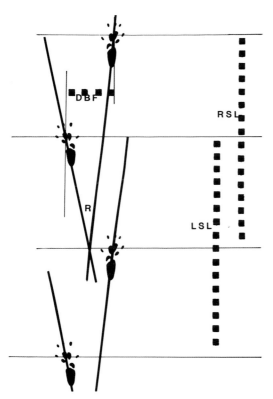

FIG. 4. Footprint illustration. A reconstruction of hindpaw prints illustrating the measurements used. Base of support (*DBF*), stride length (*RSL, LSL*) and limb rotation (*R*) are measured from the prints. This illustrates the basis for the quantitative measurements of recovery of function illustrated in Figs. 15–19. (From ref. 108, with permission.)

has certain advantages from experimental and conceptual views, and each has contributed in an important way to our understanding of some of the neurobiologic issues concerning the CNS response following spinal cord injury. One difficulty in the multiplicity of approaches, however, is the inability to make straightforward assumptions about the extent to which principles demonstrated with one approach apply uniformly to other approaches. The consequences of grafting various types of neural tissue into the damaged spinal cord have been explored under a wide range of lesion conditions. These lesion and transplantation models have been reviewed re-

cently (2,14,18,36,134–136,167), particularly in relation to the anatomic consequences of transplantation. Some of the advantages and disadvantages of the various approaches are summarized briefly here, and their contribution to our understanding of anatomic repair and recovery of function after spinal cord injury is addressed in the following discussion.

Surgical Models

One classic approach to the study of spinal cord injury has been to interrupt the pathways within the spinal cord surgically, either unilaterally (hemisection) or completely (transection). An advantage of the hemisection model is the availability of an internal comparison between intact and lesioned pathways. A disadvantage of this and other partial lesion paradigms in studies of recovery of function after spinal cord injury is that care must be taken to distinguish the contribution of the reorganization of host systems to recovery from that of transplant-mediated mechanisms. The clear advantage of transection models is that the lesion is complete, and a contribution of intact host pathways does not confound the behavioral analysis. One major disadvantage of transection models is the requirement for extensive and intensive postsurgical animal care to prevent morbidity and mortality. An additional disadvantage is the difficulty in maintaining an adequate interface between the ends of the transected spinal cord and any transplant placed within the lesion site.

In all of the studies to suggest that transplants have made a contribution to recovery of function, it is essential that the lesion be reconstructed serially to ensure that the pathways intended to be lesioned were, in fact, lesioned, and that the extent of the lesion is equivalent between transplant and lesion control groups. This has been particularly problematic in some of the transection studies, since it is quite easy to spare host fibers inadvertently; even a few spared fibers can then contribute substantially to recovery of function. In fact, some of the early controversy concerning the presence or absence of functional recovery after spinal cord injury can be attributed to inadequate verification of the nature and extent of the lesion and the unintentional sparing of pathways.

Traumatic Injury Models

More recently, a variety of traumatic compression or contusion injury models have been introduced for the study of spinal cord injury (41,67,104,139,178). One advantage cited for this approach is that such trauma yields histopathologic and pathophysiologic changes that closely resemble human spinal cord injury. The potential disadvantages include variability in the extent of injury between animals and between laboratories, and difficulty in determining which pathways are damaged and which remain to contribute to recovery of function. Most of the studies of spinal cord injury to date have examined the response of the acutely injured spinal cord. Only recently has the capacity of the chronically injured spinal cord for repair and recovery of function been examined. The studies suggest that chronically injured neurons maintain the capacity to regrow axons, if provided an appropriate environment such as PNS or fetal CNS tissue (88,91,92).

Neuronal Depletion Models

Another approach to understanding spinal cord injury and repair has been to use neurochemical or surgical approaches to deplete particular populations of neurons or their axons within the spinal cord. For example, neurochemical lesions have been used to ablate descending monoaminergic fibers to the spinal cord (8,15–19,44,120, 121,124,125). Similarly, excitotoxic lesions can ablate spinal interneurons, and neonatal axotomy of the sciatic (other peripheral)

nerve can be used to deplete the spinal cord of populations of motor neurons. The advantage here is clearly the ability to lesion specific, identified populations of cells or their processes. In studies of recovery of function care must be taken to ensure that the populations of neurons that were intended to be depleted are depleted, and that spontaneous regeneration of those populations of axons has not occurred at the time of the behavioral analysis (124,125).

TRANSPLANTATION IN THE INJURED SPINAL CORD

Intraspinal Replacement of Particular Neurons or Neurotransmitters

One approach to recovery of function after spinal cord injury has been to directly restore a more normal balance to the SPGL between excitation and inhibition. Studies of spinal cord transection (without any neural tissue transplantation) indicate that one way to improve locomotor function dramatically is to restore a pharmacologic balance between excitation and inhibition and, thereby, restore a more normal function of the SPGL. After spinal cord transection, adult cats are completely paraplegic. They are unable to support weight on their hindlimbs and are unable to step either voluntarily or in response to external stimulation, such as the passive movement of a treadmill. The noradrenergic system seems to be particularly important in initiating hindlimb-stepping movements (44,61,80,81), and administration of noradrenergic agonists or precursors can elicit such movements (5,61,80,144,145). Administration of various monoaminergic agonists and precursors indicate that the monoaminergic descending systems can modify, rather specifically, different aspects of the locomotor pattern and, in addition to altering the activity of the SPGL, can also alter the activity of the cutaneous afferent input to the spinal cord (61,80,81).

One strategy in neural tissue transplantation to enhance recovery of function after spinal cord injury has been to transplant monoaminergic neurons directly into a spinal cord that has been depleted of its normal monoaminergic innervation by surgical transection, neurochemical depletion, or both (16,19,44,50,51,63,64,120,121,130–132). Embryonic noradrenergic neurons taken from the locus coeruleus (16,44,50,51) and embryonic serotonergic neurons from the embryonic raphe nuclei (63,64,130–132) survive, differentiate, and extend axons within the denervated mature or developing spinal cord. Following transplantation of cell suspensions, or cell aggregates, or whole-tissue transplants, embryonic monoaminergic neurons extend axons up to 2 cm within the host spinal cord. Studies of transplanted raphe neurons indicate that the transplanted embryonic neurons are capable of establishing morphologically appropriate synapses with denervated targets within the spinal cord (63,130–132), such as the intermediolateral cell column, dorsal horn laminae, and ventral horn. Thus, in the serotonergic system, neural tissue transplants are able to restore specific connections to denervated targets. Transplants of noradrenergic-containing locus coeruleus neurons also project to appropriate areas of gray matter (ventral and intermediate gray) deprived of its normal noradrenergic input (16,44,50,120), but the extent to which specific synapses with host target neurons are established is uncertain. The transplants of embryonic monoaminergic neurons may be in a position to restore function to the denervated spinal cord either by a diffuse release of neurotransmitter, which can activate the SPGL pharmacologically, or by specific synaptic activation of the neural circuitry.

Descending noradrenergic systems have been implicated in various spinal functions, including regulation of nociception, autonomic reflexes, and motor activities, such as the initiation of locomotion and enhancement of flexion reflexes. Physiologic recording of flexion reflexes in rats in which normal input was depleted by 6-hydroxydopamine (6-OHDA) lesions, was compared in animals with and without transplants of fetal catecholaminergic or noradrenergic neurons (44,120). Normal levels of norepinephrine and its metabolites are restored by injections of cell suspensions of embryonic noradrenergic neurons. Animals with transplants of locus coeruleus had significantly stronger flexion reflexes than nongrafted or sham-grafted control animals (44,120). About 30% of this enhancement of reflex activity was blocked specifically by an α-adrenergic blocker. The remainder of the enhanced flexion activity may be attributed to transplanted neurons of other transmitter phenotypes. Recovery of function mediated by transplants is further supported by other studies (180) that indicate that noradrenergic transplants permit the recovery of stepping activity in rats with surgical spinal cord transection. Recovery of specific autonomic reflexes has been observed in rats with transection and transplants of serotonergic neurons. Penile erection and ejaculation are produced by spinal reflexes that are under supraspinal control (117). Reflex ejaculation was restored in transected rats receiving transplants of raphe neurons. The specificity of the recovery is suggested by the observation that lesion-only or transected rats receiving noradrenergic transplants did not recover these autonomic reflexes (130–132). Since serotonergic innervation contributes normally to locomotor as well as autonomic function, such transplants are theoretically in a position to contribute to recovery of locomotor control after spinal cord injury, although this has not been tested experimentally.

Taken together, these studies suggest that replacement of particular neurotransmitters at the level of the SPGL restores reflex and locomotor function by altering the balance between excitation and inhibition (nonspecific mechanisms) and by restoring particular suprasegmental control of the segmental circuitry directly (specific mechanisms). Additional approaches of transplanting genetically modified cells (astrocytes, fibroblasts, neuroepithelial stem cells) designed to produce specific neurotrophic factors or neurotransmitters have been explored in intracerebral-grafting approaches (47,65,66,175). Such genetically modified cells may be in a position to restore function after spinal cord injury by mechanisms similar to those just described, such as restoring particular neurotransmitters directly to the circuitry of the SPGL. This has not yet been addressed.

Another approach to restoring function after spinal cord injury involves replacing particular populations of neurons, such as motor neurons, depleted by injury or neurodegenerative disorders. One model to examine depletion of particular neuronal populations within the spinal cord has been use of excitotoxic lesioning with kainic acid to deplete spinal interneurons, sparing both afferent axons and axons of passage (122, 123). A week later, dissociated embryonic spinal cord tissue was transplanted into the lesioned spinal cord. The growth of host segmental and suprasegmental afferents into the transplant has been examined using a variety of neuroanatomic tracing approaches. It is important to recognize that this lesion model does not axotomize neurons. Thus, the anatomic growth in response to injury represents axonal sprouting of undamaged host axons, rather than regenerative growth. This difference in lesioning methods, and the difference in assessing sprouting versus regenerative growth likely accounts for some of the differences in the degree to which particular descending and segmental populations grow into the transplant after excitotoxic lesions, as compared with spinal cord hemisection or transection models. Sprouting monoaminergic axons after excitotoxic lesion (122, 123) of the adult spinal cord project throughout the entire transplant, whereas after axotomy by surgical lesions, these same populations of host axons project only short distances within the transplants (36,97,

111,135,136,139). Recovery of function has not as yet been examined in excitotoxic models of spinal cord injury. If the reestablishment of specific neuroanatomic pathways with transplanted neurons (relay) restores particular aspects of reflex or locomotor function, however, one would expect to see differences in the extent of recovery between the excitotoxic and surgical axotomy models that parallel the differences in the extent of anatomic growth of descending monoaminergic pathways into the transplants (discussed later).

Other approaches to restore particular populations of neurons have sought both to replace motor neurons and to restore the circuitry between the motor neurons in the spinal cord and their peripheral targets. Host motor neurons depleted either surgically, by the creation of a cavity within the spinal cord or by neonatal axotomy, can be replaced by embryonic spinal cord transplants or by embryonic cell suspensions enriched for motor neurons (48,49,87,158). In these experiments, investigators have sought to restore some of the segmental circuitry by providing a bridge of peripheral nerve tissue to guide regrowing axons to targets in the periphery. In both approaches, embryonic motoneurons and dorsal root ganglion neurons survive and undergo phenotypic maturation. Retrograde neuroanatomic-tracing techniques indicate that transplanted neurons are able to extend axons into the peripheral nerve segment. In experiments in which a peripheral nerve bridge was placed between host spinal cord and muscle (87), electrophysiologic stimulation of the peripheral nerve graft elicited end plate potentials. These potentials were cholinergic, suggesting that host motor neurons were able to reinnervate skeletal muscle targets. The extent to which transplanted neurons also establish functional reinnervation of target structures has not been determined.

Although much of the work on the influence of transplants on functional recovery after spinal cord injury has emphasized recovery of reflex and locomotor function, transplants also have the potential to modify the sensory activity of the spinal cord circuitry. The loss of sensory function after spinal cord injury, as well as sensory paresthesias and hyperesthesias are often as devastating an impairment as the loss of motor function. Studies of transplants of adrenal medullary chromaffin cells into the subarachnoid space can increase the levels of catecholamines and opioid peptides and decrease pain sensitivity (146–150). Studies have demonstrated that such transplants are effective in reducing sensitivity to both acute noxious stimuli and chronic pain (146–150).

Taken together, these studies suggest that one mechanism by which transplants permit recovery of function is by restoring specific suprasegmental control over spinal cord circuitry. Transplants may also alter the segmental circuitry in a nonspecific manner, permitting greater activity of SPGL than after lesion alone. Replacement of particular neuropeptides characteristic of segmental afferent input would also be in a position to alter the function of the SPGL to enhance function.

Peripheral Nerve Grafts to Repair Spinal Cord Injury

Another approach to anatomic and functional repair after spinal cord injury has been the use of transplantation strategies to bridge the lesion site. Early studies, using segments of peripheral nerve to bridge the site of a spinal cord transection or to provide an alternate route for medullary neurons to reach spinal cord levels, were important in establishing that specific mature central neurons were capable of regrowth following spinal cord injury (1,2,56,140, 141). After spinal cord transection, a bridge of peripheral nerve placed between the cut ends of the spinal cord supports the growth of dorsal root ganglion neurons, axons of propriospinal neurons, and axons of supra-

segmental origin into the peripheral nerve bridge (140,141). Although these populations of axons are able to elongate considerable distances (10–35 mm) within the peripheral nerve environment (1,2,56,140, 141), when they reenter the CNS environment, they terminate within a few millimeters of the host–graft interface. The function of these regenerated axons within the peripheral nerve bridges in the spinal cord has not been examined recently. Early studies (101,102,165) suggesting that peripheral nerve bridges were able to restore function after spinal cord injury were equivocal at best, and failed to distinguish between recovery mediated by plasticity of host systems caudal to the lesion, and failed to verify that host fibers were not spared unintentionally.

Studies of regenerating retinal ganglion axons in a PNS environment indicate that these axons are able to form extensive arborizations and form extensive synaptic connections with host tectal neurons (46, 160,171–173). These regenerated axons are capable of eliciting photically activated transsynaptic-evoked potentials in the superior colliculus (105). The extent to which axons' growth across such PNS grafts reestablishes functional connections following spinal cord injury remains to be determined. Studies by Richardson and colleagues demonstrated that recently injured neurons have considerable growth potential and revealed a great deal about some of the neurobiologic issues surrounding regrowth in the injured spinal cord. Other studies have indicated that chronically injured neurons are also capable of growth through peripheral nerve grafts (88), and this growth can be increased by the administration of exogenous nerve growth factor (89,90).

Grafts of Central and Peripheral Glia for Repair of the Injured Spinal Cord

Based largely on the studies that indicate that elements contained within peripheral nerve grafts are able to support the growth of central axons, some investigations have explored the contribution of cultured peripheral nonneuronal cells to stimulate axon growth in the injured spinal cord (20–22,58,86,114,115,126,177,179). These studies have demonstrated axons associated with the Schwann cell components within the lesion site, but the origin of the axons within the grafts have not been determined. It is likely that many of these axons are of dorsal root ganglion origin (114,115). Other studies examined the potential for combinations of cultured Schwann cells and dorsal root ganglion neurons to support the growth of corticospinal axons within a spinal cord lesion site in newborn rats (107). However, corticospinal axons did not enter the Schwann cell–dorsal root ganglion grafts. Observations that corticospinal axons are able to grow through fetal spinal cord grafts (37) after spinal cord injury at a similar stage of development suggest that perhaps some trophic or tropic influence required by corticospinal neurons is unavailable in the Schwann cell–dorsal root ganglion grafts, the growth of the dorsal root ganglion neurons may precede that of the corticospinal axons, making the Schwann cells unavailable, or perhaps the presence of neuronal elements in these transplants down-regulates growth-promoting influences in the peripheral nerve elements. Mixed populations of dissociated dorsal root ganglion neuronal and nonneuronal cells also have been used in the adult spinal cord following contusion injury (86). Whereas these mixed transplants did not lead to recovery of function, as assessed by general observations of motor activity, neither did they lead to increased deficits (86).

The ability of immature astrocytes to support axonal growth after spinal cord injury also has been examined (106,159). Immature astrocytes are able to support the growth of dorsal root axons into the spinal cord in the adult, and some of these axons form structurally normal synapses within the cord. The functional effects of such grafts, however, have not been examined. Other studies have transplanted astrocytes into the injured spinal cord (10,11) dorsal column. Although some of the labeling methods make the study difficult to interpret unambiguously, the authors suggest that the grafted astrocytes lead to functional improvement compared with lesion-only controls (10,11). They suggest that the effect on the host nervous system is indirect—that is, that the astrocytes may exert a trophic effect on host dorsal column neurons and prevent their atrophy (11).

Since some of the loss of function after spinal cord injury may represent loss of conduction in axons that remain intact (23), replacement of oligodendrocytes or Schwann cells at the site of injury might be expected to restore conduction and lead to improved function. Studies in myelin-deficient mutants indicate that transplanted oligodendrocytes or Schwann cells are capable of migrating long distances within the CNS and remyelinating axons (6,20–22, 78,113,143). To date, these studies have emphasized the anatomic repair of myelin; the functional contribution of the repaired myelin remains to be assessed. In contrast with the studies that suggest a beneficial role of oligodendrocytes in repair of demyelination of injured CNS axons, other studies have suggested that components of oligodendrocytes are inhibitory to the growth of axons (151,154,156,157), and that interfering with this inhibition leads to some modest growth of corticospinal axons, for example (151,153). The extent to which such strategies lead to improved function after spinal cord injury are currently under investigation (B. S. Bregman, E. Kunkel-Bagden, L. Schnell, and M. E. Schwab, unpublished results).

Transplantation of Fetal Spinal Cord Tissue Into the Site of Spinal Cord Injury

Another strategy to repair the injured spinal cord has been to place transplants of fetal spinal cord tissue directly into the spinal lesion site. Work from several laboratories has now established that transplants of fetal spinal cord (and other embryonic CNS tissues) survive and mature when placed into the injured spinal cord under a variety of lesion conditions (4,26,27,36,38,54,55,83, 88,91,92,95–98,122,123,127,134–137,139, 155,168). For example, after spinal cord hemisection or transection at birth or at maturity (Figs. 5 and 6), transplants of fetal spinal cord tissue survive, grow, and differentiate (26,27,39,98,135,136). Similar survival and maturation is observed under a variety of lesion paradigms, including surgical lesions and contusion injury, in both acute and chronic injury conditions. Neuroanatomic connections are established be-

tween the host CNS and the fetal tissue (whole tissue or suspension) transplants. Such transplants appear to have a wide range of effects on the host nervous system. Transplants may alter tissue oxygen tension levels in the lesion area (163). Abnormal metabolism in the spinal cord may contribute to some of the secondary pathologic changes after spinal cord injury (138). Transplants may also limit the reactive glial responses with the injured spinal cord (138). Studies of long-term injury models suggest that fetal spinal cord transplants may even reverse some of the gliosis that had developed (138). In addition, transplants provide trophic support for immature and mature axotomized neurons (28,30, 35,39). Such trophic support is able to res-

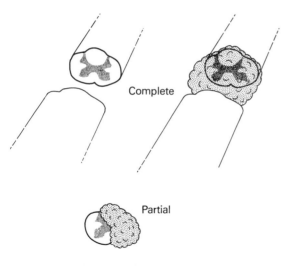

Complete

Partial

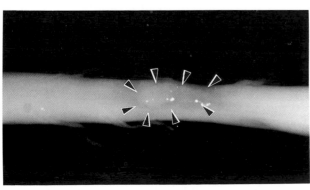

FIG. 5. Schematic diagram of the lesion-plus-transplant strategies for replacing neurons at the site of spinal cord transection or hemisection. Spinal cord lesions are made in developing or mature mammals, and transplants of fetal spinal cord placed into the lesion site. Adult spinal cord containing a transplant of fetal spinal cord tissue, approximately 2 months posttransplantation. Rostral is to the *left. Arrowheads* indicate the approximate border between transplant and host spinal cord. The transplant tissue appears more translucent than the surrounding host spinal cord.

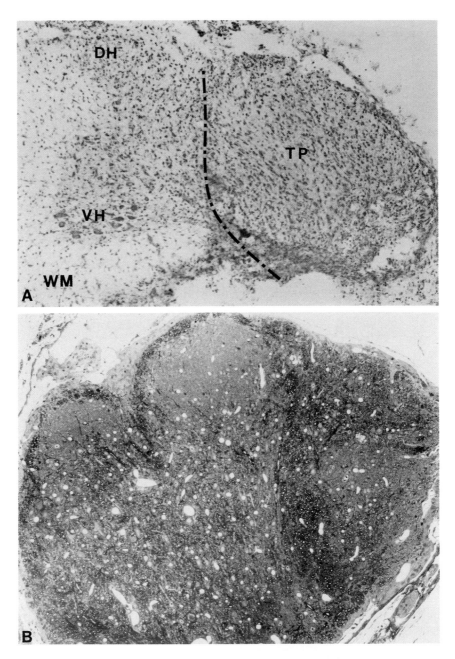

FIG. 6. Example of transplant of fetal spinal cord tissue placed into the site of a neonatal spinal cord hemisection (**A**) or transection (**B**). In both cases, the transplants develop, mature, and establish extensive areas of apposition with the host spinal cord. The host gray and white matter are visible on the *left side* of A. Border between host and transplant is indicated by *dashed line.* In B, the entire field of this photomicrograph is transplant tissue. Myelinated and lightly myelinated areas of transplant are visible.

cue permanently immature axotomized brain stem–spinal neurons from retrograde cell death (28,30,35,39) and prevent the retrograde retraction (dieback) of mature corticospinal axons after injury (37). Thus, the transplants may improve function by limiting some of the secondary consequences of spinal cord injury.

Neuroanatomic connections between the host and transplant are established. Some of the connections that have been demonstrated by neuroanatomic-tracing and immunocytochemical methods are summarized in Fig. 7. After spinal cord lesions at birth, transplants of fetal spinal cord tissue rescue immature axotomized brain stem–spinal neurons from injury-induced retrograde cell death in a target-specific manner (28,30,35). In the presence of a transplant, these rescued neurons are able to regenerate and to extend axons both into the transplant, and through it, to reach normal targets within the host spinal cord caudal to the lesion site (12,26,27,29,30). In addition, neurons within the transplant send their axons into the host spinal cord (30,39,97). Thus, after injury at birth, transplants are anatomically in a position to serve both as a bridge and as a relay (see Fig. 7). After

spinal cord injury in the adult, neurons within the transplant send their axons into the host spinal cord, and host neurons (corticospinal, raphe–spinal, coeruleospinal, intraspinal, and dorsal root) project axons into the transplant (30,37,39,40,91,92,95, 96,98,122,136,168). Axons of host origin form synapses within the transplanted tissue in both neonatal- and adult-lesioned animals (30,95–98). After injury in the adult, the transplant is in a position to serve as a relay to convey supraspinal control to the host spinal cord caudal to the injury. There is now no evidence for the ability of mature neurons to use the transplants as a bridge for injured axons to cross the lesion site.

Our model system of spinal cord lesions and transplants in newborn and adult rats provides an opportunity to identify the conditions that regulate and the mechanisms that underlie recovery of function after spinal cord injury. We hypothesize that transplants of fetal spinal cord tissue mediate recovery of function both by specific mechanisms (i.e., by permitting the regeneration of particular descending and segmental pathways) and by nonspecific mechanisms (such as providing trophic support, stimulating sprouting of host pathways, and so

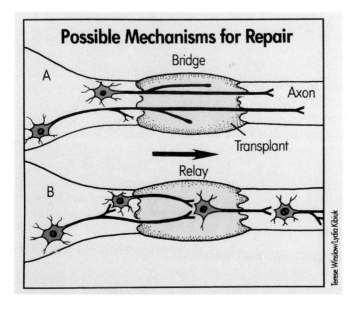

FIG. 7. Schematic diagram illustrating two potential mechanisms (*Bridge, relay*) by which transplants of fetal spinal cord tissue placed into the site of injury may repair the injured spinal cord of developing and mature mammals and mediate recovery of function. See text for description of these mechanisms.

forth). We also suggest that, although transplants of fetal spinal cord tissue mediate recovery of function after spinal cord injury in both neonatal and adult operates, they do so by different mechanisms.

The response of the immature spinal cord to injury often exhibits a greater amount of anatomic reorganization than the same injury in the adult (7,9,31–34,43,45,99,100, 103,112,116,119,152,162,170). Rerouting of late-developing pathways and a more robust axonal sprouting after neonatal lesions than observed after lesion in the adult contribute to this enhanced anatomic plasticity in the developing animal. Axonal sprouting after injury in the neonate is often a much more robust phenomenon than after injury in the adult. Axonal sprouting in the adult CNS is spatially restricted and is characterized by an increased density of an existing projection (74,76,77,79). Sprouting after lesions during development not only results in an increased density of innervation of a particular target area, but also results in an increased area of innervation. This may reflect either maintenance of exuberant projections normally present during early development, or *de novo* invasion of denervated areas by sprouting axons. Although it is generally assumed that the immature spinal cord responds to injury with greater anatomic plasticity, in fact, the response of particular spinal cord pathways to injury varies. Concomitant with greater anatomic plasticity of some pathways, in other pathways the immature neurons are more vulnerable to injury (28,31,34,35,39,40). For example, injury to the immature rubrospinal pathway results in massive retrograde cell death of axotomized red nucleus neurons, whereas injury to the mature pathway results in neuronal atrophy and increased gliosis within the nucleus, but little cell loss (31,34,129). Similarly, dorsal root axons are capable of robust sprouting after injury to the immature spinal cord, but exhibit more restricted growth in the adult after injury (74–77). The unique response of a particular pathway to spinal cord damage may reflect

the relative maturity of that pathway at the time of the damage. Different spinal cord pathways are at different relative stages of development at birth in the rat, and many continue to develop postnatally. The fibers of the corticospinal pathway, a late-developing pathway, enter and make synaptic contact within the spinal cord during the first 2 weeks postnatally (57,79). Other pathways, such as the rubrospinal, raphe–spinal, and dorsal root projections, are present at birth, but continue to mature postnatally (26,29,30). Coincident temporally with this anatomic maturation within the spinal cord is the maturation of many spinal cord reflexes and locomotion itself. The immature form of locomotion that the animals use at birth matures into the adult pattern postnatally. Therefore, both the anatomic and functional development of locomotion take place postnatally. Injury before the mature pattern of locomotion is established may have very different consequences on the loss and subsequent recovery of function than injury after the mature pattern has developed.

FACTORS INFLUENCING GRAFT–HOST INTERACTIONS IN THE SPINAL CORD

The Capacity of the Host Nervous System for Growth After Injury and Transplantation Decreases With Age

Just as the intrinsic capacity of the host CNS for axonal sprouting is more robust after lesions at birth, both the density and spatial extent of transplant-mediated growth is also much more robust after lesions at birth. This capacity for transplant-elicited growth decreases as the animal matures. This developmental decrease in the capacity of the host nervous system for growth after injury and transplantation is illustrated by the corticospinal pathway (37). Figure 8A is a schematic diagram illustrating the progressive postnatal restriction in corticospinal plasticity after lesions or le-

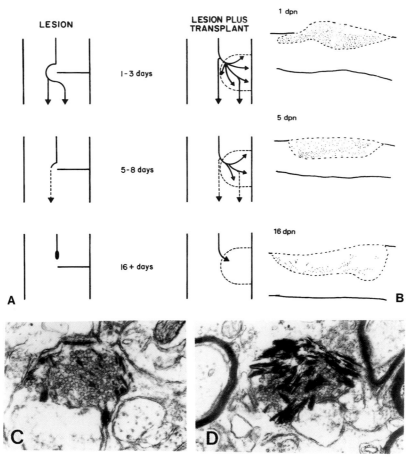

FIG. 8. A,B: Schematic diagrams of the progressive restriction of corticospinal tract plasticity with increasing age at time of lesion. See text for description. After spinal cord lesions and transplants at birth or at maturity, corticospinal axons form synapses with target structures within the transplants. **C,D**: Horseradish peroxidase (HRP) was injected into the sensorimotor cortex to label anterogradely corticospinal axons and terminals within the transplant 1 month after lesion and transplantation at birth or at maturity. Vesicles filled HRP-labeled synaptic profiles in contact with dendritic structures within the transplant are illustrated. (Modified from Refs. 30,37, with permission.)

sions plus transplants from birth to adult-hood. After spinal cord lesions between 1 and 3 days postnatal, which interrupt the terrain over which corticospinal axons grow but do not damage the axons directly, late-growng corticospinal axons take an aberrant course around the lesion site and reach normal targets throughout the caudal spinal cord. By 5 to 8 days postnatal, the normal corticospinal axons have reached all levels of the spinal cord, but have not completed synaptogenesis. After spinal cord lesions at 5 to 8 days postnatal, some im-mature corticospinal axons are able to sprout and reach targets caudal to the lesion (dashed lines). The development of the cor-ticospinal pathway is complete by 16 days postnatal. Corticospinal axotomy at 16 days of age or later throughout adulthood results in retrograde retraction (dieback) of injured corticospinal axons rostral to the le-sion site. Thus, the plasticity of the corti-cospinal tract (CST) in response to injury becomes progressively restricted as the animal and the pathway matures. At all ages (from birth through adult) the presence of a transplant of fetal spinal cord tissue at the site of injury increases the anatomic plasticity of the corticospinal tract above that observed after lesion alone. This is shown both in the schematic diagram in Fig. 8A (lesion plus transplant) and in the camera lucida tracings that accompany the schematic diagram (see Fig. 8B). The degree and extent of this transplant-mediated growth becomes restricted as the age of the animal at time of injury increases. After spinal cord injury and transplantation at birth, there is robust growth of corticospinal axons throughout the transplant. The growth is not restricted to the transplant; rather, CST axons grow into the transplant and through it to reach all spinal cord levels caudal to the lesion site. After lesions at birth, the transplant-mediated plasticity is not simply an indirect effect on the contralateral intact spinal cord, since (a) contralateral hemisection of the previously intact side does not abolish retrograde labeling of corticospinal neurons after injection of tracer into the lumbar enlargement (12), and (b) after complete transection, a variety of descending pathways cross the transplant and reinnervate the host spinal cord caudal to the transection (27; B. S. Bregman, unpublished results). After spinal cord lesion at 5 to 8 days postnatal, the density of corticospinal growth within the transplant is decreased compared with the earlier lesion, but the range of CST axonal growth still extends throughout the territory provided by the transplant. In addition, CST axons are still able to elongate throughout the spinal cord caudal to the lesion and transplant. After damage to the mature corticospinal pathway, transplants of fetal spinal cord tissue prevent the "dieback" of axotomized corticospinal axons, perhaps by providing a trophic support for the injured axons. Mature injured CST axons grow into the transplant, but the density of innervation is decreased compared with lesions earlier in development, and the

range of ingrowth is restricted to the immediate host–transplant border. Both the immature and mature injured CST axons form morphologically normal synapses within the transplant (see Fig. 8C,D), suggesting that they are in a position to influence locomotor function after spinal cord injury. The anatomic plasticity of the corticospinal pathway is accompanied by recovery of function (Fig. 9). Contact-placing responses are mediated specifically by the corticospinal tract. These responses are permanently abolished after spinal cord hemisection in the adult (31,32,57,109). The aberrant growth of the corticospinal tract after lesion at birth results in a sparing of contact-placing response, but the responses remain abnormal in their threshold and excursion (32). The presence of a transplant of fetal spinal cord tissue enhances the recovery of contact-placing beyond that mediated by mechanisms intrinsic to the host nervous system (see Fig. 9). We have

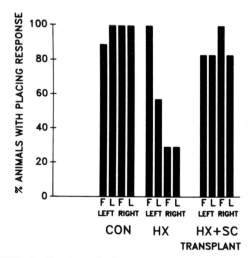

FIG. 9. Contact-placing responses are spared after spinal cord lesions at birth, but are abolished permanently after the same injury in the adult. The presence of a transplant of fetal spinal cord tissue at the site of injury enhances the recovery of contact-placing beyond that mediated by mechanisms intrinsic to the host nervous system. Transplants in the adult fail to restore contact-placing responses.

demonstrated previously that other descending pathways are also capable of robust transplant-induced growth after spinal cord injury and undergo a similar pattern of restriction with increasing age at time of injury.

Relative Contribution of Regenerating and Late-Developing Axons to Transplant-Mediated Anatomic Plasticity

Both regenerating and late-developing pathways contribute to transplant-induced anatomic plasticity after spinal cord lesions at birth (12,29,30). It was important to determine whether the axons that grow across the site of the neonatal lesion and transplant are derived from axotomized neurons and are therefore *regenerating,* or whether the axons that grow across the transplant are *late-growing* axons that have not been axotomized directly. We have used an experimental paradigm of midthoracic spinal cord lesion plus transplant at birth and temporally spaced retrograde tracing with the fluorescent tracers fast blue (FB) and diamidino yellow (DY) to address this issue. Fast blue was placed into the site of a spinal cord hemisection in rat pups that were younger than 48 hours. After 3 to 6 hours, to allow uptake and transport of the tracer, the source of fast blue was removed by aspiration, and the lesion was enlarged to an "overhemisection." A transplant of embryonic day-14 fetal spinal cord tissue was placed into the lesion site. The animals survived 3 to 6 weeks before the injection of the second tracer (DY) bilaterally into the host spinal cord caudal to the lesion plus transplant. Neurons with late-developing axons would not be exposed to the first dye (FB), but could only be exposed to the second tracer, diamidino yellow. Thus, neurons with a diamidino yellow-labeled nucleus are interpreted as "late-developing" neurons. Neurons axotomized by midthoracic spinal cord lesion at birth could be exposed to the first tracer, fast blue. If after

axotomy they regrew caudal to the transplant, they could be labeled by the second tracer as well. We interpret these double-labeled neurons as regenerating neurons. If neurons labeled with fast blue and axotomized by the spinal cord hemisection either fail to regenerate or grow into the transplant, but not caudal to it, they would be labeled only by the first dye. We have examined the pattern and distribution of single (FB or DY)- and double (FB + DY)-labeled neurons in the sensorimotor cortex, red nucleus, locus coeruleus, and raphe nuclei. The results indicate that both regenerating axons and late-growing axons project to the host spinal cord caudal to a neonatal spinal cord lesion and transplant (Fig. 10).

A similar experimental paradigm (12) was used (a) to determine the magnitude of the regeneration and (b) to test the hypothesis that the long-distance growth beyond the site of a neonatal lesion plus transplant is by late-developing neurons, whereas regenerating neurons project to spinal cord levels immediately caudal to the transplant (or simply into the transplant). We counted the number of double-labeled (regenerating), single diamidino yellow-labeled (late-growing), and single fast blue-labeled (nonbridging) neurons in the cortex, red nucleus, raphe nuclei, and locus coeruleus. By systematically varying the distance of the diamidino yellow injection site caudal to the transplant, we were able to compare the distance that injured axons regenerate with the distance that late-growing axons extend (see Fig. 10). When the diamidino yellow injection was placed within 5 mm caudal to the transplant, 24% of the neurons in the red nucleus, 32% of the neurons in the locus coeruleus, and 37% of the neurons in the raphe nuclei were double-labeled (regenerating). Although the percentage of double-labeled neurons decreased as the distance beyond the transplant increased, a substantial population of regenerating neurons was identified in each of the brain stem nuclei examined following diamidino yellow injections up to 15 mm caudal to the transplant.

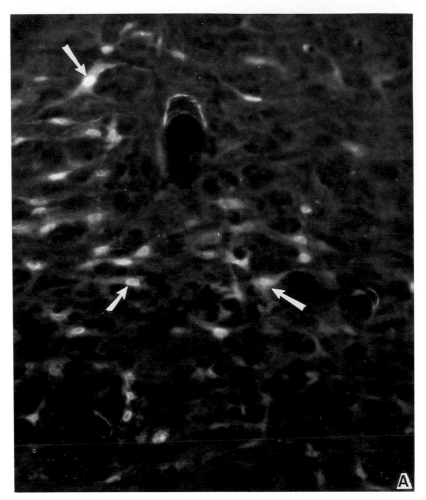

PERCENT OF DOUBLE LABELED NEURONS
FOLLOWING NEONATAL AXOTOMY

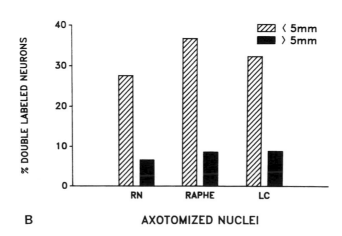

Thus, the hypothesis that the long-distance growth beyond the transplant is solely by late-developing neurons is not supported. Rather, after spinal cord lesions and transplants at birth, *both* regenerating neurons and late-developing neurons extend axons long distances (up to 15 mm) caudal to the lesion site. Surprisingly, the proportion of regenerating neurons in the red nucleus, raphe nuclei, and locus coeruleus is similar. These findings, taken together with earlier studies demonstrating a trophic influence of transplants on immature axotomized neurons, suggest that if immature axotomized neurons survive, they can regenerate.

Comparison of Anatomic Plasticity of Descending and Segmental Pathways After Lesion and Transplantation in Neonatal and Adult Operates

To compare the extent of the anatomic plasticity after spinal cord lesions and transplants between neonatal and adult operates, the anatomic changes associated with the transplants were studied by examining the fiber growth into the transplants in both groups. The effects on recovery of function are described below. The general approach for both the anatomic and functional studies is illustrated in Fig. 11. All of the data presented concerning both anatomic plasticity and recovery of function was derived from neonatal and adult operates that had equivalent lesions and transplants. Figure 12 illustrates transplants placed into the site of a spinal cord hemisection at birth (see Fig. 12A) or at maturity (see Fig. 12B).

Neonate

The labeling of several descending brain stem–spinal fiber pathways reveals many fibers throughout the extent of the transplant, similar to our observations in the corticospinal pathway (37). For example, immunocytochemical visualization of descending serotonergic (Fig. 13A) and noradrenergic fibers indicate that after spinal cord injury and transplantation at birth, these axons extend throughout the transplant territory (26,30,97,111). Immunocytochemical visualization of segmental dorsal root axons with antibodies to the calcitonin gene-related peptide (CGRP) indicates that dorsal root axons also grow into the transplant and project throughout it (30,92,95,96; Fig. 14 A–C). Thus, the transplants promote extensive growth of both the descending supraspinal fibers and the segmental dorsal root fibers into the transplant in the neonate group. Both suprasegmental (30,37; see Fig. 8) and dorsal root axons (see Fig. 14C) form synapses within the transplants, suggesting that they are in a position to mediate functional recovery.

FIG. 10. After spinal cord lesions and transplants at birth, immature axotomized brain stem–spinal neurons are rescued and regenerate to reach host spinal cord levels caudal to the transplant. **A:** Double-labeled neurons within the raphe nucleus are illustrated. **B:** The percentage of double-labeled neurons with regenerated axons in the red nucleus (*RN*), *raphe,* and locus coeruleus (*LC*) after neonatal axotomy plus transplant are illustrated. Note that the magnitude of regeneration is similar for each of the brain stem–spinal nuclei examined. Regenerated axons project not only to spinal cord levels immediately caudal to the transplant (*hatched bars*), but also project long distances beyond the transplant (up to 15 mm; *solid bars*). In the red nucleus, 28% of the axotomized neurons regenerated axons to the host spinal cord immediately caudal to the transplant, whereas 7% reached up to 15 mm caudal to the transplant. In the raphe nuclei, 37% of the axotomized neurons regenerated axons immediately caudal to the transplant, and 9% long-distances beyond it. In the locus coeruleus, 32% of the axotomized neurons regenerated axons immediately caudal to the transplant and 9% long-distances beyond it. (B, from ref. 12, with permission.)

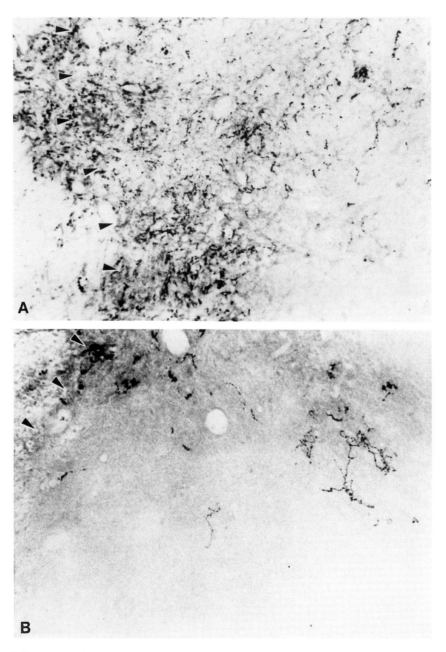

FIG. 13. Adjacent sections to those shown in Fig. 12A,B at higher power are labeled immunocyto-chemically to illustrate differences in anatomic interaction between host and transplant in neonatal (**A**) and adult (**B**) operates. Border between host and transplant is indicated by *arrowheads*. Dense projection of serotonergic axons throughout the transplant after lesion at birth (A). After similar lesion in the adult, axonal growth is restricted to the host–transplant interface (B).

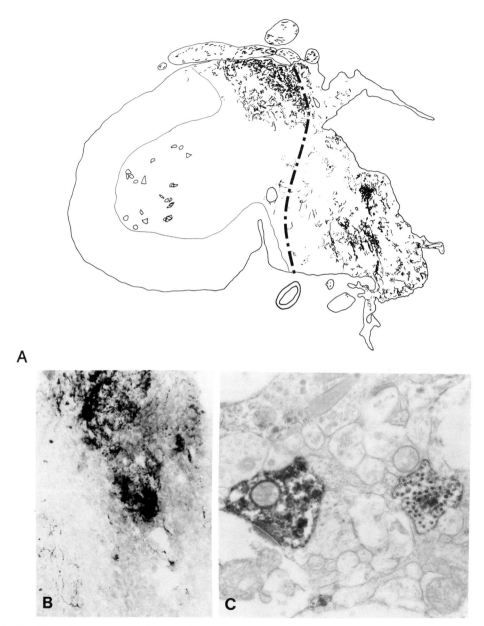

FIG. 14. Growth of segmental axons into a transplant of fetal spinal cord tissue. **A**: Camera lucida drawing of CGRP-labeled dorsal root axons. Border between host and transplant is indicated by *dashed line*. Dorsal root axons grow throughout the transplant. **B,C**: Photomicrographs of CGRP-labeled fibers within the transplant at light (B) and electron microscopic (C) levels.

lesion model does not axotomize neurons. Thus, the anatomic growth in response to excitotoxic injury represents axonal sprouting of undamaged host axons, rather than regenerative growth. Sprouting monoaminergic axons after excitotoxic lesion (122, 123) of the adult spinal cord project throughout the entire transplant, whereas after axotomy by surgical lesions, these same populations of host axons project only short distances within the transplants (97,111,136). In contrast with the growth of brain stem–spinal axons, which is restricted to the host–transplant border in the adult spinal cord, dorsal root axons (visualized with CGRP immunocytochemistry) extend throughout the transplant (30,92,95–98, 168). Both the descending and segmental afferents to the transplant establish synaptic connections with the transplanted neurons. The projection of CGRP fibers in the transplants of the adult operates, however, appears to be less dense than within the transplants of neonatal operates.

Previous studies have demonstrated that, after spinal cord injury at birth or at maturity, neurons within the transplant send axons into the host spinal cord (97,98,136) and, conversely, neurons within the host spinal cord send axons into the transplants (40,97,98,135,139). Light and electron microscopic studies indicate that host CNS axons are in synaptic contact with neurons in the transplant after spinal cord lesions at birth or at maturity and, thus, are in a position to influence the animal's motor behavior by serving as a relay for supraspinal control of spinal cord circuitry. The studies from my laboratory indicate that, after spinal cord lesions at birth, the transplants also serve as a bridge for axons to reach spinal cord levels caudal to the transplant. Transplants of fetal spinal cord tissue mediate recovery of locomotor function after spinal cord injury in newborn and adult mammals (30,44,72,93,94,108,111,164). In our laboratory, we have demonstrated that this recovery of function is dependent on the anatomic connections established be-

tween the host and the transplant, since if the transplant is intentionally isolated from the host spinal cord to prevent anatomic connections from forming, recovery fails to occur (36,108,110; B. S. Bregman and E. Kunkel-Bagden, *unpublished results*).

TRANSPLANT-MEDIATED RECOVERY OF FUNCTION

Spinal Cord Transplants Enhance the Recovery of Locomotor Function After Spinal Cord Injury at Birth

Earlier studies from my laboratory have demonstrated that transplants of fetal spinal cord tissue rescue immature axotomized neurons from retrograde cell death and support the growth of axons from the host CNS both into and through the site of injury (26,27,29,30,37,39). By using sensitive quantitative analysis of motor behavior, we also demonstrated that such transplants mediate recovery of function after spinal cord injury at birth (14,30,108). Spinal cord injury at birth leads to permanent qualitative and quantitative deficits in locomotor function. For example, the base of support is increased significantly (Fig. 15), the swing phase of locomotion is permanently hypermetric (see Fig. 3D), and hindlimb rotation is increased, among other deficits. The presence of a transplant of fetal spinal cord tissue mediates permanent recovery of function (Figs. 15 and 16) in some of these deficits. The recovery is dependent on a transplant present within the lesion site in anatomic contiguity with the host spinal cord. We suggest that the functional changes associated with the transplants are the result of the anatomic plasticity promoted by the transplants. We suggest that it is by *specific* anatomic integration into the circuitry of the host spinal cord, rather than simply through release of neurotransmitters or neurotrophic substances, that transplants of fetal spinal cord tissue promote recovery of function after neonatal spinal cord dam-

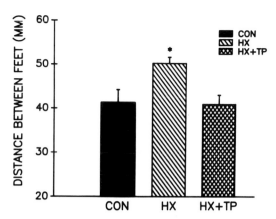

FIG. 15. Base of support: Transplants of fetal spinal cord tissue mediate recovery of locomotor function after lesions at birth. The base of support (see Fig. 4) is increased significantly (*asterisk*) after spinal cord hemisection at birth (*HX*). In animals with transplants (*HX + TP*) of fetal spinal cord tissue, the base of support was similar to that observed in control animals (*CON*). (From Ref. 108, with permission.)

age. We hypothesize that segmental, intersegmental, and suprasegmental pathways make *unique* contributions to anatomic plasticity and recovery of function after spinal cord lesions and transplants, and that their *relative contribution* to recovery *dif-*

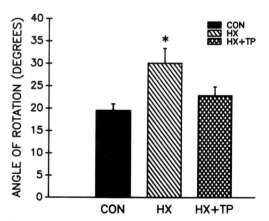

FIG. 16. Limb rotation: Limb rotation (see Fig. 4) is also increased significantly by lesion at birth. In animals with transplants, hindlimb rotation is significantly improved compared with lesion-only animals. (From ref. 108, with permission.)

fers following lesions in the adult versus lesions in the neonate. For example, after neonatal spinal cord lesion, it is likely that the transplant-mediated growth of corticospinal fibers contributes to the enhanced recovery of contact-placing responses, compared with lesion-only littermates (see Fig. 9). Contact-placing responses fail to recover after spinal cord injury in the adult; the presence of a transplant is unable to restore this function after injury in the adult. The transplants mediate recovery of both reflex and locomotor function.

Spinal Cord Transplants Mediate Recovery of Function by Permitting the Maturation of Locomotor Patterns That Are Immature at Birth

One way in which transplants mediate recovery of function after spinal cord injury at birth is by permitting the maturation of motor patterns that are immature at this stage (Fig. 17). We examined the contribution of spinal cord transplants to the development of motor function in three groups of animals: lesion-only, lesion-plus-transplant, and normal (unlesioned) littermates. Rats were tested daily for 28 days on a battery of postural reflexes and locomotion. In addition, at 8 to 12 weeks of age quantitative tests of locomotor function were assessed as described previously (108,110). Spinal cord injury at birth abolishes postural reflexes that were present. Examinations of postural reflexes in rats indicate that hemisection at birth delays, by several days, the onset and maturation of postural reflexes, such as righting, vestibular-placing, and contact-placing, which are immature at birth. The presence of a transplant prevents this lesion-induced delay in the development of these reflexes, and shifts the time course of development of sensorimotor function toward normal. If one examines the locomotor function in these three groups, for example, immature locomotion (2 weeks; see Fig. 17) is characterized by a

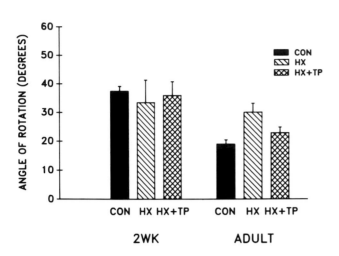

FIG. 17. One mechanism by which transplants mediate recovery of function after spinal cord injury at birth is by permitting the maturation of locomotor patterns that were immature at the time of injury. At 2 weeks of age (*2WK*), there are no differences among the control (*CON*), lesion-only (*HX*), or lesion-plus-transplant (*HX+TP*) animals in the amount of hindlimb rotation or in the base of support (not shown). When these same groups of animals are examined after they have matured (*ADULT*), the deficits in the lesion-only (*HX*) group persist. The presence of a transplant permits the maturation of hindlimb locomotor patterns, similar to that observed in the control animals.

wide base of support and excessive lateral rotation of the hindlimbs. At this stage of development, the behavior of control, lesion-only, and lesion-plus-transplant animals is identical. As the normal animal matures, the base of support and the amount of rotation decrease. After hemisection at birth, these characteristics of locomotion fail to mature, and an immature pattern persists. If a transplant is present at the lesion site, the pattern of locomotion matures similar to that in control animals (see Fig. 17, adult).

Effect of Spinal Cord Transplants on Recovery of Motor Function After Spinal Cord Lesions in Adult Animals

More recently, transplant-mediated recovery of function was assessed after spinal cord hemisection in adult rats (36,111). Footprint analysis revealed that animals with a hemisection had a significant decrease in stride length (Fig. 18). Adult operates with a transplant, however, had a stride length similar to that in control animals (see Fig. 18). This is in contrast with observations on the effect of transplants in the neonatal operates (108), since the transplant did not improve recovery of stride

length after lesions at birth (see Fig. 8; 108). This observation indicates that (a) transplants mediate recovery of function after lesions in the adult, and (b) supports our hypothesis that the mechanisms underlying recovery of function in neonatal and adult operates differ. Animals with transplants were also able to cross runways requiring accurate foot placement faster and with fewer steps than the hemisected-only animals (Fig. 19A). In these aspects of locomotor function, recovery was similar between neonatal- and adult-lesioned animals (see 108). Analysis of the lesion sites revealed that the transplant-mediated alterations in recovery were dependent on good apposition of the transplant with the host spinal cord. Although the ingrowth of corticospinal and brain stem–spinal axons from the host CNS into the transplant in the adult is less extensive than after similar lesions at birth, this anatomic plasticity may be sufficient to promote recovery of function. The transplant may serve as a relay for supraspinal control to reach spinal cord levels caudal to the lesion. The growth of dorsal root fibers into the transplant is substantial in both adult (92,95,96) and neonatal operates (30). Although there is substantial recovery of function mediated by the transplant, permanent deficits remain, and

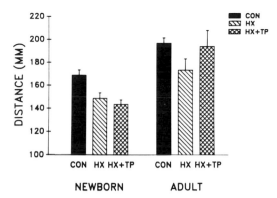

FIG. 18. Stride length (see Fig. 4): The mean (+ SEM) distance traversed by the right limb with each step cycle for each group. The distance was significantly decreased in animals with a neonatal hemisection (*HX*; *N* = 11) and hemisection plus transplant (*HX + TP*; *N* = 9) compared with controls (*CON*; *N* = 10). The adult operates also had a decrease in the distance traversed, but the presence of a transplant resulted in an increase in the distance toward control values (*CON, N* = 4; *HX, N* = 4; *HX + TP, N* = 4).

motor behavior does not return to control levels. For example, similar to our results after lesions at birth (108), the number of errors in foot placement on the grid runway was not improved by the presence of a transplant in the adult operates (see Fig. 19B). Recovery of function after contusion injury in the adult has also been observed (4,135,139,164) when using similar methods of analysis. Electrophysiologic studies indicate that several aspects of hindlimb segmental reflex function are closer to normal values in animals with transplants than in lesion-only control groups (135,139,169).

The effects of neural tissue transplants on recovery of function has recently begun to be examined after spinal cord injury in cats in several laboratories (4,93,94,135, 139). The use of cats in these transplantation studies offers several advantages for studies concerning recovery of function, since many of the electrophysiologic studies that have established much of the basis for our understanding of locomotor control have been done in cats. Howland and colleagues have examined the consequences

of neural tissue transplantation after spinal cord transection in newborn cats (93,94). Those studies suggest that, after transection at birth, the presence of a transplant of fetal spinal cord tissue at the lesion site leads to recovery of function far beyond that observed after transection alone. For example, animals with transplants develop full-weight-supported treadmill and overground locomotion. Although segmental stepping occurs after transection, neither weight support nor overground locomotion develop or recover after transection alone. During overground locomotion, cats with transplants develop patterns of limb movement that suggest coordination between forelimbs and hindlimbs occurs (93,94). It is thought that the anatomic connections made possible by the presence of the transplant contribute to this recovery (93,94).

Possible Mechanisms Underlying Recovery of Function

After lesions in the developing or mature nervous system, there is recovery of function mediated by sources intrinsic to the CNS, such as spared pathways not damaged by the lesion. The response of the spared pathways to the loss of other pathways must determine both the extent of recovery and the specific functions that recover (72). Recovery of function after spinal cord injury may involve reorganization of segmental, intersegmental, and suprasegmental pathways. Each of these sources may contribute unique aspects of the recovered behavior. There is recovery of function after spinal cord lesions in both newborn and adult cats or rats (30–34,74–76,108,109). Quantitative behavioral and kinematic analyses indicate, however, that the locomotor patterns and motor strategies used by the newborn and adult operates differ (31,33,109). This suggests that the mechanisms underlying the recovery also must differ. Differences between adult operates and neonatal operates may be

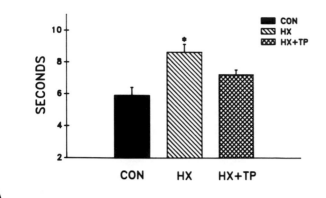

A

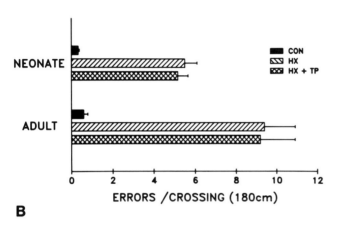

B

FIG. 19. A: The mean (+SEM) time necessary for the animals to cross the grid runway. Data from animals lesioned at maturity is illustrated. Results from animals lesioned at birth (108) was similar; in both groups the presence of a transplant permitted recovery of motor function. Animals that received a hemisection as neonates or as adults took a significantly longer time to cross the runway than the control. Both the neonatal and adult operates with a transplant (HX+TP) crossed significantly faster than the hemisected animals and were not significantly different from the control animals. **B**: The mean number of hindlimb errors crossing the grid runway in neonate and adult operates. Permanent deficits in the accuracy of locomotion persist.

partly explained by the stage of development of the behavior at the time of the lesion. At birth, locomotion in the rat is immature. Spinal cord injury in the adult interrupts the descending control of locomotor patterns that have already developed. Spinal cord injury at birth, in contrast, interrupts the descending control of locomotor patterns during their development. Spinal cord injury at birth may prevent the development of the adult pattern, and the immature locomotor pattern may persist, or a novel pattern of locomotion may develop. Deficits in the neonatal operates may reflect arrested development. Despite considerable recovery of function, permanent deficits persist.

The presence of a transplant of fetal spinal cord tissue at the injury site may restore a more normal balance among the segmental, intersegmental, and suprasegmental influences on the SPGL and permit the development or recovery of more normal patterns of locomotor function. Transplants of fetal spinal cord tissue placed into the lesion site increase the extent of recovery beyond that mediated by naturally occurring mechanisms intrinsic to the animal. A model comparing anatomic plasticity and possible mechanisms underlying recovery of function after spinal cord injury and transplantation in the neonate and the adult is illustrated in Fig. 20. The transplant may function as a bridge to enable supraspinal

NEONATE   ADULT

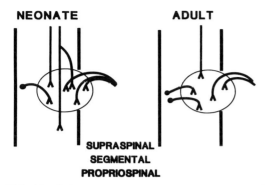

SUPRASPINAL
SEGMENTAL
PROPRIOSPINAL

FIG. 20. Schematic diagram illustrating some of the relative differences in anatomic plasticity after spinal cord lesions at birth versus that observed after lesions at maturity. See text for description of potential mechanisms underlying recovery of function in both groups.

fibers to reach caudal spinal levels, or as a relay for segmental and intersegmental input. Our evidence indicates that, after spinal cord lesion and transplant at birth, the transplant functions both as a bridge and as a relay. After lesions in the adult, anatomic evidence supports the potential for transplants to function as a relay, but not as a bridge. Since fibers in the adult grow into, but not caudal to, the transplant, their action is confined to a relay function. Therefore, the effect of the transplant may differ in neonates where a bridge function as well as a relay function may result. We hypothesize that anatomic reorganization of descending pathways plays a predominant role in transplant-mediated recovery of function after lesions at birth, whereas segmental and intersegmental pathways are primarily responsible for transplant-mediated recovery of function after lesions in the adult. These two mechanisms may have different consequences in the behavior of the animal. These differences in recovery between neonate and adult operates may reflect the contribution of different neuronal systems to the recovery in each. In the neonate after injury, the descending serotonergic, noradrenergic, and corticospinal fibers grow throughout the transplant

and beyond into the host spinal cord. The presence of the transplants allows the descending serotonergic, noradrenergic, and corticospinal fibers to traverse the lesion area and reestablish connections caudal to the lesion. This robust anatomic growth of descending pathways suggests that these fiber pathways contribute to the functional changes that accompany the fiber ingrowth in the neonatal operates. The recovery in particular functional tests by the neonatal operates only may reflect the contribution of these pathways to the recovery. The limited serotonergic, noradrenergic, and corticospinal fiber ingrowth into the transplant in the adult group after injury would suggest that these descending fiber pathways do not contribute as much to the recovery in the adult animals when compared with their contribution in the neonatal operates, or may do so less directly (i.e., by a relay).

In contrast with the suprasegmental input, the segmental dorsal root fibers grow throughout the transplant in both the neonate and adult after injury, although the growth is more robust in the neonate. The anatomic response of this fiber pathway suggests this neuronal system may contribute to recovery after injury and transplantation in both the neonate and the adult. The presence of a transplant has promoted recovery on some functional tests in both the neonatal and adult operates, for example, the grid. The improved performance on tests of locomotion requiring accurate foot placement by the neonatal and adult operates, in the presence of the transplant, may reflect the contribution of the dorsal root system to recovery in both. In addition to the contribution of the descending supraspinal fibers and the segmental afferent fibers, the propriospinal system may contribute to the recovery in the presence of the transplants (36,111,161). A greater cell loss within the spinal cord has been suggested after a neonatal hemisection than after an adult hemisection (109). The extent of damage along the rostrocaudal axis is greater after a surgical hemisection in developing than in mature animals. This greater cell loss suggests a greater loss of propriospinal neurons in the neonatal operates. The injured propriospinal neurons in the neonate and the adult may respond differently in the presence of transplants. The differences in the response of the propriospinal neurons could contribute to the differences in the recovery of particular motor functions in the neonate and the adult. The cell loss within the spinal cord in the presence of the transplants has not been examined, but in both neonatal and adult hemisected animals, the host neurons within the spinal cord do extend fibers into the transplant. The transplants could promote the reestablishment of segmental or intersegmental fiber connections within the host spinal cord and alter the recovery of function after injury.

Taken together, neural tissue transplantation strategies to repair spinal cord injury by transplantation at the lesion site or by transplantation at the level of the SPGL, suggest that replacement of particular neurotransmitters at the level of the SPGL restore reflex and locomotor function by altering the balance between excitation and inhibition (nonspecific mechanisms) and by restoring particular suprasegmental control of the segmental circuitry directly (specific mechanisms). The transplants are capable of restoring both reflex function and enhancing locomotor function beyond that achieved by mechanisms intrinsic to the host nervous system.

used to analyze the mechanisms underlying anatomic plasticity and recovery of function after spinal cord injury in the developing or mature CNS. Such an understanding is essential to provide a rational basis for future therapeutic intervention. Taken together, these studies suggest that transplants of fetal spinal cord tissue mediate recovery of function *both* by *specific mechanisms* (i.e., by permitting the regeneration of particular descending and segmental pathways) and *nonspecific* mechanisms, such as by providing trophic support. Although recovery of function is substantial, permanent deficits persist after spinal cord injury and transplantation in both neonatal and adult operates. The transplants are able to restore some, but not all, of the function lost after spinal cord injury. Combinations of interventions may be required to restore reflex, sensory, and locomotor function to more normal levels after spinal cord injury. For example, if the amount of regeneration and sprouting after injury can be increased by interventions, such as providing additional trophic or tropic influences to the injured spinal cord, or by nullifying some of the inhibitory influences that restrict growth, and such alterations in the extent of descending control are combined with strategies designed to reestablish a balance between excitation and inhibition at the level of the spinal pattern generator for locomotion, greater recovery of function may be obtained.

SUMMARY AND CONCLUSIONS

The findings reviewed here are important because they demonstrate that a variety of transplantation strategies mediate recovery of locomotor function after spinal cord injury. Analysis of recovery of function after such injury requires sensitive behavioral analysis to examine the effects of experimental interventions designed to further enhance that recovery. These studies also indicate that neural tissue transplants can be

ACKNOWLEDGMENTS

Research from my laboratory described in this review has been supported by NIH grants NS 27054 and NS 19259 and by a grant from the American Paralysis Association. Barbara S. Bregman is the recipient of an NIH Research Career Development Award (NS 01356). I thank Dr. Ellen Kunkel-Bagden for her extensive contributions to the behavioral studies of recovery of function quoted here and Dr. Holli Bernstein-Goral for her contribution to the studies of regeneration after spinal cord lesions at birth. These studies would not have been possible without the excellent technical support of Marietta McAtee, Hai Ning Dai, and Da Gao; I am indebted to them for their contributions. This review is dedicated to the memory of Dr. Michael E. Goldberger, a true scholar of the mechanisms underlying recovery of function after spinal cord injury; my teacher, my colleague, and my friend.

REFERENCES

1. Aguayo AJ, David S, Bray G. Influences of the glial environment on the elongation of axons after injury: transplantation studies in adult rodents. *J Exp Biol* 1981;95:231–240.
2. Aguayo AJ, David S, Richardson P, Bray GM. Axonal elongation in peripheral and central nervous system transplants. *Adv Cell Neurobiol* 1979;3:215–234.
3. Amassian VE, Ross RJ. Developing role of sensorimotor cortex and pyramidal tract neurons in contact placing in kittens. *J Physiol* 1978;74:165–184.
4. Anderson DK, Reier PJ, Wirth ED, Theele DP, Brown SA. Delayed grafting of fetal CNS grafts in chronic compression lesions of the adult cat spinal cord. *Restor Neurol Neurosci* 1991;2:309–325.
5. Barbeau H, Rossignol S. Recovery of locomotion after chronic spinalization in the adult cat. *Brain Res* 1987;386:84–95.
6. Baron-Van Evercooren A, Gansmuller A, Duhamel E, Pascal F, Gumpel M. Repair of a myelin lesion by Schwann cells transplanted in the adult mouse spinal cord. *J Neuroimmunol* 1992;40:235–242.
7. Barth TM, Stanfield BB. The recovery of forelimb-placing behavior in rats with neonatal unilateral cortical damage involves the remaining hemisphere. *J Neurosci* 1990;10:3449–3459.
8. Baumgarten HG, Björklund A, Lachenmayer L, Rensch A, Rosengren E. De- and regeneration of the bulbospinal serotonin neurons in the rat following 5,6- or 5,7-dihydroxytryptamine treatment. *Cell Tissue Res* 1974;152:271–281.
9. Bernstein DR, Stelzner DJ. Developmental plasticity of the corticospinal tract (CST) following mid-thoracic "over-hemisection" in the neonatal rat. *J Comp Neurol* 1983;221:371–385.
10. Bernstein JJ, Goldberg WJ. Rapid migration of grafted cortical astrocytes from suspension grafts placed in host thoracic spinal cord. *Brain Res* 1989;491:205–211.
11. Bernstein JJ, Goldberg WJ. Grafted fetal astrocyte migration can prevent host neuronal atro-

phy: comparison of astrocytes from cultures and whole piece donors. *Restor Neurol Neurosci* 1991;2:261–270.
12. Bernstein-Goral H, Bregman BS. Spinal cord transplants support the regeneration of axotomized neurons after spinal cord lesions at birth: a quantitative double labeling study. *Exp Neurol* 1993;123:118–132.
13. Björklund A. Neural transplantation—an experimental tool with clinical possibilities. *TINS* 1991;14:319–322.
14. Björklund A, Lindvall O, Isacson O, et al. Mechanisms of action of intracerebral neural implants: studies on nigral and striatal grafts to the lesioned striatum. *TINS* 1987;10:509–516.
15. Björklund A, Nobin A, Stenevi U. Regeneration of central serotonin neurons after axonal degeneration induced by 5,6-dihydroxytryptamine. *Brain Res* 1973;50:214–220.
16. Björklund A, Nornes H, Gage FH. Cell suspension grafts of noradrenergic locus coeruleus neurons in rat hippocampus and spinal cord: reinnervation and transmitter turnover. *Neuroscience* 1986;18:685–698.
17. Björklund A, Stenevi U. Regeneration of monoaminergic and cholinergic neurons in the central nervous system. *Physiol Rev* 1979;59:62–100.
18. Björklund A, Stenevi U. *Neural grafting in the mammalian CNS. Fernstrom Foundation Series, vol 5.* Amsterdam: Elsevier; 1985.
19. Björklund A, Stenevi U, Dunnett SB. Transplantation of brainstem monoaminergic "command" systems: models for functional reactivation of damaged CNS circuitries. In: Kao CC, Bunge RP, Reier PJ, eds. *Spinal cord reconstruction.* New York: Raven Press; 1983:397–413.
20. Blakemore WF, Crang AJ, Evans RJ, Patterson RC. Rat Schwann cell remyelination of demyelinated cat CNS axons: evidence that injection of cell suspension of CNS tissue results in Schwann cell remyelination. *Neurosci Lett* 1987;77:15–19.
21. Blakemore WF, Crang AJ, Patterson RC. Schwann cell remyelination of CNS axons following injection of cultures of CNS cells into areas of persistent demyelination. *Neurosci Lett* 1987;77:20–24.
22. Blakemore WF, Franklin RJM. Transplantation of glial cells into the CNS. *TINS* 1991;14:323–327.
23. Blight AR. Axonal physiology of chronic spinal cord injury in the cat: intracellular recording in vitro. *Neuroscience* 1983;10:1471–1486.
24. Blight AR. Cellular morphology of chronic spinal cord injury in the cat: analysis of myelinated axons by line sampling. *Neuroscience* 1983;10:521–543.
25. Bray GM, Aguayo AJ. Exploring the capacity of CNS neurons to survive injury, regrow axons, and form new synapses in adult mammals. In: Seil FJ, ed. *Neural regeneration and transplantation.* New York: Alan R Liss; 1989:67–78.

26. Bregman BS. Development of serotonin immunoreactivity in the rat spinal cord and its plasticity after neonatal spinal cord lesions. *Dev Brain Res* 1987;34:245–263.

27. Bregman BS. Spinal cord transplants permit the growth of serotonergic axons across the site of neonatal spinal cord transection. *Dev Brain Res* 1987;34:265–279.

28. Bregman BS. Requirements of immature axotomized CNS neurons for survival and axonal elongation after injury. In: Reier PJ, Bunge RP, Seil FJ, eds. *Neurology and neurobiology: current issues in neural regeneration research.* New York: Alan R Liss; 1988:75–87.

29. Bregman BS, Bernstein-Goral H. Both regenerating and late-developing pathways contribute to transplant-induced anatomical plasticity after spinal cord lesions at birth. *Exp Neurol* 1991;112:49–63.

30. Bregman BS, Bernstein-Goral H, Kunkel-Bagden E. CNS transplants promote anatomical plasticity and recovery of function after spinal cord injury. *J Restor Neurol Neurosci* 1991;2:327–338.

31. Bregman BS, Goldberger ME. Anatomical plasticity and sparing of function after spinal cord damage in neonatal cats. *Science* 1982;217:553–555.

32. Bregman BS, Goldberger ME. Infant lesion effect: II. Sparing and recovery of function after spinal cord damage in newborn and adult cats. *Dev Brain Res* 1983;9:119–135.

33. Bregman BS, Goldberger ME. Infant lesion effect: I. Development of motor behavior following neonatal spinal cord damage in cats. *Dev Brain Res* 1983;9:103–117.

34. Bregman BS, Goldberger ME. Infant lesion effect: III. Anatomical correlates of sparing and recovery of function after spinal cord damage in newborn and adult cats. *Dev Brain Res* 1983;9:137–154.

35. Bregman BS, Kunkel-Bagden E. Effect of target and non-target transplants on neuronal survival and axonal elongation after injury to the developing spinal cord. *Prog Brain Res* 1988;78:205–212.

36. Bregman BS, Kunkel-Bagden E. Potential mechanisms underlying transplant mediated recovery of function after spinal cord injury. In: Marwah J, Teitelbaum H, Prasat P, eds. *Neural transplantation, CNS neuronal injury and regeneration: recent advances.* Boca Raton: CRC Press; 1994;81–102.

37. Bregman BS, Kunkel-Bagden E, McAtee M, O'Neill A. Extension of the critical period for developmental plasticity of the corticospinal pathway. *J Comp Neurol* 1989;282:355–370.

38. Bregman BS, McAtee M. Neural tissue transplantation to study development and regeneration. *Neuroprotocols* 1993;3:17–27.

39. Bregman BS, Reier PJ. Neural tissue transplants rescue axotomized rubrospinal cells from retrograde death. *J Comp Neurol* 1986;244:86–95.

40. Bregman BS, Reier PJ. Neural tissue transplants modify the response of the immature spinal cord to damage. In: Althaus HH, Seifert W, eds. *Glial–neuronal communication in development and regeneration.* Berlin: Springer-Verlag; 1987:507–528.

41. Breshnahan JC, Beattie MS, Todd I, Noyes DH. A behavioral and anatomical analysis of spinal cord injury produced by a feedback-controlled impaction device. *Exp Neurol* 1987;95:548–570.

42. Brundin P, Strecker RE. Preparation and intracerebral grafting of dissociated fetal brain tissue in rats. In: Conn PM, ed. *Lesions and transplantation.* San Diego: Academic Press; 1991:305–326.

43. Bryz-Gornia WF, Stelzner DJ. Ascending tract neurons survive spinal cord transection in the neonatal rat. *J Comp Neurol* 1991.

44. Buchanan JT, Nornes HO. Transplants of embryonic brain stem containing the locus coeruleus into spinal cord enhance the hindlimb flexion reflex in adult rats. *Brain Res* 1986;381:225–236.

45. Cabana T, Martin GF. Developmental sequence in the origin of descending spinal pathways. *Dev Brain Res* 1984;15:247–263.

46. Carter DA, Bray GM, Aguayo AJ. Regenerated retinal ganglion cell axons can form well-differentiated synapses in the superior colliculus of adult hamsters. *J Neurosci* 1989;9:4042–4050.

47. Cattaneo E, McKay R. Identifying and manipulating neuronal stem cells. *TINS* 1991;14:338–340.

48. Clowry G, Sieradzan K, Vrbova G. Transplants of embryonic motoneurones to adult spinal cord: survival and innervation abilities. *TINS* 1991;114:355–357.

49. Clowry GJ, Vrbova G. Embryonic motoneurons grafted into the spinal cord of an adult rat can innervate a muscle. *Restor Neurol Neurosci* 1991;2:299–302.

50. Commissiong JW. Fetal locus coeruleus transplanted into the transected spinal cord of the adult rat. *Brain Res* 1983;271:174–179.

51. Commissiong JW. Fetal locus coeruleus transplanted into the transected spinal cord of the adult rat: some observations and implications. *Neuroscience* 1984;12:839–853.

52. Conn PM. *Lesions and transplantation.* San Diego: Academic Press; 1991.

53. Cunningham TJ, Haun F, Chantler PD. Diffusible proteins prolong survival of dorsal lateral geniculate neurons following occipital cortex lesions in newborn rats. *Brain Res* 1987;465:133–141.

54. Das GD. Neural transplantation in the spinal cord of the adult mammal. In: Kao CC, Bunge RP, Reier PJ, eds. *Spinal cord reconstruction.* New York: Raven Press; 1983:367–397.

55. Das GD. Neural transplantation in the spinal cord of adult rats. *J Neurol Sci* 1983;62:191–210.

56. David S, Aguayo AJ. Axonal regeneration after crush injury of rat central nervous system

fibres innervating peripheral nerve grafts. *J Neurocytol* 1985;14:1–12.

57. Donatelle JM. Growth of the corticospinal tract and the development of placing reactions in the postnatal rat. *J Comp Neurol* 1977;175:207–232.

58. Duncan ID, Aguayo AJ, Bunge RP, Wood PM. Transplantation of rat Schwann cells grown in tissue culture into the mouse spinal cord. *J Neurol Sci* 1981;49:241–252.

59. Dunnett SB, Björklund A. *Neural transplantation: a practical approach.* London: IRL Press; 1992.

60. Eagleson KL, Cunningham TJ, Haun F. Rescue of both rapidly and slowly degenerating neurons in the dorsal lateral geniculate nucleus of adult rats by a cortically derived neuron survival factor. *Exp Neurol* 1992;116:156–162.

61. Forssberg H, Grillner S. The locomotion of the acute spinal cat injected with clonidine i.v. *Brain Res* 1973;50:184–186.

62. Forssberg H, Grillner S, Sjostrom A. Tactile placing reactions in chronic spinal kittens. *Acta Physiol Scand* 1974;92:114–120.

63. Foster GA, Roberts MHT, Wilkinson LS. Structural and functional analysis of raphe neurone implants in denervated rat spinal cord. *Brain Res Bull* 1989;22:131–137.

64. Foster GA, Schultzberg M, Gage FH. Transmitter expression and morphological development of embryonic medullary and mesencephalic raphe neurones after transplantation to the adult rat central nervous system. I. Grafts to the spinal cord. *Exp Brain Res* 1985;60:427–444.

65. Gage FH, Buzsaki G. CNS grafting—potential mechanisms of action. In: Seil FJ, ed. *Neural regeneration and transplantation.* New York: Alan R Liss; 1991:211–226.

66. Gage FH, Kawaja MD, Fisher LJ. Genetically modified cells: applications for intracerebral grafting. *TINS* 1991;14:328–333.

67. Gale K, Kerasidis H, Wrathall JR. Spinal cord contusion in the rat: behavioral analysis of functional neurological impairment. *Exp Neurol* 1985;88:123–134.

68. Gash DM, Sladek JR. Transplantation into the mammalian CNS. *Prog Brain Res vol 78.* Amsterdam: Elsevier; 1988.

69. Goldberger ME. Partial and complete deafferentation of cat hindlimb: the contribution of behavioral substitution to recovery of motor function. *Exp Brain Res* 1988;73:343–353.

70. Goldberger ME. Spared-root deafferentation of a cat's hindlimb: hierarchical regulation of pathways mediating recovery of motor behavior. *Exp Brain Res* 1988;73:329–342.

71. Goldberger ME. Spared-root deafferentation of a cat's hindlimb: hierarchical regulation of pathways mediating recovery of motor behavior. *Exp Brain Res* 1988;73:329–342.

72. Goldberger ME. The use of behavioral methods to predict spinal cord plasticity. *Restor Neurol Neurosci* 1991;2.339–350.

73. Goldberger ME, Bregman BS, Vierck CJ, Brown M. Criteria for assessing recovery of function after spinal cord injury: behavioral methods. *Exp Neurol* 1990;107:113–117.

74. Goldberger ME, Murray M. Axonal sprouting and recovery of function may obey some of the same laws. In: Cotman CW, ed. *Neuronal plasticity.* New York: Raven Press; 1978:73–96.

75. Goldberger ME, Murray M. Recovery of function and anatomical plasticity after damage to the adult and neonatal spinal cord. In: Cotman CW, ed. *Synaptic plasticity.* New York: Guilford Press; 1985:77–110.

76. Goldberger ME, Murray M. Patterns of sprouting and implications for recovery of function. In: Waxman SG, ed. *Functional recovery in neurological disease.* New York: Raven Press; 1988:361–385.

77. Goldberger ME, Murray M, Tessler A. Sprouting and regeneration in the spinal cord. Their roles in recovery of function after spinal cord injury. In: Gorio A, ed. *Neuroregeneration.* New York: Raven Press; 1993:241–264.

78. Gout O, Gansmuller A, Baumann N, Gumpel M. Remyelination by transplanted oligodendrocytes of a demyelinated lesion in the spinal cord of the adult shiverer mouse. *Neurosci Lett* 1988;87:195–199.

79. Gribnau AAM, DeKort EJM, Dedern PJWC, Neiuwenhuys R. On the development of the pyramidal tract in the rat II. An anterograde tracer study of the outgrowth of corticospinal fibers. *Anat Embryol* 1986;175:101–110.

80. Grillner S. Some aspects of the descending control of the spinal circuits generating locomotor movements. In: Herman RM, Grillner S, Stein PSG, Stuart DG, eds. *Neural control of locomotion.* New York: Plenum Press; 1976:351–373.

81. Grillner S, Dubuc R. Control of locomotion in vertebrates: spinal and supraspinal mechanisms. In: Waxman SG, ed. *Functional recovery in neurological disease.* New York: Raven Press; 1988:425–453.

82. Guth L, Brewer CR, Collins WF Jr, Goldberger ME, Perl ER. Criteria for evaluating spinal cord regeneration experiments. *Exp Neurol* 1980;69:1–3.

83. Hallas BH. Transplantation into the mammalian adult spinal cord. *Experientia* 1982;38:699–701.

84. Haun F, Cunningham TJ. Specific neurotrophic interactions between cortical and subcortical visual structures in developing rat: in vivo studies. *J Comp Neurol* 1987;256:561–569.

85. Helgren ME, Goldberger ME. The recovery of postural reflexes and locomotion following low thoracic hemisection in adult cats involves compensation by undamaged primary afferent pathways. *Exp Neurol* 1993;123:17–34.

86. Hoovler DW, Wrathall JR. Implantation of neuronal suspensions into contusive injury sites in the adult rat spinal cord. *Acta Neuropathol* 1991;81:303–311.

87. Horvat JC, Baillet-Derbin C, Ye JH, Rhrich F, Affane F. Co-transplantation of embryonic

neural tissue and autologous peripheral nerve segments to severe spinal cord injury of the adult rat. Guided axiogenesis from transplanted neurons. *Restor Neurol Neurosci* 1991;2:289–298.

88. Houle JD. Demonstration of the potential for chronically injured neurons to regenerate axons into intraspinal peripheral nerve grafts. *Exp Neurol* 1991;113:1–9.

89. Houle JD. Regeneration of dorsal root axons is related to specific non-neuronal cells lining NGF-treated intraspinal nitrocellulose implants. *Exp Neurol* 1992;118:133–142.

90. Houle JD, Johnson JE. Nerve growth factor (NGF)-treated nitrocellulose enhances and directs the regeneration of adult rat dorsal root axons through intraspinal neural tissue transplants. *Neurosci Lett* 1989;103:17–23.

91. Houle JD, Reier PJ. Transplantation of fetal spinal cord into the chronically injured adult rat spinal cord. *J Comp Neurol* 1988;269:535–547.

92. Houle JD, Reier PJ. Regrowth of calcitonin gene-related peptide (CGRP) immunoreactive axons from the chronically injured rat spinal cord into fetal spinal cord tissue transplants. *Neurosci Lett* 1989;103:253–258.

93. Howland DR, Bregman BS, Tessler A, Goldberger ME. Transplants alter the motor development of kittens after neonatal spinal cord transection. *Soc Neurosci Abstr* 1990;16:37.

94. Howland DR, Bregman BS, Tessler A, Goldberger ME. Anatomical and behavioral effects of transplants in spinal kittens. *Soc Neurosci Abstr* 1991;17:236.

95. Itoh Y, Tessler A. Ultrastructural organization of regenerated adult dorsal root axons within transplants of fetal spinal cord. *J Comp Neurol* 1990;292:396–411.

96. Itoh Y, Tessler A. Regeneration of adult dorsal root axons into transplants of fetal spinal cord and brain—a comparison of growth and synapse formation in appropriate and inappropriate targets. *J Comp Neurol* 1990;302:272–293.

97. Jakeman LB, Reier PJ. Axonal projections between fetal spinal cord transplants and the adult rat spinal cord: a neuroanatomical tracing study of local interactions. *J Comp Neurol* 1991;307:311–334.

98. Jakeman LB, Reier PJ, Bregman BS, Wade EB, Kastner RJ, Dailey M. Differentiation of substantia gelatinosa-like regions in intraspinal and intracerebral transplants of embryonic spinal cord tissue in the rat. *Exp Neurol* 1989;103:17–33.

99. Kalil K, Reh T. Regrowth of severed axons in the neonatal CNS. *Science* 1979;205:1158–1161.

100. Kalil K, Skene JHP. Elevated synthesis of an axonally transported protein correlates with axon outgrowth in normal and injured pyramidal tracts. *J Neurosci* 1986;6:2563–2570.

101. Kao CC. Comparison of healing process in transected spinal cords grafted with autoge-

nous brain tissue, sciatic nerve and nodose ganglion. *Exp Neurol* 1974;44:424–439.

102. Kao CC, Fariello RG, Quaglieri CE, Messert B, Bloodworth JMB. Functional recovery of contused spinal cords repaired by delayed nerve grafting. *Proc Am Assoc Neurol Surg* 1977.

103. Keifer J, Kalil K. Effects of infant versus adult pyramidal tract lesions on locomotor behavior in hamsters. *Exp Neurol* 1991;111:98–105.

104. Kerasidis H, Wrathall JR, Gale K. Behavioral assessment of functional deficit in rats with contusive spinal cord injury. *J Neurosci Methods* 1987;20:167–169.

105. Kierstead SA, Vidal-Sanz M, Rasminsy M, Aguayo AJ, So KF. Electrophysiologic responses in hamster superior colliculus evoked by regenerating retinal axons. *Science* 1989;246:255–258.

106. Kliot M, Smith GM, Siegal JD, Silver J. Astrocyte-polymer implants promote regeneration of dorsal root fibers into the adult mammalian spinal cord. *Exp Neurol* 1990;109:57–69.

107. Kuhlengel KR, Bunge MB, Bunge RP, Burton H. Implantation of cultured sensory neurons and Schwann cells into lesioned neonatal rat spinal cord. II. Implant characteristics and examination of corticospinal tract growth. *J Comp Neurol* 1990;293:74–91.

108. Kunkel-Bagden E, Bregman BS. Spinal cord transplants enhance the recovery of locomotor function after spinal cord injury at birth. *Exp Brain Res* 1990;81:25–34.

109. Kunkel-Bagden E, Dai HN, Bregman BS. Recovery of function after spinal cord hemisection in newborn and adult rats: differential effects on reflex and locomotor function. *Exp Neurol* 1993;116:40–51.

110. Kunkel-Bagden E, Dai HN, Bregman BS. Methods to assess the development and recovery of locomotor function after spinal cord injury in rats. *Exp Neurol* 1993;119:153–164.

111. Kunkel-Bagden E, Dai HN, Gao D, Reier PJ, Bregman BS. Fetal spinal cord transplants alter the recovery of locomotor function after spinal cord injury. *Exp Neurol* 1993;123:3–16.

112. Lahr SP, Stelzner DJ. Anatomical studies of dorsal column axons and dorsal root ganglion cells after spinal cord injury in the newborn rat. *J Comp Neurol* 1990;293:377–398.

113. Lubetzki C, Gansmuller A, Lachapelle F, Lombrail P, Gumpel M. Myelination by oligodendrocytes isolated from 4–6 week old rat central nervous system and transplanted into the newborn shiverer brain. *J Neurol Sci* 1988;88:161–175.

114. Martin D, Delree P, Schoenen J, Rogister B, Rigo JM, Leprince P, Stevenaert A, Moonen G. Transplants of syngeneic adult dorsal root ganglion neurons to the spinal cord of rats with acute traumatic paraplegia: morphological analyses. *Restor Neurol Neurosci* 1991;2:303–308.

115. Martin D, Schoenen J, Delree P, Leprince P,

Rogister B, Moonen G. Grafts of syngenic cultured adult dorsal root ganglion-derived Schwann cells to the injured spinal cord of adult rats—preliminary morphological studies. *Neurosci Lett* 1991;124:44–48.

116. Martin GF, Xu XM. Evidence for developmental plasticity of the rubrospinal tract. Studies using the North American opossum. *Dev Brain Res* 1988;39:303–308.

117. Mas M, Zahradnik MA, Martino V. Stimulation of spinal serotonergic receptors facilitates seminal emission and suppresses penile erectile reflexes. *Brain Res* 1985;342:128–134.

118. Moorman SJ, Whalen LR. Fetal implants in the lesioned spinal cord of the rat. In: Conn PM, ed. *Lesions and transplantation*. San Diego: Academic Press; 1991:300–304.

119. Murray M, Goldberger ME. Restitution of function and collateral sprouting in the cat spinal cord: the partially hemisected animal. *J Comp Neurol* 1974;158:19–36.

120. Nornes H, Björklund A, Stenevi U. Reinnervation of the denervated adult spinal cord of rats by intraspinal transplants of embryonic brain stem neurons. *Cell Tissue Res* 1983; 230:15–35.

121. Nornes H, Björklund A, Stenevi U. Transplantation strategies in spinal cord regeneration. In: Sladek JR Jr, Gash DM, eds. *Neural transplants: development and function*. New York: Plenum Press; 1984:407–421.

122. Nothias F, Peschanski M. Homotypic fetal transplants into an experimental model of spinal cord neurodegeneration. *J Comp Neurol* 1990;301:520–534.

123. Nothias R, Cadusseau J, Dussart I, Peschanski M. Fetal neural transplants into an area of neurodegeneration in the spinal cord of the adult rat. *Restor Neurol Neurosci* 1991;2:283–288.

124. Nygren L-G, Fuxe K, Johnsson G, Olson L. Functional regeneration of 5-hydroxytryptamine nerve terminals in the rat spinal cord following 5,6-dihydroxytryptamine induced degeneration. *Brain Res* 1974;78:281–306.

125. Nygren L-G, Olson L, Seiger A. Monoaminergic reinnervation of the transected spinal cord by homologous fetal brain grafts. *Brain Res* 1977;29:227–235.

126. Paino CL, Bunge MB. Induction of axon growth into Schwann cell implants grafted into lesioned adult rat spinal cord. *Exp Neurol* 1991;114:254–257.

127. Pallini R, Fernandez E, Gangitano D, DelFa A, Olivieri-Sangiacomo C, Sbriccoli A. Studies on embryonic transplants to the transected spinal cord of adult rats. *J Neurosurg* 1989;70:454–462.

128. Polistina DC, Murray M, Goldberger ME. Plasticity of dorsal root and descending serotoninergic projections after partial deafferentation of the adult rat spinal cord. *J Comp Neurol* 1990;299:349–363.

129. Prendergast J, Stelzner DJ. Changes in the magnocellular portion of the red nucleus following thoracic hemisection in the neonatal and adult rat. *J Comp Neurol* 1976;166:163–172.

130. Privat A, Mansour H, Geffard M. Transplantation of fetal serotonin neurons into the transected spinal cord of adult rats: morphological development and functional influence. *Prog Brain Res* 1988;78:155–166.

131. Privat A, Mansour H, Pavy A, Geffard M, Sandillon F. Transplantation of dissociated fetal serotonin neurons into the transected spinal cord of adult rats. *Neurosci Lett* 1986;66:61–66.

132. Privat A, Mansour H, Rajaofetra N, Geffard M. Intraspinal transplants of serotonergic neurons in the adult rat. *Brain Res Bull* 1989;22:123–129.

133. Reese NB, Garcia-Rill E, Houle JD, Skinner RD. Modulation of locomotion through a peripheral nerve graft across a complete chronic spinal cord transection in the adult rat. *Soc Neurosci Abstr* 1991;17:938.

134. Reier PJ. Annotation. Neural tissue grafts and repair of the injured spinal cord. *J Neuropathol Appl Neurobiol* 1985;11:81–104.

135. Reier PJ, Anderson DK, Thompson FJ, Stokes BT. Neural tissue transplantation and CNS trauma: anatomical and functional repair of the injured spinal cord. *J Neurotrauma* 1992;9: S223–S248.

136. Reier PJ, Bregman BS, Wujek JR. Intraspinal transplantation of embryonic spinal cord tissue in neonatal and adult rats. *J Comp Neurol* 1986;247:275–296.

137. Reier PJ, Houle J, Jakeman L, Winialski D, Tessler A. Transplantation of fetal spinal cord tissue into acute and chronic hemisection and contusion lesions of the adult rat spinal cord. *Prog Brain Res* 1988;78:173–179.

138. Reier PJ, Houle JD. The glial scar: its bearing on axonal elongation and transplantation approaches to CNS repair. In: Waxman SD, ed. *Physiologic basis for functional recovery in neurological disease*. New York: Raven Press; 1988:87–138.

139. Reier PJ, Stokes BT, Thompson FJ, Anderson DK. Fetal cell grafts into resection and contusion/compression injuries of the rat and cat spinal cord. *Exp Neurol* 1992;115:177–188.

140. Richardson PM, Issa VMK, Aguayo AJ. Regeneration of long spinal axons in the rat. *J Neurocytol* 1984;13:165–182.

141. Richardson PM, McGuiness UM, Aguayo AJ. Peripheral nerve autografts to the rat spinal cord: studies with axonal tracing methods. *Brain Res* 1982;237:147–162.

142. Rivlin AS, Tator CH. Objective clinical assessment of motor function after experimental spinal cord injury in the rat. *J Neurosurg* 1977; 47:577–581.

143. Rosenbluth J, Hasegawa M, Shirasaki N, Rosen CL, Liu Z. Myelin formation following transplantation of normal fetal glia into myelin-deficient rat spinal cord. *J Neurocytol* 1990; 19:718–730.

144. Rossignol S. Assessment of locomotor func-

tions in the adult chronic spinal cat. In: Brown M, Goldberger ME, eds. *Criteria for assessing recovery of function: behavioral methods.* Springfield, NJ: American Paralysis Association; 1989:62–65.

145. Rossignol S, Barbeau H, Julian C. Locomotion of the adult chronic spinal cat and its modification by monoaminergic agonists and antagonists. In: Goldberger ME, Gorio Á, Murray M, eds. *Development and plasticity of the mammalian spinal cord.* New York: Springer-Verlag; 1986:323–346.

146. Sagen J, Kemmler JE. Increased levels of met-enkephalin-like immunoreactivity in the spinal cord CSF of rats with adrenal medullary transplants. *Brain Res* 1989;502:1–10.

147. Sagen J, Kemmler JE, Wang H. Adrenal medullary transplants increase spinal cord cerebrospinal fluid catecholamine levels and reduce pain sensitivity. *J Neurochem* 1991;56:623–627.

148. Sagen J, Pappas GD. Morphological and functional correlates of chromaffin cell transplants in CNS pain modulatory regions. *Ann NY Acad Sci* 1987;495:306–333.

149. Sagen J, Pappas GD, Perlow MJ. Adrenal medullary tissue transplants in the rat spinal cord reduce pain sensitivity. *Brain Res* 1986;384:189–194.

150. Sagen J, Pappas GD, Pollard HB. Analgesia induced by isolated bovine chromaffin cells implanted in rat spinal cord. *Proc Natl Acad Sci USA* 1986;83:7522–7526.

151. Savio T, Schwab ME. Lesioned corticospinal tract axons regenerate in myelin free rat spinal cord. *Proc Natl Acad Sci USA* 1990;87:4130–4133.

152. Schneider GE. Is it really better to have your brain lesion early: a revision of the "Kennard principle." *Neuropsychologia* 1979;7:557–583.

153. Schnell L, Schwab ME. Axonal regeneration in the rat spinal cord produced by an antibody against myelin-associated neurite growth inhibitors. *Nature* 1990;343:269–272.

154. Schwab M, Thoenen H. Dissociated neurons regenerate into sciatic but not optic nerve explants in culture irrespective of neurotrophic factors. *J Neurosci* 1985;5:2415–2423.

155. Schwab ME. Myelin-associated inhibitors of neurite growth. *Exp Neurol* 1990;109:2–5.

156. Schwab ME, Caroni P. Oligodendrocytes and CNS myelin are nonpermissive substrates for neurite growth and fibroblast spreading in vitro. *J Neurosci* 1991;11:2381–2393.

157. Schwab ME, Schnell L. Channeling of developing rat corticospinal tract axons by myelin-associated neurite growth inhibitors. *J Neurosci* 1991;11:709–721.

158. Sieradzan K, Vrbova G. Replacement of missing motorneurons by embryonic grafts in the rat spinal cord. *Neuroscience* 1989;31:115–130.

159. Smith GM, Miller RH, Silver J. Changing role of forebrain astrocytes during development, regenerative failure and induced regeneration upon transplantation. *J Comp Neurol* 1986;251:23–43.

160. So K-F, Aguayo AJ. Lengthy regrowth of cut axons form ganglion cells after peripheral nerve transplantation into the retina of adult rats. *Brain Res* 1985;328:349–354.

161. Stelzner DJ, Cullen JM. Do propriospinal projections contribute to hindlimb recovery when all long tracts are cut in neonatal or weanling rats? *Exp Neurol* 1991;114:193–205.

162. Stelzner DJ, Weber ED, Prendergast J. A comparison of the effect of midthoracic spinal hemisection in the neonatal or weanling rat on the distribution and density of dorsal root axons in the lumbosacral spinal cord of the adult. *Brain Res* 1979;172:407–426.

163. Stokes BT, Reier PJ. Oxygen transport in intraspinal fetal grafts—graft host relations. *Exp Neurol* 1991;111:312–323.

164. Stokes BT, Reier PJ. Fetal grafts alter chronic behavioral outcome after contusion damage to the adult rat spinal cord. *Exp Neurol* 1992;116:1–12.

165. Sugar O, Gerard RW. Spinal cord regeneration in the rat. *J Neurophysiol* 1940;3:1–19.

166. Tarlov IM. Spinal cord compression studies. III. Time limits for recovery after gradual compression in dogs. *Arch Neurol Psychiatry* 1954;71:588–597.

167. Tessler A. Intraspinal transplants. *Ann Neurol* 1991;29:115–120.

168. Tessler A, Himes BT, Houle J, Reier PJ. Regeneration of adult dorsal root axons into transplants of embryonic spinal cord. *J Comp Neurol* 1988;270:537–548.

169. Thompson FJ, Parmer R, Reier PJ. Alterations in lumbar motoneuron excitability following thoracic contusion compared to hemisection spinal cord injury. *Soc Neurosci Abstr* 1991;17:161.

170. Tolbert DL, Der T. Redirected growth of pyramidal tract axons following neonatal pyramidotomy in cats. *J Comp Neurol* 1987;260:299–311.

171. Vidal-Sanz M, Bray GM, Villegas-Perez MP, Thanos S, Aguayo AJ. Axonal regeneration and synapse formation in the superior colliculus by retinal ganglion cells in the adult rat. *J Neurosci* 1987;7:2894–2909.

172. Vidal-Sanz M, Bray GM, Aguayo AJ. Regenerated synapses present in the superior colliculus after regrowth of retinal ganglion cell axons. *J Neurocytol* 1991;20:940–952.

173. Villegas-Perez MP, Vidal-Sanz M, Bray GM, Aguayo AJ. Influences of peripheral nerve grafts on the survival and regrowth of axotomized retinal cells in adult rats. *J Neurosci* 1988;8:265–280.

174. Wall PD. Recruitment of ineffective synapses after injury. *Adv Neurol* 1988;47:387–400.

175. Whittemore SR, Holets VR, Keane RW, Levy DJ, McKay RD. Transplantation of a temperature sensitive, nerve growth factor-secreting neuroblastoma cell line into adult rats with fimbria–fornix lesions rescues cholinergic septal neurons. *J Neurosci Res* 1991;28:156–170.

176. Wrathall JR. Behavioral methods for evaluating

rats with contusive spinal cord injury: the combined behavioral score. In: Brown M, Goldberger ME, eds. *Criteria for assessing recovery of function: behavioral methods*. Springfield, NJ: American Paralysis Association; 1989:26–33.

177. Wrathall JR, Kapoor V, Kao CC. Observation of cultured peripheral nonneuronal cells implanted into the transected spinal cord. *Acta Neuropathol* 1984;64:203–212.

178. Wrathall JR, Pettegrew RK, Harvey F. Spinal cord contusion in the rat: production of graded, reproducible injury groups. *Exp Neurol* 1985; 88:108–122.

179. Wrathall JR, Rigamonti DD, Bradford MR, Kao CC. Reconstruction of the contused cat spinal cord by the delayed nerve graft technique and cultured peripheral nonneuronal cells. *Acta Neuropathol* 1982;57:59–69.

180. Yakovleff A, Roby-Brami A, Guezard B. Locomotion in rats transplanted with noradrenergic neurons. *Brain Res Bull* 1989;22:115–121.

Functional Neural Transplantation,
edited by S. B. Dunnett and A. Björklund.
Raven Press, Ltd., New York © 1994.

21

Mechanisms of Function of Neural Grafts in the Injured Brain

Stephen B. Dunnett and *Anders Björklund

*Department of Experimental Psychology, University of Cambridge,
Cambridge CB2 3EB, United Kingdom; *Department of Medical Cell Research, University of
Lund, S-223 62 Lund, Sweden*

The preceding chapters provide ample demonstration that neural grafts can influence the functional capacities of the host animal. Indeed, whereas earlier research in this field employed the techniques of neural transplantation to study the basic mechanisms of neuronal development and plasticity, the rapid increase in interest in this branch of neuroscience since the early 1980s has been stimulated, in large part, by the prospect that neural grafts can also produce functional changes and, thereby, provide the basis for development of new therapies to address the major health problems associated with neurodegenerative damage and disease in the central nervous system (CNS).

When we were first engaged in early studies of the functional effects of nigral cell transplantation in rats with nigrostriatal damage, the grafts were observed to extend new axons into the host brain over approximately the same time course that the simple motor asymmetries were compensated in tests of amphetamine- or apomorphine-induced rotation (13,56,164; see also Chapter 2). Therefore, it was natural to assume that the behavioral recovery was actually due to the anatomic growth and reinnervation. Similarly, in early neuroendocrine models, it was natural to assume that the apparent restoration of drinking following intraventricular implants of normal hypothalamic tissues in the Brattleboro rat was attributable to the returned neurohormonal secretion of vasopressin (see Chapter 18). Already the notion of different possible mechanisms of graft function began to be apparent. Perhaps, then, the reinnervation in rats bearing nigral grafts was irrelevant and the observed behavioral recovery was simply due to the graft cells secreting the deficient neurotransmitter into the host brain in the same way that pharmacologic delivery of levodopa (L-dopa) can alleviate many of the symptoms of nigrostriatal lesions in animals or Parkinson's disease in humans. Conversely, in the various neuroendocrine models, the grafts did not simply diffuse deficient neurohormones into the general blood system, but instead, were observed to give rise to extensive neurite outgrowth that reestablished rather precise specialized contacts with the fenestrated capillaries of the host median eminence (167,171).

Thus, it fairly soon became apparent that identification of the mechanisms by which the grafts exerted their effects in different model systems requires separate analysis in each case. This issue has become of increasing practical as well as theoretical importance as the techniques of neural transplantation have become considered for clinical application. For example, a major factor in the debate about the selection of alternative graft tissues in Parkinson's disease has focused around the issue of how do different graft tissues—fetal nigral grafts, adrenal autografts, or dopamine-secreting matrices—exert their effects, and what type of repair is necessary to produce sustained recovery in this particular disease state (see Chapters 3–6). Thus, if embryonic nigral grafts simply exert their effects by secreting dopamine into the host parenchyma, then other catecholamine-secreting tissues or engineered cells should be capable of providing simple and more readily available alternatives. Conversely, if reestablishment of local neuronal connections and synaptic release of dopamine underlies the greater functional effects so far achieved with nigral grafts than those achieved with adrenal grafts (in both animals and humans), then cells that simply secrete the missing neurotransmitter can have only a rather limited efficacy and we should instead focus attention on the availability of developing dopamine neurons, since at present these alone have the capacity to grow and make the appropriate connections following transplantation.

In addition to the advantages and disadvantages of different sources of tissue for

TABLE 1. *Mechanisms of graft function*

Mechanism	Example	Ref.
Nonspecific or negative effects of surgery	Tumor-like growth of graft tissues.	46,158
	Peripheral nerve grafts have leaky blood–brain barrier, allowing drugs to penetrate the brain.	161
	Induction of seizure activity.	29
Acute trophic stimulation of recovery	Adrenal grafts stimulate sprouting response in host dopamine systems.	20,48
	Astrocytes stimulate recovery from frontal cortex ablation.	110
Chronic trophic target support of host projections	Cortical grafts protect basal forebrain cholinergic neurons from retrograde degeneration.	176
	Spinal cord grafts protect red nucleus neurons from axotomy-induced degeneration.	24
Diffuse release of deficient neurochemicals	Neurohormonal release from hypothalamic grafts.	83,120
	Catecholamine-secreting polymers and encapsulated cells.	2,3,10,67, 136,202
Diffuse reinnervation of the host brain	Dopaminergic reinnervation of denervated striatum.	54,56,164
	Cholinergic reinnervation of denervated hippocampus or cortex.	14,17,144
Passive bridges	Peripheral nerve grafts permit axonal regeneration in optic nerve and spinal cord.	49,195
Active bridges	Hippocampal bridges allow regrowth of septohippocampal fibers	28,122,123
Reciprocal graft–host reinnervation	Striatal grafts restore corticostriatal and striatopallidal circuits.	51,173,199
Full reconstruction of damaged circuitry	Not yet achieved in any model system.	

From refs. 15,52, in which more detailed accounts can be found.

transplantation, analysis of the functional effects of adrenal grafts has revealed novel trophic mechanisms of graft function, including the possibility that grafts may act as a source of trophic activity to stimulate spontaneous repair processes in the host brain, in addition to the promotion of the graft cells themselves by the provision of trophic support (see 61; and Chapter 6). This, in turn, is leading to new strategies for functional transplantation, oriented primarily to the promotion of the brain's own spontaneous processes of reorganization and repair, rather than to repair by replacement of lost neurons.

In addition to the fundamental interest in understanding the basic biologic processes of neural development and plasticity, the advent of neural transplantation as a clinical technique is providing a new urgency to the task of improving the functional efficacy of neural grafts in a variety of neurodegenerative conditions (see Chapter 5). At our present stage of understanding, grafts, although generally viable, still provide only limited benefit in patients with Parkinson's disease. On the one hand, development and improvement of existing graft techniques has so far been based on empiric principles. However, more substantial long-term developments will come only through a better understanding of the mechanisms by which the grafts exert their effects, and by developing alternative strategies for repair and reconstruction, based on rational, rather than pragmatic, principles.

There have already been a number of theoretical accounts of the different mechanisms of function of neuronal grafts, each of which elucidates a basically similar range of proposed mechanisms (Table 1) (15,53, 73,79,111). In the first part of the present chapter, we provide an updated overview of the alternative mechanisms of recovery. Then, in the latter part of the chapter, we consider recent data suggesting that psychologic factors (i.e., the training and experience of the experimental animal itself) can influence the viability and functional efficacy of grafts.

NONSPECIFIC MECHANISMS

One of the first factors to be considered in analysis of graft function is whether the observed functional changes are indeed due to the inserted graft tissue itself and its direct action on the host brain. It has become apparent that in a number of experimental situations neural transplantation results in functional consequences that are best described as "nonspecific": for example, that the surgical intervention itself induces a disturbance in the host brain, independently of any direct influence of the grafted tissue.

Placebo Effects

Whereas it has always been of basic biologic importance, particular interest in the issue of graft specificity has been stimulated by attempts to understand the effectiveness of clinical adrenal grafts in the light of some anomalous observations. This issue became particularly crucial when attempts to detect or identify surviving grafts failed, even in patients for whom some functional alleviation was reported. First of all, it is extremely difficult to detect any evidence of graft activity in the living brain, either by functional imaging or by the presence of dopamine or its metabolites in the cerebrospinal fluid (CSF), although these failures could be attributed to insensitivity of the *in vivo* monitoring techniques that are presently available (5,84,169). Even more worrying, however, was that the grafts were generally found not to have survived at postmortem examination, even in patients who had apparently shown a significant degree of recovery (94,98,103,119,196).

Placebo effects have to be a major issue of concern in such clinical trials. These can apply to the medical scientists as much as to the patients themselves. The patients and their doctors are motivated to try any novel possibility to address a relentless disease, and optimism and hope are inevitable in the light of the bold and experimental nature of the therapy (127,194). Awareness of the strength of placebo effects, therefore, must be a major consideration in the design of adequate trials, with objective tests and blind ratings being used to complement patient, family, and nurses' reports and doctors' clinical evaluations. The lack of such attention in many of the patients receiving adrenal grafts has led to most of the early reports of apparently dramatic recovery now being generally disregarded.

Beneficial Nonspecific Mechanisms

Not all beneficial effects of nonsurviving adrenal grafts can be due to placebo effects. Thus, rats and mice, as well as patients, can show significant recovery, even when the grafts survive only poorly (20)(see Chapters 4 and 6). For a period, it became popular to ascribe such failures entirely to nonspecific effects of the implantation procedure (61).

Myers and others had reported, over four decades ago, that lesions of the caudate nucleus could alleviate some symptoms of Parkinson's disease, albeit only temporarily (138,139). Since the Madrazo technique for adrenal tissue implantation also involved large aspirative lesions in the head of the caudate nucleus to form the graft bed (131), it has been a matter of speculation whether the reported functional benefits were attributable to the grafted tissue or to the implantation procedure itself. However, it is probably inadequate to attribute functional recovery in these patients exclusively to the cavitation procedure, rather than to subsequent tissue implantation for two reasons. First, as discussed in more detail by Lindvall (see Chapter 5), recovery in adrenal transplant patients, in at least a few studies (104,142), may be as good using stereotaxic techniques, which cause rather little nonspecific damage, as in the initial cavitation procedure. Second, in a series of patients who were operated on with a two-stage grafting technique, benefit was not seen following creation of the initial cavity, but only after subsequent implantation of the

graft tissue (150). Rather, although adrenal grafts do not now provide a sufficiently reliable technique to warrant widespread clinical use, the reported benefits are likely to be, at least partly, due to the brief secretion of either catecholamines or to as yet unidentified trophic factors. Although trophic stimulation of growth may be only transitory, this could possibly lead to a permanent reorganization in the host brain so that the functional effects of the grafts can outlast the temporary survival of the implanted cells themselves (see Chapter 6).

More generally, although "psychosurgery" has frequently received a rather bad press (193,194), it is clear that neurosurgical interventions can have a clearly demonstrable beneficial effect, not only in situations involving removal of pathologic tissue (such as excising tumors or epileptic foci), but also to damage circumscribed areas of apparently healthy tissue to restore an imbalance in neural function, such as the successful treatment of some parkinsonian tremors by ventrobasal thalamic lesion (186). Although the caudate lesion hypothesis does not adequately characterize the recovery observed in parkinsonian patients following implantation of a variety of alternative tissues, such a mechanism is not ruled out in all cases. It is quite feasible that some beneficial transplant effects are due to additional lesions restoring balance in a disturbed neuronal network and, thereby, alleviating some of the symptoms. It would be expected that a more comprehensive functional analysis of such cases would also reveal additional deficits associated with the second lesion that were not apparent before transplantation. Once identified, it should be possible to clarify such factors, at least in experimental studies in animals, by the use of adequate control groups.

Vascular Changes and the Blood–Brain Barrier

Rosenstein and Brightman (161) have proposed a novel means by which grafts can be used to modify the functional influence of drugs given to the host animals. They showed that solid pieces of peripheral ganglia can readily survive implantation into the brain ventricles or parenchyma. In such circumstances, the capillary network of the grafts becomes connected by anastomosis into the host vascular network, but retains many of its peripheral features. In particular, the peripheral vasculature does not acquire a complete blood–brain barrier, but is permeable to many proteins. Consequently, the vasculature of peripheral ganglia grafts is "leaky" to large molecules. This provides a route by which drugs that do not cross the blood–brain barrier can be injected intravenously, penetrate through the vascular walls within the intracerebral grafts, and then diffuse directly into the host brain parenchyma. Rosenstein and Brightman provide clear demonstration of the penetration of large marker molecules, such as horseradish peroxidase into the brain by this route and propose that it may provide a more general means of enhancing drug access to identified and circumscribed targets within the brain. More generally, though, the permeability of the blood–brain barrier in neural grafts is not restricted to grafts of peripheral ganglia, but may also be seen in circumstances when viability is poor and the graft is subject to slow rejection (205). It should be emphasized, however, that viable grafts of fetal CNS tissue develop a fully mature and complete blood–brain barrier within 1 to 2 weeks after intracerebral transplantation (25,114,154,185).

Detrimental Side Effects of Neural Transplantation

Most nonspecific effects of neural transplantation are negative, rather than beneficial, and attributable to the transplantation procedure inducing further disturbance of brain function. Under this heading can be considered damage caused by the transplantation surgery itself, damage caused by growth of the graft, and the graft's exertion of an active influence on the host brain as a source of "noise."

The possibility that the neural transplantation procedure itself can cause damage to the host brain and additional functional deficits is a reasonable concern, in particular, with solid graft procedures that require creation of additional graft cavities. For example, implantation of solid tissue pieces into deeper brain sites, such as the hippocampus or caudate nucleus, requires aspirative cavities to be made through the overlying cortex and callosal fibers, which inevitably must cause some functional disturbance in its own right. Some of the side effects in many clinical trials using visual guidance with an open transfrontal approach were almost certainly attributable to the extraneous damage to overlying tissues and exposure of the ventricles (155). The introduction of stereotaxic injection of dissociated cell suspensions into deep brain sites in both animals and humans is associated with considerably fewer risks, but even then a stereotaxic approach has a small, but significant, risk of bleeding and vascular accident.

Although, under most normal circumstances, embryonic tissue grafts become well incorporated with the host brain and produce little overt disturbance, in some circumstances, the grafts can grow quite large. Ridley and colleagues have described a case in which unregulated tumor-like growth of a striatal graft led to premature death of the host animal (158), and in several other studies, normal expansion of graft volume has reached a large enough size to induce functional deficits (46,63). In addition, tumor formation is still a major issue of concern for grafts based on engineered cells and cell lines of nonneuronal origin (70,96,97,190). Such tumor-like growth may cause profound functional disturbance by compression and by producing "space-occupying lesions"; an actual tumor would be a massive drain on nutrients and metabolic resources. Thus, although it has not generally proved to be a problem when grafting in experimental animals, the theoretical possibility of tumor-formation remains a reasonable concern that has to be considered when developing clinical programs.

In other circumstances, the grafts may induce a pronounced disturbance of host brain function by a more active influence, such as acting as a focus of epileptic discharge (29) or secretion of a variety of neuroactive substances with unwanted effects. For example, adrenal grafts have been associated with a significant morbidity in human clinical trials, including the induction of sleep and psychotic disturbances (155). In rats, cortical grafts were seen to induce a long-term exacerbation of the learning deficits induced by prefrontal lesions, which was attributed to graft-derived ingrowth contributing "noise" to the complex patterns of neural activity in adjacent undamaged areas of neocortex (63). Such side effects, although considered to be nonspecific, in the sense of being unintended in terms of the planned profile of cellular replacement, nevertheless, are specific in the present sense of being mediated by active pharmacologic or neural influences by the graft on the host brain. The mechanisms of active side effects, therefore, need to be considered in the same context as the positive signs of recovery and repair in the following sections on specific mechanisms.

CONTROL PROCEDURES TO IDENTIFY THE SPECIFICITY OF GRAFT FUNCTION

The consideration of nonspecific effects, in turn, leads us to the need to consider the nature and sufficiency of alternative control procedures in studies of the effects of neural transplantation. It is not always apparent what might be the appropriate controls. For example, in any lesion and graft model, should one compare the performance of grafted animals, on the one hand, against animals with lesions alone, or against animals with lesions and sham grafts, and on the other hand, against unoperated controls, or animals with sham lesions? It depends on the questions being

asked. If we are seeking to identify the neurobiologic mechanisms and specificity of graft function, it will be most appropriate to use additional groups of animals with sham lesions and sham grafts. However, if we wish to evaluate whether we can achieve functional recovery in a particular model of brain damage and disease, the presence of any recovery in grafted animals is best evaluated in comparison against the performance of animals with lesions alone, and the degree of recovery is best compared to the performance of normal, intact animals, rather than of ones that are already compromised (albeit to a limited extent) by a series of sham lesion and sham graft procedures. Several alternatives, therefore, suggest themselves and need to be considered in each particular experimental context.

Sham Grafts

Perhaps the most obvious control procedure, akin to that employed in a lesion study, is the use of a "sham" graft, in which the full surgical procedure is followed, but excludes only the actual implantation of graft tissue. Most transplantation studies provide sham graft procedures based on injection of sterile saline or buffered medium in place of a cell suspension graft, or implantation of Gelfoam alone in place of a solid graft into the graft cavity. Sham grafts are easiest to perform, but they do not control for nonspecific influence of grafts that produce space-occupying lesions through excessive or tumorous growth following implantation, or for the influence of glial cells and other nonneuronal factors secreted by embryonic tissue grafts.

Control Tissue Grafts

A common alternative is the use of alternative tissues for implantation. Thus, for example, hippocampal and cerebellar grafts have been used as cholinergic-poor tissues to control for the cholinergic specificity of septal grafts implanted in the cortex or hippocampus. Here the control is defined in terms of a negative feature—the absence of a particular cell type—whereas in fact the tissues also differ in many other respects. In other studies, some consideration has been given to controls that are in some senses "appropriate." For example, in a study of the dopaminergic specificity of the functional effects of nigral grafts in the neostriatum, we have used raphe grafts as an alternative source of brain stem monoamine neurons and striatal grafts as an alternative source of neuronal cells appropriate to the target (58). Elsewhere we and others have compared the effects of septal, brain stem, and hippocampal grafts providing alternative sources of reinnervation or reconstruction of the subcortically deafferentated hippocampus (17,35,60,95,182). Nevertheless, in all such cases the different sources of graft tissue differ in many different respects, rather than simply the specific neurotransmitter or particular population of neurons identified as the experimental focus.

Removal of Selected Populations of Cells

A third approach to enhance the specificity of a control graft procedure is to consider the selective blockade or removal of the specific groups of cells within the graft. For example, if the functional effects of nigral grafts are specifically attributable to the dopaminergic neurons in the implants, then it should be possible to remove this particular population of neurons from the grafts before implantation. Although the selective lesioning of dopaminergic neurons in mature grafts, using the toxin 6-hydroxydopamine (6-OHDA) abolishes functional recovery, it has not been shown (at least to our knowledge) that toxic removal of the dopaminergic neurons before implantation blocks the development of recovery in the first place. Attempts to use this approach in our own laboratory, by incubating E14–15 ventral mesencephalon in 6-OHDA before grafting, have been unsuccessful; when this

is done, either (at low concentrations of 6-OHDA) the removal of dopamine neurons has been incomplete or (at higher concentrations) the survival of the whole graft has been compromised (unpublished observations). However, Doucet et al. (50) have had more success in removing the serotonin neurons selectively from ventral mesencephalic transplants by preincubation in 5,7-dihydroxytryptamine (50).

With a similar reasoning, Kesslak et al. (110) dissected grafts from the postnatal cortex under conditions that do not favor the survival of neurons, to show that the recovery provided by cortical grafts implanted into the lesioned prefrontal cortex can be sustained by glial cells alone. This evidence was a major factor in identifying trophic mechanisms of graft function (see later discussion).

Dead Tissue Grafts

A more dramatic control procedure is to kill all cells in the graft before implantation. This procedure provides a somewhat different level of specificity. In particular, if recovery is still provided by dead grafts, and entirely nonspecific effects can be ruled out by sham injections and space-occupying control implants, then the graft effects are likely to be mediated by the transient release of neuroactive compounds, such as growth factors, that have not been degraded by the procedure used to kill the cells. Kesslak et al. (109) used this strategy to show that both dead cells and soluble extracts from the separated material could yield substantial alleviation of the T-maze deficits in rats with prefrontal lesions and provided further evidence in favor of a trophic mechanism of graft function in this model.

Graft Removal

LeVere and LeVere (129) first proposed that the only clear way to determine whether the effects of a graft were not due to nonspecific effects of the transplantation surgery was to demonstrate that removal of the grafts reinstated the original lesion deficit.

The graft-removal strategy has proved an effective means of demonstrating that nigral graft effects are indeed due to a sustained influence of the grafts on the host brain. Thus, the rotational asymmetry in animals with unilateral nigrostriatal lesions, which has recovered following implantation of nigral grafts, is subsequently reinstated by removal of the grafts, by aspiration (13), rejection (27), or neurotoxic lesion (58).

Conversely, in at least two other models, removal of the grafts has not reinstated the initial lesion deficits. Thus, Stein removed cortical grafts that alleviated water maze deficits following implantation into the prefrontal cortex and found that the recovery remained (181). Similarly, Woodruff et al. (204) found that the deficits in an operant DRL task, which were alleviated by hippocampal grafts implanted into a hippocampal lesion cavity, were not reinstated when he subsequently removed the grafts. Thus, in each of these examples, the recovery could not have been dependent on the continuous presence of the grafts. LeVere and LeVere originally considered that, in these circumstances, the graft effects must be nonspecific consequences of the implantation surgery. However, more detailed analyses, in particular in the contexts of the prefrontal cortex lesion model and of adrenal grafts (see Chapters 16 and 6, respectively), have shown that trophic influences of the grafts can be provided quite specifically by the graft tissue, even if they are relatively transient, and are not dependent on the long-term survival of the graft itself. These studies also identify how, with the adrenal graft, the positive identification of specific mechanisms can be necessary to resolve the issue of the relative specificity of graft effects in a manner that was very different from that originally envisioned at the outset of experimentation.

PHARMACOLOGIC MECHANISMS

The simplest way in which a graft might provide a specific functional influence is for it to provide a long-term replacement of a deficient neurochemical by diffuse secretion or release. In such circumstances, the graft may be considered to have a pharmacologic mode of action, acting on the host brain by the same mechanism(s) than any other neuroactive drug influences brain function. The efficacy of a graft will be determined by its capacity to deliver the active molecules, at physiologic concentrations, to appropriate sites in the host brain, rather than by its precise patterns of connectivity or dynamic regulation.

Neuroendocrine Mechanisms

As described by Wood and Charlton (see Chapter 18), the first application of the techniques of intracerebral transplantation for functional studies was the use of pituitary grafts to study the hypophysiotrophic functions of the basal hypothalamus. In these early studies, first Knigge (115) and then Halasz et al. (85,86) demonstrated that pituitary grafts implanted into the third ventricle could restore sexual and growth-related functions disturbed by hypophysectomy. Subsequent workers have confirmed similar effects in a variety of neuroendocrine model systems involving the hypothalamic–pituitary axis, including genetic mutant strains (such as the Brattleboro rat and hpg mouse), in which single populations of hypothalamic neurons are deficient. In each case, a neurohormonal mode of communication is involved, either by release of hypothalamic neurohormones into the portal vessels to signal the cells of the anterior pituitary, or by release of pituitary hormones directly into the peripheral vasculature as the route of relay to the rest of the body. These various model systems, therefore, appear to be primary candidates for a pharmacologic mode of graft action in which grafted cells simply secrete the deficient neurochemical into the host parenchyma or cerebrospinal fluid to reach its distant targets either by diffusion or by uptake and transport within the vascular circulation.

One clear case of intracerebral grafts providing diffuse release of deficient substances has been in the utilization of the brain as a site of relative immune privilege to receive pancreatic islet implants in animals with experimental diabetes. Thus, for example, McEvoy and Leung showed good survival, partial restitution of insulin secretion, and restitution of normoglycemia in rats rendered diabetic with the toxin alloxan. The response was maintained for up to 34-weeks survival (135). The authors concluded from the placement of the grafts in these experiments that insulin was secreted by the graft tissue into the cerebrospinal fluid, from where it traversed into the blood circulation, thereby to regulate peripheral homeostasis. Fetal pancreas has been transplanted into a number of peripheral sites in over 1500 patients with diabetes (188). Poor survival and rejection appears to be a major factor in the relatively limited response in these pancreatic transplantation trials. Intracerebral grafting of fetal pancreatic tissues has not yet been considered in the human experiments.

The first observations of pituitary grafts in hypophysectomized rats also suggested that the grafts may have exerted their effects by relatively diffuse release of deficient neurohormones (see Chapter 18). Thus, for example, Halasz and colleagues reported that pituitary grafts in the third ventricle needed to survive to have a functional effect, but it was not necessary for them to make direct vascular contact with the median eminence (86). Nevertheless, even in these early studies, it was apparent that the effective grafts tended to be positioned in close proximity with the median eminence in the base of the third ventricle, for secreted hormones to reach the portal capillaries by diffusion. Subsequent studies of pituitary and hypothalamic grafts have indicated that functional grafts consistently

manifest the re-formation of specialized contacts with fenestrated capillaries for direct communication of hypothalamic neurons with the posterior pituitary by the portal vasculature. For example, the effectiveness of hypothalamic grafts in the hpg mouse is correlated not only with survival of gonadotropin-releasing hormone (GnRH) neurons within the grafts, but also with the re-formation of fiber connections with the median eminence (171). Conversely, placement of the grafts in the lateral ventricles, although not detrimental to graft survival or fiber outgrowth, leads to a complete absence of functional recovery (117). Thus, a general diffuse release of the active neurohormone into the cerebrospinal fluid circulation is by itself not sufficient. The precise nature of the re-formed contacts will depend on the particular model system, and can involve both the targeted outgrowth of axons from grafted hypothalamic neurons specifically toward the fenestrated capillaries of the host median eminence (37,83, 163,171), and the extension of the host capillary network into the grafts for re-formation of local contacts within the graft tissue itself (100,133,167).

Many neuroendocrine deficits can be alleviated by direct infusion of the deficient neurohormone directly into the blood circulation. For example, intravenous infusions of the antidiuretic hormone vasopressin will reverse the polyuria and polydipsia of the diabetes insipidus of the Brattleboro rat, and insulin infusions alleviate the hypoglycemia of diabetes mellitus. Therefore, it would seem plausible that neural grafts could reverse such neuroendocrine deficits by diffuse secretion of the deficient neurohormone and its uptake and distribution to targets throughout the body through the peripheral circulation. However, although there are a few circumstances when that does provide the likely mechanism, surprisingly, it is more common, at least in the hypothalamic–pituitary interactions, for the grafts to re form specialized contacts with appropriate neuronal and vascular targets, with the likelihood that communication is, in some ways, regulated and targeted, rather than any functional changes being mediated simply by a diffuse release mechanism.

Nigral and Adrenal Grafts

Many of the early studies of the survival and growth of neural grafts focused on the monoamine systems, largely because of the very practical reason that, at that time, these were the only cells for which good neurotransmitter-specific techniques for microscopic visualization were available. Studies involving transplantation of a variety of different systems—noradrenergic, serotonergic, or cholinergic grafts implanted into the hippocampus or nigral grafts implanted into the neostriatum—all revealed extensive fiber outgrowth into the host brain (13,17–19). It was therefore natural to assume, when animals bearing such grafts were first found to show good recovery from the functional deficits associated with lesions of the intrinsic monoamine systems (13,18,149), that the recovery was due to the observed re-formation of connections between the graft and host brain. However, this assumption was soon challenged.

When Freed and colleagues undertook a detailed fluorescence histochemical analysis of their surviving nigral grafts, they found that axon growth proliferated within the graft tissues in their intraventricular transplantation site, but gave rise to only rather limited ingrowth into the host neostriatum, even in some animals showing good recovery in the apomorphine rotation test (76). Measurement of dopamine content in tissue punches revealed a rather high concentration in the graft itself, but a rapid decline in the adjacent host striatum at sites other than those immediately adjacent to the ventricle. This led them to suggest that, although the grafts may have been exerting their effects by reinnervation and re-formation of synaptic contacts, an alternative mechanism based on passive diffusion of

dopamine from cells within the grafts could not be excluded, and was indeed more plausible. This could be equally effective in producing down-regulation of supersensitive dopamine receptors necessary to alleviate the rotational asymmetry induced by direct receptor agonists such as apomorphine (74). In the studies of nigral grafts, Freed was unable to determine the extent to which reinnervation contributed to the recovery. However, the situation was less equivocal in parallel studies using grafts of adrenal medulla as an alternative source of catecholamine-producing cells. Here, the grafted chromaffin cells gave rise to fine, elongated processes that grew extensively within the graft tissue, but very few fibers were seen to leave the grafts and penetrate into the host brain (75). Nevertheless, these animals showed a degree of compensation on the apomorphine rotation test similar to that seen in the rats with intraventricular nigra grafts. This led the authors to suggest that, in this instance at least, catecholamines can diffuse from the graft in sufficient quantities to reduce dopaminergic receptor sensitivity in the adjacent caudate–putamen and, thereby, to reduce apomorphine-induced rotation.

So, in this interpretation, the graft functions as a passive source for the diffuse secretion of a deficient neurotransmitter into the host neostriatum, rather than as the origin of a necessary reinnervation and one dependent on re-formation of synaptic contacts. Replacing dopamine by a living graft may provide a more efficient, stable, and long-lasting delivery of the transmitter at a physiologic concentration to selected targets within the brain than is possible with any other available drug-delivery system. Nevertheless, the fundamental mechanism is still essentially pharmacologic, the graft functioning as an efficient self-renewing "biologic minipump."

As it has subsequently turned out, the diffuse release of deficient catecholamines is only one of the mechanisms whereby adrenal grafts may exert their influence. Indeed, in some circumstances, that may be of less importance than the trophic influence exerted by adrenal tissues on an incompletely lesioned host dopamine system (see Chapter 6). Nevertheless, these early studies using adrenal graft tissues pointed to an important potential mode of action and have stimulated the development of explicit diffuse pharmacologic delivery systems for application in the brain. The viability of various dopamine delivery systems now provides the clearest evidence that a diffuse pharmacologic action can indeed provide one potential mechanism of graft function.

Dopamine Delivery Systems

A variety of different strategies are under active development for delivering dopamine or other neuroactive chemicals at a stable and prolonged level in the brain.

Direct Intracerebral Infusion of Dopamine

It has been known since the early 1970s that brief infusions of dopamine or dopamine agonists directly into the neostriatum induce motor behaviors in rats. Thus, for example, striatal infusions induce head-turning and motor biases to the contralateral side of the body (42,191), whereas infusions into the nucleus accumbens are associated with increased general locomotor activities (151,152). However, of more interest in the context of the mechanisms of graft function are the effects of long-term, stable intracerebral infusions, in particular in animals with lesions. This has been investigated in considerably less detail than might have been expected. Nevertheless, Olson et al. (146) reported that infusion of dopamine over 1 to 2 weeks into the neostriatum of rats with unilateral nigrostriatal lesions down-regulated receptor supersensitivity and alleviated the apomorphine-induced rotation asymmetry, akin to the effects of adrenal grafts implanted into the

same site, and this has subsequently been replicated by others (88,121).

Dopamine-Secreting Polymers

Crystalline dopamine can be encapsulated within a polymer matrix. Suitable polymers are now available that will dissolve slowly (over a period of months) and provide slow release of the entrapped dopamine following implantation in the brain (78,137). Moreover, such polymeric implants can exert a functional influence on host animals, similar to the recovery reported with adrenal grafts, as measured by a reduction of spontaneous and of apomorphine rotation in rats with unilateral nigrostriatal lesions (10,136,202).

Cells Engineered to Secrete Dopamine or Its Precursors

Stable delivery of dopamine or other neuroactive molecules may be best achieved either by identifying cell lines that already produce the molecules of interest (e.g., pheochromocytoma-derived PC12 cells secrete dopamine and other catecholamines), or by explicitly engineering cells or cell lines to produce them (81). Both primary cells and cell lines have been engineered to produce dopamine, its precursor L-dopa, or the synthetic enzyme tyrosine hydroxylase, and these cells are capable of increasing levels of dopamine *in vivo*, occasionally requiring an endogenous supply of cofactors (70,96,189,190,203). Moreover, engineered cells have been capable of alleviating apomorphine-, but not amphetamine-induced rotation (70,96,97,105). However, one problem in these studies is that, whereas engineered primary cells, such as fibroblasts or muscle cells, may survive for several months following transplantation without problem (70,81,105), engineered cell lines can become tumorous, showing uncontrolled growth and production of seizures within 2 weeks of transplantation (70,96,97,190).

Encapsulation of Dopamine-Secreting Cells

One approach to the problem associated with the potential uncontrolled growth of tumorigenic cells and engineered cell lines has been to encapsulate the cells in semipermeable polymer tubes. This allows entry of nutrients essential for the grafted cells to survive and the exit of small, soluble molecules (such as dopamine) into the host brain. At the same time the encapsulation not only provides a physical containment of the grafted tissue from uncontrolled growth, but in addition, protects the grafted cells from cells of the host immune system, making it possible to transplant xenografts without rejection or immunoprotection (67). Such an approach has been used to permit long-term grafting and function of a dopamine-secreting immortalized PC12 cell line (3,202), which otherwise forms tumors in the absence of encapsula-

tion (11,102). Similarly, bovine chromaffin cells survive encapsulation and secrete catecholamines *in vitro,* and they survive xenotransplantation of the capsules into rats and alleviate apomorphine rotation asymmetries *in vivo* (2). However, in this latter study, the efficacy of the encapsulated grafts was followed over only 4 weeks, and long-term survival was not evaluated in either the *in vitro* or the *in vivo* models.

These various strategies indicate that long-term diffuse delivery of dopamine into the denervated neostriatum can down-regulate receptor supersensitivity and alleviate motor asymmetries in the apomorphine rotation test. This suggests that at least some of the effects of nigral and adrenal grafts could be mediated by a relatively diffuse pharmacologic mechanism of action. However, many other aspects of nigral graft function (and perhaps also of adrenal graft function) are unlikely to involve such a diffuse mechanism. Thus, as summarized in Table 2, in contrast with the broad range of behavioral functions that are alleviated

TABLE 2. *Functional effects of alternative dopamine replacement strategies in rats with unilateral nigrostriatal lesions*

Test	Nigral grafts	Adrenal grafts	Long term dopamine infusion	Engineered cell implants	Encapsulated cell implants
Apomorphine rotation	+	+	+	+	+
Apomorphine hyperactivity	+	?	?	?	?
Amphetamine rotation	+ +	+ /0	0	0	?
Spontaneous rotation	+ +	?	?	?	?
Exploratory biases	+ +	?	?	?	?
Contralateral neglect	+ +	+ /0	?	?	?
Skilled paw use	0	0	?	?	?
Intracranial self-stimulation	+	?	?	?	?
Conditioned rotation	+ / −	?	?	?	?

+ +, complete recovery; +, partial recovery; 0, no recovery; −, negative effects; ?, not tested.

by nigral grafts (see Chapter 2), cells engineered to secrete dopamine provide a return of striatal dopamine and reduce spontaneous and apomorphine-induced rotation, but do not alleviate deficits in the amphetamine rotation test. The situation with adrenal grafts is more ambiguous. In some cases, the amphetamine rotation deficits are modestly reduced (9), whereas in others, adrenal grafts have no effect whatsoever on this impairment (26). The difference here may relate to the extent of the host lesions. In some circumstances, adrenal grafts provide only a diffuse release of dopamine, whereas in other situations the host system is sufficiently spared to be responsive to trophic actions of the graft (8). By contrast, adrenal grafts do not provide any significant alleviation on some other tests against which nigral grafts are effective, such as contralateral somatosensory neglect (71).

These observations suggest that a variety of different mechanisms apply to different grafts, even ones that are designed as alternative strategies for dopamine replacement in the dopamine-denervated forebrain: some grafts may effectively alleviate a selected subset of deficits primarily by the pharmacologic mechanism of diffuse dopamine replacement. They restore normal sensitivity to dopamine receptors and provide a tonic background level of dopaminergic activation of the intrinsic neurons of the neostriatum. However, this appears to provide a restitution of function to only a limited subset of symptoms. A more extensive profile of recovery requires regulated synaptic transmitter release and perhaps a more complete reorganization of dopaminergic connections within the host striatum. This may be provided either from grafted embryonic nigral neurons or by reorganization within host systems spared by the initial lesions. A more detailed characterization of the extent and limitations of recovery that may be achieved by the simpler pharmacologic mechanisms is clearly needed. However, the model systems that

would allow such an analysis—such as the novel implant systems for tonic dopamine delivery—have so far been studied only on a limited range of functional tests (see Table 2).

TROPHIC MECHANISMS

The preceding discussion has alluded to several experiments that suggest that grafts can provide a trophic influence on intrinsic host systems to stimulate reorganization within the damaged brain or to counteract secondary damage associated with toxic or traumatic brain injury. Although trophic mechanisms are also pharmacologic, in the sense that the graft provides diffuse secretion of neuroactive molecules, the mechanisms of recovery involves a reorganization and return of functional activity within the intrinsic neural circuits of the host brain itself, rather than the graft contributing directly to that functional activity in the behaving animal.

Graft-Derived Stimulation of Recovery

Trophic mechanisms of graft action were first suggested by the studies of Stein and colleagues, with the demonstration of recovery on T-maze alternation tasks after implantation of cortical tissues into bilateral aspiration lesion sites in the prefrontal cortex (126). As reviewed by Kolb and Fantie (see Chapter 16), several lines of evidence suggest that this recovery is not dependent on the continued presence of the graft; rather, the grafts appear to stimulate spontaneous recovery processes within the host brain. In this situation, once the intrinsic reorganization had taken place, removal of the graft did not influence the continued improved performance of recovered rats (181). A comparable alleviation of complex-learning deficits by hippocampal grafts, which is not abolished even when the grafts are subsequently removed, has been seen in other studies using bilateral aspirative le-

Growth Factor-Secreting Cografts

Grafted neurons, like all others in the developing nervous system, are likely to depend on a variety of growth factors to regulate their survival, and to stimulate and direct axon outgrowth. Thus, for example, adrenal chromaffin cells are normally dependent on the availability of NGF for survival and phenotypic differentiation (187, 192), and there is now good evidence to indicate that intracerebral administration of NGF may promote the survival, differentiation, and long-term function of adrenal grafts both in rats and monkeys (for review see 61). For example, Strömberg et al. (184) have observed that extended infusion of NGF improved the survival of catecholamine fluorescent cells within adrenal grafts in the striatum and was associated with an improvement in the duration of functional recovery of the host animals in the apomorphine rotation test.

An alternative to making repeated injections or continuous infusion through implanted cannulae to deliver trophic factors into the vicinity of the transplant is to use cografts as a source of trophic factors for other graft tissues. This approach has been applied to promote the survival and differentiation of adrenal chromaffin cells. Thus, for example, cotransplantation with C6 glioma cells yielded an almost fourfold increase in the numbers of surviving chromaffin cells in adrenal grafts, and the grafted cells formed more extensive processes (12). Parallel biochemical measurements indicated a shift in the capacity of the grafted adrenal cells to secrete dopamine, rather than norepinephrine or epinephrine. Another source of peripheral tissue rich in NGF is the peripheral nerve. Cotransplantation of adrenal medulla tissues with sections of sciatic or sural nerve (either as autografts or allografts) has promoted adrenal graft survival and fiber extension in monkeys (87,118,197), rats (77), and mice (48).

Thus, it appears that trophic factor-secreting cografts can yield a detectable improvement in the viability of intracerebral neural transplants. However, the present techniques are almost certainly not optimal. In particular, the available tissues for cografts provide only modest levels of NGF supplementation. Cells specifically engineered to secrete trophic factors may be more efficient, and initial studies along these lines have given promising results. For example, Cunningham et al. (44) obtained a significant increase in survival and fiber extension in adrenal chromaffin cells cografted with astrocytes engineered to produce NGF, and Ernfors et al. (68) found a similar increase in the survival and fiber outgrowth of fetal septal cholinergic neurons cografted with NGF-secreting 3T3 cells. Needless to say, a long-term strategy designing cells with particular profiles of growth-promoting activity must take account of the broader spectrum of factors to which neuronal cells respond, rather than focusing on NGF alone.

REGENERATIVE MECHANISMS

Whereas the preceding sections confirm the hypothesis that a variety of alternative mechanisms can mediate graft function, there remain many situations for which the replacement of lost neuronal connections still provides the most plausible mechanism of graft-derived recovery in brain-damaged animals. In earlier accounts (15) we distinguished, on the one hand, between grafts that provided a diffuse reinnervation of the host brain, and from which the release of neurotransmitter was tonic and unregulated (see Fig. 1A–C), and on the other hand, grafts that established reciprocal connections with the host brain, and so were effective by reconstruction of damaged neuronal circuits (see Fig. 1D and 2). Although there is a clear logical distinction between these alternatives, it turns out that individual cases are seldom so clear-cut. Rather, in most situations in which there is observable outgrowth from grafted neurons, the elec-

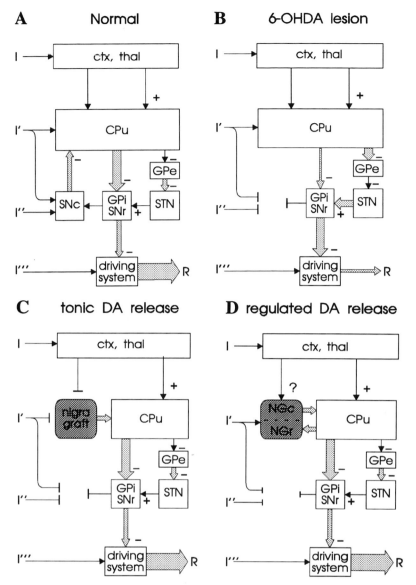

FIG. 1. A proposed model of nigral graft function in the dopamine (*DA*) deafferentated neostriatum (*CPu*). **A:** Motor responses are elicited from a set of brain stem-driving systems (for example, the subthalamic and brain stem locomotor nuclei) that are activated by two major striatal outputs structures, the globus pallidus (*GP*) and substantia nigra pars reticulata (*SNr*). The GP and SNr, in turn, are under inhibitory control from the CPu. The nigrostriatal DA neurons in the substantia nigra pars compacta (*SNc*) regulate the functional state of the CPu and its responsiveness to inputs from the cortex (*ctx*) and thalamus (*thal*) to control the selection and initiation of motor programs. Removal of the DA inputs to the CPu by a 6-hydroxydopamine (6-OHDA) lesion (**B**) results in an increased threshold for motor responses (*R*) to diverse activating sensory, limbic, or cortical inputs (*I–I'''*). One potential mechanism of nigral grafts (*NG*) action is to provide a tonic release of DA into the deafferentated CPu, normalizing the threshold for motor responses (**C**). In fact, it appears that in addition to this tonic influence, nigral grafts develop a degree of internal organization and are subject to regulatory control both from some ascending systems (*I'*) and feedback from striatal neurons onto both the dendrites and presynaptic terminals of the grafted dopaminergic neurons (**D**). Note that the *plus* and *minus* signs symbolize the net effect of a projection on the functional activity in the target structure, and do not necessarily indicate the excitatory or inhibitory nature of the synapse itself. The sizes of the *arrows* denote proposed changes in these net functional influences. (Redrawn from ref. 15, with permission.)

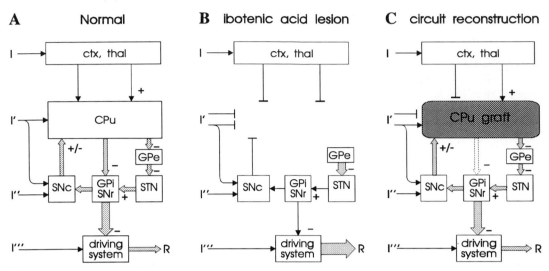

FIG. 2. A proposed model of striatal graft function in the ibotenic acid-denervated neostriatum (*CPu*). See Fig. 1 legend for abbreviations and principles of organization in the intact system. Destruction of the intrinsic neurons of the CPu by ibotenic acid results in loss of inhibitory control of the CPu and SNr, disinhibiting of the motor-driving system, denoted by an increased motor response (*R*) to activating inputs *I'''* (**B**). Striatal grafts reinstate the striatal inhibitory control of the GP and (in some cases) the SNr (**C**). In addition, the striatal grafts also come under the regulatory control of ascending inputs (*I'*, *SNc*) and receive projections from systems (cortex and thalamus) that guide the selection and initiation of motor programs within the striatal circuits. (Redrawn from ref. 15, with permission.)

trophysiologic activity, neurotransmitter release, and postsynaptic activation elicited from those neurons, all are subject to host regulation to a greater or lesser extent. Consequently, whereas we need to distinguish between logical alternatives (see Table 1), in practice, the requirement is to subject each graft model to detailed individual analysis; the outcome is often quite complex.

Tonic Reinnervation

Evidence for the importance of fiber outgrowth providing tonic reinnervation of the host brain has been most obvious in cases of grafts of brain stem catecholamine, indoleamine, and cholinergic systems implanted into deafferentated target areas in the forebrain, such as the neostriatum, cortex, and hippocampus. Many of the early studies of graft function were based on such

models, which have been well described in several of the preceding chapters (see Chapters 2, 4, 10–13). In all of these model systems, the grafts are seen to provide an extensive fiber reinnervation of the host brain. Moreover, reinnervation seems to be a necessary condition for, and to correlate with, functional recovery in the host animals. For example, in our early studies of recovery of animals bearing nigral grafts, the degree of recovery in individual animals correlated better with the extent of fiber reinnervation into the denervated striatum than with the size and number of dopamine cells surviving within the grafts themselves (13). Moreover, the topographic distribution of reinnervation, rather than its density alone, is critical in the profile and degree of functional recovery (14,55).

In the septohippocampal system also, we have seen a good correlation between the degree of recovery in a maze-learning task and the extent of cholinergic reinnervation in the hippocampus (60). However, this study provided the first indications of the need for caution in drawing a simple conclusion: although the cholinergic reinnervation was necessary for functional alleviation, it was not by itself sufficient. Thus, although recovery was seen only in animals with good grafts, there were a few instances in which animals with good grafts showed no indication of significant recovery. This led us to suggest that the formation of other connections in conjunction with the cholinergic reinnervation may be necessary to restore maze performance. Indeed, subsequent electrophysiologic studies have indicated that septal grafts may form reciprocal septohippocampal connections sufficient to maintain an effective theta rhythm (28), and such reciprocal connections may be required for good restitution of behavioral function.

Of particular note in each of these model systems is that the grafts are effective even though they are placed in an ectopic location. Thus, in these studies, the nigral grafts have been placed into the deafferentated neostriatum and the septal grafts into the deafferentated hippocampus or neocortex to obtain functional effects (54,95). This corroborates the underlying hypothesis that it is terminal reinnervation per se that is the necessary level of reconstruction for functional recovery.

A noteworthy common feature of such grafts is that they all involve cells of the isodendritic core, which is characterized by a small number of cells producing a widespread and highly-branched innervation of large forebrain areas. These neuronal systems, as individual components of the classic reticular formation, are all thought to exert a relatively diffuse regulatory control over their targets. Whereas, the target areas themselves subserve a variety of complex functions, based on processing high-order patterned information within highly organized point-to-point connections, this complex organization is not disturbed by the experimental subcortical lesions. Rather, the grafted neurons must provide only a rather diffuse reinnervation to provide reactivation of the targets and, thereby, enable them to return to a more normal level of function. Thus, as discussed in detail elsewhere (16), the grafts can provide recovery of complex functions (such as are involved in spatial navigation, learning, or memory) by enabling otherwise intact neuronal circuitries in the cortex, hippocampus, and basal ganglia to return to normal function. In particular, it should be kept in mind that recovery in the performance of complex cognitive tasks in these graft models does not imply that the grafts are actually reconstructing the primary neuronal circuits mediating those cognitive functions.

Additional Regulated Control

Although nigral and septal grafts have occasionally been considered to provide the best examples of grafts providing a diffuse, tonic reinnervation, evidence is accumulating in both models that the graft-derived reinnervation is regulated to a certain extent by the host brain.

The most direct means to monitor the functional activity of a diffuse reinnervation is to monitor transmitter turnover *in vivo*. Thus, Nilsson et al. (143,144) used microdialysis probes to monitor acetylcholine release from septal grafts implanted in the hippocampus of animals with fimbria–fornix lesions. As expected from previous postmortem biochemical studies, the grafts restored a normal baseline level of acetylcholine turnover, which was shown, by potassium and tetrodotoxin infusions, to be dependent on normal axonal impulse flow. More importantly for the present discussion, acetylcholine release from the grafts appeared to be regulated by the host brain, since acetylcholine overflow was increased both by direct electrical stimulation of the lateral habenula and by stress induced either by handling or immobilization of the animals. Similarly, acetylcholine release in the graft-reinnervated hippocampus increased during motor activity (swimming), and this effect was abolished when the axonal connections between the graft and the host were severed by a knife cut (143). The authors concluded that "despite their ectopic location, [the septal grafts] can become functionally integrated with the host brain and that the activity of the transplanted cholinergic neurons can be modulated from the host brain during ongoing behavior" (144). To identify the source of the host influence over the grafts, a combination of anatomic techniques were used to demonstrate ingrowth of septal, hippocampal, serotonin-positive, and tyrosine hydroxylase-positive axons growing into the grafts. In a subsequent study, Leanza et al. (128) have obtained pharmacologic evidence that noradrenergic and dopaminergic afferents to the grafts, originating in the brain stem of the host, exert a regulatory control over the grafted septal cholinergic neurons.

The anatomic basis of a similar host regulation of nigral grafts has been apparent for a long time (see Fig. 1C, D). At the ultrastructural level, nonimmunoreactive axon terminals have been seen to make contact with the tyrosine hydroxylase–immunoreactive processes of grafted nigral dopamine neurons in functionally recovered rats, both within the grafts and, more particularly, with dendrites extending into the host neostriatum (39,132,145). Moreover, Doucet et al. (50) have used immunocytochemical methods and phaseolus vulgaris leucoagglutinin (PHA-L) tracing to demonstrate ingrowth of both serotonin and cortical fibers into nigral grafts. It is also likely that the graft-derived dopamine fiber outgrowth is subject to local presynaptic regulation within the host striatum, since opiate receptors, which are believed to be located on nigral terminals and are lost after nigrostriatal lesion, are restored over the area of reinnervation following implantation of nigral grafts (172). Thus, the machinery ap-

pears to be present for the host brain to be capable of regulating the activity of dopaminergic neurons in nigral grafts, both at the level of the cell bodies within the grafts and at the presynaptic terminals in the host brain.

In vivo microdialysis has been used to show that dopamine turnover can be restored to near-normal levels in the immediate vicinity of grafts, that turnover is responsive to pharmacologic modulation, and that dopamine metabolism is probably subject to a degree of autoregulation to maintain normal levels of synthesis and turnover (159,183,206). In a recent microdialysis study, Cenci et al. (36) have shown that dopamine release from nigral grafts implanted into the nucleus accumbens and anteromedial frontal cortex is increased during rewarded behavior (eating) and following mildly stressful stimulation (handling), although the magnitude of the responses was less than normal. By contrast, graft-derived transmitter release was unaffected by forced immobilization, which is a powerful activator of cortical dopamine release in the intact animal. These observations indicate that the grafted dopaminergic neurons can be activated during ongoing behavior, but their functional integration with the host brain is clearly incomplete. It seems possible, therefore, that the inability of the grafted nigral neurons to release adequate amounts of dopamine in certain behavioral contexts could explain, at least partly, the limited improvement of more complex adaptive behaviors, such as exploration and hoarding, seen after transplantation into corticolimbic structures.

Thus, although nigral and septal grafts were initially considered as prototypical examples of models in which the graft exerted a functional influence by providing a diffuse reinnervation and tonic synaptic reactivation at denervated receptors, even in these cases a degree of host regulation appears to apply. The necessity of that additional level of regulation for graft function remains unknown. Perhaps the clearest case for graft function being mediated by its outputs alone is provided by a quite different model system, that of retinal grafts replacing afferent visual inputs to the tectum in blinded rats. Lund and colleagues have used several strategies to show that such grafts are functional (41), including the observations that they are capable of transducing light inputs and relaying that information to the host brain to restore the pupillary reflex in the eyes from which the optic nerve has been cut (113). This model system provides clear demonstration, at both the anatomic and functional levels, of unidirectional relay by graft axons of afferent information into the host brain, with little apparent reciprocal regulation.

Reconstruction of Reciprocal Graft–Host Connections

Although several model systems provide clear evidence for reciprocal connections between the graft and the host brain, usually it has not proved possible to conclude that such a level of reconstruction is necessary for their functional efficacy. Thus, for example, as discussed in Chapter 3, it has been hypothesized that the limits of recovery with intrastriatal nigral grafts are to a great extent due to their ectopic location. Although, there is considerable effort underway to provide full reconstruction of the nigrostriatal pathway, taking advantage of a variety of bridging, growth-promoting, or developmental processes to enhance long-distance growth from nigral grafts implanted into the ventral mesencephalon (4,62), effective reconstruction in that circuitry has not yet been achieved with a sufficient degree of reliability to evaluate the working hypothesis with any conviction. In other model systems, such as implantation of embryonic Purkinje cells into the cerebellum of mutant Purkinje cell degeneration (pcd) mice, there has been good evidence for the rather precise incorporation of the

grafted cells into the tightly organized neuroanatomic circuitry of the developing cerebellum (178,179), but such grafts have not yet been subjected to rigorous functional analysis.

One model system that has been considered to provide evidence suggesting a functional mechanism dependent on reciprocal graft–host connections is that provided by striatal grafts implanted into the excitotoxically lesioned neostriatum in an animal model of Huntington's disease (15; see Fig. 2). As reviewed in Chapter 7 and elsewhere (199), striatal grafts establish extensive connections, both to and from the host brain, that to a varying extent reproduce all the major inputs and outputs of the intact neostriatum. Although striatal grafts comprise nonstriatal as well as striatal tissues, importantly for any functional influence the striatal cells aggregate into patches within the grafts, and the normal inputs and outputs are established within that striatal compartment. Moreover, such grafts can restore function on a variety of behavioral tests (51). That fact by itself would not be sufficient to determine whether the reciprocal connectivity was necessary for graft function, which is suggested by several additional observations.

First, whereas damage in the nigrostriatal dopamine system, whether made experimentally in animals or by an intrinsic disease process in humans, can be alleviated by drugs such as L-dopa or bromocriptine, it has not been possible to provide any fundamental pharmacologic amelioration of deficits in Huntington's disease or with experimental striatal lesions. This indicates that whereas a simple pharmacologic mode of action has to be considered as a possible mechanism for nigral grafts a similar action is less plausible for striatal grafts.

Second, the neostriatum receives its primary inputs from the whole neocortical mantle and provides a major route for cortical selection, initiation, and control over voluntary action. Lesions within the neostriatum, whether by the experimental injection of excitotoxins in animals or by Huntington's disease in humans, produce frontal cognitive dysfunctions that are believed to reflect a "disconnection" syndrome of the prefrontal cortex from subcortical motor control (147). Consequently, any therapeutic strategy must be oriented to reconnection of disrupted corticostriatopallidal and corticostriatonigral circuits, which striatal grafts seem to provide, at least at the anatomic level (see Fig. 2). Notably, striatal grafts have been as effective in relieving deficits on classic frontal cognitive tasks, such as delayed alternation, as on simple motor hyperkinesias (101).

Third, although the replacement of a single dopamine input to a dopamine denervated striatum may appear *a priori* to be a simpler goal to achieve than reconstruction of damaged striatal circuits after lesions of all intrinsic striatal neurons, in fact striatal grafts have yielded recovery on tests of skilled paw-reaching that have been largely resistant to amelioration by nigral grafts (59,65,140). This initially counterintuitive result is understandable if this task is dependent on the striatal relay of afferent information that is provided by the homotopic striatal grafts, but not by ectopic nigral grafts (see Chapter 3).

Fourth, although the issue of topography has not yet been studied in detail, striatal grafts must be substantially located within the striatum, but close to the pallidum, to subserve a functional effect on both cognitive maze-learning tasks and on locomotor activity tests, whereas grafts located predominantly in the globus pallidus itself are without substantial effect (101). This suggests that target reinnervation alone is insufficient to exert a functional effect, but is compatible with the graft needing to be placed in a location where it can attract cortical (or other) afferents.

Finally, several studies have undertaken to investigate the relay of afferent and efferent information in striatal grafts directly. Thus, Sirinathsinghji et al. (173) used push–pull perfusion to monitor γ-aminobutyric acid (GABA) release from striatal graft axons projecting to the globus pallidus (and substantia nigra). Striatal lesions abolish GABAergic projections to the pallidum and result in almost total loss of extracellular pallidal GABA turnover. Not only is baseline GABA turnover restored (to approximately 35% of the normal level) in rats bearing striatal grafts, but also so is the increased release induced by pharmacologic activation of host dopamine afferents to the grafts. Moreover, in a recent microdialysis study, Campbell et al. (30) have obtained pharmacologic evidence of both dopaminergic and glutamatergic (probably cortical) regulation of GABA release from the intrastriatal striatal grafts. Thus, both nigrostriatal and corticostriatal inputs may participate in the regulation of the graft-derived outputs.

Bridge Grafts

A particular aspect of using grafts for reconstructing neural circuits in the damaged brain has arisen in the use of bridge grafts. This mechanism of function was originally conceived in terms of the grafted tissue providing a substrate for axon growth, in particular in the context of permitting central axons to regenerate across a barrier to reinnervate a denervated target. A classic example of this type of regeneration is the use of an implanted segment of sciatic nerve to bridge a transection of the spinal cord (49), and further examples of bridging the transected fiber bundles of the nigrostriatal pathway, the optic tract, and the spinal cord are well described in Chapters 3, 17, and 20.

Bridge grafts of this first type have concentrated on providing good substrates for growth of axons of the host brain, allowing them to regrow over distances that are not achieved by spontaneous regenerative processes in the mature mammalian CNS. Thus, a major focus has been on the use of peripheral nerve grafts in the CNS, since this tissue is known to provide a good substrate for spontaneous regeneration in the PNS (69). This has led to an active field of research seeking to identify the critical components of PNS that are conducive to CNS axon regeneration, and the development of purer strategies for promoting CNS regeneration, such as blocking the activities of inhibitory molecules (165,166) or using artificial bridges coated in Schwann cells, basal lamina, or extracellular matrix molecules, such as laminin or fibronectin, to enable growth of damaged axons to distant targets *in vivo* (62,99,116,124,148,170,207). Gage and Buzsaki (79) designate bridge grafts of this first type, involving placement of tissues or other materials into the cavity between cells of origin and their targets as a substrate for promoting axonal regeneration, as *passive bridges*.

They also identify a second type of bridge graft, which they designate *active bridges* (79). These typically involve use of embryonic CNS tissues for the bridge graft and have been most actively investigated in the septohippocampal system and in the spinal cord (123,157). Here, the situation is more complicated than for passive bridges because, in addition to providing a substrate for host axons to reinnervate distant targets, the embryonic neuronal tissues that compose the grafts provide a target for direct innervation from the host brain and the neurons within the grafts can, in turn, innervate the host (22,122,156,157). Consequently, bridge grafts of this second type appear capable of reconstructing reciprocal connections between the graft and host brain rather than serving simply as passive bridges for host axon growth. In addition, although most attempts to reconstruct spinal damage with neural transplants have been without functional effects (for fuller discussion, see Chapter 20), there have been a few instances for which the grafts appear to be functional in a number of tests of simple locomotor function (23,82,125). However, whether that recovery is actually mediated through the incorporation of the graft tissue within reconstructed neuronal circuits within the spinal cord, or is due to a less specific process involving enhancement of anatomic plasticity within the damaged host cord, remains a matter for considerable debate (82,125).

PSYCHOLOGIC FACTORS IN GRAFT FUNCTION

Up to this point, the mechanisms of graft function have been considered in terms of the patterns of anatomic connectivity or neurochemical influence between the grafted cells and the host brain. However, although not yet well studied, a number of lines of evidence are accumulating to suggest that graft efficacy needs to be considered in psychologic as well as structural terms, in that the training and experiences of the animal can have a substantial influence on the functional efficacy of a neural transplant.

Environment

The first, and simplest, level of analysis of the role of psychologic factors on the growth, connectivity, and functional efficacy of a neural graft relates to influences of the animal's environment. It has been well established that richness or poverty of an animal's environment can influence developmental processes in neocortex, so that, for example, raising an animal in an enriched environment results in detectable increases in thickness and in the density of synaptic connections in the neocortex (162). Moreover, providing rats with an enriched environment can enhance the rate and extent of recovery after brain injury (47,106,198). Several groups, therefore, have asked whether similar experiences could modify the growth, connectivity, and functional efficacy of neuronal grafts implanted in the brain. In the first such study, after making fimbria–fornix lesions followed by implants of cholinergic-rich septal grafts into the hippocampus, we housed rats either in small groups in standard laboratory rat cages *(impoverished)* or as a large colony in a large wire-mesh monkey cage filled with climbing frames, branches, tubes, shelves, and other objects *(enriched)* (64). Although there were no significant differences in graft survival or volume, the density of acetylcholinesterase-stained fibers in the hippocampus was significantly higher at 4 weeks after grafting. By 10 weeks, outgrowth had reached a similarly high level in all animals. Thus, enrichment appeared to enhance the initial rate of fiber outgrowth, but not the final extent of reinnervation, which stabilized at a close to normal asymptotic level in all animals.

Kelche and colleagues have adopted this same fimbria–fornix lesion and septal graft paradigm to investigate further whether enriched housing conditions can lead to improved functional recovery (107). Therefore, they housed control, lesion, and grafted animals in either enriched or standard environments before training in the Hebb–Williams series of maze-learning tasks, first at 2 months and then again at 10 months after surgery. Although grossly impaired in contrast with the sham-operated control animals, the lesioned and grafted rats did not differ on the short-term test. However, when retested at 10 months, there was a significant improvement in the grafted rats housed in the enriched environment. By contrast, the grafts did not, by themselves, yield recovery in the rats reared under standard housing conditions. As in the 10-week evaluation in the previous study, the extent of cholinergic fiber outgrowth did not differ between the two grafted groups when assessed after the 10 month tests. Thus, improved reinnervation alone is unlikely to account for the benefit provided by the enriched environment, suggesting that both regrowth and appropriate experience are required for substantial recovery in these rather complex maze tasks (see following section "Learning to Use the Transplant").

Conditioning Effects

A second area for which psychologic factors can influence graft effects lies in the influence of previous experience on an animal's response to training stimuli which, in turn, can alter the ways grafted animals respond in tests of recovery. This issue has been most apparent in considering the extent to which changes in responsiveness of animals with nigrostriatal lesions and nigral grafts in drug tests of activity and rotation are attributable to (a) pharmacologic factors (such changes in receptor sensitivity), or (b) psychologic factors (such as changes in learning and reinforcement processes).

The first concern for such processes influencing behavioral test scores came from the analysis of rotational responses in animals that had received bilateral 6-OHDA lesions and unilateral nigral grafts in infancy. Snyder-Keller and Lund (174) found that such animals would rotate contralateral to the grafts, when activated by a tail-pinch stressor, only if they had previously been tested with amphetamine, whereas naïve, grafted animals showed little turning response. They, therefore, suggested that amphetamine treatment is necessary to "prime" a graft to render it functionally effective.

The ability to modify rotational responding by associative conditioning was first demonstrated by Carey (31–33). He gave rats with unilateral 6-OHDA lesions repeated injections of apomorphine in one of two environments, and similar exposure to the other environment without any drug injection. As expected, the drug induced contralateral rotation wherever tested. He then gave the same rats an injection of saline: they rotated in the contralateral direction if placed in the environment in which they had previously been given apomorphine, but did not rotate if placed in the other environment. Thus, the rats established a conditioned (Pavlovian) association between the experience of the drug and the environment in which the drug response was tested which would modify performance when subsequently reexposed to that environment, even in the absence of the drug. Carey went on to demonstrate that the conditioned rotation response to the saline injections in trained animals was not blocked by antagonism of the dopamine receptors, indicating that the conditioning process was independent of changes in the receptor supersensitivity that underlie the primary rotational response to apomorphine in 6-OHDA-treated rats (34).

In one set of experiments designed to assess whether such conditioned associations may also influence the response of grafted animals, Reading studied the effects of conditioned hyperactivity. In an as yet unpublished study (see Chapter 8), he first demonstrated that 6-OHDA lesions of the ventral striatum abolished both amphetamine-induced and conditioned hyperactivity in photocell cages. As in previous studies (38,57,141), nigral grafts were very effective in restoring the drug-induced response. However, the same animals showed no detectable restitution whatsoever in the conditioned response in the same apparatus. This dissociation corroborates Carey's speculation that the conditioning process is independent of primary changes in the dopamine receptors, and highlights the limitation of graft-induced restitution of conditioned behaviors.

More encouraging results were obtained by Annett et al. (6), using the standard rotation paradigm to test rats with unilateral 6-OHDA lesions and intrastriatal nigral grafts (Fig. 3). They gave animals injections of amphetamine in different test environments before treatment with saline in one. Two separate effects were identified: First, repeated injections of amphetamine produced a progressively greater response in the animals. Thus, animals with unilateral 6-OHDA nigrostriatal lesions showed greater ipsilateral rotation response on each consecutive trial. In this particular experiment,

as is often true with such grafts (1,56,93), the grafts were all effective not only in completely counteracting the lesion-induced asymmetry, but produced an "overcompensation" (i.e., turning in the contralateral direction). Moreover, the contralateral rotation in grafted animals was at progressively higher rates on each consecutive trial (6). This apparent progressive "sensitization" of the amphetamine response is unremarkable and has been described many times before (e.g., 26,58). More interesting was the clear demonstration of conditioning of the rotation response. Thus, when given saline in an environment (e.g., rotation test bowls) in which they had not received any other previous treatment, neither lesioned nor grafted animals showed any rotation, whether or not they had received amphetamine in a different environment. By contrast, parallel groups of rats that had received a series of tests with amphetamine in the rotation bowls were then injected with saline in these rotation bowls: they turned in the same direction under saline as they had previously under amphetamine—lesioned animals turned ipsilaterally under saline and graft animals turned contralaterally. Moreover, the rate of turning by the individual graft animals under saline correlated with their degree of overcompensation on the earlier amphetamine test. Most importantly, it was not the previous experience of amphetamine *per se* that modified the response of lesioned or grafted animals, which would be so if the influence was primarily pharmacologic; rather, the animals' responses were modified by experience in a discrete environment and were specific to that environment, indicative of an effect that was truly due to a conditioning process.

These studies demonstrate that an animal's response can be modified or even determined by associative conditioning to stimuli in its environment, and such a process can account for both the priming of stress-induced rotation (174) and the onset

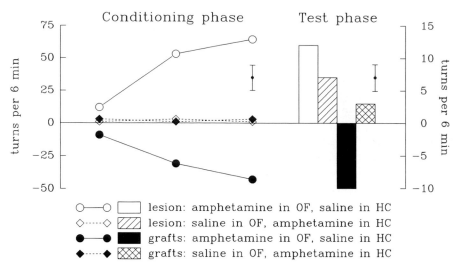

FIG. 3. The functional responses of animals with unilateral 6-hydroxydopamine (6-OHDA) lesions and nigral grafts is influenced by conditioning processes. Subgroups of rats with lesions alone and rats with additional nigral grafts received repeated injections of amphetamine, given either in an open-field arena (*OF*) or in their home cages (*HC*). On alternate training days the animals received saline injections in the other environment. The rotation response to amphetamine became sensitized with repeated injections (**left panel**). On the test day, all animals were simply placed in the open field without receiving any additional injections. Animals that had received amphetamine in the open field on previous training days now rotated spontaneously in the same direction—lesion rats to the ipsilateral side, and grafted rats to the contralateral side—whereas animals that had received the same number of amphetamine injections, but given in the home showed only limited turning (**right panel**). (Redrawn from ref. 6, with permission.)

of rotation in saline-treated animals (6). A similar conditioning process could equally account for the apparent sensitization of rotation after repeated doses of amphetamine and is likely to contribute to that phenomenon, but this does not rule out pharmacologic changes in receptor sensitivity also playing a major role, either owing to repeated receptor stimulation or simply with the passage of time.

Learning to Use the Transplant

The importance of training has recently become apparent in a quite different context. In a series of influential studies, Lund and colleagues have demonstrated that retinal transplants can establish connections with the host tectum to restore a functional retinotectal projection. Thus, for example,

retinal grafts placed over the tectum can detect a light stimulus and relay that information to the host brain in sufficient detail to maintain a simple reflex circuit, such as the pupillary response, both in neonatal and mature rats (112,113,130). This raised the question of whether the light stimulus was perceived and used as a visual stimulus *per se*—was the input from the graft restoring some aspect of "sight"—or was it simply an initially neutral stimulus with no intrinsic meaning to the animals?

Although the question might appear almost philosophic, these investigators have started to address this difficult issue in a series of elegant studies using the principles of associative conditioning and transfer of learning to identify how rats used the newly established inputs originating from light stimuli applied to retinal grafts (41). Their experimental preparation involved removing one eye from rat pups at birth, and at the same time transplanting embryonic retinae onto the tectal surface. Once the rats had matured and the grafts had established projections to the host tectum, the overlying parietal bone was removed to expose the transplants. The viability of the graft was first confirmed by determining whether the pupil constricted to shining light onto the retinal graft, before fixing a Perspex window into the skull over the graft so that it could subsequently be illuminated (40). A patch could then be put over the window so that the intact eye alone could be exposed to light stimuli, or conversely a patch could be placed over the intact eye so that the graft alone could be exposed to light stimuli.

The simplest test of visual function in the rats bearing retinal grafts was of the tendency of normal rats to avoid bright lights in an open field. Disappointingly, when placed into a large arena in which one-third was shaded, the rats would spend most of their time in the dark segment when the good eye was exposed, but moved through all parts of the arena equally when only the retinal transplant was exposed (108). This suggested that the rats did not use the information transduced by the grafts in the particular open-field situation, but it is not informative about whether that information was nevertheless present. To address the latter question, Coffey et al. (40) trained rats to lever-press for food reward in an operant chamber. They then trained the rats in a conditioned suppression paradigm in which they received periodic footshocks predicted by a bright light as a warning signal. Normal rats quickly learn the conditioned response to suppress lever-pressing and freeze in response to the warning signal. In this test, the rats with retinal grafts could indeed learn to suppress, responding on presentation of the visual stimulus, not only when trained through the good eye, but also when the eye was patched and when the only illumination was detected through the transplant. This suggests that the animals can indeed learn to use the light as a discriminable stimulus when the motivational conditions are strong, as in this test involving footshock.

Once the animals had undergone training in the conditioned suppression test, they were retested in the open-field arena. Now, the grafted animals spent most of the time in the shaded segment, whether tested using the normal eye or with only the retinal graft exposed (108). This suggested that, although the animals had not initially interpreted graft stimulation as light (to be avoided), they could be trained to interpret the information relayed from the graft appropriately, that is, they had to "learn to use the transplant." On the first test the visual information was relayed to the tectum, but the animal could not interpret the signal and so did not use it. After training in the conditioned suppression task, the retinal inputs acquired meaning for the animal, which could then be used to guide behavior. Nevertheless, this does not by itself resolve what exactly training had taught the rats. On the one hand, the animal may have learned that the signal transduced by the grafted retina was indeed light, and that the animal now avoided the open area of the arena as an inbuilt response to bright visual stimuli. On the other hand, the rat may simply have learned in the course of the conditioned suppression training that the stimulus is significant, associated with aversive consequences, and to be avoided. In this second interpretation, the light stimulus transduced by the graft remains arbitrary, rather than of an essentially visual nature. A preliminary indication that if animals are trained on the conditioned suppression task using the graft, learning does not transfer to the normal eye and *vice versa* (130) suggests that the latter interpretation may be favored, but this issue will require more detailed investigation to be resolved properly. For example, the two alternative interpretations of what the animal has learned produce opposite predictions if the animals are trained on an appetitive task with the visual information predictive of food reward before being tested in the open-field test. Here, the light stimulus would be associated with positive, rather than aversive, consequences. Consequently, when tested in the open arena, the rats would still spend most of their time in the shaded segment of the arena if they have learned to interpret the neutral stimulus as a bright light in the visual modality, but they should now spend more time in the open segment if simply treating the stimulus as a positive stimulus in a not specifically visual modality.

Further evidence of rats' need to learn how to use the transplants comes from a study of striatal grafts to alleviate rats' deficits in a visual choice–reaction time task (134) (Fig. 4). In this test, Mayer et al.

trained rats to make rapid contralateral head-turn responses to brief lateralized flashes of light (i.e., turn right to a left stimulus, turn left to a right stimulus). This is a complex and rather unnatural sensorimotor response for rats, but they are nevertheless able to learn the task with extended training. The rats were then divided into three groups to remain as sham-operated controls, or to receive either unilateral ibotenic acid lesions of the neostriatum alone or lesions plus additional striatal grafts. After allowing 6 months for recovery, growth, and incorporation of the grafts, the animals were retested over 3 weeks on the reaction time task. Whereas the controls rapidly reattained their initial levels of performance, the lesioned animals were seriously

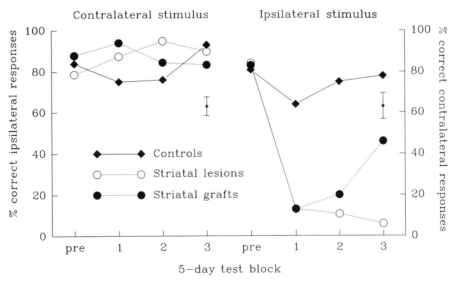

FIG. 4. Animals with ibotenic acid lesions and striatal transplants need to "learn to use the transplant" before the functional effects are apparent. All animals were trained on a complex reaction time task in which they had to respond on the opposite side to the visual stimulus: a left nose-poke in response to a right stimulus and a right nose-poke in response to a left stimulus. Six months after lesion and graft surgery, all animals were returned to the task. The lesions produced a major disruption in the animals ability to initiate a response in the contralateral direction (relative to the lesion) when the stimulus was on the ipsilateral side, but did not influence the responses to a contralateral stimulus (since both afferent and efferent projections cross over between the brain and the periphery, this pattern of results indicates that the lesion deficit is response-based, rather than due to a sensory or attentional impairment). The grafted animals were initially as impaired as the rats with lesions alone, but they showed substantial improvement with 3 weeks of additional training, indicating that they had to relearn the rather unnatural sensorimotor habit required by the task for the graft to be effective. (Data reanalyzed from ref. 134, with permission.)

impaired on the task, having lasting impairments in the reaction time to initiate contralateral responses and a strong bias to respond to the ipsilateral side whatever stimulus was presented. Although the grafted animals showed a similar impairment when first retested, their performance improved dramatically with training and by the end of 3 weeks of testing both the reaction time and response bias deficits converged on a normal level of performance. The 6-months survival posttransplantation was probably sufficient for anatomic reconstruction to achieve an asymptotic level of growth and reformation of connections, but was not by itself sufficient for functional recovery. Rather, the animals required additional training with relevant experience for them to be able to utilize the graft and for it to become functionally effective in this complex sensorimotor coordination task.

CONCLUSIONS

The essential conclusion, not just of this chapter, but of the whole book, is that there is no single or simple answer to the question: How do grafts work? Rather, it has become apparent that there are a multiplicity of different ways in which grafted tissues can influence the host brain and the function of the host animal. The extent and pattern of interaction between the graft and host brain depends not just on such obvious structural or anatomic factors as the nature of the underlying deficit, the tissue that is implanted, and the extent of reciprocal connections that happen to be formed between the graft and the host brain, but also on more subtle aspects, such as the total glial, vascular, pharmacologic, and growth factor environment of the grafted tissue. Moreover, the extent and limitations of functional recovery substantially depend on the selection of tests to characterize the animals' deficits. Finally, it is increasingly becoming clear that psychologic factors, including the role of the sensory environment, and the opportunities for relearning

knowledge, acquiring experience, and reacquiring motor skills, also play an important role in graft-derived recovery, even though such factors are even less tangible and more difficult to characterize than the anatomic incorporation of the grafts.

REFERENCES

1. Abrous DN, Torres EM, Annett LE, Reading PJ, Dunnett SB. Intrastriatal dopamine-rich grafts induce a hyperexpression of Fos protein when challenged with amphetamine. *Exp Brain Res* 1992;91:181–190.
2. Aebischer P, Tresco PA, Sagen J, Winn SR. Transplantation of microencapsulated bovine chromaffin cells reduces lesion-induced rotational asymmetry in rats. *Brain Res* 1991; 560:43–49.
3. Aebischer P, Tresco PA, Winn SR, Greene LA, Jaeger CB. Long-term cross-species brain transplantation of a polymer-encapsulated dopamine-secreting cell line. *Exp Neurol* 1991; 111:269–275.
4. Aguayo AJ, Björklund A, Stenevi U, Carlstedt T. Fetal mesencephalic neurons survive and extend long axons across peripheral nervous system grafts inserted into the adult rat striatum. *Neurosci Lett* 1984;45:53–58.
5. Ahlskog JE, Tyce GM, Kelly PJ, Van Heerden JA, Stoddard SL, Carmichael SW. Cerebrospinal fluid indices of blood–brain barrier permeability following adrenal–brain transplantation in patients with Parkinson's disease. *Exp Neurol* 1989;105:152–161.
6. Annett LE, Reading PJ, Tharumaratnam D, Abrous DN, Torres EM, Dunnett SB. Conditioning versus priming of dopaminergic grafts by amphetamine. *Exp Brain Res* 1993;93:46–54.
7. Bankiewicz KS, Plunkett RJ, Mefford I, Kopin IJ, Oldfield EH. Behavioral recovery from MPTP-induced parkinsonism in monkeys after intracerebral tissue implants is not related to CSF concentrations of dopamine metabolites. *Prog Brain Res* 1990;82:561–571.
8. Becker JB, Curran EJ, Freed WJ, Poltorak M. Mechanisms of action of adrenal medulla grafts: the possible role of peripheral and central dopamine systems. *Prog Brain Res* 1990; 82:499–507.
9. Becker JB, Freed WJ. Adrenal medulla grafts enhance functional activity of the striatal dopamine system following substantia nigra lesions. *Brain Res* 1988;462:401–406.
10. Becker JB, Robinson TE, Barton P, Sintov A, Siden R, Levy RJ. Sustained behavioral recovery from unilateral nigrostriatal damage produced by the controlled release of dopamine from a silicone polymer pellet placed into the denervated striatum. *Brain Res* 1990;508:60–64.

11. Bing G, Notter MFD, Hansen JT, Gash DM. Comparison of adrenal medullary, carotid body and PC12 cell grafts in 6-OHDA lesioned rats. *Brain Res Bull* 1988;20:399–406.

12. Bing G, Notter MFD, Hansen JT, Kellogg C, Kordower JH, Gash DM. Cografts of adrenal medulla with C6 glioma cells in rats with 6-hydroxydopamine-induced lesions. *Neuroscience* 1990;34:687–697.

13. Björklund A, Dunnett SB, Stenevi U, Lewis ME, Iversen SD. Reinnervation of the denervated striatum by substantia nigra transplants: functional consequences as revealed by pharmacological and sensorimotor testing. *Brain Res* 1980;199:307–333.

14. Björklund A, Gage FH, Stenevi U, Dunnett SB. Intracerebral grafting of neuronal cell suspensions. VI. Survival and growth of intrahippocampal implants of septal cell suspensions. *Acta Physiol Scand [Suppl]* 1983;522:49–58.

15. Björklund A, Lindvall O, Isacson O, Brundin P, Wictorin K, Strecker RE, Clarke DJ, Dunnett SB. Mechanisms of action of intracerebral neural implants—studies on nigral and striatal grafts to the lesioned striatum. *Trends Neurosci* 1987;10:509–516.

16. Björklund A, Nilsson OG, Kalén P. Reafferentation of the subcortically denervated hippocampus as a model for transplant-induced functional recovery in the CNS. *Prog Brain Res* 1990;83:411–426.

17. Björklund A, Stenevi U. Reformation of the severed septohippocampal cholinergic pathway in the adult rat by transplanted septal neurons. *Cell Tissue Res* 1977;185:289–302.

18. Björklund A, Stenevi U. Reconstruction of the nigrostriatal dopamine pathway by intracerebral transplants. *Brain Res* 1979;177:555–560.

19. Björklund A, Stenevi U, Svendgaard N-A. Growth of transplanted monoaminergic neurones into the adult hippocampus along the perforant path. *Nature* 1976;262:787–790.

20. Bohn MC, Cupit L, Marciano F, Gash DM. Adrenal grafts enhance recovery of striatal dopaminergic fibers *Science* 1987;237:913–916.

21. Bohn MC, Kanuicki M. Bilateral recovery of striatal dopamine after unilateral adrenal grafting into the striatum of the 1-methyl-4-(2'-methylphenyl)-1,2,3,6-tetrahydropyridine (2'CH₃-MPTP)-treated mice. *J Neurosci Res* 1990;25:281–286.

22. Bregman BS. Spinal cord transplants permit the growth of serotonergic axons across the site of neonatal spinal cord transection. *Dev Brain Res* 1987;34:265–279.

23. Bregman BS, Bernstein-Goral H, Kunkel-Bagden E. CNS transplants promote anatomical plasticity and recovery of function after spinal cord injury. *Restor Neurol Neurosci* 1991;2:327–338.

24. Bregman BS, Reier PJ. Neural tissue transplants rescue axotomized rubrospinal cells from retrograde death. *J Comp Neurol* 1986;244:86–95.

25. Broadwell RD, Charlton HM, Ebert P, Hickley WF, Villegas JC, Wolf AL. Angiogenesis and the blood–brain barrier in solid and dissociated cell grafts within the CNS. *Prog Brain Res* 1990;82:95–101.

26. Brown VJ, Dunnett SB. Comparison of adrenal and fetal nigral grafts on drug-induced rotation in rats with 6-OHDA lesions. *Exp Brain Res* 1989;78:214–218.

27. Brundin P, Widner H, Nilsson OG, Strecker RE, Björklund A. Intracerebral xenografts of dopamine neurons: the role of immunosuppression and the blood–brain barrier. *Exp Brain Res* 1989;75:195–207.

28. Buzsaki G, Gage FH, Czopf J, Björklund A. Restoration of rhythmic slow activity (theta) in the subcortically denervated hippocampus by fetal CNS transplants. *Brain Res* 1987;400:334–347.

29. Buzsaki G, Masliah E, Chen LS, Horvath Z, Terry R, Gage FH. Hippocampal grafts into the intact brain induce epileptic patterns. *Brain Res* 1991;554:30–37.

30. Campbell K, Kalén P, Wictorin K, Lundberg C, Mandel RJ, Björklund A. Characterization of GABA release from intrastriatal striatal transplants: dependence on host-derived afferents. *Neuroscience* 1993;53:403–415.

31. Carey RJ. A conditioned anti-parkinsonian drug effect in the hemi-parkinsonian rat. *Psychopharmacology* 1986;89:269–272.

32. Carey RJ. Conditioned rotational behavior in rats with unilateral 6-hydroxydopamine lesions of the substantia nigra. *Brain Res* 1986;365:379–382.

33. Carey RJ. Application of the unilateral 6-hydroxydopamine rat model of rotational behavior to the study of conditioned drug effects. *J Neurosci Methods* 1988;22:253–261.

34. Carey RJ. Dopamine receptors mediate drug-induced but not Pavlovian conditioned contralateral rotation in the unilateral 6-OHDA animal model. *Brain Res* 1990;515:292–298.

35. Cassel JC, Kelche C, Will B. Time-dependent effects of intrahippocampal grafts in rats with fimbria–fornix lesions. *Exp Brain Res* 1990;81:179–190.

36. Cenci MA, Kalén P, Duan W-M, Björklund A. Transmitter release from transplants of fetal ventral mesencephalon and locus coeruleus in the rat frontal cortex and nucleus accumbens: effects of pharmacological and behavioral activating stimuli. *Brain Res* 1994;641:225–248.

37. Charlton HM. Neural grafts and the restoration of pituitary and gonadal function in hypogonadal (HPG) mice. *Ann Endocrinol* 1987;48:378–384.

38. Choulli K, Herman JP, Rivet JM, Simon H, Le Moal M. Spontaneous and graft-induced behavioral recovery after 6-hydroxydopamine lesions of the nucleus accumbens in the rat. *Brain Res* 1987;407:376–380.

39. Clarke DJ, Brundin P, Strecker RE, Nilsson OG, Björklund A, Lindvall O. Human fetal dopamine neurons grafted in a rat model of Parkinson's disease: ultrastructural evidence for

synapse formation using tyrosine hydroxylase immunocytochemistry. *Exp Brain Res* 1988; 73:115–126.

40. Coffey PJ, Lund RD, Rawlins JNP. Retinal transplant-mediated learning in a conditioned suppression task in rats. *Proc Natl Acad Sci USA* 1989;86:7248–7249.
41. Coffey PJ, Lund RD, Rawlins JNP. Detecting the world through a retinal implant. *Prog Brain Res* 1990;82:269–275.
42. Costall B, Naylor RJ. Specific asymmetric behaviour induced by the direct chemical stimulation of neostriatal dopaminergic mechanisms. *Naunyn-Schmiedebergs Arch Pharmacol* 1974; 285:83–91.
43. Cuello AC, Garofalo L, Kenigsberg RL, Maysinger D. Gangliosides potentiate in vivo and in vitro effects of nerve growth factor on central cholinergic neurons. *Proc Natl Acad Sci USA* 1989;86:2056–2060.
44. Cunningham LA, Hansen JT, Short MP, Bohn MC. The use of genetically altered astrocytes to provide nerve growth factor to adrenal chromaffin cells grafted into the striatum. *Brain Res* 1991;561:192–202.
45. Cunningham TJ, Haun F, Chantler PD. Diffusible proteins prolong survival of dorsal lateral geniculate neurons following occipital lesions in newborn rats. *Dev Brain Res* 1987;37:133–141.
46. Dalrymple-Alford JC, Kelche C, Cassel JC, Toniolo G, Pallage V, Will BE. Behavioral deficits after intrahippocampal fetal septal grafts in rats with selective fimbria–fornix lesions. *Exp Brain Res* 1988;69:545–558.
47. Dalrymple-Alford J, Kelche C, Eclancher F, Will B. Preoperative enrichment and behavioral recovery in rats with septal lesions. *Behav Neural Biol* 1988;49:361–373.
48. Date I, Felten SY, Felten DL. Cografts of adrenal medulla with peripheral nerve enhance the survivability of transplanted adrenal chromaffin cells and recovery of the host nigrostriatal dopaminergic system in MPTP-treated young adult mice. *Brain Res* 1990;537:33–39.
49. David S, Aguayo AJ. Axonal elongation into peripheral nervous system "bridges" after central nervous system injury in adult rats. *Science* 1981;214:931–933.
50. Doucet G, Murata Y, Brundin P, Bosler O, Mons N, Geffard M, Ouimet CC, Björklund A. Host afferents into intrastriatal transplants of fetal ventral mesencephalon. *Exp Neurol* 1989; 106:1–9.
51. Dunnett SB. Functional analysis of neural grafts in the neostriatum. In: Björklund A, Aguayo AJ, Ottoson D, eds. *Brain repair.* Basingstoke: Macmillan; 1990:355–373.
52. Dunnett SB. Neural tissue transplantation. In: Greenwood RJ, Barnes MP, McMillan TM, Ward CD, eds. *Neurological rehabilitation.* London: Churchill Livingstone; 1993:93–109.
53. Dunnett SB, Björklund A. Mechanisms of function of neural grafts in the adult mammalian brain. *J Exp Biol* 1987;132:265–289.

54. Dunnett SB, Björklund A, Schmidt RH, Stenevi U, Iversen SD. Intracerebral grafting of neuronal cell suspensions. IV. Behavioral recovery in rats with unilateral 6-OHDA lesions following implantation of nigral cell suspensions in different forebrain sites. *Acta Physiol Scand [Suppl]* 1983;522:29–37.
55. Dunnett SB, Björklund A, Stenevi U, Iversen SD. Grafts of embryonic substantia nigra reinnervating the ventrolateral striatum ameliorate sensorimotor impairments and akinesia in rats with 6-OHDA lesions of the nigrostriatal pathway. *Brain Res* 1981;229:209–217.
56. Dunnett SB, Björklund A, Stenevi U, Iversen SD. Behavioral recovery following transplantation of substantia nigra in rats subjected to 6-OHDA lesions of the nigrostriatal pathway. 1. Unilateral lesions. *Brain Res* 1981;215:147–161.
57. Dunnett SB, Bunch ST, Gage FH, Björklund A. Dopamine-rich transplants in rats with 6-OHDA lesions of the ventral tegmental area. 1. Effects on spontaneous and drug-induced locomotor activity. *Behav Brain Res* 1984;13:71–82.
58. Dunnett SB, Hernandez TD, Summerfield A, Jones GH, Arbuthnott GW. Graft-derived recovery from 6-OHDA lesions: specificity of ventral mesencephalic graft tissues. *Exp Brain Res* 1988;71:411–424.
59. Dunnett SB, Isacson O, Sirinathsinghji DJS, Clarke DJ, Björklund A. Striatal grafts in rats with unilateral neostriatal lesions. III. Recovery from dopamine-dependent motor asymmetry and deficits in skilled paw reaching. *Neuroscience* 1988;24:813–820.
60. Dunnett SB, Low WC, Iversen SD, Stenevi U, Björklund A. Septal transplants restore maze learning in rats with fornix–fimbria lesions. *Brain Res* 1982;251:335–348.
61. Dunnett SB, Mayer E. Neural grafts, growth factors and trophic mechanisms of recovery. In: Hunter AJ, Clarke M, eds. *Neurodegeneration.* New York: Academic Press; 1992:183–217.
62. Dunnett SB, Rogers DC, Richards SJ. Nigrostriatal reconstruction after 6-OHDA lesions in rats: combination of dopamine-rich nigral grafts and nigrostriatal bridge grafts. *Exp Brain Res* 1989;75:523–535.
63. Dunnett SB, Ryan CN, Levin PD, Reynolds M, Bunch ST. Functional consequences of embryonic neocortex transplanted to rats with prefrontal cortex lesions. *Behav Neurosci* 1987; 101:489.
64. Dunnett SB, Whishaw IQ, Bunch ST, Fine A. Acetylcholine-rich neuronal grafts in the forebrain of rats: effects of environmental enrichment, neonatal noradrenaline depletion, host transplantation site and regional source of embryonic donor cells on graft size and acetylcholinesterase-positive fiber outgrowth. *Brain Res* 1986;378:357–373.
65. Dunnett SB, Whishaw IQ, Rogers DC, Jones GH. Dopamine-rich grafts ameliorate whole

body motor asymmetry and sensory neglect but not independent limb use in rats with 6-hydroxydopamine lesions. *Brain Res* 1987;415: 63–78.

66. Eagleson KL, Cunningham TJ, Haun F. Rescue of both rapidly and slowly degenerating neurons in the dorsal lateral geniculate nucleus of adult rats by a cortically derived neuron survival factor. *Exp Neurol* 1992;116:156–162.

67. Emerich DF, Winn SR, Christenson L, Palmatier MA, Gentile FT, Sanberg PR. A novel approach to neural transplantation in Parkinson's disease: use of polymer encapsulated cell therapy. *Neurosci Biobehav Rev* 1992;16:437–447.

68. Ernfors P, Ebendal T, Olson L, Mouton P, Strömberg I, Persson H. A cell line producing recombinant nerve growth factor evokes growth responses in intrinsic and grafted central cholinergic neurons. *Proc Natl Acad Sci USA* 1989;86:4756–4760.

69. Fawcett JW. Factors responsible for the failure of structural repair in the central nervous system. In: Hunter AJ, Clark M, eds. *Neurodegeneration.* New York: Academic Press; 1992; 81–96.

70. Fisher LJ, Jinnah HA, Kale LC, Higgins GA, Gage FH. Survival and function of intrastriatally grafted primary fibroblasts genetically modified to produce L-DOPA. *Neuron* 1991;6: 371–380.

71. Freed WJ. Functional brain tissue transplantation: reversal of lesion-induced rotation by intraventricular substantia nigra and adrenal medulla grafts, with a note on intracranial retinal grafts. *Biol Psychiatry* 1983;18:1205–1267.

72. Freed WJ, Cannon-Spoor HE, Krauthamer E. Intrastriatal adrenal medulla grafts in rats: long-term survival and behavioral effects. *J Neurosurg* 1986;65:664–670.

73. Freed WJ, de Medinaceli L, Wyatt RJ. Promoting functional plasticity in the damaged nervous system. *Science* 1985;227:1544–1552.

74. Freed WJ, Ko GN, Niehoff DL, Kuhar MJ, Hoffer BJ, Olson L, Cannon-Spoor HE, Morihisa JM, Wyatt RJ. Normalization of spiroperidol binding in the denervated rat striatum by homologous grafts of substantia nigra. *Science* 1983;222:937–939.

75. Freed WJ, Morihisa JM, Spoor E, Hoffer BJ, Olson L, Seiger Å, Wyatt RJ. Transplanted adrenal chromaffin cells in rat brain reduce lesion-induced rotational behavior. *Nature* 1981; 292:351–352.

76. Freed WJ, Perlow MJ, Karoum F, Seiger Å, Olson L, Hoffer BJ, Wyatt RJ. Restoration of dopaminergic function by grafting of fetal rat substantia nigra to the caudate nucleus: long-term behavioral, biochemical, and histochemical studies. *Ann Neurol* 1980;8:510–519.

77. Freed WJ, Willingham G, Heim R. Effects of adrenal medulla and sciatic nerve cografts in rats with unilateral substantia nigra lesions. *J Neural Transplant Plast* 1992;3:159–167.

78. Freeze A, Sabel BA, Saltzman WM, During MJ, Langer R. Controlled release of dopamine from a polymeric implant: in vitro characterization. *Exp Neurol* 1989;103:234–238.

79. Gage FH, Buzsaki G. CNS grafting: potential mechanisms of action. In: Seil FJ, ed. *Neural regeneration and transplantation.* New York: Alan R Liss; 1989:211–226.

80. Gage FH, Fisher LJ, Jinnah HA, Rosenberg MB, Tuszynski MH, Friedmann T. Grafting genetically modified cells to the brain—conceptual and technical issues. *Prog Brain Res* 1990;82:1–10.

81. Gage FH, Wolff JA, Rosenberg MB, Xu L, Yee JK, Shults C, Friedmann T. Grafting genetically modified cells to the brain: possibilities for the future. *Neuroscience* 1987;23:795–807.

82. Garcia-Rill E, Houle JD, Reese NB, Skinner RD. Modulation of locomotion by a nerve graft across a spinal transection in rat. *Restor Neurol Neurosci* 1992;4:419–424.

83. Gash D, Sladek JR, Sladek CD. Functional development of grafted vasopressin neurons. *Science* 1980;210:1367–1369.

84. Guttman M, Burns RS, Martin WRW, Peppard RF, Adam NJ, Ruth TJ, Allen G, Parker RA, Tulipan NB, Calne DB. PET studies of parkinsonian patients treated with autologous adrenal implants. *Can J Neurol Sci* 1989;16:305–309.

85. Halasz B, Pupp L, Uhlarik S, Tima L. Growth of hypophysectomized rats bearing pituitary transplants in the hypothalamus. *Acta Physiol Acad Sci Hung* 1963;23:287–292.

86. Halasz B, Pupp L, Uhlarik S, Tima L. Further studies on the hormone secretion of the anterior pituitary transplanted into the hypophysiotrophic areas of the rat hypothalamus. *Endocrinology* 1965;77:343–355.

87. Hansen JT, Fiandaca MS, Kordower JH, Notter MFD, Gash DM. Striatal adrenal medulla/sural nerve co-grafts in hemiparkinsonian monkeys. *Prog Brain Res* 1990;82:573–580.

88. Hargraves RW, Freed WJ. Chronic intrastriatal dopamine infusions in rats with unilateral lesions of the substantia nigra. *Life Sci* 1987; 40:959–966.

89. Haun F, Cunningham TJ. Cortical transplants reveal CNS trophic interactions in situ. *Dev Brain Res* 1984;15:290–294.

90. Haun F, Cunningham TJ. Specific neurotrophic interactions between cortical and subcortical visual structures in developing rat: in vivo studies. *J Comp Neurol* 1987;256:561–569.

91. Hefti F. Nerve growth factor promotes survival of septal cholinergic neurons after fimbrial transections. *J Neurosci* 1986;6:2155–2162.

92. Hefti F, Will B. Nerve growth factor is a neurotrophic factor for forebrain cholinergic neurons: implications for Alzheimer's disease. *J Neural Transm* 1987;309–315.

93. Herman JP, Choulli K, Le Moal M. Hyperreactivity to amphetamine in rats with dopaminergic grafts. *Exp Brain Res* 1985;60:521–526.

94. Hirsch ED, Duyckaerts C, Javoy-Agid F, Hauw J-J, Agid Y. Does adrenal graft enhance

recovery of dopaminergic neurons in Parkinson's disease? *Ann Neurol* 1990;27:676–682.

95. Hodges H, Allen Y, Kershaw T, Lantos PL, Gray JA, Sinden J. Effects of cholinergic-rich neural grafts on radial maze performance of rats after excitotoxic lesions of the forebrain cholinergic projection system. 1. Amelioration of cognitive deficits by transplants into cortex and hippocampus, but not into basal forebrain. *Neuroscience* 1991;45:587–607.

96. Horellou P, Brundin P, Kalén P, Mallet J, Björklund A. In vivo release of DOPA and dopamine from genetically engineered cells grafted to the denervated rat striatum. *Neuron* 1990;5:393–402.

97. Horellou P, Lundberg C, Lebourdelles B, Wictorin K, Brundin P, Kalén P, Björklund A, Mallet J. Behavioral effects of genetically engineered cells releasing DOPA and dopamine after intracerebral grafting in a rat model of Parkinson's disease. *J Physiol (Paris)* 1991;85:158–170.

98. Hurtig H, Joyce J, Sladek JR, Trojanowski JQ. Post mortem analysis of adrenal–medulla-to-caudate autograft in a patient with Parkinson's disease. *Ann Neurol* 1989;25:607–614.

99. Ide C, Osawa T, Tohyama K. Nerve regeneration through allogeneic nerve grafts, with special reference to the role of the Schwann cell basal lamina. *Prog Neurobiol* 1990;34:1–38.

100. Inoue H, Kohsaka S, Otani M, Toya S, Tsukada Y. The effect of arcuate nucleus transplantation on the development of the anterior pituitary in monosodium glutamate-treated rats. *Neurosci Res* 1986;3:555–567.

101. Isacson O, Dunnett SB, Björklund A. Graft-induced behavioral recovery in an animal model of Huntington disease. *Proc Natl Acad USA* 1986;83:2728–2732.

102. Jaeger CB. Immunocytochemical study of PC12 cells grafted to the brain of immature rats. *Exp Brain Res* 1985;59:615–624.

103. Jancovic J, Grossman R, Goodman C, Pirozzolo F, Schneider L, Zhu Z, Scardino P, Garber AJ, Jhingran SG, Martin S. Clinical, biochemical, and neuropathologic findings following transplantation of adrenal medulla to the caudate nucleus for treatment of Parkinson's disease. *Neurology* 1989;39:1227–1234.

104. Jiao SS, Ding YJ, Zhang WC, et al. Adrenal medullary autografts in patients with Parkinson's disease. *N Engl J Med* 1989;321:324–325.

105. Jiao SS, Gurevich V, Wolff JA. Long-term correction of rat model of Parkinson's disease by gene therapy. *Nature* 1993;362:450–453.

106. Kelche C, Dalrymple-Alford J, Will B. Effects of postoperative environment on recovery of function after fimbria–fornix transection in the rat. *Physiol Behav* 1987;40:731–736.

107. Kelche C, Dalrymple-Alford J, Will B. Housing conditions modulate the effects of intracerebral grafts in rats with brain lesions. *Behav Brain Res* 1988;28:287–295.

108. Kentridge RW, Shaw C, Aggleton JP. Amygdaloid lesions and stimulus-reward associations in the rat. *Behav Brain Res* 1991;42:57–66.

109. Kesslak JP, Brown L, Steichen C, Cotman CW. Adult and embryonic frontal cortex transplants after frontal cortex ablation enhance recovery on a reinforced alternation task. *Exp Neurol* 1986;94:615–626.

110. Kesslak JP, Nieto-Sampedro M, Globus J, Cotman CW. Transplants of purified astrocytes promote behavioral recovery after frontal cortex ablation. *Exp Neurol* 1986;92:377–390.

111. Kimble DP. Functional effects of neural grafting in the mammalian central nervous system. *Psychol Bull* 1990;108:462–479.

112. Klassen H, Lund RD. Retinal transplants can drive a pupillary reflex in host rat brains. *Proc Natl Acad Sci USA* 1987;84:6958–6960.

113. Klassen H, Lund RD. Retinal graft-mediated pupillary responses in rats: restoration of a reflex function in the mature mammalian brain. *J Neurosci* 1990;10:578–587.

114. Klausen BS, Swenson RS, Zimmer J, Castro AJ. Fetal neocortical transplants in rats—blood–brain barrier development and partial permeability to IgG in long surviving grafts. *Restor Neurol Neurosci* 1992;4:393–400.

115. Knigge KM. Gonadotrophic action of neonatal pituitary glands implanted in the rat brain. *Am J Physiol* 1962;202:387–391.

116. Knoops B, Ponsar C, Hubert I, Van den Bosch de Aguilar P. Axonal regeneration after peripheral nerve grafting and fibrin–fibronectin-containing matrix implantation on the injured septohippocampal pathway of the adult rat: a light and electron microscopic study. *Restor Neurol Neurosci* 1993;5:103–117.

117. Kokoris GJ, Silverman AJ, Zimmerman EA, Perlow MJ, Gibson MJ. Implantation of fetal preoptic area into the lateral ventricle of adult hypogonadal mutant mice: the pattern of gonadotropin-releasing hormone axonal outgrowth into the host brain. *Neuroscience* 1987;22:159–167.

118. Kordower JH, Cochran E, Penn RD, Goetz CG. NGF-like trophic support from peripheral nerve for grafted rhesus adrenal chromaffin cells. *J Neurosurg* 1990;73:418–428.

119. Kordower JH, Cochran E, Penn RD, Goetz CG. Putative chromaffin cell survival and enhanced host-derived TH-fiber innervation following a functional adrenal medulla autograft for Parkinson's disease. *Ann Neurol* 1991;29:405–412.

120. Krieger DT, Perlow MJ, Gibson MJ, Davies TF, Zimmerman EA, Ferin M, Charlton HM. Brain grafts reverse hypogonadism of gonadotropin releasing hormone deficiency. *Nature* 1982;298:468–471.

121. Kroin JS, Kao LC, Zhang TJ, Penn RD, Klawans HL, Carvey PM. Dopamine distribution and behavioral alterations resulting from dopamine infusion into the brain of the lesioned rat. *J Neurosurg* 1991;74:105–111.

122. Kromer LF, Björklund A, Stenevi U. Innervation of embryonic hippocampal implants by re-

generating axons of cholinergic septal neurons in the adult rat. *Brain Res* 1980;210:153–171.

123. Kromer LF, Björklund A, Stenevi U. Regeneration of septohippocampal pathway in adult rats is promoted by utilizing embryonic hippocampal implants as bridges. *Brain Res* 1981; 210:173–200.

124. Kromer LF, Cornbrooks CJ. Transplants of Schwann cell cultures promote axonal regeneration in the adult mammalian brain. *Proc Natl Acad Sci USA* 1985;82:6330–6334.

125. Kunkel-Bagden E, Bregman BS. Spinal cord transplants enhance the recovery of locomotor function after spinal injury at birth. *Exp Brain Res* 1990;81:25–34.

126. Labbe R, Firl A, Mufson EJ, Stein DG. Fetal brain transplants: reduction of cognitive deficits in rats with frontal cortex lesions. *Science* 1983;221:470–472.

127. Landau WM. Artificial intelligence: the brain transplant cure for parkinsonism. *Neurology* 1990;40:733–740.

128. Leanza G, Nilsson OG, Björklund A. Functional activity of intrahippocampal septal grafts is regulated by catecholaminergic host afferents as studied by microdialysis of acetylcholine. *Brain Res* 1993;618:47–56.

129. LeVere TE, LeVere ND. Transplants to the central nervous system as a therapy for brain pathology. *Neurobiol Aging* 1985;6:151–152.

130. Lund RD, Radel JD, Coffey PJ. The impact of intracerebral retinal transplants on types of behavior exhibited by host rats. *Trends Neurosci* 1991;14:358–362.

131. Madrazo I, Drucker-Colín R, Díaz V, Martínez-Mata J, Torres C, Becerril JJ. Open microsurgical autograft of adrenal medulla to the right caudate nucleus in two patients with intractable Parkinson's disease. *N Engl J Med* 1987; 316:831–834.

132. Mahalik TJ, Finger TE, Strömberg I, Olson L. Substantia nigra transplants into denervated striatum of the rat: ultrastructure of graft and host interconnections. *J Comp Neurol* 1985; 240:60–70.

133. Matsumoto A, Murakami S, Arai Y, Osanai M. Synaptogenesis in the neonatal preoptic area grafted into the aged brain. *Brain Res* 1985; 372:363–367.

134. Mayer E, Brown VJ, Dunnett SB, Robbins TW. Striatal graft-associated recovery of a lesion-induced performance deficit in the rat requires learning to use the transplant. *Eur J Neurosci* 1992;4:119–126.

135. McEvoy RC, Leung PE. Transplantation of fetal rat islets into the cerebral ventricles of alloxan-diabetic rats. *Diabetes* 1983;32:852–857.

136. McRae A, Hjorth S, Mason DW, Dillon L, Tice TR. Microencapsulated dopamine (DA)-induced restitution of function in 6-OHDA denervated rat striatum in vivo: comparison between two microsphere excipients. *J Neural Transplant Plast* 1991;2:165–173.

137. McRae-Degueurce A, Hjorth S, Dillon DL, Mason DW, Tice TR. Implantable microencapsulated dopamine (DA): a new approach for slow release DA delivery into brain tissue. *Neurosci Lett* 1988;92:303–309.

138. Meyers R. The modification of alternating tremors, rigidity and festination by surgery of basal ganglia. *Assoc Nerv Ment Dis Proc* 1942;21:602–665.

139. Meyers R. Surgical experiments in therapy of certain "extrapyramidal" diseases: current evaluation. *Acta Psychiat Neurol [Suppl]* 1951; 67:1–42.

140. Montoya CP, Astell S, Dunnett SB. Effects of nigral and striatal grafts on skilled forelimb use in the rat. *Prog Brain Res* 1990;82:459–466.

141. Nadaud D, Herman JP, Simon H, Le Moal M. Functional recovery following transplantation of ventral mesencephalic cells in rats subjected to 6-OHDA lesions of the mesolimbic dopaminergic neurons. *Brain Res* 1984;304:137–141.

142. Neal JH, Apuzzo MLJ, Waters C. Stereotactic adrenostriatal autografts for parkinsonism: rationale, techniques and observations. *Prog Brain Res* 1990;82:683–691.

143. Nilsson OG, Björklund A. Behavior-dependent changes in acetylcholine release in normal and graft-reinnervated hippocampus: evidence for host regulation of grafted cholinergic neurons. *Neuroscience* 1992;49:33–44.

144. Nilsson OG, Kalén P, Rosengren E, Björklund A. Acetylcholine release from intrahippocampal septal grafts is under control of the host brain. *Proc Natl Acad Sci USA* 1990;87:2647–2651.

145. Nishino H, Ono T, Takahashi J, Kimura M, Shiosaka S, Yamasaki H, Hatanaka H, Tohyama M. The formation of new neuronal circuit between transplanted nigral dopamine neurons and non-immunoreactive axon terminals in the host rat caudate nucleus. *Neurosci Lett* 1986;64:13–16.

146. Olson L, Strömberg I, Herrera-Marschitz M, Ungerstedt U, Ebendal T. Adrenal medullary tissue grafted to the dopamine-denervated rat striatum: histochemical and functional effects of additions of nerve growth factor. In: Björklund A, Stenevi U, eds. *Neural grafting in the mammalian CNS.* Amsterdam: Elsevier; 1985: 505–518.

147. Öberg RGE, Divac I. "Cognitive" functions of the neostriatum. In: Divac I, Öberg RGE, eds. *The neostriatum.* New York: Plenum Press; 1980:291–313.

148. Paino CL, Bunge MB. Induction of axon growth into Schwann cell implants grafted into lesioned adult rat spinal cord. *Exp Neurol* 1991;114:254–257.

149. Perlow MJ, Freed WJ, Hoffer BJ, Seiger Å, Olson L, Wyatt RJ. Brain grafts reduce motor abnormalities produced by destruction of nigrostriatal dopamine system. *Science* 1979;204: 643–647.

150. Pezzoli G, Motti E, Zechinelli A, Ferrante C, Silani V, Falini A, Pizzuti A, Mulazzi D, Bar-

atta P, Vegato A, Villani R, Scarlato G. Adrenal medulla autograft in 3 parkinsonian patients: results using two different approaches. *Prog Brain Res* 1990;82:677–682.

151. Pijnenberg AJJ, Honig WMM, van der Heyden JAM, van Rossum JM. Effects of chemical stimulation of the mesolimbic dopamine system upon locomotor activity. *Eur J Pharmacol* 1976;35:45–58.

152. Pijnenberg AJJ, van Rossum JM. Stimulation of locomotor activity following injection of dopamine into nucleus accumbens. *J Pharm Pharmacol* 1973;25:1003–1005.

153. Plunkett RJ, Bankiewicz KS, Cummins AC, Miletich RS, Schwartz JP, Oldfield EH. Long-term evaluation of hemiparkinsonian monkeys after adrenal autografting or cavitation alone. *J Neurosurg* 1990;73:918–926.

154. Pollack IF, Lund RD. The blood–brain barrier protects foreign antigens in the brain from immune attack. *Exp Neurol* 1990;108:114–121.

155. Quinn NP. The clinical application of cell grafting techniques in patients with Parkinson's disease. *Prog Brain Res* 1990;82:619–625.

156. Reier PJ, Bregman BS, Wujek JR. Intraspinal transplantation of embryonic spinal cord tissue in neonatal and adult rats. *J Comp Neurol* 1986;247:275–296.

157. Reier PJ, Perlow MJ, Guth L. Development of embryonic spinal cord transplants in the rat. *Dev Brain Res* 1983;10:201–219.

158. Ridley RM, Baker HF, Fine A. Transplantation of fetal tissues. *Br Med J* 1988;296:1469.

159. Rioux L, Gaudin DP, Bui LK, Grégoire L, DiPaolo T, Bédard PJ. Correlation of functional recovery after a 6-hydroxydopamine lesion with survival of grafted fetal neurons and release of dopamine in the striatum of the rat. *Neuroscience* 1991;40:123–131.

160. Rosenberg MB, Friedmann T, Robertson RC, Tuszynski M, Wolff JA, Breakefield XO, Gage FH. Grafting genetically modified cells to the damaged brain: restorative effects of NGF expression. *Science* 1988;242:1575–1578.

161. Rosenstein JM, Brightman MW. Circumventing the blood–brain barrier with autonomic ganglion transplants. *Science* 1983;221:879–881.

162. Rosenzweig MR, Bennett EL, Diamond MC. Chemical and anatomical plasticity of the brain: replications and extensions. In: Gaito J, ed. *Macromolecules and behavior.* New York: Appleton-Century-Croft; 1972:205–278.

163. Saitoh Y, Gibson MJ, Silverman AJ. Targeting of gonadotrophin releasing hormone axons from preoptic area grafts to the median eminence. *J Neurosci Res* 1992;33:379–391.

164. Schmidt RH, Björklund A, Stenevi U, Dunnett SB, Gage FH. Intracerebral grafting of neuronal cell suspensions. III. Activity of intrastriatal nigral suspension implants as assessed by measurements of dopamine synthesis and metabolism. *Acta Physiol Scand [Suppl]* 1983;522:19–28.

165. Schwab ME. Myelin-associated inhibitors of neurite growth and regeneration in the CNS. *Trends Neurosci* 1990;13:452–456.

166. Schwab ME, Kapfhammer JP, Bandtlow CE. Inhibitors of neurite growth. *Annu Rev Neurosci* 1993;16:565–595.

167. Scott DE, Sherman DM. Neuronal and neurovascular integration following transplantation of the fetal hypothalamus into the third cerebral ventricle of adult Brattleboro rats. I. Neurological transplants. *Brain Res Bull* 1984;12:453–467.

168. Sharp FR, Gonzalez MF. Fetal cortical transplants ameliorate thalamic atrophy ipsilateral to neonatal frontal cortex lesions. *Neurosci Lett* 1986;71:247–251.

169. Shults CW, O'Connor DT, Baird A, Hill R, Goetz CG, Watts RL, Klawans HL, Carvey PM, Bakay RA, Gage FH, U HS. Clinical improvement in parkinsonian patients undergoing adrenal to caudate transplantation is not reflected by chomogranin-A or basic fibroblast growth factor in ventricular fluid. *Exp Neurol* 1991;111:276–281.

170. Silver J, Ogawa MY. Postnatally induced formation of the corpus callosum in accallosal mice on glia-coated cellulose bridges. *Science* 1983;220:1067–1069.

171. Silverman AJ, Zimmerman EA, Gibson MJ, Perlow MJ, Charlton HM, Kokoris GJ, Krieger DT. Implantation of normal fetal preoptic area into hypogonadal mutant mice: temporal relationships of the growth of gonadotrophin-releasing hormone neurons and the development of the pituitary/testicular axis. *Neuroscience* 1985;16:69–84.

172. Sirinathsinghji DJS, Dunnett SB. Disappearance of the m-opiate receptor patches in the rat neostriatum following lesioning of the ipsilateral nigrostriatal dopamine pathway with 1-methyl-4-phenylpyridinium ion (MPP$^+$): restoration by embryonic nigral dopamine grafts. *Brain Res* 1989;504:115–120.

173. Sirinathsinghji DJS, Dunnett SB, Isacson O, Clarke DJ, Kendrick K, Björklund A. Striatal grafts in rats with unilateral neostriatal lesions. II. In vivo monitoring of GABA release in globus pallidus and substantia nigra. *Neuroscience* 1988;24:803–811.

174. Snyder-Keller AM, Lund RD. Amphetamine sensitization of stress-induced turning in animals given unilateral dopamine transplants in infancy. *Brain Res* 1990;514:143–146.

175. Sofroniew MV, Dunnett SB, Isacson O. Remodeling of intrinsic and afferent systems in neocortex with cortical transplants. *Prog Brain Res* 1990;82:313–320.

176. Sofroniew MV, Isacson O, Björklund A. Cortical grafts prevent atrophy of cholinergic basal nucleus neurons induced by excitotoxic cortical damage. *Brain Res* 1986;378:409–415.

177. Sofroniew MV, Pearson RCA. Degeneration of cholinergic neurons in the basal nucleus following kainic acid or *N* methyl-ᴅ-aspartic acid ap-

plication to the cerebral cortex in the rat. *Brain Res* 1985;229:186–189.

178. Sotelo C, Alvarado-Mallart RM. Reconstruction of the defective cerebellar circuitry in adult Purkinje cell degeneration mutant mice by Purkinje cell replacement through transplantation of solid embryonic implants. *Neuroscience* 1987;20:1–22.

179. Sotelo C, Alvarado-Mallart RM, Gardette R, Crepel F. Fate of grafted embryonic Purkinje cells in the cerebellum of the adult "Purkinje cell degeneration" mutant mouse. I. Development of reciprocal graft–host connectivity. *J Comp Neurol* 1990;295:165–187.

180. Springer JE, Collier TJ, Sladek JR, Loy R. Transplantation of male mouse submaxillary gland increases survival of axotomised basal forebrain neurons. *J Neurosci Res* 1988;19: 291–296.

181. Stein DG. Transplant-induced functional recovery without specific neuronal connections. *Prog Res Am Paral Assoc* 1987;18:4–5.

182. Stenevi U, Björklund A, Svendgaard N-A. Transplantation of central and peripheral monoamine neurons to the adult rat brain: techniques and conditions for survival. *Brain Res* 1976;114:1–20.

183. Strecker RE, Sharp T, Brundin P, Zetterström T, Ungerstedt U, Björklund A. Auto-regulation of dopamine release and metabolism by intrastriatal nigral grafts as revealed by intracerebral dialysis. *Neuroscience* 1987;22:169–178.

184. Strömberg I, Herrera-Marschitz M, Ungerstedt U, Ebendal T, Olson L. Chronic implants of chromaffin tissue into the dopamine-denervated striatum. Effects of NGF on graft survival, fiber growth and rotational behavior. *Exp Brain Res* 1985;60:335–349.

185. Swenson RS, Shaw P, Alones V, Kozlowski G, Zimmer J, Castro AJ. Neocortical transplants grafted into the newborn rat brain demonstrate a blood–brain barrier to macromolecules. *Neurosci Lett* 1989;100:35–39.

186. Tasker RR. Surgery for Parkinson's disease. In: Morley TP, ed. *Current controversies in neurosurgery.* Philadelphia: WB Saunders; 1976: 411–418.

187. Tischler AS, Perlman RL, Nunnemacher G, Morse GM, DeLellis R, Wolfe HJ, Sheard BE. Long-term effects of dexamethasone and nerve growth factor on adrenal medullary cells cultured from young adult rats. *Cell Tissue Res* 1982;225:525–542.

188. Tuch BE. Clinical results of transplanting fetal pancreas. In: Edwards RG, ed. *Fetal tissue transplants in medicine.* Cambridge: Cambridge University Press; 1992;215–237.

189. Uchida K, Ishii A, Kaneda N, Toya S, Nagatsu T, Kohsaka S. Tetrahydrobiopterin-dependent production of *l*-DOPA in NRK fibroblasts transfected with tyrosine hydroxylase cDNA: future use for intracerebral grafting. *Neurosci Lett* 1990;109:282–286.

190. Uchida K, Takamatsu K, Kaneda N, Toya S,

Tsukada Y, Kurosawa Y, Fujita K, Nagatsu T, Kohsaka S. Synthesis of l-3,4-dihydroxyphenylalanine by tryosine hydroxylase cDNA-transfected C6 cells: application for intracerebral grafting. *J Neurochem* 1989;53:728–732.

191. Ungerstedt U, Butcher LL, Butcher SG, Andén N-E, Fuxe K. Direct chemical stimulation of dopaminergic mechanisms of the neostriatum of the rat. *Brain Res* 1969;14:461–471.

192. Unsicker K, Krisch B, Otten U, Thoenen H. Nerve growth factor-induced fiber outgrowth from isolated rat adrenal chromaffin cells: impairment by glucocorticoids. *Proc Natl Acad Sci USA* 1978;81:2242–2246.

193. Valenstein ES. *Brain control.* New York: John Wiley & Sons; 1973.

194. Valenstein ES. *Great and desperate cures.* New York: Basic Books; 1986.

195. Vidal-Sanz M, Bray GM, Villegas-Perez M-P, Aguayo AJ. Axonal regeneration and synaptic formation in the superior colliculus by retinal cells in the adult rat. *J Neurosci* 1987;7:2894–2907.

196. Waters C, Itabashi HH, Apuzzo MLJ, Weiner LP. Adrenal to caudate transplantation—postmortem study. *Mov Disord* 1990;548:248–250.

197. Watts RL, Bakay RAE, Herring CJ, Sweeney KM, Colbassani HJ, Mandir A, Byrd LD, Iuvone PM. Preliminary report on adrenal medullary grafting and co-grafting with sural nerve in the treatment of hemiparkinsonian monkeys. *Prog Brain Res* 1990;82:581–591.

198. Whishaw IQ, Zaborowski JA, Kolb B. Postsurgical enrichment aids adult hemidecorticate rats on a spatial navigation task. *Behav Neural Biol* 1984;42:183–190.

199. Wictorin K. Anatomy and connectivity of intrastriatal striatal transplants. *Prog Neurobiol* 1992;38:611–639.

200. Will B, Hefti F. Behavioral and neurochemical effects of chronic intraventricular injections of nerve growth factor in adult rats with fimbria lesions. *Behav Brain Res* 1985;17:17–24.

201. Williams LR, Varon S, Peterson GM, Wictorin K, Fischer W, Björklund A, Gage FH. Continuous infusion of nerve growth factor prevents basal forebrain neuronal death after fimbria-fornix transection. *Proc Natl Acad Sci USA* 1986;83:9231–9235.

202. Winn SR, Wahlberg L, Tresco PA, Aebischer P. An encapsulated dopamine-releasing polymer alleviates experimental parkinsonism in rats. *Exp Neurol* 1989;105:244–250.

203. Wolff JA, Fisher LJ, Xu L, Jinnah HA, Langlais PJ, Iuvone PM, O'Malley KL, Rosenberg MB, Shimohama S, Friedmann T, Gage FH. Grafting fibroblasts genetically modified to produce *l*-DOPA in a rat model of Parkinson disease. *Proc Natl Acad Sci USA* 1989;86: 9011–9014.

204. Woodruff ML, Baisden RH, Nonneman AJ. Transplantation of fetal hippocampus may prevent or produce behavioral recovery from hip-

pocampal ablation and recovery persists after removal of the transplant. *Prog Brain Res* 1990;82:367–376.

205. Young MJ, Rao K, Lund RD. Integrity of the blood–brain barrier in retinal xenografts is correlated with the immunological status of the host. *J Comp Neurol* 1989;283:107–117.

206. Zetterström T, Brundin P, Gage FH, Sharp T, Isacson O, Dunnett SB, Ungerstedt U, Björklund A. In vivo measurement of spontaneous release and metabolism of dopamine from intrastriatal nigral grafts using intracerebral dialysis. *Brain Res* 1986;362:344–349.

207. Zhou FC. Connectivities of the striatal grafts and laminin guiding. *Prog Brain Res* 1990; 82:441–458.

Subject Index